TEACHING ELEMENTARY HEALTH SCIENCE

Third Edition

The Jones and Bartlett Series in Health Sciences

Aging, Health and Society
Kart/Metress/Metress

Basic Law for the Allied Health Professions
Cowdrey

Basic Nutrition: Self-Instructional Modules
Stanfield

The Birth Control Book
Belcastro

Contemporary Health Issues
Banister/Allen/Fadl/Bhakthan/Howard

Drugs and Society, Second Edition
Witters/Venturelli

First Aid and Emergency Care Workbook
Thygerson

Weight Management the Fitness Way
Dusek

Fitness for Health
Thygerson

Health and Wellness, Third Edition
Edlin/Golanty

Interviewing and Helping Skills for Health Professionals
Cormier/Cormier/Weisser

Introduction to Human Disease, Second Edition
Crowley

Introduction to Human Immunology
Huffer/Kanapa/Stevenson

Introduction to the Health Professions
Miller-Allan

Medical Terminology (with *Self-Instructional Modules*)
Stanfield/Hui

Principles and Issues of Nutrition
Hui

Sexuality Today
Nass/Fisher

Teaching Elementary Health Science, Third Edition
Bender/Sorochan

Writing a Successful Grant Application, Second Edition
Reif-Lehrer

TEACHING ELEMENTARY HEALTH SCIENCE

Third Edition

STEPHEN J. BENDER
Professor of Health Science
San Diego State University

WALTER D. SOROCHAN
Professor of Health Science
San Diego State University

JONES AND BARTLETT PUBLISHERS
Boston • Portola Valley

Editorial, Sales and Customer Service Offices
Jones and Bartlett Publishers
20 Park Plaza
Boston, MA 02116

Printed in the United States of America
10 9 8 7 6 5 4 3 2

Library of Congress Cataloging-in-Publication Data

Bender, Stephen J.
  Teaching elementary health science / by Stephen J. Bender & Walter
  D. Sorochan.—Rev. 3rd ed.
    p. cm.
    Sorochan's name appears first on the earlier eds.
    Includes bibliographies and index.
    ISBN 0-86720-411-7
    1. Health education (Elementary)—United States.   I. Sorochan,
  Walter D. II. Title.
  LB1587.A3B45 1988
  372.3′7′0973—dc19   88-21788
                                                          CIP

ISBN 0-86720-411-7

Production and typesetting: Editing, Design & Production, Inc.
Designer: Russell Schneck Design
Copyeditor: Kate Daly
Cover design: Rafael Millán
Cover illustration: FPG Int./Mark Kozlowski
Part and chapter opening illustrations: H. Armstrong Roberts, Inc.

To all those prospective elementary teachers who will, we hope, benefit from this book.

Contents

Preface

The Surgeon General's landmark report on health promotion and disease prevention entitled *Healthy People* (U.S. Department of Health, Education and Welfare, 1979) recommends that the nation's health goals include a comprehensive program of school health education. The report indicates that schools may well be the richest source of behavior change with respect to those health matters that are directly related to an unhealthful lifestyle. Among the report's many recommendations is that comprehensive school health education include the dissemination of up-to-date knowledge dealing with the causes of disease, especially as they relate to the personal decisions we make concerning smoking, alcohol, drug use, exercise, and sexual activity.

The third edition of *Teaching Elementary Health Science* was developed with the Surgeon General's thoughts in mind. New emphasis has been placed upon those areas cited in the report as being major factors affecting the nation's health. Each area of preparation deemed essential to the development of a competent elementary health educator has been updated in terms of contemporary theory.

To assist the elementary school teacher in accomplishing this goal, the third edition of *Teaching Elementary Health Science* is divided into five parts. Part I examines the many meanings of health and suggests a two-dimensional model of well-being in order to describe optimal well-being.

Part II discusses how children grow and attain health and the typical developmental tasks and physical problems of elementary school children. Emotional and behavioral problems of elementary school youngsters are emphasized. Concluding Part II is a chapter concerning the general guidelines for emergency care. Part II focuses exclusively on the child.

Part III addresses the relationship of health education to the elementary school curriculum. The role of the elementary teacher in the school health program and the elementary health education curriculum are discussed.

Part IV deals solely with elementary health instruction. In this section the reader is provided with detailed chapters concerning the conceptual approach, behavioral objectives, learning experiences, evaluation, and finally, lesson planning, all of which provide a basis for Part V.

Part V devotes eleven chapters to teaching about health. In each chapter an overview of the content is followed by examples of lesson plans. The eleven topics, highly relevant to elementary school age children, are the human body, emotional and social health, drugs, tobacco, alcohol, environmental conservation, nutrition, dental health, safety, disease, and family living. Although the lesson plans are not comprehensive, they provide an excellent basis from which to develop a complete lesson.

Last but certainly not least, we wish to express our sincere appreciation to all those who helped make this book a reality. It is our profound hope that many will benefit from its contents.

San Diego, California S.J.B.
January, 1989 W.D.S.

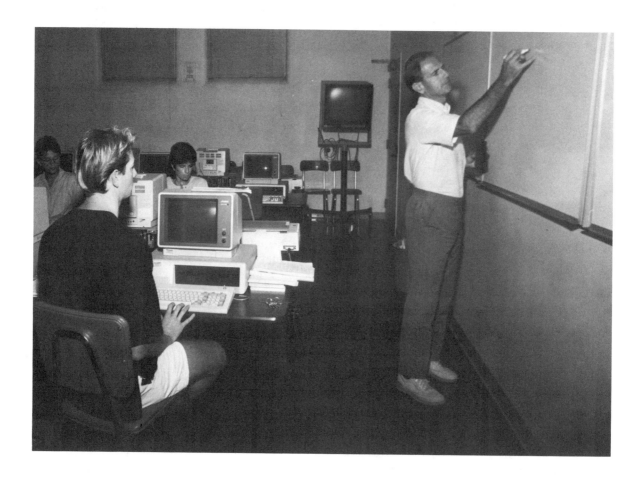

Stephen J. Bender, H.S.D., M.P.H.
Professor of Health Science
San Diego State University

Stephen J. Bender was born and reared in the upstate New York community of Rochester. He received his Bachelor of Science degree in health science from the State University of New York, Brockport, in 1966. He completed the Master of Science degree at Indiana University, Bloomington, in 1967 and the Doctor of Health Science degree at the same university in 1969. A year of post-doctoral study at UCLA in 1982 culminated in the M.P.H. degree in behavioral science.

Dr. Bender's first professional appointment was as an Assistant Professor of Health Science at Memphis State University in Memphis, Tennessee. In 1970 he accepted an appointment in the Department of Health Science at San Diego State University, where he is now a Professor of Health Science. During his tenure at SDSU, Dr. Bender has served as the Campus Ombudsperson for two years, as Chair of the Department of Health Science for two years, as and the first Director of the Division of Health Promotion in the Graduate School of Public Health. He is the author or coauthor of five health science texts and numerous periodical articles. Dr. Bender's most recent research interest and publication record have centered on violence and its relationships to public health.

An avid sportsman, Professor Bender plays golf, runs, and takes tours by bicycle.

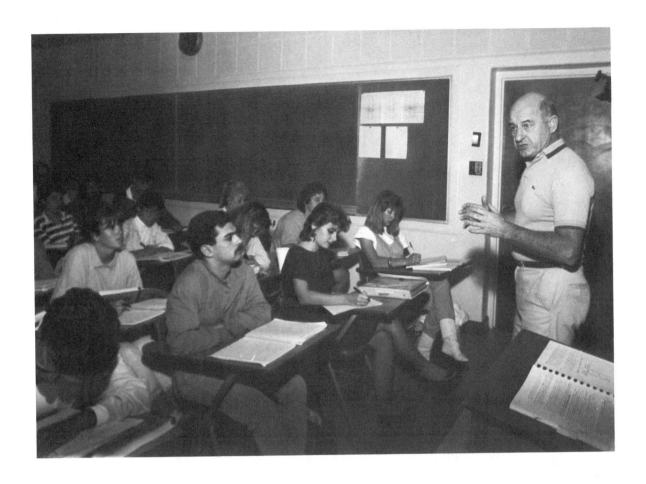

Walter D. Sorochan, H.S.D., M.P.H.
Professor of Health Science
San Diego State University

Walter D. Sorochan was born in Lamont, Alberta, and reared in a farming community near Vancouver, British Columbia. He received his undergraduate degree in biology and physical education from the University of British Columbia in 1952. After receiving his Teacher Training Diploma in 1953, he taught for a year in Kamploops, British Columbia.

After receiving his Master of Science degree from the University of British Columbia, he taught and coached for six years at the junior and high school levels in Vancouver.

Dr. Sorochan taught health education at Bemidji State College, Bemidji, Minnesota, in 1962, and thereafter accepted an appointment at Eastern Kentucky University, where he taught health education from 1963 to 1968. During this time, he worked on his terminal degree at Indiana University, Bloomington, receiving his Doctor of Health Science degree in 1969. Since then, he has been teaching at San Diego State University, where he is now Professor of Health Science. After a year of postdoctorate study at UCLA, he received his M.P.H. degree in behavioral science in 1983.

Although his lifestyle has mellowed with age, he continues to exercise regularly, enjoys dancing and the theater, and is an avid sports fan. As a hobby, he plays in and leads a big band dance orchestra. In the 1970's Dr. Sorochan was instrumental in focusing national attention on lifestyle and health promotion through his articles and texts. He is author or coauthor of five health education texts and numerous articles.

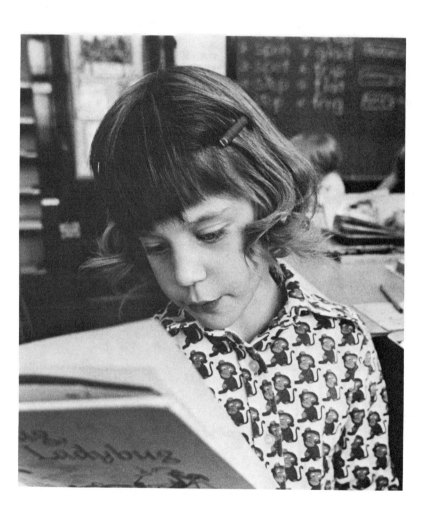

Part One

The Concept of Health

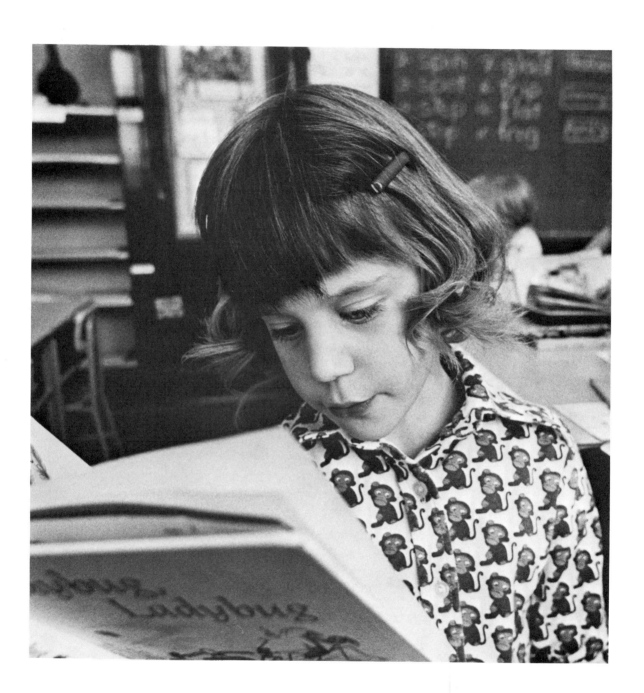

Chapter 1

The Meaning Of Health

INTRODUCTION

Why should elementary school teachers be concerned about teaching for health? The observation that most people today die of self-inflicted behaviors suggests that such deaths can be prevented. One approach to such prevention is to begin formal health education at the elementary school level. Teachers can help children learn and practice health enhancement behaviors. To facilitate such an approach, teachers need to have a good working knowledge of health. More important, teachers should be models of optimal wellness in order to assist children in emulating good health habits. The first prerequisite is for prospective elementary school teachers to understand the concept of health and the factors that influence the ability to attain and maintain optimal well-being. This chapter provides the theoretical foundation for such an understanding.

THE CONCEPT OF HEALTH

Although good health is difficult to define, the most widely accepted definition is that proposed by the World Health Organization (WHO, 1947): "Health is a state of physical, mental and social well-being and not merely the absence of disease or infirmity." This description is somewhat incomplete and can be misleading, for health is not a state but better perceived as the result of a dynamic ever-changing adaptive process that is the body's adjustments to internal and external stressors. This hypothesis of adjustment is supported by Bernard and Cannon's theory of homeostasis, which implies that the body is constantly striving for stability and balance. The body state may be perceived as fluctuating through different levels of wellness as it strives for homeostasis. This idea was proposed as levels of well-being by the President's Commission on the Health Needs of the Nation (Dunn, 1957); as gradations of health by Rogers (Rogers, 1960); expanded into levels of wellness by Dunn (1961); and evolved into an ecological model of health and disease by Hoyman (Hoyman, 1962). The

theory of levels of wellness is more comprehensive than previous theories in that it provides a health status continuum for various stages of illness up to death, or no health at all. Wellness, according to the stepladder notion, implies that one's level of well-being may fluctuate from time to time. Figure 1.1 illustrates the well-known observation that one's health may vary from a high level of wellness through minor to major illness. However, this theory does not provide a comprehensive picture of health or account for various components that make up well-being.

Five fitness components of health have been identified by the American Association for Health, Physical Education and Recreation. Contrary to the statement of the World Health Organization's perception of three fitness components (physical, mental, social), this health model adds two components for a total of five (see Figure 1.2): physical, emotional, social, spiritual and

FIGURE 1.1
Levels of wellness. The levels of well-being extend from zero wellness (death) at one end of a continuum to optimal wellness at the other end.

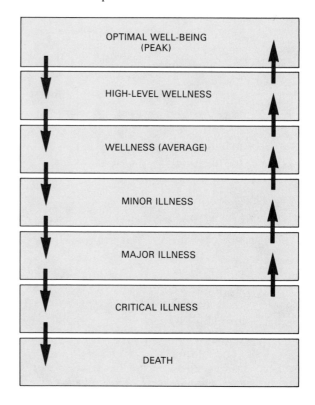

cultural. Each component identifies a different dimension of wellness.

These components are characterized as follows:

1. Physical fitness (function of body systems and processes):
   a) efficient functioning of body systems and organs
   b) high level of immunity
   c) adequate regular diet
   d) adequate muscular strength
   e) adequate neuromuscular coordination, balance and flexibility
   f) appropriate body density and weight
2. Emotional fitness (feelings, thoughts, social behaviors, identity)
   a) coping successfully with stressors
   b) feeling good about self (self-image)
   c) feeling good about others
   d) accepting reality
   e) maintaining self-discipline and self-control
   f) maintaining emotional stability
   g) accepting responsibility for behavior and social roles
   h) establishing and maintaining commitments
3. Social fitness (interacting with others)
   a) having 5 to 10 intimate friends
   b) socializing frequently with friends, relatives, and others
   c) accepting responsibility for others
   d) making new friends
   e) having friends of all ages
4. Spiritual fitness (inner strength to live)
   a) having hope
   b) having the will to live and do
   c) aspiring for excellence and better things in life
   d) having ambition to achieve and accomplish
   e) having the courage to take calculated risks and face the unknown
5. Cultural fitness (being involved and identifying with community)
   a) contributing to betterment of community life
   b) involvement in civic organizations
   c) playing and acting to please others
   d) attending cultural and social events
   e) sharing artistic talents and abilities with others
   f) accepting responsibility for public office

Although these fitness components have been exemplified as separate entities, normally they are inseparable, interdependent parts of the whole. For example, physical fitness is conceived as a prerequisite for all the remaining types of fitness and is easiest to identify. It is not possible for a person with a high degree of physical fitness but low social fitness or low spiritual fitness to have optimal well-being. All five kinds of fitness complement one another and all are responsible for contributing to the quality of lifestyle. Each expresses a distinct dimension of wellness. The characteristics of each of the components of fitness reflect American values (Mitchell, 1984).

Superimpose the concept of fitness components in Figure 1.2 over the concept of levels of wellness in Figure 1.1 to create a health grid. Each level of wellness comprises five components of fitness. This health grid is illustrated in Figure 1.3. If one or more of the five components of fitness drops, the level of wellness also drops. The converse is also true.

The two theories of health—levels of wellness and components of fitness—collectively present a much more comprehensive concept of health than the definition by the World Health Organization.

We hope the preceding discussion provides a more nearly complete understanding of the

FIGURE 1.2

Five fitness components of well-being conceptualized as continuous, interrelated and interdependent. Fitness components as a theory characterize one dimension of health only.

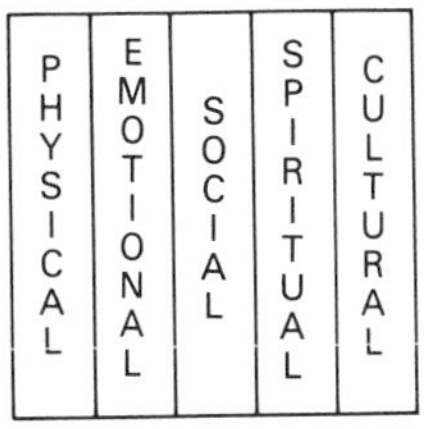

PHYSICAL	EMOTIONAL	SOCIAL	SPIRITUAL	CULTURAL

FIGURE 1.3

Theory of fitness components superimposed over theory of levels of wellness. Each type of fitness fluctuates interdependently, modifying the levels of other types of fitness, and of course raising or lowering the whole level of well-being.

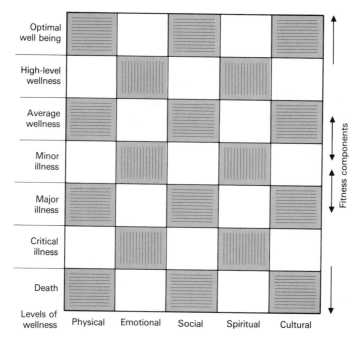

meaning of health. Health, while difficult to define, can be thought of as a dynamic, ever-changing phenomenon based upon the interaction of the five components of fitness and the levels of well-being. Health is more than a state of well-being in the absence of disease. To attain optimal well-being requires a conscious effort to harmonize the components of fitness at an optimal level. To achieve optimal well-being is difficult. Success on the road to high-level wellness is dependent upon the ability to harness the many determinants that affect one's health.

DETERMINERS OF OPTIMAL WELL-BEING

Our initial discussion has centered on developing an understanding of health as a concept. To attain optimal well-being is quite commendable; to maintain well-being is a lifelong task that is not without its ups and downs.

Why are some of us more successful than others in attaining and reasonably maintaining optimal well-being? The variance of success among the general population can be attributed to the influence of five major factors that dramatically affect one's quest for optimal well-being (see Figure 1.4). The five major variables:

- Human biology (heredity, function of organs and systems, immunity, maturation, aging)
- Physical and social environment (food, shelter, air, noise, water, soil, chemicals, other living things, cultural demands, interpersonal relationships)
- Lifestyle (knowledge, attitudes, and behavior)
- Health care system (organization of, availability of, access to appropriate health care—drugs, doctors, dentists, hospitals, voluntary agencies, insurance coverage)
- Political and economic reinforcements for health (legislation, political policy, availability of financial resources)

FIGURE 1.4

Five determiners of personal health conceptualized as a theoretical model for the United States.

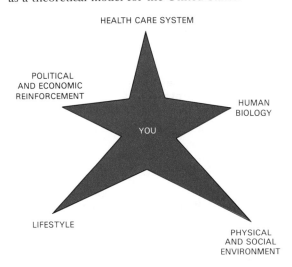

Much debate centers on how much each determiner of health influences the ability to achieve and maintain optimal well-being. As with any controversy, there are as many theories as there are vested interests. Suffice it to say that each determiner makes a unique and essential contribution to health. A brief description of the five determiners follows:

Human Biology[1]

Since we are born with the genetic makeup of our parents, there is little we can do to change biological traits. Some of us are fortunate to inherit traits that contribute to good health; others are less fortunate. Some inherit a predisposition to allergies, diabetes, and other body disorders. However, those affected often can reduce the risks from their genetic defect through health-enhancing behavior.

Physical and Social Environment[2]

The wastes of industry and general living are dumped into the air, water, and soil on the assumption that Mother Nature will absorb these wastes and neutralize them over time. Given ample time, Mother Nature has the ability to disperse and neutralize these wastes. When we dump wastes faster than Mother Nature can get rid of them, these wastes pile up and poison the environment. We and other living things come in contact with wastes such as air, water, soil, and noise pollutants. The consequences of such exposure are discomfort, irritability, respiratory disabilities, aggravation of genetic disability, accidents, low sperm count, miscarriages, birth defects, and cancer. We have also increased the use of chemicals in our food. Thus, by harnessing technology we have polluted our environment.

Just as important as our physical environment is our social environment. Forces with strong underlying social bases—such as nurturance and parenting, discipline, education, culture, religion, social identification, social acceptance, friends, family, community, and play—all combine to shape one's approach to health matters.

Lifestyle[3]

Lifestyle has a dramatic influence on health. A classic example of this may be found in the United States (Fuchs, 1986) by comparing the health of populations of the two neighboring states of Nevada and predominantly Mormon Utah. While similar in many ways, these populations have very different patterns of health behavior. The population of Utah as a whole has fewer illnesses and chronic diseases than the

---

[1]The following references affirm this determiner: Conrad, 1979; Dubos, 1961; Dunn, 1961; Hoyman, 1962; LaLonde, 1974; McKeown, 1978; McKinley and McKinley, 1977; Williams, 1976.

---

[2]The following references affirm this determiner: Conrad, 1979; Dubos, 1961; Dunn, 1961; Hoyman, 1962; Knox, 1977; McKeown, 1977; Williams, 1973.

[3]The following references affirm this determiner: Belloc, 1973; Dubos, 1970; Etzioni, 1972; Fuchs, 1986; Haggerty, 1977; McCamy and Presley, 1975; Mitchell, 1984; Selye, 1974; Sorochan, 1974.

population of Nevada. Fuchs (9:17) argues that the explanation for this difference is to be found in the lifestyle of each population.

Additional research suggests that changes in lifestyle can and do contribute to better health. Recent data from the National Center for Health Statistics and the National Heart, Lung and Blood Institute show that our health has indeed been changing for the better (*Nutrition Action,* September 1984:4). Heart disease deaths have declined by an astounding 36 percent between 1968 and 1983, probably because of reduced smoking, dietary changes, increased physical activity, and improved medical care for the population at highest risk. Likewise, stroke deaths have declined by 51 percent between 1968 and 1983, most likely because of antihypertension medications and dietary changes. Life expectancy has increased by 3.1 years in the 1970's (JAMA, 1982, 247 or 877). These few examples provide evidence that effective lifestyle changes can be made by individuals who practice poor health behaviors.

Health Care Systems[4]

Everyone needs medical care at one time or another. We need medical services for vaccinations, checkups, advice, and healing when hurt or sick. On occasion a person needs to be hospitalized for a serious illness, diagnostic tests, or surgery.

Increasing numbers of people in the United States are dissatisfied with the medical care they receive. Frequent complaints include the poor quality of care, excessive suffering through treatment, and overcharging. As with any service, the quality of medical care varies dramatically.

Often the patient lacks understanding of what the medical profession and physicians can and cannot do. Many patients do not understand their rights and responsibilities and how to enhance their own healing.

Although we spend more money per capita on health care than any other country and have the best medical technology, our health care system has not prolonged life in the United States significantly in the past 30 years (Knowles, 30: 37; McKinley and McKinley). Nor has more spending provided better individual health. This is reflected in the most sensitive and popular public health indicator of the general health of a country—the infant mortality rate (IMR). The IMR of 11 for the United States in 1982 was worse than that of 11 other countries that spend less on their health care system than we do. There are several reasons for this. Most of the bad things that happen to people are beyond the reach of medicine. While our medical care system has focused on treating the sick, it has overlooked helping well people to maintain their health. Most people dying today do not die of lack of treatment but of their own bad habits.

Another reason why life has not been prolonged has to do with the changing nature of disease itself in this country since 1900. Most people before 1900 died of communicable waterborne respiratory diseases. Because communicable diseases are environmentally or microbically caused, control measures in the past have focused on treatment. By contrast, chronic diseases of today are caused by deleterious life styles. Unfortunately, much of today's medical practice is still geared to treatment rather than to prevention or health promotion. Thus, although good medical care is available, it fails to prevent diseases of poor habits, and the victims tend to die prematurely.

Thus, although our health care system is excellent, it does not control the health of people today. This is because most chronic diseases are affected more by behavior than by the quality of health care available. The significant gains in people living beyond 50 years of age at the turn of this century were due to improvements in sanitation and better nutrition; the gains took place before the advent of antibiotics and surgical advancements (McKeown, 1978; McKinley and McKinley, 1977; Vickery, 1978). Likewise, today significant gains in improving health and extending life beyond age 75 are dependent on personal habits and behaviors more than on the health care system.

---

[4]The following references affirm this determiner: Illich, 1976; Knowles, 1977; LaLonde, 1974; Gray, 1982.

Political and Economic Reinforcement for Health[5]

Politics can play a major role in determining health. Politicians may pass legislative measures to protect the health of the public when it may be or is threatened. Although governments have a responsibility to safeguard the health of their people, acceptance of responsibility varies. A classic example was the reduction of the risk of alcohol-related cirrhosis through political intervention in England during World War I. The British tax on alcohol was reinforced by restricted hours of sale, reducing availability. Consumption fell, and with it deaths from cirrhosis—from 10.3 per 100,000 people in 1914 to 4.5 per 100,000 in 1920. Following World War I, regulations governing alcohol were relaxed, but taxes on it continually increased. In 1926 the death rate for cirrhosis was 3.1 per 100,000, and it has remained at this level in England since 1926 (Knowles, 1977:77; McDermott and Hough, 1979:77).

The reduction in the risk of alcohol-related cirrhosis in England after World War I can be contrasted to the same period in the United States. During the U.S. wartime legislative prohibition of alcohol, the U.S. death rate for cirrhosis fell from 11.8 per 100,000 in 1916 to 7.1 per 100,000 in 1920. This rate lasted through 1932, the end of prohibition. In 1973, the U.S. death rate rose to 16.0 per 100,000, five times the rate for cirrhosis in England (Knowles, 1977:77).

It has been demonstrated in Australia that a national law making seat belt use mandatory can considerably lower automobile fatalities (Knowles, 1977:77). A marked reduction of automobile-related fatalities and injuries in the United States during the 1974 oil crisis suggests that the reduction of speed limits (from 70 mph to 55 mph) produced the decline (Knowles, 1977:77).

Another example of political influence on health at the national level occurred when Congress inadvertently contributed to smoking by millions of persons by legislating free cigarettes to servicemen during World War I and World War II. Upon request of the military, the government contracted for the entire output of Bull Durham cigarettes in the spring of 1918 (Heimann, 1960). By providing free cigarettes, the government habituated thousands of servicemen to tobacco. Millions have subsequently died of lung cancer.

Economics is also strongly linked to quality of health. In the United States, one of the most striking features of the distribution of disease is its relationship to poverty. Poverty influences health; that is, the poorer the population, the more sick people there are, and the higher the death rates. Syme and Berkman (1976) studied the relationship of social class to sickness. They found that life in the lower class may compromise disease defense systems and engender greater vulnerability to disease and that those who are poor are more likely to be unhealthy because of inadequate nutrition, insanitary living conditions, substandard housing, exposure to accidents and violence, and lack of preventive medical care. Levels of mortality decline and life expectancy rises with higher levels of income (Brenner and Mooney, 1983). This is true throughout the world. Availability of money is a definite determiner of health. Lack of money (or purchasing power) limits one's options for food, housing, medical care, health education and ability to function optimally.

IMPLICATIONS FOR THE PROSPECTIVE ELEMENTARY SCHOOL TEACHER

Each of the aforementioned determiners of health significantly affect one's health status. For the purposes of our discussion as prospective elementary school teachers, we will want to focus on factors that are most amenable to change. For

---

[5] The following references affirm this determiner: Brenner and Mooney, 1983; Brown, 1984; Chossudovsky, 1983; Elling, 1981; Enthoven, 1970; Glasser, 1965; Gray, 1982; Gregory and Piche, 1983; Heimann, 1960; Knowles, 1977; McDermott and Hough, 1979; Mintz and Cohen, 1977; Navarro, 1981, 1984; USDHHS, 1981; Rudov and Santangelo, 1979; Ryan, 1976; Syme and Berkman, 1976; Terris, 1980.

example, teachers can not change heredity. Therefore, while human biology includes heredity as a major determiner of health, we are better advised to concentrate our efforts on factors that we stand the best chance of influencing.

Mortality and morbidity data for the United States clearly indicate that the leading causes of death for all age groups are closely related to lifestyle. Therefore, we surely want to emphasize appropriate health behaviors to young children. Behavioral learning experiences should be based upon the fact that individuals are personally responsible for their own health promotion, risk reduction, and disease prevention.

On the other hand, it is important to understand how other factors, often beyond a person's control, may radically alter the level of well-being.

REFERENCES AND BIBLIOGRAPHY

Antonovsky, Aaron, *Health, Stress and Coping (GRS)* (San Francisco: Jossey-Bass, 1980).

Ardell, Donald B. *High Level Wellness* (New York: Bantam Books, 1979).

Belloc, Nedra B. "Relationship of health practices and mortality." *Preventive Medicine* 2 (1973) pp. 67-81.

Brenner, Harvey M., and Ann Mooney. "Unemployment and Health in the Context of Economic Change," *Social Science and Medicine* 17,16 (1983) 1125-1138.

Brown, Lester. *State of The World* (New York: W.W. Norton, 1984):32-34.

Cadwalader, Mary H. "Early Warnings of Future Disaster." *Smithsonian* (May 1974):27-29.

Chossudovsky, Michel. "Underdevelopment and the Political Economy of Malnutrition and Ill Health," *International Journal of Human Services,* 13:1 (1983):69-83.

Conrad, Fran. "Society May Be Dangerous to Your Health," *Science for the People* (March/April 1979):14-38.

Conrad, Peter. "Who Gets Sick? The Unequal Social Distribution of Disease," *The Sociology of Health and Illness* (1981).

Dubos, Rene. "Health and Creative Adaptation." *Human Nature* (January 1978):74-82.

Dubos, Rene. *Mirage of Health* (Garden City, New York: Doubleday, 1961).

Dunn, H.L. *High Level Wellness* (Washington, D.C.: Mt. Vernon Printing Co., 1961).

Dunn, H.L. "Points of Attack for Raising the Levels of Wellness," *Journal of the American Medical Association* (July 1957).

Elling, Ray H. "The Capitalistic World-System and International Health," *International Journal of Health Services,* 11:1(1981):21-51.

Enthoven, Alain. "Shattuck Lecture: Cutting Cost without Cutting the Quality of Care." *The New England Journal of Medicine* 298:22 (June 1, 1978):1229-1238.

Etzioni, Amitai. "Human Beings Are Not Very Easy to Change after All," *Saturday Review* (June 3, 1972).

Fuchs, Victor, "A Tale of Two Cities," *The Health Economy* (Cambridge, Mass.: Harvard University Press, 1986): 196-199.

Glasser, William. *Reality Therapy* (New York: Harper & Row, 1965).

Gray, Alastair. "Inequities in Health. The Black Report: A Summary and Comment," *International Journal of Health Services* 12:3 (1982):349-373.

Gregory, Joel W. and Victor Piche. "Inequality and Mortality: Democratic Hypotheses Regarding Advanced and Peripheral Capitalism," *International Journal of Health Services* 13:1 (1983):89.

Haggerty, Robert J. "Changing Life Styles to Improve Health," *Preventive Medicine* 6 (1977):276-289.

Heimann, Robert K. *Tobacco and America.* (New York, McGraw-Hill, 1960):226-265.

———, "HH Starts Push for Cancer Prevention," *The Nation's Health* (April 1984):8.

Hoyman, H. S. "Our Modern Concepts of Health," *Journal of School Health* (September 1962):253.

Illich, Ivan. *Limits to Medicine.* (Toronto: McClelland & Stewart, 1976).

———, *Journal of the American Medical Association* (1982) 247-248.

Johnson, Donald D. "Listen to Your Body," *Newsletter: Society of Prospective Medicine* 1:3 (May 1978).

Kahn, Carol, "If I Die Tomorrow It Ain't Going to Be My Fault," *Family Health* (February 1978):43-45.

Kaplan, et al. "Social Support and Health," *Medical Care* (supplement):25 (1977) 47-58.

Kluger, Mathew J. "The Importance of Being Feverish, *Natural History Magazine* (January 1976):147-150.

Knox, E. G. "Foods and Diseases," *British Journal of Preventive and Social Medicine* 31 (1977):71-80.

Knowles, John H. *Doing Better and Feeling Worse* (New York: W.W. Norton, 1977):77.

Kugler, Hans J. *Dr. Kugler's Seven Keys to a Longer Life* (New York: Stein and Day, 1978).

Lalonde, Marc. *A New Perspective on the Health of Canadians* (Ottawa, Canada: The Queen's Printer, 1974).

Levine, J. D. "Pain and Analgesia: The Outlook for More Rational Treatment" *Annals of Internal Medicine* 100:269 (1984).

Maslow, Abraham H. "A Theory of Metamotivation: The Biological Routing of the Value Life," *Journal of Humanistic Psychology* (Fall 1967).

Maslow, Abraham H. *Eupsychian Management* (Homewood, Ill.: Dorsey Press, 1965).

Maslow, Abraham H. *Religions, Values and Peak Experiences* (Columbus: Ohio State University Press, 1964).

Maslow, Abraham H. *Toward a Psychology of Being* (New York: Van Nostrand Reinhold, 1968).

Mayo, Rollo. *Man's Search for Himself* (New York: American Library, 1967).

Mathison, David A. "On Hay Fever and Other Bedeviling Allergies," *Executive Health* (July 1977):6.

McCamy, John C., and James Presley. *Human Life Styling: Keep Whole in the Twentieth Century* (New York: Harper & Row, 1975).

McDermott, F.T., and D.E. Hough. "Reduction in Road Fatalities and Injuries after Legislation for Compulsory Wearing of Seat Belts: Experience in Victoria and the Rest of Australia," *British Journal of Surgery*, Vol. 66 (1979):518-521.

McKeown, Thomas. "Determinants of Health," *Human Nature* (April 1978):60-67.

McKinley, John B., and Sonja M. McKinley. "The Questionable Contribution of Medical Measures to the Decline of Mortality in the United States in the Twentieth Century," *Milbank Memorial Fund Quarterly* (Summer 1977): 405-428.

McLuhan, Marshall. "Playboy interview: Marshall McLuhan," *Playboy* (March 1969).

Mintz, Morton, and Jerry S. Cohen. *Power Inc.* (New York: Bantam Books, 1977): 198-201; 227-242; 252-269; 292-303; 312-315; 368-375.

Mitchell, Arnold. "Nine American Values and Lifestyles," *The Futurist* (August 1984):4-14.

Navarro, Vincent. "A Critique of the Ideological and Political Positions of the Willy Brandt Report and the WHO Alma Ata Declaration," *Social Science Medicine* 18:6 (1984): 467-474.

Navarro, Vincent. *Imperialism, Health and Medicine* (Farmingdale, N. Y.: Baywood Publishing, 1981).

____, "New Health Data Testify to Benefits of Improved American Lifestyles," *Nutrition Action* (September 1984):4.

____, "Risk-Factor Prevalence Survey—Utah," *Morbidity and Mortality Weekly Report*, USDHHS, June 5, 1981, 253, 254, 259.

Reisfeld, Ralph A., and Barry D. Kahan. "Markers of Individuality," *Scientific American* (June 1972):208-217.

Rogers, E. S. *Human Ecology and Health* (New York: MacMillan, 1960).

Rosen, G. *A History of Public Health* (New York: M.D. Publications, 1958).

Rudov, Melvin H., and Nancy Santangelo. *Health Status of Minorities and Low-Income Groups:* DHEW Publication No. 79-627 (Washington, U. S. Printing Office, 1979).

Ryan, William. *Blaming the Victim* (New York: Vintage Books, 1976).

____, "Scientific Data Confirm Exercising Lengthens Life," *San Diego Union* (July 27, 1984).

Selye, Hans. *Stress without Distress* (Philadelphia: Lippincott, 1974).

Selye, Hans. *The Stress of Life* (New York: McGraw-Hill, 1959).

Simonton, Carl O. *Getting Well Again* (New York: Bantam Books, 1981).

Sorochan, Walter D. "Health Concepts as a Basis for Orthobiosis," *The Journal of School Health* (December 1968): 673-682.

Sorochan, Walter D. "Life Style as an Approach to Health," *California School Health* (July 1974): 36-38.

Syme, Leonard S., and Lisa F. Berkman. "Social Class, Susceptibility, and Sickness," *American Journal of Epidemiology* (1976):1-8.

Terris, Milton. "The Three World Systems of Medical Care: Trends and Prospects," *World Health Forum* 1(1,2) (1980):78-86.

____, *U. S. Congressional Record*, Washington, U. S. Printing Office (August 24, 1976): H8975.

USDHHS Working Group. *Report of the Working Group on Critical Patient Behavior in the Dietary Management of High Blood Pressure* (Bethesda: National Institutes of Health, 1982).

Vickery, Donald M. *Lifeplan for Your Health* (Reading: Addison-Wesley, 1978).

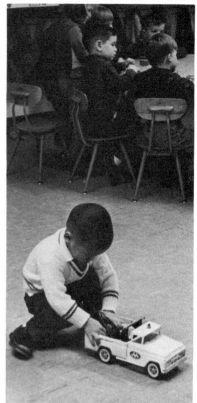

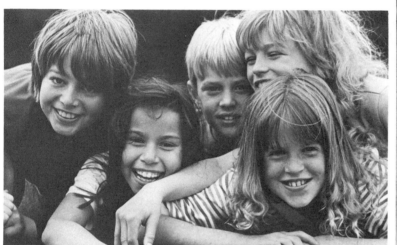

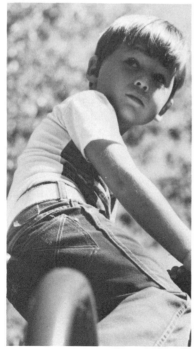

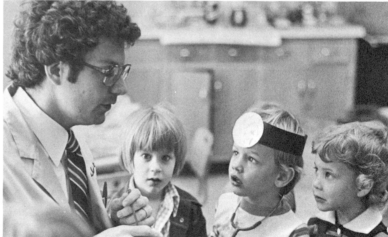

Part Two

The Health of the Elementary School Age Child

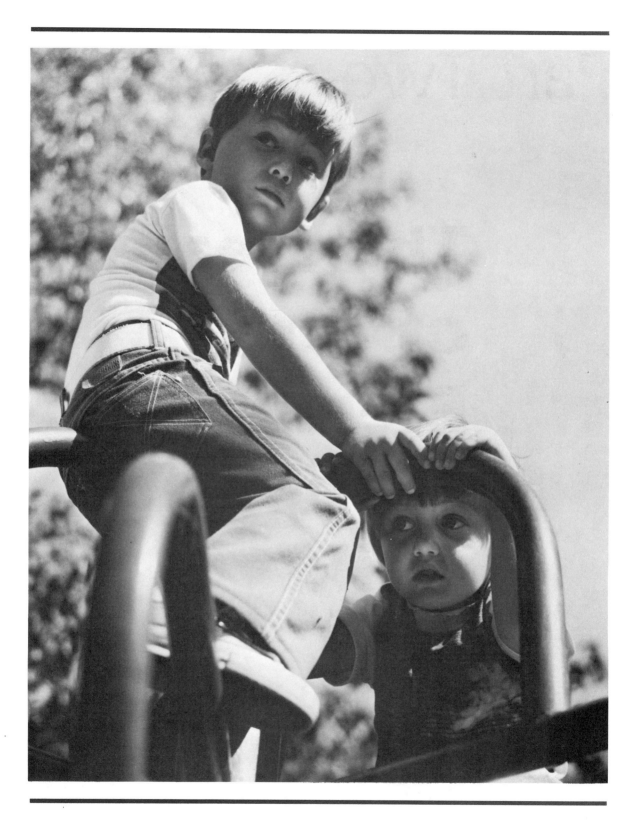

Chapter 2 Growth and Development

HOLISTIC DEVELOPMENT: OVERVIEW

Childhood, an adorable stage of life, has been referred to as the latency period, a relatively quiescent and untroubled time for children ages 6 to 12. Excepting fatal accidents, death rates for children ages 6 to 12 are extremely low; involvement with the legal political system is limited, and severe problems of emotional disorders are rare. In a sociological sense this developmental period may be more accurately described as a "learning-the-ropes" period rather than as a latency period. It is a time when the child begins to cope with autonomy and a continuously expanding world. Before this time, the child was essentially a homebody whose culture was confined largely to the family and to informal friendship groups. After entering school, the child comes into sustained contact with persons other than the immediate family. He or she cannot escape the need to learn more with great speed in order to facilitate relations with strangers. The classroom is the child's first constant and highly organized group experience. Children become most aware of the necessity for learning and communicating and of the need for interpersonal, intellectual, and physical skills.

Preadolescence is when the first signs and early warnings of personal and social inadequacies stemming from home life become evident and visible to others in the community. During the elementary school years many children reveal for the first time the physical and behavioral problems that lead to their being tagged as "good or bad" and as "smart or dumb." On the other hand, the absence of psychiatric and behavioral symptoms in childhood virtually guarantees that a child will not be sociopathic as an adult (Freeman and Jones, 1971). During this time new health-maintenance habits and behaviors are developed. Such health habits become the habits of life.

The attitudes that children pick up in school not only determine much of their early success or failure, but also influence the rest of their educational careers and adult attitudes toward work, responsibility, self, and later life in general. According to Erikson (1959, 1963), childhood is a crucial period for the development of a "sense of identity." An identity is structured through "industry" during childhood; it is through work that the child acquires a sense of duty and achievement. The child makes subconscious commitments to both of these, thereby evolving an identity.

Perhaps equally important to structuring an identity and learning the three Rs is the child's need for standards of moral conduct and ethical behavior. The school setting offers unlimited supportive experiences for clarifying as well as acquiring values.

Teachers should observe children at all times of the school day and as they progress from grades one through six. During this time children's physical growth is slow, and their mental growth appears to go on quietly. By middle childhood the ability to understand and to express self has progressed remarkably. In late childhood the reasoning becomes better, and this allows progress from premoral selfish to conventional adolescent values.

In addition to observing children's physical and mental growth, teachers will observe the children's state of health. They will note that children get sick less and less as they progress into late childhood. They also take better care of themselves, for they have learned many safe ways to live. Even so, almost every day teachers will observe children with health, learning, and living problems. Such problems can be readily corrected or modified when the problem is in its emergent stage and when children are most amenable to adjustment and change.

During their elementary school years boys and girls try out their own abilities and interests and begin to gain self-confidence and self-reliance. Although they still need and count on the friendly care and backing of their parents and family, they manage more and more of their own affairs. While becoming self-reliant, self-directing, and self-motivated, children still need appreciating attention, love, and sympathy.

Children love to play. Play not only makes friends, but also expresses self, maintains physical fitness, and clarifies values of life. Play, as activity, is also essential for the physical development of the body. It is through physical activities and play that the child acquires the good balance, gracefulness, coordination, muscular strength, and physical stamina that are the foundations of adult health and life. For example, children of ages six to ten delight in hopscotch and jacks. The intricate rhythm of skipping rope and the body control required in tumbling, gymnastics, and skating give children the thrill of adventures and also the exhilarating feeling of body control and management.

Children can't get enough of games that emphasize physical alertness—chasing, climbing, dodging. Swinging, whether from a safe swing, a rope, or a vine in the woods, gives children a chance to feel and identify their kinesthetic senses. Tag, run-sheep-run, cops and robbers, and other games in which there is a chance to avoid capture appeal to children. Turning handsprings; balancing on a beam; bouncing a ball; catching, throwing, and batting a ball are all physical skills demanding control of big skeletal muscles.

While playing, children create their own rules and insist on playing by the rules. They enforce moral virtues of honesty and fair play much more harshly than a teacher does. Their play entails trying out values by which to play and live. These games and trying-out experiences are critical, for they have great developmental meaning and payoff for maturity. All children need to play!

Once children, especially those in the primary grades, have acquired good control over their bodies, they have a great deal of energy for learning and social skills and for developing their partially perfected abilities. Just as children's play develops their skeletal muscles and physical well-being, their efforts in learning to read and write demand exact adjustments of the smaller muscles and development of hand-eye coordination.

School-age children delight in putting their hands to work. With initiative and furor, children construct things—carts, kites, airplanes, and boats—weave, tie knots, carve, and cut out paper dolls with varying degrees of success. Intermediate-level children are very industrious. They like to work and to do things, finding it emotionally satisfying to accomplish things with

their minds and bodies. It is through work that children discover how to become successful, feel good about themselves, and feel confident enough to "try it again."

Children try out new things. Experimentation challenges children to try out all of their senses. They discover the tastes of new foods and sweet grass and the pungent odors of perfume, flowers, and pine needles. They feel a kitten's fur, finger paint, and sift sand through their fingers. They burrow into snow and haystacks and fling themselves down slides. They enjoy going barefoot and feeling mud squish between their toes.

Children like guessing games, riddles, and jokes. Table games help children to learn that someone must be a loser.

Eating is a joy, although children tend to gobble. They get hungry between meals and snack—often on junk foods, thereby acquiring faulty eating habits.

Children often observe parents, teachers, and adolescents taking medicines, smoking tobacco and marijuana cigarettes, drinking alcoholic beverages, and abusing drugs. Such observations arouse their curiosity about habit-forming substances and medicines. Such curiosity motivates them to discover for themselves what it's like to be drunk and to inhale tobacco smoke. Ideally, such experimentation will satisfy children's curiosities before they drift into self-destructive behaviors.

Elementary school children are very conscious of the clothes that other children wear. Children want to look like their classmates.

Sometimes boys will be intolerant of girls, and girls will snub boys. Boys learn to become conscious of masculinity, girls of femininity. Boys learn to like looking and feeling rough, careless, and scruffy; girls often acquire the opposite characteristics.

Children are beautiful; they are naive and unspoiled, zestful, and playful, and they have boundless energies. They are eager to learn and discover, and they have undeveloped talents and abilities. Teachers are fortunate to be able to help children structure the foundations of life. Watching and helping children develop into unique, well-adjusted, successful personalities has to be one of the greatest rewards and joys of being a teacher.

This brief overview of the elementary school child has emphasized that children develop in many ways—physically, emotionally, socially, and morally—and gradually mature into healthy adult personalities. Although these developments are readily available, they may be overlooked by the insensitive teacher because such developments occur simultaneously and instantly. Their holistic development is founded on their need to: (1) fulfill biological, safety, social, ego, and intellectual needs; and (2) develop skills for fulfilling these human health needs. In essence, children attain optimal well-being when they develop skills that allow them to fulfill these basic needs. Conversely, children unable to develop skills to fulfill most of their basic health needs suffer from minor illnesses and personality disorders. They are unable to become effective learners and succeed in adult life.

DEVELOPMENTAL TASKS

The preceding generalizations about the development of elementary school children reflect a "holistic" development. Such development is affected by not only the child's nutrition, genetic potentials, physical activity, and physical environment, but also the social milieu. Social and peer-group pressures greatly influence children's behaviors and habits. One such behavioral conditioner is the sociocultural environment. A culture creates aspirations: feeling a need to learn to read and write, to ride a bicycle or skateboard, to play team sports, to play a musical instrument, to go to college, to become a doctor or stock car racer, to drive a car, to drink soft drinks, to chew gum, to drink beer, to smoke cigarettes, and so on.

By making children feel these needs, society "forces" them to behave in certain ways. The culture determines the manner in which children meet these socially defined, or developmental, needs. These developmental needs have been identified as socially expected behaviors, which Havighurst (1953, p. 2) refers to as "developmental tasks":

A developmental task is a task which arises at or about a certain period in the life of the individual, successful achievement of which leads to his happiness and to success with later tasks, while failure leads to unhappiness in the individual, disapproval by society, and difficulty with later tasks.

The developmental tasks of elementary school children can be summarized as:

1. learning physical skills necessary for ordinary games and activities;
2. building wholesome attitudes toward oneself as a growing organism;
3. learning to get along with peers;
4. learning an appropriate masculine or feminine role;
5. developing fundamental skills in reading, writing, and calculating;
6. developing concepts necessary for everyday learning;
7. developing a conscience, morality, and a scale of values;
8. achieving personal independence;
9. developing attitudes toward social groups and institutions.

Origin of Developmental Tasks

Developmental tasks arise from (1) the physiological process of maturation; (2) social expectations; and (3) the child's personal values and aspirations. Some tasks arise mainly as a result of physical maturation: learning to walk, to control elimination, to skip, to throw and catch a ball, and to write. Other tasks are developed mainly from the cultural pressures of society: learning to read, to participate as a responsible citizen in society, and to assume appropriate sex roles. Still others grow out of personal values and aspirations: choosing and preparing for a vocation. Most developmental tasks arise from all three forces working together. For example, before a child can ride a bicycle, she or he must: (1) see others doing so (perceive a value and evolve an aspiration for attaining it); (2) feel pressure from peers and parents (social pressure); and (3) have reached a certain level of neuromuscular maturity (physiological) (see Figure 2.1). Many sociohygienic tasks have similar origins.

The major developmental tasks for children and adolescents ages 0 to 18 are schematically illustrated in Figure 2.2. This illustration identifies the developmental tasks of middle childhood (ages 6 to 12) as well as those that precede and follow this period.

Basis for Evolving Developmental Tasks

The key to understanding developmental tasks is to understand Erikson's theory of the development of a healthy personality (human life stages). Erikson (1963) has identified eight major life stages. For our purposes here, the most important stage of personality development is the fourth stage—becoming competent and acquiring skills. This stage coincides with the developmental tasks of middle childhood (ages 6 to about 12).

Developmental tasks evolve from three developmental thrusts in the child. First, the child is thrust out of the home and into the peer group by entering school. Second, while at school, the child is thrust physically into the world of games and work requiring neuromuscular skills. Third, the school thrusts the child into the world of adult concepts, logic, symbolism, and communication. At the beginning of school, the child has all the potentials for realizing these possibilities. All developmental tasks have implications for optimal well-being and style of living.

FIGURE 2.1
Example of how a developmental task (e.g., learning to ride a bicycle) originates.

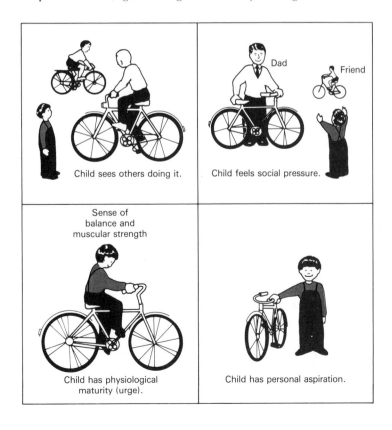

FIGURE 2.2

The characteristics and continuity of developmental tasks for ages 0 to 18. The horizontal dimension of each task is a measure of the amount of development taking place. The vertical dimension of each task indicates the age at which development in such a task occurs.

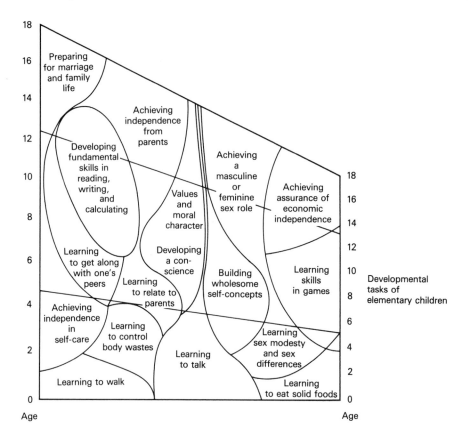

This is so because the child develops as a whole person—physically, emotionally, socially, culturally, and intellectually. Thus developmental tasks, because of their biological-sociocultural nature, are also developmental tasks for optimal well-being. The child needs to be well (healthy) in order to master the skills needed for abundant living and to be able to mature into a well-adjusted adult.

Developmental tasks occur at all ages. Society expects the child to master the tasks appropriate to its age level. These tasks should be considered as active goals that all children, consciously or unconsciously, strive to achieve.

The number of developmental tasks for each stage is arbitrary. Thus a major task may be broken down into small tasks. Consider, for example, the child learning locomotion (a major developmental task). The minor tasks involved are as follows: The *infant* learns to sit up, crawl, stand, and walk; the *child* learns to walk, run, jump, skip, and ride a bicycle; eventually, the *adolescent* learns to drive a car. Furthermore, major developmental tasks may be broken into sequential and progressively smaller tasks. This has special significance for the selection of content for well-being by elementary school teachers.

All of the tasks to be learned constitute healthful and satisfactory growth in our society. They are the things children must learn if they are to be judged, and to judge themselves, as reasonably happy and successful persons.

The timing of a developmental task is identical to the emergence of Erikson's life stages (1959, 1963). Failure to mature fully at one stage of development causes partial or complete failure to progress and to develop in the subsequent stages. Arrest of one or more developmental processes (physical, emotional, and social) upsets the functional harmony of the whole child, who eventually becomes a defective or deprived adult. Thus all development proceeds by critical steps—"critical" being characteristic of turning points or moments of decision between progress and regression. As a turning point, crisis should be interpreted as a crucial period of increased vulnerability and heightened potential and therefore a source of adjustment or maladjustment. Once a process or a part of it has been suppressed, it cannot develop at a later time. Such incomplete development hinders the development of future stages, so that a child often adjusts by evolving personality and behavioral aberrations during childhood, adolescence, and/or adulthood. Chapters 3, 4, and 5 provide more insight into such consequences—physical and psychoemotional-social problems.

GROWTH AND DEVELOPMENT
Definition of Terms

Three terms—growth, development, and maturity—are often used synonymously to describe the progress of the child toward adulthood. In reality, the terms are different, though inseparable; none takes place alone. *Growth* refers to quantitative changes—increases in size and structure. It indicates actual increase in size of either a part of the body or the whole organism. A child grows in height and weight, and his or her brain increases in size.

Development, by contrast, refers to changes that are qualitative in nature. Development, as an organization of all the parts that growth and differentiation have produced, implies the overall process of change. An increase in height is growth; an increase of small-muscle coordination in the fingers is development. Development depends in part on physical maturation—on

growth. Development may also refer to emotional and social behavior.

Maturity marks the end of growth and development. However, when applied to children, it is used to connote potentiality. It is most often used to identify that process of inner growth and development by which the individual moves toward the attainment of his or her uppermost physical, emotional, intellectual, and social potentialities. It is a sort of ripening. Maturity also refers to growth and development that have reached their ceiling or that are greater than expected for a child at a given age. A five-year-old child who resembles a seven-year-old in behavior is said to be "mature for his or her age." The term may be used to describe either growth or development at any stage. For example, the child's ability to control elimination is dependent on development of the sphincter muscles. When these are fully developed, at about three years, the child can begin to control elimination like other individuals.

The complex processes of growth, development, and maturation should be viewed as products of heredity, environment, self-concept, and cultural expectations. When the child is mature physically, emotionally, and socially, she or he is also ready to learn. Learning occurs most efficiently when the child is sufficiently mature for a particular learning experience.

Principles of Growth and Development

All growth and developmental processes of children, when studied in detail over a long time, follow basic patterns. These patterns reflect physical, emotional (psychological), social, intellectual, and behavioral traits of the whole child. All normal children tend to follow a general sequence of growth and development characteristic of their species and of their cultural group. Development follows a pattern that is little influenced by experience. The child matures when he or she is ready to mature. Such generalizing patterns are referred to as principles.

Teachers should use these principles as guidelines for understanding children, their growth and development, what to expect of them, and when to expect it, as well as for handling children effectively. The following principles should be helpful to teachers:

1. *Growth is patterned.* Although some children mature early and others late, each child has a unique pattern that unfolds at a characteristic rate.

2. *Growth is sequential.* Growth follows an orderly and predictable sequence, which in general is the same for all individuals. When age differentials are ignored, the growth pattern for boys and girls is the same. One stage leads to the next. Deviations from the sequence provide clues to growth difficulties.

3. *Growth is cyclic.* Rapid growth is usually followed by an intervening period of slow, steady growth and development. These cycles are readily apparent in the curve of the growth of the body as a whole. Human life proceeds by stages. Each stage is distinguished by a dominant feature that gives the period its unity and its uniqueness.

4. *Developmental rates vary.* Developmental rates are unique for boys and girls. After age ten, the growth rate for girls changes and is about two years ahead of that for boys. The tempo of development is not even. The feet, hands, and nose, for example, reach their maximum developmental level early in adolescence, whereas the lower parts of the face and shoulders are slower in reaching theirs. Likewise, the heart, liver, and digestive systems grow slowly in childhood but rapidly during the early adolescent years.

5. *Developmental patterns show wide individual differences.* Each child's growth and development are unique. Children reach puberty at different ages. Because of genetic influences, each part of the body has its own particular rate of growth and development. Each child follows a predictable pattern in a way and at a rate that are unique. Physical

development depends partly on heredity and partly on environmental factors such as food, emotional stress, and so on. Personality development is influenced by attitudes and social relationships.

6. *Each stage of development has characteristic traits.* Each body system develops at its own rate. Each body trait has its own unique developmental rate and characteristics helping to identify the child's behavioral, chronological, and maturational levels. The developmental pattern is affected not so much by what the child can accomplish as by the way in which he or she behaves.

7. *Development is a product of the interaction of the child with his or her environment.* Growth and development are genetically, socioculturally, and environmentally determined.

8. *The body tends to maintain a state of equilibrium,* called homeostasis. The body strives to maintain a constant internal environment despite changing conditions, whether internal or external.

9. *There is unity in growth patterns.* The child grows physically, emotionally, socially, morally, intellectually as a whole being. All aspects of the child's development are interrelated. The stage of maturity in one trait affects the development of others. There is a marked relationship between sexual maturing and patterns of interest and behavior. Desirable traits complement one another and tend to go together.

10. *Development is continuous.* Cellular growth continues from conception to death. Likewise, emotional, social, spiritual, cultural, creative, and intellectual potential exists and may be developed to high levels toward self-actualization. Because development is continuous, what happens at one stage has an influence on the stage that follows.

11. *Development proceeds from general to specific responses.* A baby sits before she or he walks. A child learns words that are ab-

stract, like "doggie," before he or she calls the dog a specific name, like "Brownie."

12. *Development comes from maturation and learning.* Development of physical, emotional, and intellectual traits, for example, comes partly from an intrinsic maturing of those traits and partly from exercise and experience on the part of the child.

GROWTH CYCLES

Growth in height and weight reflects general physical progress in development of body systems and processes. It is an indication of progress toward the child's optimal well-being and maturity. Height and weight are only outward indicators of growth and development, for there is no correlation between body size and well-being. The organs and body systems within the body are also increasing in size and are developing their unique functions at their own speed.

Increases in height and weight progress at a slow rate for ages 6 to 12. Weight increases average approximately four to seven pounds a year, whereas height increases two or more inches a year (see Figure 2.3). From ages 5 to 10 years, boys are generally taller than girls. Then there is a short period, from ages 10 to 14, when girls exceed boys in height. In general, children show a much steadier rate of gain in height than they do in weight.

Growth and development are rhythmic, not regular. A child does not gain a given number of pounds annually or grow a given number of inches. Studies of growth and development have revealed that there are four distinct periods of growth—two characterized by slow growth and two by rapid growth. These periods are depicted by growth in height cycles in Figure 2.4. From birth to 2 years, there is rapid growth. This is followed by a period of slow growth up to puberty, or sexual maturing, which usually begins between the eighth and eleventh years. From then until 15 or 16 years, there is once again rapid growth. This in turn is followed by a period

FIGURE 2.3
Average height of 6- to 19-year-old boys and girls.

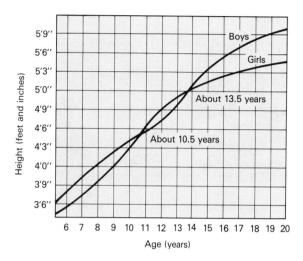

of fairly abrupt tapering off of growth to the time of full adult maturity.

The growth cycle for elementary school children is identified by the (b) cycle curve in Figure 2.4. This is a period of slow growth and is preceded by the infancy cycle. Because outward

FIGURE 2.4
The three cycles of growth in height: (a) infancy cycle; (b) childhood cycle; (c) adolescent cycle.

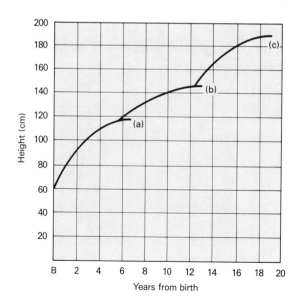

manifestations are presumed to mirror inner maturation, height and weight are often taken as indices of growth and normal well-being in general.

In general, the body systems are increasing in size and are developing their unique functions at their own rate of speed. The increments of growth and development for each body system will be discussed in greater detail under the corresponding sections.

INCREMENTS OF GROWTH AND DEVELOPMENT

The measurement of various body organs at regular intervals during their periods of growth and development reveals certain trends in the rate of change common to all normal children. Table 2.1 presents such a summary. Such measurements may also be plotted on a graph to provide a visual summary of the growth and development of the various parts of the body. This has been done in Figure 2.6.

Four types of growth curves (A, B, C, D) are illustrated in Figure 2.5. Curve A represents growth and development of the lymphoid type (thymus, tonsils, adenoids); curve B, that of the central nervous system (brain, nerves); curve C, that of the body as a whole (respiratory, digestive, muscular, skeletal, excretory, and cardiovascular systems); curve D, that of the reproductive, or genital, system. The growth curves for height and weight resemble the C, or general type, curve in Figure 2.5.

Development of Body Systems

The Central Nervous System

Neural maturity precedes the maturity of all other body systems. Because of its genetic endowment, the nervous system initiates the growth and development of the rest of the body. Neural maturity sets the stage for muscular development, which in turn allows psycho-emotional-social maturity to develop in the child. Brain growth is rapid during infancy and early childhood but slows down after 5 years of age. Brain weight in 10-year-olds is as great as that of adults (see Table 2.1). Nerve fibers in the brain areas are nearly mature by about 5 years of age, thus equipping the child for complex learning in school.

The growth of the central nervous system is most rapid in the first three years after birth, then slows down during childhood. This growth pattern of the nervous system is illustrated by curve B in Figure 2.6. Such early postnatal

TABLE 2.1
Average Weights (in Grams) of Organs at Different Ages.

	Newborn	1 Yr	6 Yr	Puberty	Adult
Brain	350	910	1200	1300	1350
Heart	24	45	95	150	300
Thymus	12	20	24	30	0-15
Kidneys (both)	25	70	120	170	300
Liver	150	300	550	1500	1600
Lungs (both)	60	130	260	410	1200
Pancreas	3	9	—	40	90
Spleen	10	30	55	95	155
Stomach	8	30	—	80	135

From G. H. Lowrey, *Growth & Development of Children*, 7th edition. Copyright © 1978 by Year Book Medical Publishers, Inc., Chicago. Used by permission.

FIGURE 2.5

Curves of organ growth drawn to a common scale by computing their values at successive ages in terms of their total (average) postnatal increments.

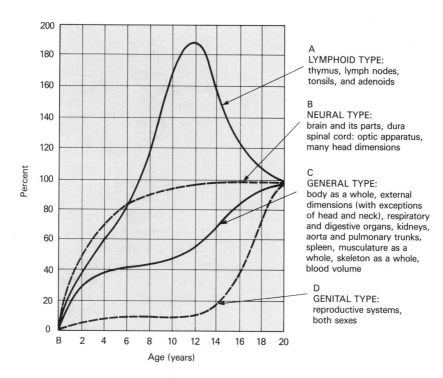

A
LYMPHOID TYPE:
thymus, lymph nodes,
tonsils, and adenoids

B
NEURAL TYPE:
brain and its parts, dura
spinal cord: optic apparatus,
many head dimensions

C
GENERAL TYPE:
body as a whole, external
dimensions (with exceptions
of head and neck), respiratory
and digestive organs, kidneys,
aorta and pulmonary trunks,
spleen, musculature as a
whole, skeleton as a whole,
blood volume

D
GENITAL TYPE:
reproductive systems,
both sexes

growth consists primarily of the development of immature cells present at birth. Most of the special senses are well developed at birth, although their association with higher centers comes about gradually during early life. The eyeball, for example, reaches adult size at about 12 to 14 years of age. However, since there is continuous growth and development of the eyes, vision does not assume adult level until after the middle of childhood. The eyes are not biologically "ready" for reading in most cases before the sixth year. That is, the fine coordination required of the eye muscles for moving rapidly over a page of print is achieved partly as a result of nerve and muscle growth. Furthermore, most children are naturally farsighted in early childhood. Their eyes take time to become normal-sighted and become best adapted to reading at about 8 years of age.

The ear is fully developed at birth. Both the inner and middle ear have reached nearly adult proportions. The main difference in ear structure between the infant and the grown adult is in the Eustachian tube. In children this tube connects the ear with the throat and is a short, wide, straight passage. As a result, the young child is continuously threatened with ear infections which develop in the throat.

From ages 3 to 10, neuromuscular coordination and skills are developed. These are discussed briefly in the section on the muscular system.

Glandular (Endocrine) System

The glandular system, largely through specific hormones, regulates growth and development of the body in general. Hormones govern maturation. These concepts are not readily apparent from the organ growth curves in Figure 2.6. All four types of curves probably represent some kind of glandular growth and function at one time or another. The numerous glands begin to influence body functions at various ages. Collectively, endocrine glands have a dynamic

FIGURE 2.6

Secondary ossification centers, showing average time of appearance.

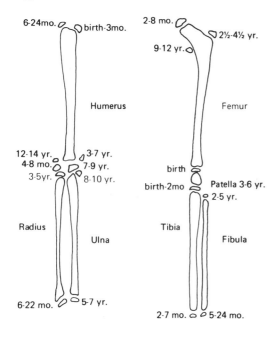

effect on the body. They regulate not only body growth and development during childhood, but also the functioning of body systems throughout life.

Four glands of internal secretion are concerned primarily with the regulation of growth: the pituitary, the thyroid, the gonads, and the adrenal cortex. Although the function of all the glands is determined by heredity, such function is often altered by nutrition and by physical and socioeconomic environments. All the glands reinforce and complement one another. Their synergistic action is essential for normal growth, development, and maturation.

The master gland in the body is not the pituitary gland. The pituitary is regulated by the hypothalamus (master gland) in the brain and directs the function of the other glands. Indirectly, the pituitary hormone influences growth of the skeleton, the muscles, and the viscera. General body size depends on the output of somatotropin, the principal growth hormone that also controls the pituitary gland. The gonadotropic hormone of the pituitary initiates and regulates growth and differentiation of the gonads.

It also has a modifying effect on the metabolism and affects the growth pattern of the child.

The thyroid gland reinforces the work of the pituitary gland. It exerts a profound influence on growth and development of bones and governs the rate at which energy is used up.

The adrenal cortex, located at the tip of the kidneys, secretes hormones that promote metabolism and aid the body in stress adaptation. Cortin, the principal secretion of the adrenal cortex, affects the rate of maturation. There is a rapid decrease in the size of the adrenal glands after birth. Then they increase rapidly in size up to age 5, slow down in growth from 5 to 11 years, and then increase in size rapidly up to 16 years. Until growth in size has increased, there will be less adrenalin secreted. This has a marked influence on emotional states in childhood.

The gonads control the growth and development of the organs of reproduction and growth. Gonadal hormones bring about epiphyseal closure in bones and thus terminate growth. When gonadal secretion is inadequate when normal epiphyseal closure should occur, the limbs may continue to grow in length, so that height becomes excessive, and body proportions may become abnormal.

The reproductive organs grow very little during early childhood, but develop rapidly from about age 10 to 14. This is illustrated in Figure 2.5 by curve D. It is at this time that sex hormones bring about secondary sexual characteristics. The girl begins to ovulate, and the boy is capable of producing spermatozoa. Sexual development shows marked male and female differences. The cultural impact of sexual expectation creates disparities of skills between boys and girls.

Awareness of the growth and development of the glandular system in elementary school children is most important for teachers. Many emotional and adjustment problems stem from the child's inability to cope with glandular changes. Changing sexual development creates different and new roles, needs, and interests for boys and girls at various age levels. Such changes impose on the child numerous emotional stresses and adjustments. Children may in turn project their personal problems on their peers, parents, and teachers. Thus many emotional and health problems, as discussed in Chapters 3 and 4, initially stem from the effects of glandular growth and development on the child.

Skeletal System

Skeletal development and maturity follow a unique pattern. This is illustrated in Figure 2.6 by the C, or general type, curve. In general, bone growth is rapid in the first five years and at puberty, when bones begin to harden, or ossify. Bone growth and ossification during childhood (ages 5 to 10) are slow, with various bones ossifying at various ages.

Children of different racial and geographic backgrounds have different skeletal developmental rates. In general, the stage of osseous maturation correlates well with weight, height, and sexual development. That is, the child whose height and weight are less than average for age also has repressed bone maturation. A greater variation of this is found in girls. Longitudinal studies reveal that a boy or girl with advanced skeletal maturation will reach physiological maturity at an earlier chronological age than one with a relatively slow degree of maturation.

In comparison with the bones of the adult, the bones of the child contain a greater part of water and soft proteinlike materials and a considerably lesser portion of mineral substances. Likewise, the skeletal constituents contain much more cartilage and fibrous tissue during the early years. Therefore, the bones of the child are more pliable and elastic than those of the adult. Although this characteristic is desirable in that fracture is less likely, it does provide more opportunity for deformity and imperfection, since the bones resist less successfully the many stresses and strains of muscles and tissues.

From studying a series of X-ray pictures of a child's skeletal system as he or she matures, we can predict the sequence of physical maturation. We become aware that the bones in a young child are not firmly grown together. This is illustrated in Figure 2.6 by the time schedule of appearance of ossification centers in the arms and legs. Figure 2.7 presents the normal maturation of the bones of the hands and feet in both sexes. Note the great amount of space between the ends of the bones. The amount of space is inversely pro-

FIGURE 2.7

Ossification centers of the hands and feet, showing time of appearance. Note the wide range of "normal." (Modified from Scammon in *Morris' Human Anatomy* and reproduced with permission from Caffey, J.: *Pediatric X-Ray Diagnosis,* 6th edition, Vol. 2. Copyright © 1972 by Year Book Medical Publishers, Inc., Chicago.)

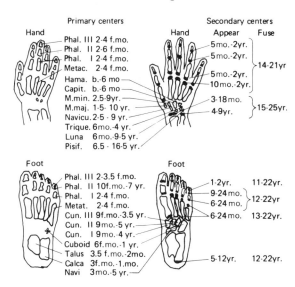

f.mo. = fetal months,   mo. = postnatal months,   yr. = year

portional to age. Infant cartilage is gradually replaced by ossification of bone. Ossification, or fusion of the growth line of bones (epiphysis), follows a fairly definite pattern and time schedule from birth to maturity. The duration of the cartilaginous stage is a rough measure of the relative speed of general body development.

The number of teeth at given stages of development is another gauge of growth, development, and maturity. Figure 2.8 shows that tooth eruption follows the familiar pattern already illustrated by height and weight curves. The curve has a slow beginning, rapid acceleration, with a slowing down between ages 9 and 10, followed by a second rapid growth between ages 11 and 13.

A child entering school at 6 has usually lost some of his or her early teeth. At 6 years of age the child has 1 or 2 permanent teeth; at 8 years, 10 or 11; at 10 years, 14 or 16; at 12 years, 24 or 26; and at 13, 27 or 28. Growth of teeth is thus a continuing process.

There are individual differences in the time

FIGURE 2.8

The eruption of teeth as a form of growth and development. (From Cecil V. Millard, *Child Growth and Development in the Elementary School Years,* Lexington, Mass.: D.C. Heath, 1958, p. 83.)

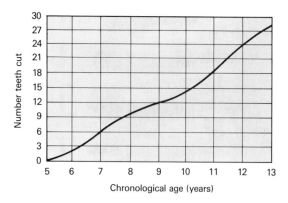

required for growth and in the ages at which teeth appear. Girls cut their teeth a little earlier than boys do. Normally, as teeth appear, the jaw also grows so as to adjust to the number of teeth that it must accommodate.

Loss of teeth mars the child's appearance and makes him or her feel self-conscious. The child may become emotional about losing teeth and project such feelings toward others at this time.

Muscular System

Gain in musculature in childhood is related to the growth of other organs, systems, and tissues. As shown in Figure 2.6, there are two rapid rates of muscle growth in general. One occurs before the age of 5 and the other after the age of 10. During the elementary school interval, there is less muscular growth taking place. Instead, muscular development replaces growth.

At birth, muscle fibers are present in an undeveloped state. No new muscle fibers develop after birth, but the ones that are present change in size, shape, and composition. Muscles increase in size by growth in length, breadth, and thickness of the fibers. With muscle growth comes an increase in body weight. Up to 5 years of age, muscles grow in proportion to the increase in body weight. The large skeletal muscles, as used for locomotion, become well developed. After the age of 5, the smaller and finer muscles, which

control the child's ultimate strength and manipulative capacities, begin to develop. During this primary period, there is a rapid spurt in muscle growth, at which time the child's weight gain is approximately 75 percent muscle weight. Now, as the small muscles develop, the child's ability to coordinate his or her body increases. As the child enters fourth grade, muscle development continues slowly until about age 10.

In general, as size and weight of muscle tissue increase, strength also increases. From age 3 on, a child's strength grows, doubling at about 11. It doubles again between 12 and 16 years of age. Because muscular development is relatively slow, the greatest increases in muscular strength take place during puberty. In boys and girls up to the age of 10, there is no difference in muscular strength. However, after this period, muscular strength increases much faster in boys than in girls.

Exercise and physical activities seem to stimulate muscular growth (size) and development (neuromuscular coordination). The elementary child's need to move about is thought to be directly related to the building up of muscular tension resulting from physical growth. Activity not only relieves such tension and brings on a feeling of general well-being, but also stimulates further growth and development of large and small muscles. In addition to these benefits, exercise of large muscles helps to regulate body systems and processes. Exercise is thus essential to muscle growth and neuromuscular development.

From ages 3 to 10, neuromuscular coordination and manipulative skills are developed. During the first four or five years of life, the child gains control over gross movements—those involving the large muscle areas of the body used in walking, running, swimming, and bicycling. After 5 years of age, major development takes place in the control of finer coordinations—the neuromuscular development of the smaller muscle groups used in grasping, throwing and catching balls, writing, and using tools. Such neuromuscular maturity precedes learning and is related to the child's emotional and social adequacy. In general, girls mature more rapidly than boys do. Many neuromuscular differences between sexes, such as boys' greater proficiency in throwing a ball, are attributable to cultural influences. The changes in coordination during this time continue to follow the principle of movement toward increasing complexity. There are increases in speed, dexterity, and coordination ability for social purposes.

Cardiovascular System

Heart growth and development are characterized by two rapid growth spurts: between ages 1 and 5, and between ages 9 and 16 years. During the elementary school years, the heart grows slowly. When compared with overall body size, the heart is smallest at 7 years of age. Heart growth keeps pace with general body growth and development, as shown by curve C in Figure 2.6.

Growth of the heart occurs at rapid increments after the first year. Such growth is summarized in Table 2.2. By age 5 it has increased fourfold; by age 9, sixfold.

The heart rate is quite variable throughout the life of the child. Rates differ only slightly between sexes. Table 2.2 lists the average heart rates obtained from several sources for children at rest but not sleeping.

Blood pressure in a child may vary greatly from day to day, and the increase in blood pressure that occurs with age is not constant from year to year. In other words, each child has his or her developmental pattern. Table 2.2 presents the normal systolic blood pressures for various ages.

The growth in caliber of the arteries and veins seems related to the volume or weights of the regions to which they supply blood.

The child's heart is vulnerable to the stresses of life. Although heart growth keeps pace with general body growth and development, it is not ready to support all the activities in which the child's body participates, in addition to the growth and developmental needs of the body as a whole. Since it grows slowly during the early school years, the many activities imposed on it must be interspersed with periods of rest. Physical fatigue is nature's way of slowing the child down and protecting him or her from overworking the heart. A child who gets tired will naturally stop for rest. Teachers should keep these principles in mind when planning work and physical activities for their students.

Respiratory System

Growth and development of the respiratory system follow curve C, as shown in Table 2.3. With increased muscular mobility comes concomitant stress on development of the lungs after birth. Although the number of air pockets, or alveoli, is the same at birth as in adulthood, the increase in respiratory exchange of gases is dependent on the growth in size of undeveloped alveoli as well as on the development of capillaries around each air sac to facilitate gaseous exchanges. As these changes take place, the oxygen-carrying capacity of the body increases with an increase in the number of red blood cells. Thus the lungs grow rapidly between birth and about age 5 and again with the advent of adolescence.

The young child breathes air by movement of the diaphragm until ages 5 to 7. Thereafter, the costal and other chest muscles begin to help out. The rate and depth of breathing are ex-

TABLE 2.2
Comparison of Heart Growth and Development from Birth to Adolescence, Averaged for Both Sexes.

	Birth	1 Yr	5 Yr	7 Yr	9 Yr	10-16 Yr
Heart size compared to birth		2×	4×	5×	6×	7×-20×
Heart weight (g)	20-24	38-45	82-90	100	125	135-220
Heart rate (at rest)	150	110-115	100	95	90-95	82-85
Average systolic blood pressure (mm Hg)	52	96	99	105	110	115-120

TABLE 2.3
Summary of Variations in Respiration with Age.

	Birth	*1 Yr*	*5 Yr*	*10 Yr*	*20 Yr*
Lung weight (increases as compared to birth)	1	3×			20×
Respiratory rates (min)	30-80	20-40	20-25	17-22	15-20
Tidal air (cc)	19	48	175	320	500

tremely variable in children (see Table 2.3). From studying this table, we can generalize that variations in respiration occur with changes in age. Respiration becomes slower, deeper, and more regular as the child gets older. Sexual differences in breathing are negligible during childhood. Lungs increase in size by the use of more latent alveoli, thus increasing the volume of tidal air. It is during this time of alternating growth and development of the respiratory system that the child is most susceptible to respiratory infections.

Excretory System

Kidney growth is most rapid in infancy and during childhood. The kidney is five times its birth size by age 5 and ten times its birth size by age 10. Bladder and bowel control in most children begins at about 2 years, when the sphincter muscles in the anus and bladder have matured and the child assumes willful control of these muscles. Such control is complete in most children when they enter school. In general, the excretory system follows the general growth curve up to 5 years, then a slow growth period during the elementary school period, and then an accelerated growth period during adolescence.

With the excretory system maturing at about 5 years, the entire body is brought into a higher state of homeostasis.

Lymphatic System

This is the protective system of the body and includes lymph nodes and tissue and the thymus gland. The number of lymph nodes and the amount of lymphoid tissue are considerable at birth. These increase steadily during childhood but undergo a relative reduction after puberty. Such lymphoid growth is illustrated in Figure 2.6. Tonsils, adenoids, and especially the thymus gland undergo marked hypertrophy from ages 5 to 10 years, then atrophy to adult size. The hypertrophy of these structures is a normal physiological process.

The maximal development of these tissues during the time when acute infections of the respiratory and alimentary tracts are most common and during the period of greatest increase in weight and height has led to the conclusion that they are a part of a natural defense mechanism. The lymphatic system plays an important part in evolving body immunity during early and middle childhood. Formation of antibodies takes place in part or completely within this system. During infancy and childhood, lymphoid tissues characteristically respond to infection by rapid swelling and hyperplasia (increase in size of tissue). Hyperplasia is especially notable in the thymus gland.

The gradual building up of antibodies in the body reaches a peak at about 12 to 15 years of age. The buildup of such immunity also enhances homeostasis.

Digestive System

Growth of the digestive system follows curve C as illustrated in Figure 2.6. It is most rapid before the child enters school and during adolescence. There is a slow, gradual growth period while the child attends elementary school. In general, the digestive organs tend to resemble adult organs in appearance with advancing age.

Summary of Physiological Development

In general, physiological development is sequential, continuous, and unique. Body systems are interrelated in both function and development. The child must mature physically before developing emotionally and socially. However, physical growth and development do not take place in a vacuum. They are nurtured by the child's environment.

REFERENCES AND BIBLIOGRAPHY

Anderson, C. L. *School Health Practice* (St. Louis: C. V. Mosby, 1960).

Blackfan, Kenneth D. *Growth and Development of the Child*, Report of the Committee on Growth and Development, White House Conference on Child Health and Protection (New York: Century, 1933).

Dinkmeyer, Don C. *Child Development* (Englewood Cliffs, N.J.: Prentice-Hall, 1965).

Erikson, Erik H. "Identity and the Life Cycle," *Psychological Issues* (1959).

———. *Childhood and Society* (New York: Norton, 1963).

Faculty of University School. *How Children Develop* (Columbus: Ohio State University Press, 1964).

Freeman, Howard E., and Wyatt C. Jones. *Social Problems: Causes and Controls* (Chicago: Rand McNally, 1971), 287-288.

Gordon, Ira J. *Human Development* (New York: Harper & Row, 1962).

Guyton, Arthur C. *Textbook of Medical Physiology* (Philadelphia: Saunders, 1966).

Havighurst, Robert J. *Developmental Task and Education* (New York: Longman, Green, Arnold, 1953).

Hettinger, Theodor. *Physiology of Strength* (Springfield, Ill: Charles C Thomas, 1961).

Hurlock, Elizabeth B. *Child Development* (New York: McGraw-Hill, 1964).

Millard, Cecil V. *Child Growth and Development in the Elementary School Years* (Boston: D. C. Heath, 1958).

Nemir, Alma. *The School Health Program* (Philadelphia: Saunders, 1965).

U.S. Department of Health, Education, and Welfare. *Perspectives on Human Deprivation: Biological, Psychological and Sociological* (Washington, D.C.: U. S. Government Printing Office, 1968).

U.S.H.E.W. *Your Child from Six to Twelve* (Bronxville, N.Y.: Child Care Publishers, 1962).

Vincent, Elizabeth L., and Phyllis C. Martin. *Human Psychological Development* (New York: Ronald Press, 1961).

Watson, Ernest H., and George H. Lowrey. *Growth and Development of Children* (Chicago: Year Book Medical Publishers, 1962).

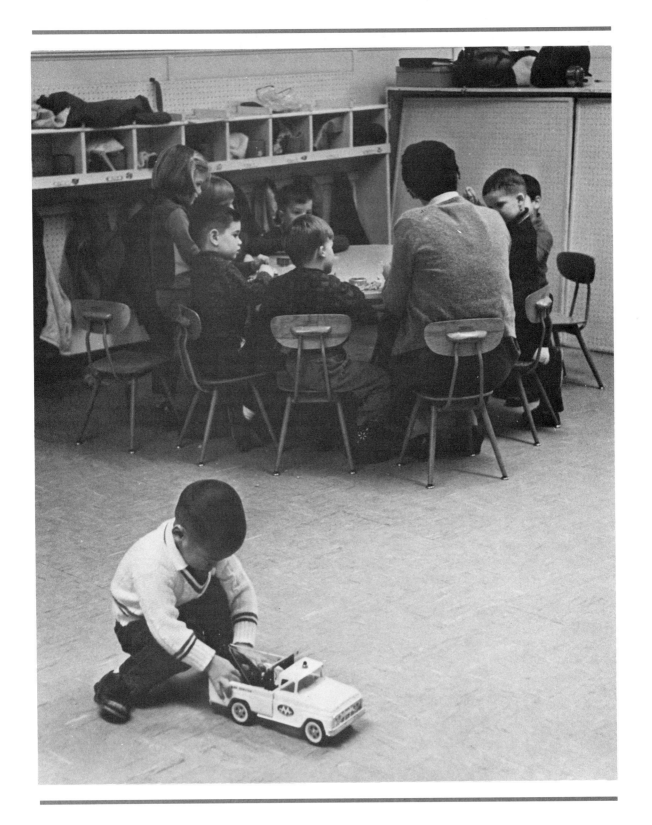

Chapter 3　Emotional-Social Development

INTRODUCTION

Children disturbed with the normal problems of growing up often have difficulty in learning. If not resolved, their troubles—physical, emotional, and social tensions, anxieties, and frustrations—may become masked and later may erupt as antisocial behavior. With each new group of kindergartners, some may be expected to develop serious emotional handicaps before completing the sixth grade. Such children, whose troubles are often unrecognized when they start school, develop learning difficulties, which in turn contribute to disciplinary problems and to dropping out. It is estimated that between 10 percent and 25 percent of elementary school children have emotional problems and maladjustments requiring psychiatric help. On the basis of these estimates, there must be, on the average, about three to eight emotionally handicapped children in each elementary classroom. At least one child in each classroom needs immediate psychiatric help.

Such children are problems not only to themselves, but also to their peers and teachers. They often disrupt the classroom and exact a disproportionate amount of the teacher's time and energy. The risk that disturbed children in today's classrooms may become delinquent as adolescents or emotionally (mentally) ill as adults is substantial. More than 20 million Americans are mentally sick today. More than half of the adults consulting doctors have complaints related to emotional disturbances. Emotional illness is the major public health problem in this country today. The extent of such disorders may be put into better perspective when emotional disorders are interrelated to include drug abuse and misuse, alcoholism, delinquency and crime, sexual aberrations, eating disorders, smoking, boredom and depression, and other deviant behavior.

Physical problems such as asthma, poor posture, obesity, poor vision, and poor hearing all pose primary handicaps for the child. Likewise, family problems such as a bad home life, one-parent households, parental neglect, sibling rivalry, child abuse, lack of constructive home responsibilities, living in poverty, and lack of close emotional relationships with either parent or both may constitute primary behavioral handicaps for the child. In addition to physical and family problems, the immediate social environment may spawn primary handicaps of an emotional nature for the child. For example, not being able to socialize with friends, not belonging to a group, being the only one without a bicycle, and other social and economic inequities may give the sensitive child a feeling of deprivation and inadequacy.

When these and other social and family problems are not corrected, are not properly compensated for, are not resolved, or are not reinforced to the satisfaction of the child's immediate physical, emotional, and social needs, the child will feel insecure, rejected, and inadequate. Such a child often tries to cope with these feelings by adapting the original handicap to his or her social environment. Such forms of adaptation often result in secondary health problems such as emotional disorders and disturbances, disobedience, disrespect for law and order, dishonesty and cheating, promiscuity, eating disorders, and other forms of bizarre and self-destructive misbehavior. Other environmental conditions that may create discipline problems are class size and grade level, the size of the school system, the availability of community services, transporting of children by bus, and the school's administrative policies. Misbehavior arising out of unfavorable conditions in these areas often has origins beyond the teacher's sphere of influence. Psychiatrists recognize these and other misbehaviors as unsuccessful attempts to fulfill the basic human needs to feel adequate and to love and to be loved.

DIFFICULTY IN INTERPRETING EMOTIONAL WELL-BEING

Emotional disturbances and abnormal behaviors are difficult to define. Various terms are used to describe them: mental illness, learning disabilities, behavioral problems, emotional disorders, emotional blocks, aberrations, social misbehaviors, psychopathologies, metapathologies, psychosomatic disturbances, psychoneurotic disorders, adjustive reactions, personality problems, maladjustments, and emotional handicaps. As symptoms, these may be secondary to a physical or a medical condition, although the etiology remains obscure. These terms denote conditions of tension or nervousness characterized by deviations in thinking, feeling, and acting. The more severe the disorder, the more radical are the disturbances, until the individual becomes almost incapable of adjusting to life.

The variety of terms used as references to emotional well-being reflects the confusion among the professional groups and the lay public. Emotional well-being appears to be interpreted as feelings (emotional), thinking (psychological), actions (adjustments), behaviors (social), and self-esteem (image). A very thin line often exists between normality and abnormality. More often than not, it is a qualitative difference. Many people cross this line several times during their lives. Emotionally well persons tend to adapt to changes and conditions. Thus no person remains completely well adjusted for any great length of time. Adults are expected to conform to social standards of emotional behavior. On the other hand, children are in the process of trying to fulfill their biological, psychological, emotional, and social needs. Many of their coping experiences are of a first-time nature. Therefore, children may pass back and forth over the normal-abnormal line several times a month. Their coping is often of a trial-and-error approach that is more readily tolerated in them than in adults. As with adults, the key to interpreting such coping behavior is whether the child is able to maintain a balanced and realistic orientation between needs and social expectations.

In conclusion, we should be aware that emotional well-being, like well-being itself, cannot be defined. Instead, it should be conceptualized. Various concepts and indices of the spectrums of emotional well-being and behavior are discussed in the next section.

CONCEPT OF EMOTIONAL WELL-BEING

Emotional well-being was conceptualized in Chapter 1 as feelings and thoughts reinforcing identity. We suggested that this state is characterized by the ability to cope successfully with the stresses of daily living; be flexible in all social situations; feel worthwhile and adequate as a person; feel content and happy; feel a sense of accomplishment and self-realization; face up to and accept reality; feel worthwhile as a member of society; have emotional stability; exercise self-discipline and self-confidence; accept responsibility for one's behavior and social roles; feel good about self and others; have worthwhile hobbies and recreational interests; have an adequate self-image; and be able to give, express, and accept love. Such feelings and thoughts may be interpreted as comprising an index of positive emotional well-being to be found among adults. Many of these traits may also be recognized in children (see Figure 3.1).

At the other end of the spectrum of well-being are emotional disturbances (see Figure 3.2). An emotionally disturbed child can be characterized as follows:

1. Seeming inability to learn that cannot be satisfactorily explained by intellectual, sensory, or health factors;
2. Unsatisfactory relationship with peers and teachers;
3. Tendency to exhibit inappropriate behavior in normal circumstances;
4. Feeling of general unhappiness or depression;
5. Tendency to develop physical symptoms or fears in relation to personal or school problems.

Other indices may also be applied to the bipolar spectrum of emotional well-being and emotional illness. Erik Erikson (1964, 1968) has taken this approach in outlining human maturational life cycles. Thus, emotionally mature children have developed a sense of trust, autonomy (self-image), initiative, and self-assertion; they are industrious (have competence), accept responsibility, are interested in doing productive work, and feel adequate; they have evolved a self-identity (personal role image). Conversely, emotionally immature children often develop the opposite feelings and behaviors: mistrust, shame and doubt, guilt and overaggression, inferiority (inadequacy), and identity diffusion.

FIGURE 3.1
A few characteristics of the emotionally disturbed child.

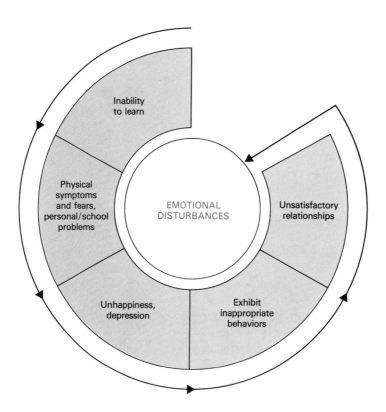

Emotional well-being may also be considered a component of a sound personality. The indices of a "healthy, multi-valued personality" have been abstracted by Rucker *et al.* (1969) from Adler, Fromm, Blotz, Horney, Rank, Sullivan, Rogers, Maslow, Allport, and Jourard. Their collective thinking suggests that healthy persons have the following characteristics:

1. They acknowledge *personal responsibility* for their own actions (high rectitude status).
2. They are *self-reliant* (high status of self-respect). They are more independent in solving their problems than are average or ill persons.
3. They deal *with their environment* in a creative manner (enlightenment and skill). They use their own skills and understanding to do things necessary for their health and happiness.

4. Their *concepts about other people are realistic* and are not distorted by experience. Such people are aware of these relationships and that their beliefs about themselves and other people are accurate (enlightenment and skill).
5. They have *social feeling* (love and respect). Such persons are identified with humanity. The unhealthy person concentrates on competing for power in order to escape from feelings of insecurity, whereas the healthy person is free to love and to respect others.
6. They tend to *realize their latent potentials* in everyday activities (skills). They are not afraid to try out new ways of doing things for fear of failure (with consequent loss of respect).
7. They tend to *see reality as it is* and to be comfortable in their relationship with it. Such persons can more easily distin-

FIGURE 3.2
Characteristics of a healthy personality.

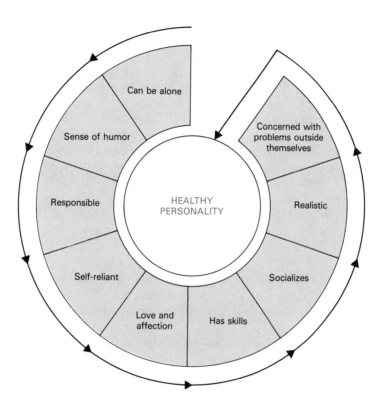

guish between the true and the false, the honest and the dishonest person. They do less wishful thinking than emotionally ill persons. They have less fear of the unknown and thus are relatively free to create new ways of doing things and to try them out with confidence (self-respect and skill).

8. They *think and often act spontaneously.* While inwardly despising the conventional, they will often accept it in order to avoid hurting people. Such persons can thus be said to have a social consciousness that forces them to think before they may act unconventionally (rectitude).

9. They are *concerned with problems outside themselves* rather than with self, in contrast to insecure people (rectitude, enlightenment, and skill). As adults, such people are concerned with the basic is-

sues of life and work in the broadest frame of reference in thinking about values and their achievement.

10. They can be *alone without discomfort* (self-respect). Such people even have more need of solitude or privacy than the "average" or ill person, who is usually uncomfortable when alone.

11. They continue to *get pleasure from the beauty of their environment throughout life.* They respond aesthetically and with pleasure to a beautiful flower, even though they have seen one almost exactly like it many times before (high status of aesthetic skill). This attitude of continuing appreciation is an index of good mental health.

12. They have *democratic personalities.* They demand that all values be shared. This is an index of high rectitude status. They will learn from the experiences of any

person of good character regardless of political belief, class, religious persuasion, or nationality (respect and affection). They treat people courteously, have respect for people on the basis of merit rather than on family or other unearned status. They are ethical in their interpersonal relationships. They demand that others have the same access to values that they demand for themselves (rectitude).

13. They are *able to distinguish between means and ends* (enlightenment and skill). They always place the goals they seek above the means by which they seek to achieve them. This trait may often be displayed in the judicious management of personal finances.

14. They have an *unholistic sense of humor* (respect), do not laugh at misfortunes of others, and do not attempt to make people laugh by hurting others. Such people, however, are quick to see the humor in the errors of human beings in general, such as trying to feel important when this feeling is not justified. They can laugh at their own mistakes. Their humor is spontaneous rather than planned (well-being).

15. They *offer intelligent and responsible resistance* to many aspects of the cultural mold (rectitude). They conform with many of the observable symbols of conventionality, but are really not conventional in the dependent sense. They accept conventional practices only to the degree to which they think they are good.

People with these personality characteristics have mature values guiding their behavior. Such persons are positive, purposeful, enthusiastic, and proud.

The indices of a healthy, multivalued personality are reinforced by the characteristics of people with good mental health as outlined by the National Association for Mental Health (1965). Such people feel comfortable about themselves; feel right about other people; and are able to meet life's demands.

Feelings and thoughts are often fused into overt actions and behavior. Consequently, understanding, interpreting, and identifying behavioral problems in children becomes a complex and difficult task when the child's thoughts and feelings, as reactions to tensions and anxieties, are masked by and transformed into overt actions and behaviors. Such behaviors are usually not perceived as being related to emotions. Because of this lack of association, teachers are often unable to recognize the early symptoms of emotional disturbance or the latent signs of maladjustment and misbehavior. As a result, disturbed children may be overlooked by a teacher and receive no assistance until their problems become so acute that they attract the attention of clinical or law enforcement agencies.

The variety of behavioral problems teachers encounter in school requires them to make some discriminatory judgments and interpretations. It is quite important that teachers be able to distinguish forms of behavior that are harmful or destructive to the child and/or to society from those that are temporary and that are consequences of environmental upsets, are by-products of normal growth, or are expressions of emotional release. Also, they must be able to predict which characteristics may be outgrown and which can be expected to become worse and lead to serious behavioral problems.

These judgments are not always easy to make. However, various research and clinical reports reveal certain clusters of symptoms to be indicators of chronic maladjustment. The following list, adapted by Kaplan (1959) from a compilation made by the Minneapolis Public Schools, indicates some of the behavioral *characteristics commonly associated with serious adjustment problems:*

1. *Nervous behavior:* habitual twitching of muscles, scowling, grimacing, twisting the hair, continuous blinking, biting or wetting the lips, nail biting, stammering, blushing or turning pale, constant restlessness, frequent complaints of minor illnesses, head banging, nervous finger movements, frequent crying, rocking the body, frequent urination.

2. *Emotional overreactions and deviations:* undue anxiety over mistakes, marked dis-

tress over failures, absentmindedness, daydreaming, meticulous interest in details, refusal to take part in games, refusal to accept any recognition or reward, evasion of responsibility, withdrawal from anything that looks new or difficult, chronic attitude of apprehension, lack of concentration, unusual sensitivity to all annoyances (especially noises), inability to work if distracted, lack of objective interests, frequent affectations and posturing, inappropriate laughing, uncontrolled laughing or giggling, explosive and emotional tone in argument, tendency to feel hurt when others disagree, unwillingness to give in, shrieking when excited, frequent efforts to gain attention, sudden intensive attachments to people (often older), extravagant expressions of any emotion.

3. *Emotional immaturity:* inability to work alone, tendency to cling to a single intimate friend, inability to rely on own judgment, unreasonable degree of worry over grades, persistent inferiority feelings, unusual self-consciousness, inability to relax and forget self, excessive suspiciousness, overcritical of others, too docile and suggestible, persistent fears, indecision, compulsive behavior, hyperactivity.

4. *Exhibitionist behavior:* teasing, pushing or shoving other pupils, trying to act tough, trying to be funny, wanting to be overconspicuous, exaggerated courtesy, marked agreement with everything the teacher says, continual bragging, frequent attempts to dominate younger or smaller children, inability to accept criticism, constant efforts to justify self, frequent blaming of failures on accidents or on other individuals, refusal to admit any personal lack of knowledge or inability, frequent bluffing, attempting either far too little or far too much work.

5. *Antisocial behavior:* cruelty to others, bullying, abusive or obscene language, undue interest in sex (especially efforts to establish bodily contact), telling offensive stories or showing obscene pictures, pro-

found dislike of all school work, fierce resenting of authority, bad reaction to discipline, general destructiveness, irresponsibility, sudden and complete lack of interest in school, truancy.

6. *Psychosomatic disturbances:* reversals or complications in toilet habits, enuresis, constipation, diarrhea, excessive urination, eating disorders,* nausea or vomiting when emotionally distressed, various aches and pains.**

Most teachers will recognize many of these characteristics as appearing in the behavior of normal children. Whenever combinations of these symptoms appear frequently and consistently or are not outgrown in time, however, the teacher should suspect a serious problem. A child may also be suspected of having an adjustment problem whenever his or her behavior is exaggerated beyond what is customary for youngsters of that age.

Emotional-social well-being may also be interpreted according to Erikson's theory of the development of a healthy personality, or human life stages. Erikson has proposed eight emotional-social development stages, as summarized in Table 3.1. In order to develop into a well-adjusted adult, a child needs to progress through the various stages in positive rather than negative ways. Stage four, concerned with acquiring competence and skills, occurs from ages 6 to 12 and is therefore of direct concern to elementary school teachers because the teacher can help children to acquire the sociohygienic skills of life. Many of the later skills of life are rooted in and are dependent on mastery of the sociohygienic skills in the formative years of the child's life. The preceding stages are also relevant, but the elementary school teacher is not in a position to help the child during them. The focus of attention in this chapter, therefore, centers on the stage relevant to the elementary school child and school teacher.

---

*For a more detailed discussion of eating disorders refer to Appendix E.

**This listing is from pp. 283-284 in *Mental Health and Human Relations in Education* by Louis Kaplan. New York: Harper & Row, 1959.

TABLE 3.1
Erikson's Stages of Human Development.

Age	Stage	Characterization of Stage	Value Strengths
0-1	oral-sensory	basic trust vs. shame	hope and drive
2-3	muscular-anal	autonomy vs. shame, doubt	willpower and self-control
4-5	locomotor-genital	initiative vs. guilt	purpose and direction
6-12	latency	industry vs. inferiority	competence and method
13-19	puberty and adolescence	identity vs. role confusion	fidelity and devotion
20-30	young adulthood	intimacy vs. isolation	love and affiliation
30-64	adulthood	generativity vs. stagnation	care and production
65+	maturity	ego integrity vs. despair	wisdom and renunciation

Adapted from Epigenetic Chart from *Childhood and Society*, 2nd Edition, Revised, by Erik H. Erikson.

The first three stages of life as outlined by Erikson should prepare the child for the fourth period. It is to be hoped that by the time the child attends school, he or she has successfully progressed through all of the developmental stages. Thus the child will have developed hope and trust from security as an infant; will have developed a will from autonomy at two and three years of age; and will have picked up purposefulness from his or her initiative play during ages four and five. The child is ready to acquire skills that will help him or her to become socialized and a self-realizing person.

In addition to these behavioral and emotional concepts, the teacher should be aware of the possibility of value deprivation in some elementary school children. Such a condition appears when the new values of today are in conflict with the traditional values of the child. The values that normally guide the child in making decisions about his or her behavior may appear irrational, abnormal, and without purpose. Maslow (1967) interprets this condition as "valuelessness." The feelings of such children are described as a lack of something to believe in and to be devoted to, amorality, rootlessness, anhedonia, anomie, emptiness, hopelessness, and other metapathologies. No doubt today's rapid and numerous changes of technology have affected our lifestyles dramatically. People unable to cope successfully with changes have been described by Toffler (1970) as being in a state of "future shock." A modern concept of emotional well-being would be incomplete without an appreciation of human value needs and an understanding that a person's physical, emotional, social, spiritual, and cultural needs and reactions are mediated by his or her value needs.

Finally, the picture of emotional and social well-being would be incomplete without an awareness of Maslow's hierarchy of human needs (1967, 1968). Children, like adults, have basic human needs (see Chapter 1). Hountras (1961, p. 99) points out that people who have been satisfied in their basic needs throughout their lives, particularly in their earlier years, develop exceptional power to withstand present and future thwarting of these needs. They have strong, healthy character structures as a result of satisfaction and fulfillment of their basic human health needs. Children have a strong motivation to fulfill physiological, safety preservation, social love, and status, or ego (emotional), needs. Fulfillment of these needs early in life optimizes well-being and a happy and well-functioning person. Acquisition of many skills early in life increases the child's facility for more adequately fulfilling these needs in adulthood.

EMOTIONAL PROBLEMS
Etiology

Physical problems and the feelings and thoughts that children use in their attempts to cope with stress are not the only conditions causing emotional disturbances and misbehaviors. Teachers and schools may unknowingly contribute to the adjustment difficulties of children. The etiology of behavioral problems has traditionally been viewed as stemming from factors such as rejection, marital discord, and adverse parental attitudes that begin early in the child's life. The family has always been assumed to be the cause of tensions within the child that influence his or her interpersonal relationships and perception of self and others and impair his or her effectiveness in learning and in behavioral control. Such a child has been referred to as "emotionally disturbed." Because this model has focused attention on personality development, it has failed to consider why some children do not do well in school. Significantly, assessment of the child's areas of competence or weakness in skills has been left out. The interactions between the child's competence levels and the demands made by the school situation have not been taken into account. Nonetheless, the root cause of an emotional problem is often masked by precedent physical or social skills that may be undeveloped or lacking.

The latency stage in Erikson's theory has important implications for elementary school teachers. Characterized by the child's learning to become industrious, this stage requires teachers to help the child develop numerous skills and competencies in these skills. This stage coincides with entrance into school and lasts until about the age of 12. It is a prelude to entering adult life and the world of work. The child sublimates previous feelings of "making" people respond by direct attack and instead learns to win recognition by producing things. Work provides the child with the satisfaction of doing and teaches him or her the pleasure of work completion. Along with work, play not only helps the child learn to share things with others, but also fulfills the needs to be useful, to feel a sense of involvement from participation in the group, and to feel able to do well and to make things with quality. The child garners prestige and status and structures his or her self-image by becoming self-reliant in work and play, receiving self-esteem and joy from the social recognition of the things produced. The variety of skills mastered helps

to reinforce the child's need to feel adequate. She or he is motivated to face new tasks with confidence and anticipated pleasure. Thus successful work-play experiences in the elementary school help the child to structure self-esteem and a wholesome personality. It is vital for teachers to nurture children's competence in many different kinds of skills. Development of such skills is a prerequisite to the development of not only emotional well-being, but also readiness to learn.

The danger of the primary school stage is that the child may encounter more failures than successes at work. Such failure may be a consequence of immature development in the preceding preparatory life stages. Then, too, family life may not have prepared the child for school life, or school life may fail to sustain that which the child has already learned to do well. Discouragement with work deters the child from identifying with significant modelers of jobs. Besides tool skills, the child needs to develop competencies in physical play, social values, and emotional, hygienic, and learning skills. All of these skills are dependent on the maturity of neuromuscular, glandular, and other body systems. Lacking these skills when he or she needs them will make the child feel incompetent in work or play or dissatisfied with his or her status among peers in the work-play context. Such a child may develop a sense of inadequacy and inferiority, which may become a lifelong hindrance.

The damaging effects of such emotional deprivation may be reflected in the child's behavior. He or she may withdraw from involvement with other children (a possible carry-over into adult life). Lack of emotional warmth toward the child at these critical times may also stifle his or her intellectual growth. If the teacher provides only intellectual stimulation, autism, or a state of "emotional refrigeration," may result, in which the child has no interest in people. A warm, emotional classroom atmosphere generated by a perceptive teacher is crucial in nurturing the emotional development of all children.

Children lacking essential skills readily fall victim to acquire poor self-esteem, inadequacy, and emotional disorders. They are unable to function optimally in school and society. They become poor learners and "early losers" in life.

If this negative development continues, they become nonfunctioning or low-performing adolescents and adults. There are millions of people with these disorders in this country. Inability to function is the number-one social health problem today. Many adults who do work do so at a low level of proficiency, and many others are unhappy in their work.

Teachers have the marvelous opportunity to help children develop competencies in health, work, and life skills during this critical elementary school period. If such skills are not developed at the time, they will probably not be developed later on. The child grows into a "skills-deprived adult," unable to function adequately in society. Thus it is vital that teachers nurture children's competence in many different kinds of skills—health and life maintenance, self-discipline, values and social skills, the three R's, and just learning to work and accomplish things. Personal competence means that one can accomplish something with a high level of quality and to the satisfaction of others. Personal skills are essential for optimal mental health.

Research supports the view that many emotionally disturbed children have moderate to severe cognitive motor deficits. Such children are especially vulnerable to failure and maladjustment, showing symptoms of anxiety, avoidance, low achievement, low motivation, poor self-concept, low frustration tolerance, and poor emotional control. Research also indicates that at least 40 percent of children identified by their teachers as having moderate to severe behavioral problems also show signs of gross inadequacy in cognitive, perceptual, or motor-skill development.

Rubin (1970) develops these ideas in his "social competence" model, which he feels can help teachers to identify maladjusted children. The model emphasizes effective functioning in school as a measure of the child's ability to function in society (see Figure 3.3). Academic failure or inability to learn effectively may thus be a manifestation of a lack of proper emotional, social, or physical (motor) skills. Collectively, lack of such skills programs a child for failure. If the teacher were to backtrack from the observed behavior (e.g., academic failure), he or she would probably discover a tertiary (emotional), secondary (social), or primary (physical) problem at the root of the observed failure (see Figure 3.3). The success track suggests that progressive development of essential physical, social, and emotional skills prepares the child to not only succeed in life, but also learn effectively. Both models (success and failure) point out that academic failure and inability to function in life may have hidden, or latent, causes.

The primary grades construct a crucial social environment in which to establish momentum toward development of essential life skills. These skills provide reinforcers for positive emotional, social, and intellectual development. The intermediate grades become an extension of the kind of momentum and enthusiasm generated in the primary grades. Ideally, the child has received continual satisfaction and pleasure from successfully coping with skills and so is capable of integrating his or her feelings, thinking, and behavior. When a child has not achieved satisfactorily the developmental tasks of his or her age level, we can expect to observe symptoms of emotional maladjustment. Violent drives and frustrations of this stage remain dormant (latent) only to explode and become "the storm of puberty"—the next step in the life cycle.

Awareness of the etiology of emotional disturbances has implications for teachers and schools in planning appropriate early programs that adapt to individual differences in cognitive, perceptual, social, hygienic, value, emotional, and motor skills. In different grades different demands for achievement should be made, and different skills should be required for adequate and challenging performances. Rubin (1970, p. 491) illustrates this approach as follows:

In the primary grades when materials are presented in a concrete fashion, there is a high dependence on visual perception, eye-hand coordination, and visual and auditory memory. By the time the child reaches the third or fourth grade, it is assumed that basic skills have been acquired and there is then an increasing demand on conceptual skills. In social studies and science the child is asked to read to gain facts and ideas and see the relationships between these. In arithmetic, story problems call upon the

FIGURE 3.3

A personal-social competence model illustrating failure/success in the classroom. **a,** success track; **b,** failure track.

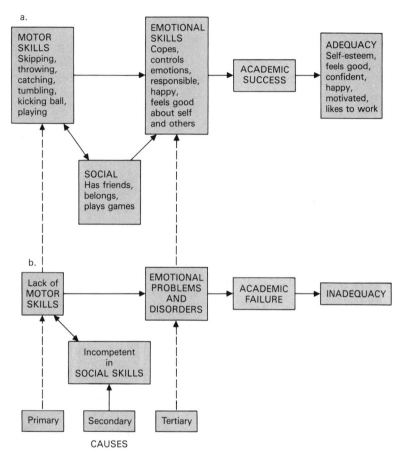

child's learned number facts but the method for the solution of the problem must be inferred. There are some children successful in the primary grades who learn well by rote, make perceptual discriminations easily, and have adequate visual and auditory memory who, lacking adequate conceptual skills, experience frustration in the later elementary grades.*

Despite the fact that handicapped children may tend to have more than their share of emotional and learning problems, with proper help and training they are capable of becoming happy and useful persons. Studies have shown that a handicap will not stop a youngster from achieving vocational success and social acceptance, provided he or she develops the appropriate skills and the ability to work harmoniously with others. This suggests that schools can best serve the emotionally disturbed child by helping him or her gain social acceptance, by promoting his or her feelings of personal adequacy, and by encouraging him or her to develop his individual potential as fully as possible. In addition, provisions must be made for helping such a child to achieve satisfying personal and social adjustments. The disturbed child needs to be shown

*From Eli Z. Rubin, "A Psycho-Educational Model for School Mental Health Planning," originally published in Community Mental Health Journal, Vol. 6, No. 1, February, 1970.

how to cope with everyday problems and how to retain a flexible attitude toward life in general.

General Symptoms of Emotional Problems

Teachers should be aware that a child's feelings and thoughts about self and others may evolve into primary emotional disturbances. If these are not resolved, they may be transformed into more serious secondary disorders, such as maladjustments and antisocial behavior. The classroom teacher does not need to discriminate between the symptoms of each of these disturbances in order to identify children with such problems. Instead, emotionally disturbed and maladjusted children may have similar overt symptoms that are easily observable.

Children may be suspected to be emotionally disturbed and maladjusted when they exhibit a group of the following general symptoms that constitutes a syndrome of emotional disturbance.

Appearance

1. Physically tense body
2. Worried look
3. Overweight/underweight
4. Sudden change in appearance or personality
5. Pallor
6. Rapid breathing
7. Depression
8. Untidy appearance

Behavior

1. Infantile speech
2. Nail biting
3. Thumb sucking
4. Temper tantrums
5. Daydreaming
6. Restlessness
7. Frequent accidents or near-accidents
8. Overtalkative
9. Highly excitable
10. Tattler
11. Overdaring or excessively shy
12. Overaggressive
13. Overdomineering
14. Excessive bragging
15. Overanxious to secure approval
16. Teases other children constantly
17. Cruelty to other children and animals
18. Marked hostility
19. Overinterest or complete indifference in sex matters
20. Easily upset
21. Extreme sensitivity to criticism
22. Resistance to authority
23. Poor sportsmanship
24. Constant quarreling with others
25. Always a spectator
26. Inability to relate to others
27. Inability to make decisions
28. Low achievement motivation
29. Low frustration tolerance
30. Poor emotional control
31. Clumsiness in fine or gross motor movements
32. Impatience
33. Inability to solve or face problems
34. Stuttering
35. Cheating
36. Lying
37. Frequent lateness
38. Frequent absence or truancy
39. Frequent breaking of school rules
40. Nonacademic achievement
41. Jealous of others
42. Bizarre behaviors and expressions
43. Cigarette smoking and drug abuse
44. Running away from home
45. Hyperactivity
46. Preoccupation with own problems

Typical Complaints

1. Being picked on
2. Others are cheating
3. Afraid of failure
4. Feeling inadequate and lack of confidence
5. Poor self-concept
6. Headache

7. Sore eyes
8. Has no friends
9. Can't be on time
10. Doesn't care about school
11. Doesn't want to go home (after school is dismissed)
12. Insomnia
13. Phobias
14. No one cares
15. Often suffers from excessive fatigue
16. Difficulty in concentration
17. Hopelessness
18. Unable to make decisions
19. Cannot solve simple problems

Suggestions for Helping Children with Emotional Problems

1. Give child recognition when appropriate and possible.
2. Be friendly and warm but firm.
3. Be a good listener.
4. Create a warm, friendly atmosphere in the classroom.
5. Call students by name.
6. Ask for volunteer helpers.
7. Involve wallflowers.
8. Demand everyone's attention before teaching.
9. Respond to inattention, disorder, and disobedience in classroom through body language. Do so quickly (evolve self-discipline).
10. Give clear and explicit directions.
11. Provide for intrinsic instead of extrinsic rewards and behavioral reinforcements.
12. Arrange for frequent rest periods.
13. Arrange for a balance of rest, sleep, and exercise.
14. Encourage interests such as hobbies, art, crafts, drama, music.
15. Allow for individual differences in academic assignments.
16. Provide for more successes than failures.
17. "Do with the child" certain complex tasks and then gradually withdraw. Show the child how to work.
18. Emphasize each child's developing emotional self-control and self-discipline.

Remedial Approaches

The primary responsibility of the classroom teacher to maladjusted and emotionally disturbed children should be to identify them early. In addition, the teacher should provide a climate favorable to the development of optimal emotional well-being. However, the teacher should refrain from correcting deep-seated behavioral problems without having the necessary training in therapy. In making such an attempt, the teacher may intensify a child's problem. After identifying an emotionally disturbed or maladjusted child, the teacher should refer the child to the proper professional or school authorities.

REFERENCES AND BIBLIOGRAPHY

Epstein, M.H., and D. Cullinan. "Depression in Children," *Journal of School Health* (1986):55(7):10-12.

Erikson, E. *Childhood and Society* (New York: Norton, 1964).

———. *Identity, Youth and Crisis* (New York: Norton, 1968).

Frick, S.B. "Diagnosing Boredom, Confusion and Adaptation in School Children," *Journal of School Health* (1985): 55(7): 254-257.

Hamberger, L.K. and J.M. Lohr. *Stress and Stress Management* (New York: Springer-Verlag, 1984).

Hountras, P.T. *Mental Hygiene* (Columbus, Ohio: Charles E. Merrill, 1961).

Maslow, A.H. "A Theory of Metamotivation: The Biological Rooting of the Value-life," *Journal of Humanistic Psychology* (Fall 1967):93-126.

———. *Toward a Psychology of Being* (New York: Van Nostrand Reinhold, 1968).

Mental Health (New York: National Association for Mental Health, 1965).

Moore, R.S. and D. Moore. "When Education Becomes Abuse: A Different Look at the Mental Health of Children," *Journal of School Health* (1986):56(2):73-75.

Rubin, E.Z. "A Psycho-Educational Model for School Mental Health Planning." *Journal of School Health* (November 1970):489-493.

Rucker, R., V.C. Arnspiger, and A.J. Brodbeck. *Human Values in Education* (Dubuque, Iowa: Wm. C. Brown, 1969).

Selye, H. "The Stress Concept: Past, Present, and Future," In *Stress Research*, C.L. Cooper (ed.)(New York: John Wiley & Sons, 1983).

Weil, A. *Health and Healing* (Boston: Houghton Mifflin, 1983).

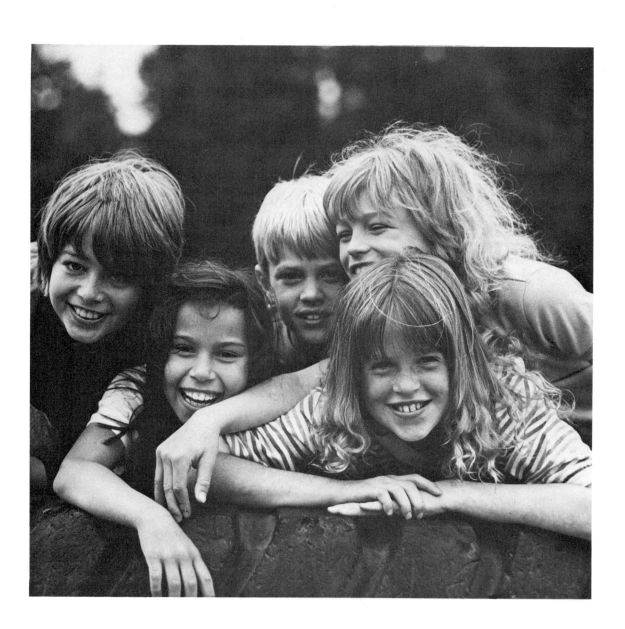

Chapter 4   Health and Developmental Problems of the Child

INTRODUCTION

The vast majority of elementary school children are able to fulfill their culturally expected tasks, resolve their needs, and continue to mature satisfactorily. However, a few children do encounter difficulty in fulfilling these tasks and are unable to achieve satisfactorily in school because of specific health impediments. Such children are therefore in need of special help and counseling services. In this chapter we deal with the most common health problems and disorders of school children. In addition to providing background information about the nature of a health problem, we will describe symptoms of the problem and outline suggestions for helping the child.

The prudent teacher should be aware that the child is a whole being, bringing to school all of his or her problems and feelings. Helping the child to overcome his or her problems is, in fact, rendering an integral service to the child in the school. This approach ideally complements the efforts of the parents at home.

The physiological health problems of elementary school children can be grouped into four broad categories:

1. Physiological disorders
   a) vision
   b) hearing
   c) teeth
   d) posture
2. Metabolic disorders
   a) overweight or underweight
   b) diabetes
3. Neurological disorders
   a) epilepsy
4. Communicable diseases and allergies
   a) communicable (respiratory)
   b) rheumatic fever
   c) allergies

These are the problems and disorders that occur most often in elementary school children and that most elementary school teachers will sooner or later encounter in the classroom.

All of these problems are important because they have the potential to evolve into grave emotional problems for the child. The danger of emotional problems is that they may often interfere with the child's ability to:

1. learn effectively
2. mature physiologically, psychologically, and sociologically so as to fulfill the developmental tasks and progress from one maturational life stage cycle to another
3. develop a wholesome, balanced personality
4. maximize potential for self-actualization
5. mature into a responsible member of society
6. graft roots for a proper lifestyle, or orthobiosis

A child may be considered to have a health problem or disorder if she or he cannot, within limits, play, learn, work, or do the things that peers can do. Teachers should be aware that all children will have health problems to some degree. Indeed, all adults encountered some degree of emotional-social-physical problems or aberrations in their childhoods as part of the natural process of growing up.

Most adults eventually outgrew their childhood health problems, learned to cope with these problems and the realities of life, and became responsible and productive adults. On the other hand, a few adults never outgrow their childhood health problems, because they failed to receive proper attention and guidance. Their handicap escalated into a disabling lifetime health problem. About 15 percent to 20 percent of the people in our society have thus become socially dependent. A greater proportion function at work and in society at a lower level of existence, unable to realize their potentialities. Although they are unhappy and feel frustrated and unfulfilled, they perform their family and social roles, albeit in diminished ways. Such results have implications for elementary health education.

Teachers should also be aware that a continuing health problem may persist for years as a handicap that can interfere with the child's learning and maturation. Such children lose years that are difficult, if not impossible, to reclaim. Unable to progress satisfactorily from one maturational stage to another, they can develop serious emotional and personality disorders and become socially maladjusted. Later, as adolescents and adults, they often "cop out" of school and society. One wonders whether elementary school teachers could have been instrumental in preventing or changing the destiny of such persons.

Before the child can learn, he or she must be physically, emotionally, and socially well. To ensure such well-being, the teacher's role is simply to locate, through observation, children in the class who may have unusual and peculiar symptoms, signs, appearances, or behaviors. It would be wrong for the teacher to diagnose the problem, much less prescribe medical treatment or therapy. These are medical concerns. The teacher's primary responsibility is to discover

such children and then, with the guidance of professional personnel, help them to overcome their problems. Such a preventive approach can be extremely rewarding in that perhaps teachers' greatest happiness accrues from helping children, seeing them mature successfully, and sharing their happiness with them.

A useful technique for helping the teacher identify children with growth and development problems is the Wetzel grid. The grid shown in Figure 4.1 (adapted from Grueninger, 1961; *The AAU-Wetzel Grid Growth Project;* Wetzel, 1941) is made up of 9 physique channels and 20 isodevelopmental levels for assessing a child's growth and development. When weight, height, and age are plotted on the grid over time, they project a profile of the child's progress. The grid summarizes the physical growth and developmental

FIGURE 4.1

Variations and progress in growth and development of children. (Francis Miller, *Life Magazine* and *Time*, Inc.

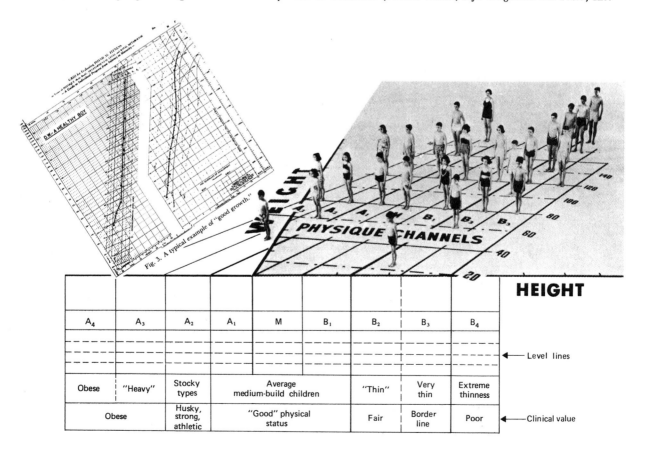

progress attained, forecasts the progress to follow, and affords a means of judging individual performance by comparison with standardized guidelines of achievement. The grid makes appropriate allowances for the great individual physical differences that are commonly found among children of the same age. Such age differences are also illustrated in Figure 4.1. Teacher observations and suspicions about the physical health and behavior of a child may be checked by use of the Wetzel grid. The grid is also an aid to justifying referrals and follow-ups.

TECHNIQUE OF OBSERVATION

Teacher observation is still the best and most reliable way to identify children's health problems and disorders. The child spends a large part of the day with the teacher. The child's life in the school reveals his or her reactions and feelings to others. It is also in the physical and social environment of the school that many changes in the child's appearance and behavior take place. Because of familiarity with the pupils, the teacher is in a strategic position to observe and to detect variations that may indicate a child's deviations from normal development, maturation, and well-being.

The teacher should observe children for health problems at the beginning of each school year. The sooner children with problems are noticed, the sooner they may be helped and the greater the likelihood of their achieving well in school. Observations should be conducted at different times of the day. Each child should be observed under different kinds of stress. Teachers should watch children while they play at recess, noon hour, during physical education class, and after school; while they eat lunch; while they study in the classroom; and while they participate in social activities. The pupil's well-being may change from minute to minute or from hour to hour or from day to day. Teachers must be constantly on the alert for these changes.

The teacher should act like a detective, observing the child for:

1. physical-personal appearance;
2. behavior; and
3. complaints about how the child feels or is.

Each of these factors will provide many clues about the child's possible problem. The Wetzel grid would be especially helpful with respect to the first item above.

Observation of a single symptom or clue does not mean that the child has a health problem or disorder. Nor does a single observation of unusual behavior indicate something is wrong with the child. It is only when the symptom or the unusual behavior recurs over a long period that the teacher should suspect that something is wrong. Health problems are expressed as recurring symptoms and interrelated behaviors. Collectively, these form an identifiable syndrome. Thus once having located a child with a possible problem, the teacher must reconfirm any suspicions. The teacher should observe the appearance and behavioral syndrome in the child for two to four weeks. If the child does not outgrow the problem or resolve the disorder during this period, the teacher should refer the child for further examination and proper attention. Specific referral and follow-up steps are suggested at the end of this chapter.

PHYSIOLOGICAL DISORDERS

The physiological disorders most often encountered with developing children and which the teacher can detect through observations are (1) poor vision, (2) defective hearing, (3) dental caries, and (4) poor posture. If not corrected, these initial problems may manifest themselves in secondary emotional and behavioral disorders.

Vision

Vision is the child's most precious sense. The preschooler's eyes allow the child to explore and to relate to the surrounding physical and social world. Upon entering school, the child discovers that he or she must begin to use vision as an instrument through which to learn. As the child progresses, the eyes sensitize the mind to the complexities of the larger world. Without the eyes the world takes on a dark sensuality and mars the child's development and progress. Defective vision may account for slow scholastic achievement, impairment of normal psychosocial progress, and numerous emotional problems. The earlier visual defects are identified and corrected, the greater the child's chances for a normal life.

Some 80 percent of the work a child does in the elementary school is built around visual acuity within arm's reach. It is important that visual difficulties be corrected as early as possible in the primary grades. Some 20 percent to 25 percent of school children have eye defects. School surveys show that fewer than half of the children who need glasses have them.

Normal seeing involves both eye and brain development. Young children are normally farsighted and see large objects, large print, and pictures fairly well. The eye and its muscles need to be trained to adjust to close work. Eye muscles especially need to mature in order for visual acuity to be considered normal.

The most common visual difficulties have to do with refraction errors. In the eye without refractive error, parallel light rays focus on the retina. Objects at a distance of 20 feet project rays that are so nearly parallel that they focus on the retina without any accommodation on the part of the eye. Because of this natural phenomenon, this distance has been accepted as a measure of normal vision acuity, or emmetropia. A child has 20/20 vision if he or she can see at 20 feet what other children with normal vision can see at 20 feet.

Four main eye defects prevail among elementary school children. The child may be nearsighted or farsighted or have astigmatism or poor binocular or two-eyes vision, such as double vision (strabismus).

Myopia

Variations in refraction are referred to as refraction errors (see Fig. 4.2). If parallel light rays come to a focus before reaching the retina,

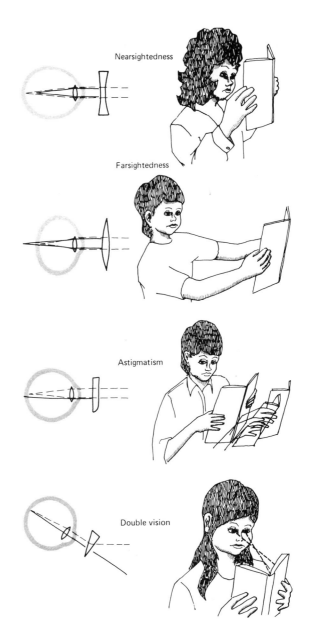

FIGURE 4.2
Four main types of defects of the eyes and the lenses needed to correct these conditions.

the image is formed in front of the retina, a condition called myopia, or shortsightedness. Although the myopic eye cannot focus distant objects distinctly on the retina, near objects are focused sharply. Because of this accommodation, the child may develop the habit of holding objects close to the eyes, as when reading a book. Often, the child compensates for nearsightedness by "squeezing" the eyelids together. This symptom may be observed by the teacher as squinting or frowning.

Hyperopia

On the other hand, if the rays reach the retina before coming to a focus, the condition is called hyperopia, or farsightedness (see Figure 4.2). The image is formed behind the retina. About 80 percent of children are born with hyperopia, 5 percent with myopia, and about 15 percent with emmetropia (normal vision).

The teacher should be aware that the refractive status of the eye is continually changing; hence the elementary school child is most susceptible to eye and reading problems. There is a need to assess the child's visual acuity from time to time.

Astigmatism

Another possible refractive condition of the eye is astigmatism (see Fig. 4.2). The curvature of the lens or cornea or both may vary so that light rays are refracted, or bent, differently. The result is a blurred image on the retina. The child with astigmatism tends to frown and hold work near.

Strabismus

This condition occurs when one eye looks in a different direction from the other eye and is caused by lack of small–eye muscle coordination. That is, one eye fixates and the other eye turns out when an object is brought near the eyes. There is a lack of clear vision, lack of single vision, and lack of coordination between clearness and singleness of vision. Hence this disorder is often referred to as cross-eyes. On inspection of the eyes, the teacher will notice a slight "crossing" of the eyes. This is more noticeable when the child is fatigued or under great emotional stress.

Color Blindness

A less frequently occurring optical disorder is color blindness. This is a sex-linked characteristic among boys; girls are almost never affected. Most of these children have difficulties distinguishing between red and green. Children who have difficulty in identifying colors in the classroom may be confused about traffic signals.

Eye Infections

Another problem the teacher should be aware of is common infection of the eye. A stye is an infection of a hair follicle in the lower eyelid and is characterized by swelling, pain, tenderness, and redness. In most cases a core of pus gradually develops. A similar infection in the upper eyelid is referred to as a shalazion. Such infections often erupt from eye strain and irritation. Excessive redness of the thin mucous membrane, or conjunctiva, lining the eyelids and eyeball may be due to irritation or infection of the blood vessels in the conjunctiva. This condition is referred to as conjunctivitis. Such irritation may be caused by smoke, dust, smog, excessive glare from the sun, snow, or bright light, or it may be associated with colds, hay fever, or allergies.

General Symptoms of Eye Problems

No one single physical symptom, behavior, or emotional disorder identifies the child with an eye problem. Usually, there is more than one telltale symptom when the child has seeing or learning difficulty. A syndrome of behaviors, when observable in the child, helps the teacher to suspect that the child may have an eye problem. The following physical symptoms and behavioral conditions, occurring usually as syndromes, will help teachers in locating children with eye problems:

A. *Appearance*
   1. *Lids:* crusting, swollen, red; skin at outer corner cracked

2. *Eyes:* sunken, protruding, crossed, blood-shot, styes, watery, presence of discharge, swelling, irregular pupils

B. *Behavior*
1. Attempts to brush away blur
2. Blinks continually when reading
3. Cries frequently
4. Has frequent temper tantrums
5. Holds the book far away from face when reading
6. Holds face close to the page when reading
7. Holds body tense when looking at distant objects
8. Reads for only a brief period without stopping
9. Reads when should be at play, as compensation
10. Rubs eyes frequently
11. Squints when reading
12. Screws up face when looking at distant objects
13. Shuts or covers one eye when reading
14. Thrusts head forward to see distant objects
15. Tilts head to one side when reading
16. Poor alignment in penmanship
17. Tends to look cross-eyed when reading
18. When reading, frequently moves book farther away and closer
19. When reading, tends to lose place on the page
20. In reading and spelling confuses o's with a's; e's with o's; n's with m's; h's, n's, and r's; f's with t's
21. Makes guesses from a quick recognition of parts of the word in easy reading material
22. Prone to accidents; stumbles over objects in path or fails to appreciate height of steps, gets fingers caught in machines, etc.
23. Frowns
24. Dislikes tasks requiring sustained visual concentration

25. Unusual fatigue after completing a visual task
26. Uses finger or marker to guide eyes
27. Says words aloud or lip-reads
28. Moves head rather than eyes while reading
29. Has difficulty in remembering what is read
30. Has poor hand-eye coordination, as in catching a ball or skipping rope

C. *Typical complaints*
1. Headaches
2. Nausea, dizziness
3. Burning, pain, itching of eyes
4. Blurring of vision at any time
5. Sensitive to light
6. Cannot see well

Suggestions for Helping the Child with Vision Problems

1. Rearrange seating plan to accommodate students with vision problems.
2. Rearrange pupils' and teacher's desks so pupils do not face the light.
3. Provide adjustable desk tops to ensure better light on work, no glare.
4. Permit child to sit where necessary to obtain best view.
5. Provide adequate lighting; replace burned-out lights in classroom; avoid glare and shadow.
6. Always provide clean blackboards; use yellow chalk on gray-green or blue-green color; avoid glare.
7. Provide clean, pastel-colored walls and white ceilings to avoid glare.
8. Select reading materials to ensure clear type and pictures; adequate spacing between lines, words, and letters; adequate margins; good-quality paper with non-glossy finish.
9. Teacher's writing on chalkboard should be large and clear.
10. Amount of homework assigned should be limited for all children, but especially for those with severe visual loss.

Hearing

After the eyes, our ears are probably the second most important sense we have. Not only do we learn by hearing, but we also learn to understand the sounds we hear. In addition, our sense of balance is in the inner ear. A child's hearing defect often leads to speech disorders, communication gaps, and emotional disturbances.

It is estimated that 1 out of 20 Americans has some degree of hearing loss, with about 0.6 percent of the school population having educationally significant losses. Hidden ear damage threatens as many as 1 in 10 American youngsters. Some 400,000 children begin school each year handicapped by unrecognized hearing loss. The elementary classroom teacher can expect to find about two children in the classroom with a hearing problem in one or both ears. Most children with hearing loss acquire it gradually.

Hearing difficulties can be divided into two classes: (1) *conduction hearing losses,* associated with the conductive structures of the outer or middle ear; and (2) sensorineural hearing losses, associated with the ear's sensory receptors in the middle ear or fibers of the auditory nerve. Relatively few of the hearing problems found in children of school age are of the sensorineural type. Sometimes both conductive and sensorineural losses are present, in which case the impairment is termed *"mixed."*

The most common cause of conductive impairment involving the outer ear is an accumulation of ear wax that blocks the canal. Conductive disorders of the middle ear are a more serious matter. Almost all middle ear disease in childhood is due to malfunction of the Eustachian tube. A watery fluid, or transudate, may fill the air space of the Eustachian tube, resulting in pain and high fever. This condition is identified as *otitis media.*

Children with hearing losses may be described as either hard of hearing or deaf. The *hard of hearing* are those in whom the loss of hearing is educationally significant, but whose residual hearing is functional for acquiring language—often with a hearing aid. The *deaf* are those whose sense of hearing is insufficient for understanding speech. Fortunately, most pupils are no more than hard of hearing.

Profound deafness is usually identified in early infancy. Any hearing impairment acquired before language has been mastered affects the entire child, not just the sense of hearing. Mild to moderate hearing loss is difficult for parents to detect. Often it is recognized only after several years of school. Meanwhile, it handicaps the growth of the child—at the age when speech, thought development, learning, and social relationships all depend on normal hearing. Because a hearing loss reduces or cuts off normal acquisition of language, hearing-impaired pupils not only tend to score less as a group on tests of intelligence, personality, adjustment, and social competence than those with normal hearing, but also are most likely to be underachievers academically.

General Symptoms of Ear Problems

The teacher should be cognizant of any or all of the following conditions in a child:

A. *Appearance*
   1. Discharge or odor from an ear
   2. Strained facial expression
   3. Cotton in ear
   4. Favoring one ear over the other
   5. Appears mentally retarded
B. *Behavior*
   1. Difficulty in talking and pronouncing
   2. Inability to localize sound
   3. Turning head to one side when spoken to
   4. Persistently inattentive
   5. Asks questions repeatedly
   6. Fails to answer or answers incorrectly when called on
   7. Watchful of the teacher
   8. Slurs word endings
   9. Speaks loudly
   10. Turns volume up on radio or TV
   11. Watches lips of other pupils as they speak
   12. Slow learner
   13. Written work better than oral work

14. Looking at someone else's work before starting assignment
C. *Typical complaints*
   1. Earache
   2. Ringing or noise in ear
   3. Inability to hear
   4. "Speak louder"
   5. "Repeat the question, please"

Suggestions for Helping the Hard-of-Hearing Child

1. Face the pupil as much as possible.
2. Move around the room as little as possible while carrying on a conversation.
3. Secure the child's attention before addressing him or her.
4. Talk slowly and enunciate clearly.
5. Ask child to clarify or repeat what you said.
6. Prescribe advance reading on the subject to be discussed in class.
7. Appoint a "buddy" to help the hard-of-hearing child.
8. Develop understanding and awareness in the pupils in the classroom toward the hard-of-hearing child.
9. Place child near front of room.
10. Avoid competing and distracting noises (air conditioners, fans) in classroom.

Dental Problems

Dental cavities occur more frequently in school children than any other disorder or health problem. About 95 percent to 99 percent of all children suffer from dental problems. The times of greatest carious activity are at ages 5 to 8 in the primary teeth and 12 to 18 in the permanent set.

Good, healthy teeth are essential to the child for several reasons. They provide the hard chewing surfaces so necessary for the mastication and proper digestion of food. Teeth are also necessary for good speech, and they mold the contour of the lower part of the face. Teeth also help to project the child's appearance and personality. Good breath accompanies healthy teeth. Loss of several teeth, dental caries, poorly aligned teeth (malocclusion), and bad breath (halitosis) may interfere with the child's development and achievement in school. More important, these disorders often are masked by emotional disturbances.

Dental Caries

The most common defect of the teeth is decay. The causes of dental decay include inherited susceptibility to caries, poor nutrition during the years that teeth are being calcified, prevalence of acid-forming bacteria in the mouth, and eating too many sweets and starches. Decay is initiated by bacteria acting on carbohydrates. Research indicates that acids form within five minutes after sweet foods are eaten. Harmful acid levels build up within 15 minutes. The acids produced by fermentation combine with saliva in the mouth to cause erosion of tooth enamel. Calcified tissue is destroyed, and a small cavity, or hole, is started. When the decay is limited to enamel and dentin, the tooth is sensitive to heat, cold, and sweets. When the pulp is involved, a toothache develops. When the nerve is destroyed, pain ceases.

Halitosis, or Bad Breath

This may indicate that the child is in poor health. The causes of bad breath may be dental caries, poor dental habits, strong-smelling food, gastric disorders, or infected mouth and/or gum tissues.

Malocclusion

Poorly aligned teeth may be caused by heredity, loss of a primary tooth and drifting of adjoining teeth toward the empty space, chronic mouth breathing, poor oral habits such as thumb or finger sucking, impacted teeth, or congenital problems such as cleft palate.

Malocclusion interferes with proper cleansing of teeth, disturbs chewing, increases the likelihood of injury to protruding teeth, and alters appearance. Such conditions may cause unfortunate psychological and social effects. Often "buck teeth" become an emotional stigma for life.

Gum Infections

Gingivitis is inflammation of gum tissue; the gums appear red and swollen, feel tender, and tend to bleed if pressure is applied. The condition occurs most often when oral hygiene and dental care are neglected. Faulty brushing neglects to agitate bacteria and prevent plaque formation. Failure to remove plaque, a sticky bacterial deposit, from the teeth near the gum line leads to the formation of calculus, or tartar. Removal of this calculus by the dentist, as in cleaning teeth, is important in avoiding gum trouble.

Neglected gingival disease may result in an advanced disease called *pyorrhea*.

General Symptoms of Tooth and Mouth Problems

A. *Appearance*
 1. Cavities in mouth
 2. Excessive tartar at necks of teeth
 3. Malocclusion
 4. Irregular teeth
 5. Bleeding or inflamed gums
 6. Swollen jaw
 7. Cracking of lips and corners of mouth
B. *Behavior*
 1. Keeps mouth closed, refrains from smiling
 2. Sensitive about missing teeth
 3. Does not brush teeth regularly
 4. Speech defect
 5. Difficulty in mastication
 6. Thumb sucking
 7. Rubs gums
 8. Constant picking of teeth
C. *Typical complaints*
 1. Toothache
 2. Sensitivity to hot, cold, or sweets
 3. Complaint about sore gums
 4. Mouth feels sore
 5. Others don't want to play with him or her

Suggestions for Helping the Child with Dental Problems

1. Provide time to brush teeth after snacks and lunches.
2. Have those children who do not brush teeth in school rinse mouth out with water.
3. Discourage eating of sweets and drinking sugared soft drinks.
4. Discourage finger sucking.
5. Demonstrate proper brushing technique.

Posture Problems

Postural habits established in the early years carry over to adulthood, with corresponding difficulties of vertical alignment and body movement. Various studies have found a significant association between poor posture and numerous physical, mental, and emotional disorders. Children with habitually poor posture have been observed to be more susceptible to diseases, to tire easily, to be underweight, to be self-conscious, to have hearing defects, to be restless, to be timid, and to have a greater incidence of asthma. Actually, 70 percent to 80 percent of all children and adults have varying degrees of postural malalignment.

Fortunately, most childhood postural disabilities may be corrected with a minimum of difficulty. When body mechanics improve in children with postural problems, there is almost always a corresponding improvement in health, physical efficiency, school work, and the child's self-image.

Good standing posture may be interpreted as an imaginary straight line (plumb line), projected through the (1) earlobe, (2) center of the shoulder, (3) hip joint, (4) just behind the kneecap, and (5) through the outside ankle on the floor (see Figure 4.3). A child's posture may be subjectively appraised as either normal or deviating from the normal by observing where the plumb line falls relative to the child's five body landmarks.

In addition to the posture from the side, the

child's lateral body alignment should be assessed. The alignment of the head, neck, shoulder blades, spine, and hips should be balanced (see Figure 4.4). Feet should naturally point straight ahead while standing and walking.

One observable posture defect is usually accompanied by one or more defects located in other parts of the human frame. For example, lordosis (exaggerated curve in the lumbar region, giving the appearance of a hollow back), is usually accompanied by such compensatory deviations as forward head, cervical lordosis, round shoulders, flat chest, knees bent backward, or flat feet.

General Symptoms of Posture Problems

A. *Appearance*
1. Head tilted forward, chin-in appearance
2. Exaggerated front-to-back spinal curves
3. Lateral spinal curves (scoliosis); one shoulder lower than the other
4. Flat-chestedness
5. Flat feet (no arch)
6. Cramped toes
7. Ptosis (protruding stomach) (obesity)
8. Losing balance
9. Hands and shoulder-joint leaning in front of ears and hips

B. *Behavior*
1. Slouching forward
2. Lack of energy
3. Withdrawal from strenuous activity
4. Clumsy and uncoordinated
5. Desire to go barefoot or take off shoes
6. Restlessness
7. Changing sitting positions

C. *Typical complaints*
1. Sore feet
2. Sore back
3. Fatigue
4. Lack of sports skills

Suggestions for Helping the Child with Postural Defects

1. Encourage all children to sit and walk properly.
2. Feet flat on floor when sitting.
3. Keep head up, chest out.
4. Use backrest of chairs so that buttocks and back are resting against backrest.
5. Provide many stretch periods, interspersed with corrective exercises.
6. Encourage coordination and graceful movements.

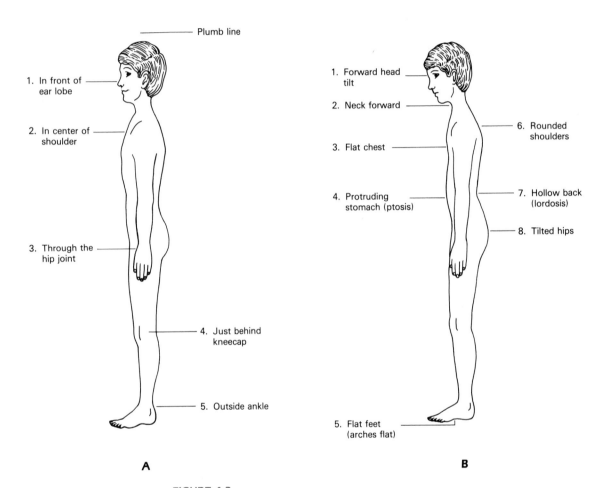

Plumb line

1. In front of ear lobe

2. In center of shoulder

3. Through the hip joint

4. Just behind kneecap

5. Outside ankle

A

1. Forward head tilt

2. Neck forward

3. Flat chest

4. Protruding stomach (ptosis)

5. Flat feet (arches flat)

6. Rounded shoulders

7. Hollow back (lordosis)

8. Tilted hips

B

FIGURE 4.3
a, Side view of good posture and body alignment with imaginary straight line, or plumb line. **b,** Side view of poor posture and malalignment of body and observable posture defects.

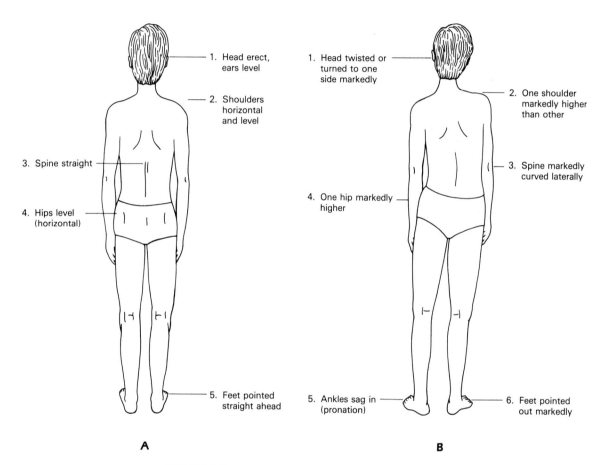

1. Head erect, ears level
2. Shoulders horizontal and level
3. Spine straight
4. Hips level (horizontal)
5. Feet pointed straight ahead

1. Head twisted or turned to one side markedly
2. One shoulder markedly higher than other
3. Spine markedly curved laterally
4. One hip markedly higher
5. Ankles sag in (pronation)
6. Feet pointed out markedly

A

B

FIGURE 4.4

a, Back view of good posture and body alignment with postural landmarks. **b,** Back view of poor posture, malalignment of body, observable postural defects.

METABOLIC DISORDERS

Two related metabolic disorders often handicapping children and adults are overweight and diabetes. Overweight is often a manifestation of diabetes. These are also interrelated conditions in that both disorders are suspected of having a common origin. Teachers need to anticipate such disorders in children.

Overweight and Obesity

Next to dental caries, obesity is probably the most prevalent health disorder in the United States. Approximately 20 million Americans are overweight or obese. Some 20 percent of elementary school age children are overweight or obese. The teacher must be concerned about overweight and obese children, for obvious reasons.

Fat children tend to remain fat as adults. Adults who were excessively heavy children have more difficulty in losing excess weight and in maintaining fat loss than do people who become obese as adults.

Obesity is the presence of excess adipose tissue in ratio to total body weight, which includes bony structure, muscular tissue, and body fluids as well as fat tissues. A normal child should have average weight for his or her height, sex, and physiological maturity. A child with 15 percent or more in excess of average weight may be considered to be overweight. A child with 30 percent or more in excess of average weight may be considered to be obese. Overweight and obese children are less active physically than nonfat children, tend to be withdrawn, and often copy the faulty eating habits of their obese parents.

The psychological aspects of obesity (see Chapter 3) are most complex. Obesity and overweight expose youngsters to difficult situations and damaging pressures. The child's ability to adapt and cope with problems, and his or her self-image may all be part of the obesity syndrome. Many obese children and adults have been found to be unhappy and frustrated, although they may not associate such feelings with their disorder.

Obesity runs in families, and children most susceptible to this disorder have genetic and cultural predispositions. Obesity developing before age 10 has a somber prognosis for eventual weight reduction. At least a third of all fat adults were overweight children. A fat person tends to remain fat. Weight-reduction programs for such people have not been effective.

Obesity at any age is a hazard to well-being. It interferes with normal body functions; increases the risk of developing certain diseases, such as diabetes and heart disease; has a detrimental effect on established diseases; and has adverse psychological reactions on the child. Obese adults tend to die sooner than do persons of normal weight. For these many reasons, the teacher's role in the classroom includes preventing obesity in the students.

Warning signs of obesity are somewhat more difficult to recognize in children than in adults. In general, any change in the developmental channel in a child's auxodrome (as in the Wetzel grid) is cause for careful medical examination. Postpubertal obesity is sometimes mistaken in its early stages for the normal "filling out" of early adulthood. Such a condition may be temporary, in which case there is no need to bring this to the attention of the child. On the other hand, the condition may persist and become irreversible if the child moves toward passivity, inactivity, and overeating.

General Symptoms of Overweight and Obesity

A. *Appearance*
   1. Fat and excess weight
   2. Ptosis (protruding abdomen)
   3. Padded waistline
   4. Large body frame
   5. Clumsy gait
B. *Behavior*
   1. Withdrawn from participation in physical activities
   2. Inactive
   3. Eats a lot
   4. Lazy and apathetic
   5. Self-conscious

C. *Typical complaints*
1. Difficulty in normal breathing
2. Exercises too difficult
3. Play is too long—need rest

Suggestions for Helping the Child with a Weight Problem

1. Become interested in the child as a human being.
2. Provide challenging alternatives to coping with problems of living.
3. Relate to child's emotional needs.
4. Involve the child in a lot of physical activity and exercise.
5. Discourage nibbling, snacking, and overeating.
6. Help child to identify his or her own self-image.
7. Allow for rest periods, but do not let rest become apathy.
8. Arrange social activities that are fun for everyone.
9. Help the child to meet many new friends.

Diabetes

Many elementary school children may be potential diabetics. They may have diabetes and not know it, or this metabolic disorder may develop as time goes on. It is estimated that 1 American in 50 has diabetes and that 1 child in 2500 under the age of 15 suffers from this disturbance. The incidence of diabetes in the average elementary school is less than 1 percent. The classroom teacher's role in identifying the diabetic child is very important because diabetes runs in families. Nearly 50 million Americans are believed to be capable of transmitting diabetes to their offspring, although most "carriers" are themselves free of the condition.

Unfortunately, the first signs of diabetes often go unnoticed. The affected child and his or her parents may not be aware of the condition until well after the process has begun and the child is gravely ill. Diabetes is usually more severe in children than in adults.

Diabetes is a hereditary metabolic disorder in which the body is unable to break down and use food properly. This defect results in increased amounts of sugar in the blood and in the urine. The condition is aggravated when the pancreas cannot regulate the secretion of insulin. Insulin regulates the storage and use of the body's sugar, or glucose.

Diabetes mellitus may involve two opposite reactions, referred to as *diabetic coma* and *insulin shock*. Diabetic coma occurs when the pancreas fails to produce sufficient insulin. Because the child's ability to use and store glucose is impaired, extra glucose accumulates in the blood (hyperglycemia) and is excreted in the urine. When the body is not using sugar normally, fat is burned to supply energy; this forms ketone bodies, which are acid. Even though the body makes every effort to neutralize them, eventually they produce acidity in the blood and other body fluids.

Insulin shock occurs when too much insulin is administered. Body sugar is used up very quickly, and the blood sugar may drop far below normal—a severe hypoglycemic state.

Both types of diabetic reaction may be controlled by a carefully maintained program of diet, exercise, and medication. There is no known cure for diabetes. However, when diabetes is controlled, the diabetic child can lead a normal life.

Diabetes may be detected by testing for the amount of sugar in the urine or in the blood. A medical examination is required to confirm the presence of diabetes.

General Symptoms of Diabetes

The signs and symptoms for diabetic coma and insulin shock are different and need entirely different treatment. Although it is not the teacher's job to diagnose or treat, awareness of the signs and symptoms will help the teacher to observe for potential diabetes and to recognize the needs of known diabetics in the classroom. Chapter 5 discusses emergency care for acute diabetic incidents.

		Diabetic coma	Insulin shock
A.	*Appearance*		
	1. Skin	Red, dry, flushed	Moist, pale (cold sweat)
	2. Breath	Fruity color (acetone)	Normal
	3. Tongue	Dry	Moist
	4. Fever	Frequent	Absent
	5. Tremor	Absent	Frequent
	6. Convulsions	None except when lapsing into coma	In last stages
	7. Vomiting	Common	Rare
	8. Breathing	Deep and labored	Normal to rapid, shallow
	9. Pulse	Weak and rapid	Full and normal
B.	*Behavior*		
	1. Alertness	Drowsy	Excited
	2. Attention	Inattentive	Inattentive
	3. Walking	May stagger	Lacks coordination
	4. Irritability	Incoherent as drunk person	Irritable
C.	*Typical complaints*		
	1. Thirst	Intense	Absent
	2. Urination	Frequent	Not affected
	3. Hunger	Absent	Intense
	4. Activity	Sluggish	Tires easily
	5. Vision	Dim	Double vision (blurred)
	6. Headache	Yes	Yes
D.	*Clinical*		
	1. Onset	Slow to gradual	Sudden
	2. Sugar in urine	Large amounts	Absent or slight
	3. Improvement	Gradual	Rapid following administration of carbohydrate

Be aware that the child who knows that he or she is diabetic will be aware of the symptoms. On the other hand, the child who is unaware of having diabetes will not be conscious of the symptoms. Such a child may not have pronounced symptoms, and the first sign will probably go unnoticed.

The symptoms listed in tabular form indicate that the disease is active. Children with latent diabetes may not have all of the symptoms. The general indicators—excessive thirst, frequent urination, overweight, constant hunger, loss of weight, fatigue, drowsiness, vision changes, and a history of diabetic relatives—should be clues for the observant teacher.

Suggestions for Helping the Child with Diabetes

1. Through conferences, involve the entire family in the management of the disease.
2. Help the child adhere to the treatment plan.
3. Do not demand too much.
4. Do not allow the class to focus attention on the child.
5. Encourage the child to participate in normal play as much as possible.
6. Make the child feel adequate at all times.
7. Help the child to become self-accepting.
8. Help the child to check weight regularly.
9. Help the child to follow medical advice regarding the amount of exercise and physical activity that may be safe for him or her.
10. Make sure the child eats regularly in school.
11. Insist that the child follow a medically prescribed diet.
12. Make sure the child avoids strenuous exercise immediately before meals, since this is the period of lowest blood sugar levels.
13. Don't overtreat the child, who simply has different eating requirements from other people.

NEUROLOGICAL DISORDERS
Epilepsy

Elementary school teachers will not very often encounter an epileptic child. A teacher who does come in contact with such a child is often psychologically unprepared to deal with the disease. The teacher's initial shock is often so overwhelming that it creates adjustment problems for the child. For these reasons epilepsy is dealt with in this chapter. (See also Chapter 5.)

A child with epilepsy can lead a normal, healthy life. However, a convulsive seizure in school is often dramatic and frightening for the teacher and the pupils. The epileptic child becomes more self-conscious and ashamed of his or her condition. Lack of understanding and failure of social adjustment by the pupils and teachers cause the development of an unwarranted social stigma toward the epileptic child. The epileptic child has emotional, physical, and social needs similar to those of other children.

Epilepsy is not a disease, but rather a sign or symptom. It results from an underlying neurological disorder; a seizure occurs when a group of brain cells becomes overactive and the well-ordered cooperation within the brain breaks down. This overactivity may remain in one area or spread to other areas of the brain. Most seizures do not last longer than two minutes. After the seizure has ended, harmonious activity is restored among the brain cells.

Convulsions are much more frequent in children than in adults. The exact cause is not known for certain. In some children the brain cells seem to be more than usually sensitive to chemical irritation. In other children seizures may be caused by any of the following: brain damage before, during, or shortly after birth; infections of the brain (encephalitis and meningitis); emotional disturbance; metabolic disorders (hypoglycemia); tetanus; temper tantrums; overdose of drugs such as aspirin and tobacco; inhalation of gasoline or alcohol fumes; snake bites; allergies. Everyone is capable of having a seizure if his or her brain cells are irritated enough.

There are at least two million known epileptics in the United States. Between 10 percent and 20 percent of the population may be latently epileptic. About 1 in every 400 school children may be expected to have epilepsy. The predisposition to epilepsy may well be inherited.

The age of onset of epilepsy varies and is important in determining the resulting psychological changes. Approximately one eighth of epileptic persons begin to have attacks between the ages of 1 and 3, and approximately 75 percent between 12 and 20. About 70 percent of epileptics are gripped by only one type of seizure; the remaining 30 percent have two or more types.

At present the seizures of 80 percent to 90 percent of children and adults can be controlled by a healthful lifestyle and with medication. In many cases the seizures disappear.

Epileptic children often need to take medication to control their convulsions. Such therapy may dull the child's responses just enough so that special learning problems occur. Memory may be affected. Such children may need to have restricted or limited participation in physical education and social activities in the school. All of these social conditions may affect the emotions and thinking of the epileptic child. Such children have numerous emotional and personality problems, secondary handicaps in that they interfere with learning. Emotional disturbances or difficult behaviors in a child with seizures do not usually result from the seizures themselves.

Despite what it may seem when a child has a convulsion, he or she does not suffer any pain. Despite the violent movements, deep and slow breathing, breath holding, paleness, or blueness, the unconscious child is not going to die and is unlikely to suffer any serious damage to the brain or body. The teacher should also remember that a convulsion will be over in a few minutes and can never harm the onlooker.

General Symptoms

There are five types of epileptic seizures. Each has a specific pattern and identifiable symptoms. However, the teacher need only be able to observe for the possibility of epilepsy and recognize a mild seizure or a warning attack, or aura, so only general symptoms are presented here. Diagnosis and prognosis are medical matters. Therefore, the symptoms for grand mal are presented separately from the rest of the seizures. The following symptoms suggest the possibility of epilepsy:

	Grand mal	Petit mal/ psychomotor convulsions (occur most frequently)
A.	*Appearance*	
	1. Aura (felt by child)	
	Tingling skin	Staring
	Tension	Confusion
	Blinking eyes	Blinking eyes
	Staring	Rage/anger
	Confusion	Sluggishness
	Loss of consciousness (1-2 min)	
	2. Convulsions	
	Eyes roll up	Slight jerking
	Difficulty in breathing	of arms and legs
	Muscles tighten	Chewing movement with mouth
	Frothing at mouth	Stares into space
	Pale bluish skin	Temporary blackout
	Convulsions begin with cry,	
	Jerky movement of whole body	
	Possible involuntary urination and defecation	
	3. After convulsions	
	Deep coma	Sleep
	Noisy breathing	
B.	*Typical complaints*	
	1. Aura stage	
	Feeling of fear	Abdominal pains
	Unpleasant odors	Headache
	Funny sounds	Spots before eyes
	Spots before eyes	Buzzing and ringing in ears
		Dizziness
	2. Upon waking	
	Confused	
	Headache	Inability to
	Feeling malaise	remember what
	Feeling nausea	happened

Suggestions for Helping the Child with Epilepsy

1. If a child has a seizure, administer suggested first aid procedures. (See Chapter 5.)
2. Help the child to be active by adhering to the commonsense rule of "nothing in excess."
3. Encourage the child to interact with peers.
4. Limit participation in body-contact sports and swimming.
5. Discourage riding a bicycle until the child is declared free of seizures.
6. Avoid overprotection.
7. Reassure the child that all is well.
8. Keep the child mentally active.
9. Provide the usual amount of discipline.
10. Encourage regulated physical activity.
11. Encourage regular meals.
12. Provide for rest periods.
13. Help the child to take medication regularly as directed by a physician.
14. Avoid emotional stresses.
15. Do not let the child become fatigued.
16. Help the child feel worthwhile.
17. Give the child recognition.
18. Encourage a wholesome, regular diet.
19. Encourage the child to establish regular bowel habits.

DISEASES AND ALLERGIES
Communicable Diseases

Communicable diseases today are not the threat to the survival of the child they were prior to 1940. With the advent of antibiotics and the use of immunizations, serious bacterial and viral complications have been greatly reduced. However, viral infections such as colds and influenza are still not under control.

Communicable diseases are those in which the causative microbes may pass or be carried from one person to another either directly or indirectly. The usual childhood diseases are caused by bacteria or viruses. Almost all children are exposed to respiratory infections early in childhood. Ideally, they build natural immunity to the invading organism or have their inherited immunity reinforced when exposed to a communicable disease.

Respiratory

About 46 percent of the common childhood diseases fall into the respiratory group and occur when the child attends elementary school. An ill child becomes physically debilitated and does not attend school regularly. Although effective immunizations are available for most communicable diseases, with the exception of colds and influenzas, most elementary school children are susceptible to chicken pox, diphtheria, German measles, Rubella (three-day measles), mumps, whooping cough or pertussis, streptococcal infections of the respiratory tract, poliomyelitis, and tetanus. The symptoms of these diseases are common and similar in nature. Most states require that parents have the child immunized for most of these diseases before the child enters kindergarten or the first grade. The teacher should observe the students for general symptoms of illness. The child with several or many of these symptoms should be suspected of illness and referred immediately to the school nurse, principal, and/or the parents.

General Symptoms of Communicable Diseases

A. *Appearance*
1. Flushed face
2. Nasal discharge
3. Persistent sneezing
4. Persistent coughing
5. Profuse sweating
6. Watery eyes
7. Red throat
8. Swollen glands
9. Rash or skin eruption
10. Diarrhea
11. Earache
12. Nausea or vomiting
13. Pallor

B. *Behavior*
1. Loss of appetite
2. Lack of interest in playing
3. Irritability and restlessness (illness, fatigue, hunger)

C. *Typical complaints*
1. Sore throat
2. Headache
3. General body soreness
4. Difficulty swallowing (sore throat)
5. Dizziness
6. Stiff neck
7. Chills, fever
8. Pain
9. Fatigue
10. Itchiness

Suggestions for Helping the Child with a Communicable Disease

1. Arrange to have the child lie down in the first aid room.
2. Arrange to transport the child home.
3. Keep surveillance for other sick children.
4. Instruct pupils on proper use of handkerchief during a cough or sneeze.
5. Insist that the child wash hands and face with soap and water after using toilet.
6. Help the child to catch up on missed school work.
7. Enforce the practice of keeping hands and unclean articles away from the eyes, ears, nose, mouth, genital areas, scratches, and sores.
8. Encourage voluntary immunizations.

Rheumatic Fever

Most heart disease in childhood is the result of rheumatic fever, which usually begins between ages 5 and 15. It causes more longtime crippling illness in children than does any other disease. Although rheumatic fever is no longer the threat it once was, it has a way of repeating itself, and each attack increases the chances for heart damage.

Rheumatic fever occurs as a sequel of streptococcal infection. The initial illness starts with a group A streptococcal infection (strep throat, streptococcal tonsillitis, or scarlet fever) that occurs about four weeks before the onset of rheumatic fever. Not all tonsillitis is streptococcal, and only about 1 percent to 3 percent of such streptococcal infections are followed by rheumatic fever.

Because of this one- to four-week interval between the streptococcal infection and the onset of rheumatic fever, it is possible to prevent rheumatic fever. If not treated in time, rheumatic fever can cause extensive and permanent disabilities and a shortened life. Teachers can help to identify pupils with suspected streptococcal infections and follow suggested preventive procedures as a way of intervening in the rheumatic fever cycle.

The final phase of rheumatic fever occurs when the streptococcal toxins irritate the heart-valve areas on the left side of the heart, causing inflammation of the surrounding tissue. A fever usually accompanies the inflammation. The inflammation subsides in about two to three weeks, and a scar is formed in place of the inflammation. The scarring interferes with the proper opening and closing of the heart valve, hence with the normal flow of blood through the heart. This chronic condition is referred to as rheumatic heart disease.

Rheumatic fever is a recurrent disease. Streptococcal infection can precipitate a recurrence in 25 percent to 30 percent of children with a history of rheumatic fever. About 90 percent of the first attacks occur in the age group 5 to 15. The age of peak risk seems to be about 8 to 10 years.

The signs and symptoms listed below do not necessarily indicate rheumatic fever; they do, however, signal the need for a visit to a physician.

General Symptoms of Rheumatic Fever

A. *Appearance*
  1. Pallor
  2. Unexplained nosebleeds
  3. Sore throat
  4. Running nose and frequent colds
  5. Twitching or jerky motions
B. *Behavior*
  1. Failure to gain weight
  2. Unusual restlessness
  3. Irritability
  4. History of rheumatic fever or strep throat
  5. Behavior and personality changes
  6. Decreasing accomplishment in school
C. *Typical complaints*
  1. Poor appetite
  2. Unexplained fever
  3. Pain in joints of arms and legs

Suggestions for Helping a Child with Rheumatic Fever

1. Involve the child in classroom activities.
2. Provide rest periods.
3. Allow slow progressive involvement in activities after the child has recovered from streptococcal infection.
4. Direct the child into creative activities.

Allergies

An allergic child is hypersensitive to one or more substances harmless to most children. About 1 child in 10 is allergic to something. For children under 15 years of age, one in five may suffer a major allergy, and normally it can be expected that four out of five allergic conditions will appear before the age of 15. Childhood is when people are most sensitive to substances in their environment. Certain types of food, house dust, animal dander, feathers, cosmetics, soaps, medicines, and even sunlight may cause reactions in the body. Such substances can be swallowed or inhaled, come into contact with the skin, or be injected, as with drugs. Predisposition to allergies may be inherited, or they may be induced, but all are usually complicated by psychosomatic factors. Children with emotional problems who are overworked or under stress tend to be more susceptible to allergies. The emotional aspect of allergies is not understood at present.

There are many types of allergy. The teacher should observe allergic reactions as illnesses in children. The most common types are nasal allergy, hay fever, asthma, food or intestinal allergies, and skin allergies.

Nasal allergy is characterized by swelling of the mucous membranes of the nose, watery secretions resulting in a runny or stuffed-up nose, and red and itchy conjunctiva with tearing. Sneezing is a dominant sign.

Hay fever is a seasonal nasal allergy to pollens from trees, weeds, and grasses. Such sensitivity usually starts in childhood. About 1 child in 20 may be expected to have sensitivity to hay fever. About one child in three who suffers from hay fever will develop asthma.

Asthma is characterized by swollen mucous membranes of the bronchial tubes in the lungs, the presence of a sticky mucus in the tubes, and a spasm of the muscle surrounding the tube. The result is a narrowed air passage obstructed by mucus, causing difficulty in breathing. Since there are at least three million people in the United States with asthma, the classroom teacher can expect to find 1 child of 50 with asthma. Asthma is the most serious of the allergies.

Food allergies are caused by sensitivity to one or more foods. The symptoms, which can appear shortly after the food is eaten, may affect the skin, the digestive tract, or the respiratory system.

Skin allergies are caused by the contact of certain substances on the skin, such as the oil resin from the leaves of the poison ivy plant. Allergic conditions may also be caused by insect or sea-animal stings.

Children vary in their reactions to allergies. Such reactions are seldom fatal, but they are always distressing, and the discomfort interferes with work, sleep, recreation, and naturally the learning process.

General Symptoms of Allergy

A. *Appearance*
  1. Wheezing
  2. Running nose
  3. Red eyes
  4. Nausea or vomiting
  5. Skin rash
  6. Inflammation of skin—redness, oozing
  7. Shock
B. *Behavior*
  1. Nose rubbing
  2. Nose wrinkling
  3. Sneezing
  4. Self-consciousness
  5. Absence from school
  6. Inability to participate in strenuous activities
C. *Typical complaints*
  1. Insomnia
  2. Difficulty in breathing
  3. Headache
  4. Difficulty in hearing
  5. Loss of appetite
  6. Abdominal pain
  7. Itchy skin

Suggestions for Helping the Child with Allergies

1. Encourage the child to participate in activities and play.
2. Avoid stressful conditions and situations that bring about allergic symptoms.
3. Arrange day for breathing exercises.
4. Perform prescribed exercises with asthmatics.

Skin Problems

Everyone, including elementary school children, is susceptible to skin problems. Although skin disorders are often approached as specific disorders, they are often a part of or mask other diseases (measles, scarlet fever, cold, or fever), emotional disorders, allergies, and insect bites. A great deal of clinical confusion about skin disorders appears to exist. The best advice for teachers is to look for rashes, boils, warts, ringworm, and acne on any part of the child's body, then follow the suggested referral procedures outlined at the end of this chapter.

SUGGESTED REFERRAL AND FOLLOW-UP PROCEDURES

Specific teacher responsibilities for helping a child with a health problem or behavioral disorder include the following:

1. *Check* the medical, family, school, and life history files of each child at the beginning of each school year. Observe for written symptoms and signs.
2. *Observe* for physical, emotional, and social deviations and manifestations (see Table 4.1). Relate these to the academic progress. Is the child progressing normally in school and toward maturity? Does the child enjoy optimal well-being? Do any of the signs and symptoms noted in the history file recur? How often and under what conditions? Make notes of the appearance, behavior, and complaints of the child.
3. *Confirm* your original observations by further detection over two or four weeks. Is the child outgrowing these and adapting, or are these health problems and behavioral disorders becoming established patterns?
4. *Refer* the child suspected of a problem or disorder for medical examinations and proper attention. Use the proper channels in the school for such referrals. The school nurse is

the logical person to assume referral responsibilities from the teacher. The teacher should confide his or her observations and suspicions to the school nurse, the child's parents, and the principal.

5. *Follow up* on the referral:
   a) *Receive* from the physician and school nurse a medical appraisal and an evaluation of the referral.
   b) Then *visit* with the school nurse, physician, and parents and decide with them on the initiation of a *corrective program.* Emphasis in such a program must be placed on the handicap of each child. The teacher is probably the best person to *coordinate* the corrective program, being in daily contact with the child.
   c) *Administer* the school aspect of the corrective program. Consult with the parents, physician, nurse, and others periodically.
   d) *Evaluate* and record the progress the child is making as the year progresses. This should be done three or four times during the school year.

These suggested steps should be followed by all prudent and responsible teachers. No doubt, most school districts already have similar approaches for dealing with the health problems and disorders of children. The teacher should realize that the most important aspect of the corrective program will be the carry-over value that such a program may have for the child. Improved well-being should result in improved learning as well as in a well-adjusted, responsible, and self-actualizing adult.

TABLE 4.1
Techniques for observation.

1. Conduct initial observation on each child at beginning of school year.
2. Observe child at different times of the day.
3. Observe child during different stress situations (play, recess, physical education period, lunch, etc.).
4. Observe for
   a) physical appearance
   b) unusual behavior
   c) complaints
5. Observe for a syndrome of appearances, behaviors, feelings, and complaints. These should be interrelated and recurring.
6. Confirm your observation and suspicions over two to four weeks.

REFERENCES AND BIBLIOGRAPHY

Allergy, Pamphlet No. 168 (Washington, D.C.:U.S. Public Health Service).

The AAU-Wetzel Grid Growth Project, NEA Service Inc., 100 West Third Street, Cleveland, Ohio.

Barrows, Howard S., and Eli S. Goldensohn. *Handbook for Parents* (Epilepsy) (New York: Ayerst Laboratories, Ltd.).

Betts, Emmett Albert. *Visual Readiness for Reading* (St. Louis: American Optometric Association).

Crowley, Leonard V. *Introduction to Human Disease,* Second Edition (Boston: Jones and Bartlett Publishers, 1988).

Current Information on Epilepsy (Washington, D.C.: The Epilepsy Foundation).

Dental Health Facts for Teachers (Chicago: American Dental Association).

Facts About Diabetes (New York: American Diabetes Association).

Grueninger, Robert M. *Don't Take Growth for Granted* (NEA Service Inc., 100 West Third Street, Cleveland, Ohio, 1961), 1-16.

Guyton, Arthur C. *Textbook of Medical Physiology* (Philadelphia: Saunders, 1986).

Handbook for the Asthmatic (New York: Allergy Foundation of America).

Heart Disease in Children, Pamphlet EM-56 (New York: American Heart Association).

The Skin and Its Allergies (New York: Allergy Foundation of America).

Teacher's Guide to Vision Problems (St. Louis: American Optometric Association).

Wetzel, Norman C. *Instructional Manual for Use of the Grid for Evaluating Physical Fitness* (NEA Service Inc., Cleveland, Ohio, 1941).

What Teachers Should Know About Children with Heart Disease, Pamphlet EM-25 (New York: American Heart Association).

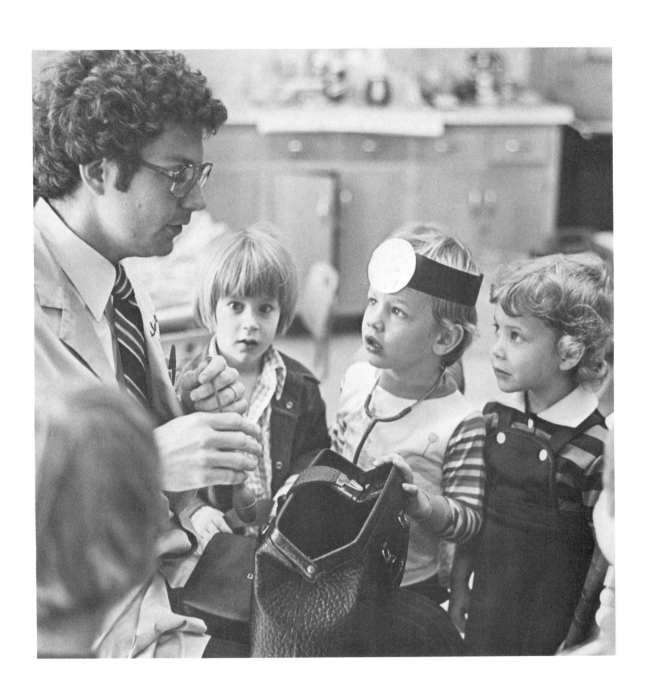

Chapter 5

Guidelines for Emergency Care

INTRODUCTION

One of the seriously neglected aspects in the preparation of elementary school teachers on a national basis is their training and skill in emergency care in the classroom. Perhaps the most traumatic moment for a teacher occurs when a student has been seriously injured or has taken ill while under the teacher's jurisdiction. With such thoughts in mind, the paramount question is whether or not the teacher is capable of performing reasonably and prudently when faced with a life-or-death emergency. If the answer is no, it is imperative to make an effort to prepare, because accidents are by far the leading cause of death among children.

The Standard Red Cross First Aid Course is excellent. Such a course makes it apparent that there is little one can do in most emergency-care situations. However, skill in administering even minimum emergency care may be the difference between life and death for a seriously injured or sick child.

BASIC PHILOSOPHY

Emergency care is aid administered immediately and temporarily to the victim of an accident or sudden illness. This care most often ceases as soon as trained medical help can be obtained. The definition implies that the victim has a serious injury or illness. This is not always the case. The vast majority of accidents and illnesses that confront the elementary-school teacher in the daily routine are minor and require a minimum of treatment. It is when a major catastrophe strikes that the teacher must be prepared to administer first aid to the victim. The teacher is not only morally responsible for the care of an injured student, but also perhaps legally.

LEGAL IMPLICATIONS

Specific responsibilities and liability for school accidents and illnesses vary from state to state. It is highly recommended that as soon as possible after being appointed, the fledgling teacher learn the specific rules and regulations regarding emergency care in the school system. In some states certain circumstances constitute liability for teachers in injury cases. A teacher can actually be sued and, if found negligent, ordered to personally pay damages. In other states teachers can be held responsible for accidents, although they are not necessarily held financially liable. However, negligence in such a situation is often excellent grounds for dismissal. Particular note should be made of the fact that suits attempting to hold teachers financially liable for injuries to students have never been more numerous. Moreover, the damages sought by such suits are in most cases staggering. The teacher who is sued and found negligent could conceivably spend a lifetime stymied by financial remuneration for a negligence incident which, in the vast majority of cases, could have been avoided.

Teachers, in essence, assume the role of a parent while students are under their care. The teacher is legally and morally expected to protect and care for each youngster in the classroom. Taking into consideration the fact that the average American family has only two children to care for and the elementary teacher is expected to effectively supervise some 35 or 40 youngsters each school day, it is not difficult to envision the occurrence of emergencies despite the best-laid plans. Children will be children, and any time large numbers of children are assembled, it is inevitable that emergency-care situations will arise.

In a broad sense every teacher should always anticipate foreseeable risks, no matter what activity the students are performing. Therefore, the teacher must take reasonable steps to prevent the foreseeable risks from becoming a reality and must certainly warn the youngsters about those risks that for whatever reason cannot be reduced or averted. In addition, the teacher also has the legal responsibility and duty to aid any student who might become injured or ill during the school day. This responsibility also implies that by rendering first aid, the teacher will not increase the severity of the injury or illness.

In the event that a child should be injured or stricken with illness while in school, the teacher should always report the incident in writing. Most school systems have a standard form to be completed by the attending teacher should an emergency situation occur. An example of such a form is the "Standard Student Accident Report Form" (Figure 5.1), which is suggested as a model accident report form by the National Safety Council.

Understanding and insight of this nature will be most beneficial should the new teacher ever be a defendant in a liability suit. The accused teacher who is found negligent in one or all aspects of liability stands an excellent chance of being found remiss in terms of his or her responsibilities and will surely be forced to endure some rather unpleasant and embarrassing consequences.

Theoretically, then, it would appear that every prospective teacher should be skilled in the basic procedures of emergency care. Unfortunately, this is not at all the case in many teacher-education programs. Because the consequences can be so devastating, the failure to provide adequate training does seem paradoxical.

EMERGENCY-CARE PROCEDURES

Every school has, or certainly should have, a written set of procedures for handling both major and minor emergency-care situations. Again, the new teacher has the responsibility to become familiar with these procedures. The following portion of "Suggested School Health Policies and Procedures for Emergency Care," prepared by Brennan and Crowe (1981), exemplifies the type of written plan that every school should possess regarding the handling of emergency-care situations.

Suggested Policies and Procedures for School Medical Emergencies*

Policies

1. The responsibilities of the school in terms of emergency care are to:
   a) Give *immediate* care.
   b) Notify parents.

---

*The material in this section is adapted from Brennan and Crowe's *Guide to Problems and Practices in First Aid and Emergency Care*, DuBuque, Iowa: Wm. C. Brown Co.

   c) See that the child is placed under the care of either the parents or a physician designated by them.
2. *All* members of the school faculty, school bus drivers, custodians, and lunch room personnel should be trained to administer emergency care of injuries and sudden illness.
3. *Every* member of the school faculty, school bus drivers, custodians, and lunch room personnel *should* have in their possession an up-to-date emergency care manual or guide for quick reference.
4. *At least one* person in the school should be *skilled* in administering all aspects of emergency care. All teachers should possess the minimum of a multimedia standard first aid certificate.
5. In the event of an emergency, the degree of injury or illness or availability of professional help will determine who shall be responsible. The order of preference is:
   a) School nurse
   b) Trained school personnel assigned first-aid duties. (See item 4 above.)
   c) Individual teachers with basic emergency care procedures.
   Keep in mind that if *none* of these people listed are available, *you* will have to skillfully attend to the victim at that precise moment until trained assistance arrives.
6. First aid equipment and supplies should be located in a strategic area in the school.
7. Every school employee should be aware of the location and availability of first aid equipment and supplies.
8. The first aid room should be under the supervision of a designated person, preferably the school nurse.
9. Every faculty member, employee, and student should have on file in the first aid room a notification card in case of injury or sudden illness. This card will be filled out at the beginning of the school year and should include
   a) The name, address, and phone number of the person to be notified

FIGURE 5.1
Accident report form.

1. Name _____ Home Address _____	
2. Schools _____ Sex M ☐ F ☐ Age _____ Grade or classification _____	
3. Time accident occurred. Hour _____ A.M. _____ P.M. Dates _____	
4. Place of Accident: School Building ☐ School Grounds ☐ To or from School ☐ Home ☐ Elsewhere ☐	

5.			DESCRIPTION OF THE ACCIDENT
NATURE OF INJURY	Abrasions _____ Amputations _____ Asphyxiation _____ Bite _____ Bruise _____ Burn _____ Concussion _____ Cut _____ Dislocation _____ Other (specify) _____	Fracture _____ Lacerations _____ Poisoning _____ Puncture _____ Scalds _____ Scratches _____ Shock _____ Sprain _____	How did accident happen? What was student doing? Where was student? List specifically unsafe acts and unsafe conditions existing. Specify any tool, machine or equipment involved. _____ _____ _____
PART OF BODY INJURED	Abdomen _____ Ankle _____ Arm _____ Back _____ Chest _____ Ear _____ Elbow _____ Eye _____ Face _____ Finger _____ Other (specify) _____	Foot _____ Hand _____ Head _____ Knee _____ Leg _____ Mouth _____ Nose _____ Scalp _____ Tooth _____ Wrist _____	_____ _____ _____ _____ _____ _____ _____ _____ _____

6. Degree of Injury Death ☐ Permanent Impairment ☐ Temporary Disability ☐ Nondisabling ☐	
7. Total number of days lost from school: _____ (To be filled in when student returns to school)	

Part B. Additional Information on School Jurisdiction Accidents

8. Teacher in charge when accident occurred (Enter name) _____ Present at scene of accident: No _____ Yes _____

9.	
IMMEDIATE ACTION TAKEN	First aid treatment _____ By (Name): _____ Sent to school nurse _____ By (Name): _____ Sent home _____ By (Name): _____ Sent to physician _____ By (Name): _____ Physician's Name: _____ Sent to hospital _____ By (Name): _____ Name of hospital: _____

10. Was a parent or other individual notified   No _____ Yes _____ When _____ Hour _____

   Name of individual notified: _____ By whom? (Enter name): _____

11. Witnesses: 1. Name _____ Address _____

   2. Name _____ Address _____

12.	Specify Activity	Specify Activity	Remarks
LOCATION	Athletic field _____ Auditorium _____ Cafeteria _____ Classroom _____ Corridor _____ Dressing rooms _____ Gymnasium _____ Home Econ. _____ Laboratories _____	Locker _____ Pool _____ Sch grounds _____ Shop _____ Showers _____ Stairs _____ Toilets and washrooms _____ Other (specify) _____	What recommendations do you have for preventing other accidents of this type? _____ _____ _____ _____

b) Preferred physician and hospital
c) For students, a permit signed by a parent, allowing the school to call the designated physician or dentist directly in case a parent cannot be reached

10. The phone numbers of the following persons and services should be posted conspicuously near each school telephone:
    a) School nurse
    b) Fire station
    c) Police station
    d) Hospital or ambulance service
    e) Poison control center
11. Every school employee should be required to fill out a standard sickness and accident report after every incident. This report should be kept in the principal's office and should include
    a) Names of persons concerned
    b) Time and date of incident
    c) Location
    d) Nature of accident or illness
    e) Witnesses
    f) Disposition of the case
12. No sick or injured child should ever be sent home if unaccompanied by a responsible person or when a responsible person is not at home.
13. Parents or guardians should be notified as calmly and as early as practicable. Every assistance should be given them in caring for their children.
14. These policies should be evaluated at the end of each school year and revised in light of the evaluation.

Procedures

1. Care of minor injuries
   In elementary grades the classroom teacher stresses the importance of cleanliness of minor wounds, washes the injured areas with soap and water, and applies the sterile dressings. Bus drivers, custodians, and lunch room personnel should also be trained in first aid and have supplies handy.

2. Care of major injuries and sudden illness
   a) Immediately summon sufficient help to do the following *simultaneously:*
      (1) Administer first aid.
      (2) Notify school administrator.
      (3) Notify parents.
      (4) Call physician.
   b) Render immediate care:
      (1) Stop external bleeding (know pressure points).
      (2) Start artificial respiration in cases of asphyxia (stoppage of breathing).
      (3) Care for shock.
      (4) Do not move a person suspected of neck or back injury.
      (5) Leave the unconscious person alone (no attempt to arouse or give liquids).
   c) Be able to render care for common emergencies such as:
      (1) Fainting
      (2) Unconsciousness
      (3) Epileptic seizures
      (4) Insulin shock
      (5) Foreign bodies in eye
      (6) Foreign bodies in air passage
      (7) Foreign bodies in food tube
      (8) Convulsions
      (9) Snake bite
      (10) Burns
      (11) Insect bites and bee stings

3. Specific care of injuries and sudden illness
   a) Clean cut:
      (1) Wash around area with soap and water.
      (2) Apply an antiseptic, preferably hydrogen peroxide. Avoid such substances as alcohol and iodine; they injure tissue.
      (3) Apply sterile dressing.
   b) Dirty wound:
      (1) Cleanse around wound with soap and water.
      (2) Cleanse with alcohol to remove dirt.
      (3) Apply antiseptic—allow to dry.

(4) Apply sterile dressing.
c) Dog bite:
   (1) Wash with water and soap.
   (2) Apply antiseptic (see 3-a-2 above).
   (3) Apply sterile dressing.
   (4) Refer to family doctor.
   (5) Report to police and try to find dog.
d) External bleeding:
   (1) Apply pressure with compress.
   (2) Elevate wound.
   (3) If bleeding persists, apply digital pressure.
   (4) As a last resort, apply tourniquet.
e) Fainting:
   (1) Lay flat on back and elevate the feet.
   (2) Rest, with supervision.
f) Burns:
   (1) First degree—skin reddened but unbroken. Apply cold water. Seek medical attention.
   (2) Second and third degree—skin and tissues broken. Apply cold water. Seek medical attention.
g) Foreign body in eye:
   (1) Wash with warm boric acid solution.
   (2) Apply loose dressing.
   (3) Refer to family doctor.
h) Epileptic seizure:
   (1) Lay on back and loosen clothing.
   (2) Do *not* restrain patient's movements.
   (3) Do not force a pad into the mouth.
   (4) Allow child to rest following seizure.
   (5) Refer to family doctor.
i) Fractures:
   (1) Do not move the part.
   (2) Immobilize injured part.
   (3) Call parent to take child to family doctor if possible.

In addition to the school's planned emergency-care program, there are also standard first aid measures with which every teacher should absolutely and unequivocally be familiar. The following thoughts and techniques provide insight into the handling of some of the most serious emergencies that might confront a teacher.

Serious Bleeding

Wounds come in all sizes and shapes. Depending on the type and location of the wound, bleeding may or may not be an extremely important factor. Severe bleeding is one of the most urgent conditions requiring emergency care. The loss of a great deal of blood in a short time is a tremendous shock to a child's system, not to mention the emotional repercussions. If the wound involves a major artery, a child could bleed to death in less than a minute.

Immediate action is imperative. These steps should be methodically performed without delay. Controlling serious bleeding encompasses one to four measures, depending on the location and severity of the wound:

1. *Elevate the wound.* Unless there is evidence of a fracture, it is good practice to elevate the bleeding portion of the body as high above the heart as possible. Because it is more difficult for the heart to pump blood up, the blood pressure in the area of the elevated wound is lessened, which enhances further control measures. If at all possible, elevation should be immediately implemented with any type of bleeding, regardless of severity.
2. *Apply direct pressure.* The combination of elevation and direct pressure will, in the vast majority of cases, effectively control hemorrhage. To apply direct pressure, cover the wound with a sterile compress and steadily apply pressure to the injured area. If a sterile gauze compress is unavailable, a clean towel, shirt, pillow case, sweater, or jacket can be used. If there is nothing available to use as a compress, apply direct pressure with the hand. However, any time a compress is available, it should be used. (See Figure 5.2.)
3. *Apply arterial pressure.* If hemorrhaging is

so severe that the combination of elevation and direct pressure to the wound does not control the loss of blood, "digital pressure" must be applied. In theory, this approach is relatively simple: One presses on a specific point on the arm or leg to compress the main artery supplying blood to the afflicted portion of the body. There is one recommended pressure point on each arm and leg—where the artery is near the skin and a bone.

Because pressure-point use tends to stop circulation to the injured limb, this method should be employed only when absolutely necessary, and in conjunction with direct pressure and elevation. It is best to have assistance, if possible, when employing all three techniques simultaneously. In addition, pressure-point use should be discontinued as soon as possible; however, one should always be ready to reapply the pressure if profuse, uncontrollable bleeding should recur.

Two accepted pressure points can be easily located and employed to control most bleeding (see Figure 5.3). It is useful to locate these points on oneself or a friend just for practice. Prior knowledge

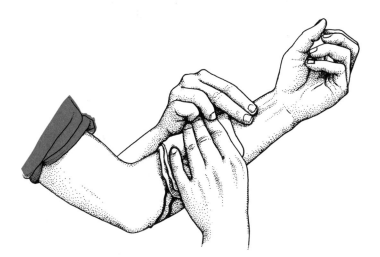

FIGURE 5.2
Applying direct pressure to a wound and elevating the wound above the victim's heart.

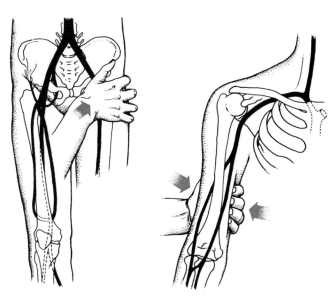

FIGURE 5.3
Proper hand positions for applying brachial and femoral pressure.

of their location eliminates indecision and fumbling if such action should be needed. Slight pressure with the index finger in each of the areas depicted in Figure 7.3 will yield a pulse. This pulse signifies that you have located the pressure point.

For a severely bleeding arm wound, apply pressure (along with direct pressure and elevation) over the brachial artery, forcing the artery against the arm bone. This pressure point is on the inside of the arm in the groove between the biceps and triceps (the large muscle masses of the upper arm). Pressure is best applied by grasping the victim's upper arm midway between the armpit and the elbow, with your thumb on the outside of the victim's arm and your fingers on the inside. Using the flat of the fingers (not the fingertips), press toward your thumb to compress the artery and stop the blood flow.

For a severely bleeding leg, pressure is best applied to the femoral artery in the pelvic area. This pressure point is on the front of the thigh just below the middle of the crease of the groin, where the artery crosses over the pelvic bone on its path to the lower leg. Pressure is best applied by placing the heel of the hand over the pressure point and then leaning forward over your straightened arm to apply pressure against the underlying bone.

It is difficult to conceive of a situation in which the combination of direct pressure, elevation, and digital pressure would not control bleeding. However, one additional technique warrants mentioning, especially because of the many misconceptions that have plagued it for years.

4. *Employ a tourniquet as a last resort.* Only as a *last resort* would one even entertain the thought of applying a tourniquet. The tourniquet stops all blood flow to an extremity (the only place a tourniquet can be applied) and can cause the loss of that limb due to lack of circulation. One would be hard pressed to cite a situation in

which use of a tourniquet might be justified. Perhaps if many children were very seriously injured, one might quickly apply a tourniquet to an injured child and then move on to another victim. Or perhaps the complete amputation of a limb might justify the use of a tourniquet. In short, a tourniquet should be applied only when there appears to be no other practical approach. Figure 5.4 illustrates the proper application of a tourniquet.

FIGURE 5.4

Tourniquet application. a, wrap twice around arm and tie half knot; b, place "windlass" over half knot; c, finish knot and turn windlass to tighten; d, secure windlass with tails of tourniquet.

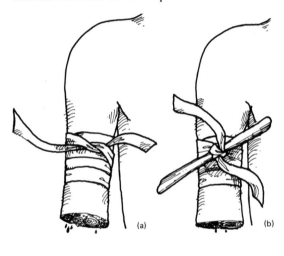

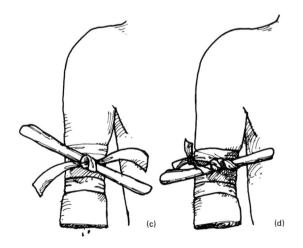

Stoppage of Breathing

Breathing can cease for many reasons: a drug overdose, lack of oxygen, electrical shock, toxic gases, a heart attack, or a blow to the head. In such a situation immediate action is called for. The chances of reviving an individual who has stopped breathing decrease with each passing minute. The person deprived of oxygen for four minutes or longer will undoubtedly suffer irreparable brain damage or death even if cardiopulmonary resuscitation is started at that time.

As with serious bleeding, the teacher cannot afford to wait for medical help. He or she must act immediately if a child's life is to be saved. Often death may be prevented if the victim's breathing and heartbeat can be restored and maintained until professional medical assistance arrives. Cardiopulmonary resuscitation (CPR) is designed to do just this, and it can be performed with a minimum of training by nearly anyone.

Cardiopulmonary resuscitation should be started as soon as possible after breathing stops. Several guidelines should be followed:

1. If you encounter a person with a death-like appearance, you should first *determine whether the victim is truly unresponsive.* This can be accomplished by simply tapping or gently shaking the shoulder of the victim. Ask in a loud voice, "Are you okay?" If the victim is unresponsive, immediately shout for help (see Figure 5.5a and b).

2. The next step is to *open the victim's airway.* Next to quick action, the most important factor in rescue breathing is an unobstructed air passage. The jaw of a non-breathing victim relaxes, and the tongue drops back so that it blocks the trachea (windpipe). To ensure a clear airway to the victim's lungs, lay the victim down face up. Then, with one hand on the victim's forehead and the fingertips of your opposite hand under the bony portion of the jaw near the chin, tilt the victim's head, keeping the mouth open. This process is the *head-tilt/chin-lift* technique (see Figure 5.5c and d).

3. You are now ready to *determine whether the unresponsive victim is breathing.* Continuing to maintain an open airway, place your ear over the victim's mouth and listen as well as feel for any sign of breathing. Also observe the victim's chest for the rise and fall of respiration. The victim who is breathing should be closely monitored until professional assistance arrives (see Figure 5.5e).

4. If the victim is *not* breathing, without delay, you must *give the victim two full slow breaths.* Maintain the open airway; pinch the nostrils closed; seal the victim's mouth with your mouth and breathe into the victim twice for 1 to 1.5 seconds at a time. You should observe the victim's chest rise as you breathe out and then fall when you stop (see Figure 5.5f).

5. Now, *check the victim for a pulse.* Continuing to maintain an open airway, locate the victim's Adam's apple by sliding your fingers along the near side of the victim's neck. Feel for a carotid pulse. Perform this procedure in no more than 5 to 10 seconds (see Figure 5.5g).

6. Keep shouting for help. As soon as someone comes, have him or her call for emergency medical services.

    For the unresponsive victim who is *not breathing* but who *does exhibit a pulse,* immediately employ *rescue breathing.* Proper procedure for *rescue breathing only:*
    a) Maintain an open airway.
    b) Pinch the nostrils closed.
    c) Seal the victim's mouth with yours.
    d) Breathe into the victim's mouth once every five seconds.
    e) Watch the victim's chest rise and fall.
    f) Continue rescue breathing for one minute (12 breaths), then reassess.

7. After the first minute of rescue breathing, you should *reassess the victim's circulation.* Continuing to maintain an open airway, once again locate the victim's carotid pulse. The reassessment should be completed in five seconds or

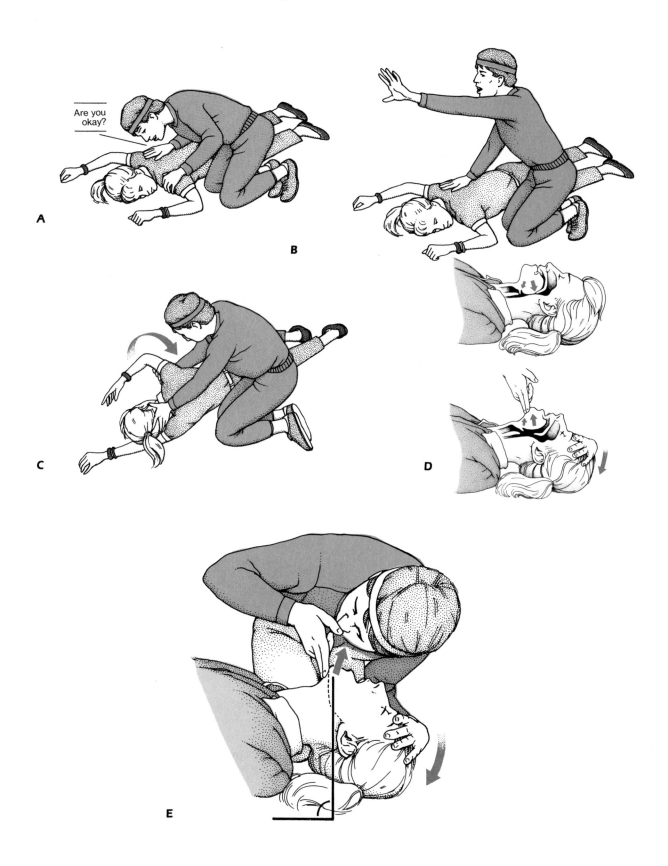

A

B

C

D

E

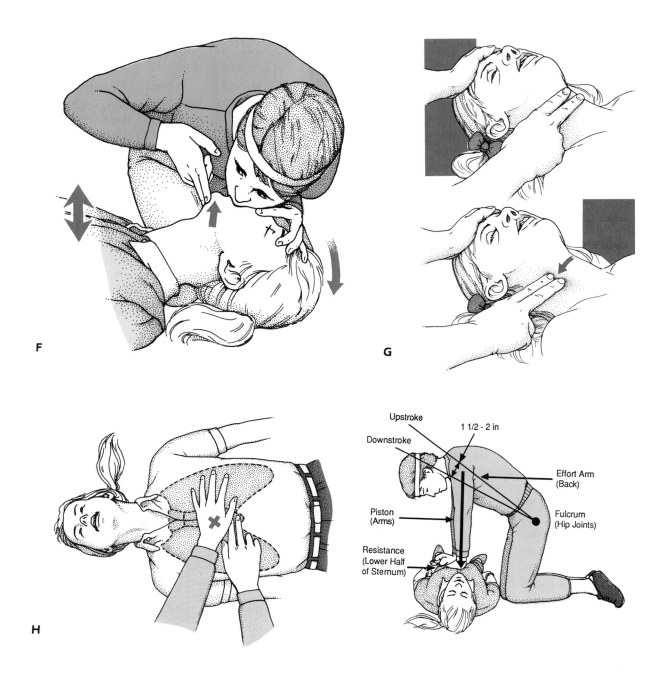

FIGURE 5.5

Cardiopulmonary resuscitation. a, determining responsiveness; b, calling for help; c, positioning the victim; d, opening the airway by tilting the head and lifting the chin; e, determining breathlessness; f, mouth-to-mouth rescue breathing; g, determining pulselessness; h, external chest compression.

less. If a pulse is found, rescue breathing *only* should be continued.

8. If at any time *no pulse is found*, begin cardiopulmonary resuscitation (CPR) at once. When no pulse is present, rescue breathing only is futile.

When you have provided the victim with two full slow breaths while maintaining an open airway and closed nostrils, you are ready to apply chest compressions, which provide the victim with circulation (see Figure 5.5h).

9. To apply proper compressions, from your kneeling position quickly locate the victim's substernal notch, where the breastbone separates to form the rib cage. Measure up one finger width above the notch and place the heel of one hand directly over the sternum, or breastbone. Place your second hand on top of your first, keeping your fingertips off the victim's chest (see Figure 5.5h).

Apply compression, keeping your elbows straight and over the victim's sternum. Compress the victim's chest 1½ to 2 inches. Make each compression and release smooth. Be sure not to lift your hands off the victim's chest when you release. Maintaining proper hand position enhances proper technique. Provide 15 compressions in 9 to 11 seconds, followed by two full slow breaths in 4 to 7 seconds. Remember to maintain an open airway and pinch the victim's nostrils closed for respiration. You should administer 80 to 100 chest compressions per minute during CPR (see Figure 5.5h).

10. After you have administered one minute of CPR to a nonbreathing, pulseless victim (4 cycles of 15 compressions and 2 ventilations), you should recheck for a pulse (see item 5). Spend no more than 5 seconds searching for a carotid pulse.

11. If the victim still lacks a pulse, continue with CPR. Reassess every few minutes. If a pulse becomes evident but the victim is still not breathing, revert to the *rescue breathing only* (item 6).

Contemporary thinking is that one-rescuer CPR is the only technique that should be taught to the general public. If a second lay rescuer who is trained in CPR arrives on the scene, the suggested procedure is that the two rescuers take turns. The two-rescuer procedures that were once taught to the general public are now taught only to health care providers and professional rescuers.

12. The CPR procedure for infants and young children is similar to that used on older children and adults with a few exceptions.

CPR for infants up to 1 year old:
1) Be careful not to hyperextend the baby's neck when employing the head-tilt/chin-lift technique to open the infant's airway.
2) Seal the baby's mouth and nose with your mouth.
3) Check for a pulse in the brachial artery on the inside of the baby's upper arm.
4) Use your fingers rather than the heels of your hands to apply chest compression. Draw an imaginary line between the baby's nipples and place two or three fingers on the sternum one finger's width below the imaginary line. The compressions should be ½ to 1 inch deep. Your fingers should stay in contact with the infant's sternum during the release. Give at least 100 compressions per minute.

CPR for the child between the ages of 1 and 8:
1) Use the *heel of one hand only* for chest compression.
2) Chest compressions should be 1 to 1½ inches deep.

Obstructed Airway—Choking

The most frequent cause of obstruction of the airway is a large piece of poorly chewed food. The obstruction can be either partial or complete. Emergency care for the choking victim is relatively simple (see Figure 5.6). If the victim can cough, speak, and breathe, it is best not to interfere. However, if the victim *is conscious* but *cannot* cough, speak, or breathe, quick action is called for:

1. *Shout for help* to alert someone who can seek medical assistance.
2. *Perform* the *Heimlich maneuver*:
   a) Stand behind the victim.
   b) Wrap your arms around the victim's waist.
   c) Make a fist with one hand and place the thumb side against the victim's abdomen above the navel and below the sternum.
   d) Grasp your fist with the other hand.
   e) Press with quick upward thrusts.
   f) Deliver each thrust with enough vigor to expel the obstruction.
   g) Keep repeating the thrusts until the object is expelled or until the victim loses consciousness (see Figure 5.6a).

For an unconscious victim with an obstructed airway, you must implement additional emergency care procedures:

3. Lay the *victim flat and face up* as quickly as possible.
4. *Shout for help*.
5. *Check for foreign objects* in the victim's mouth and throat by performing a *finger sweep*. Put your thumb in the victim's mouth and lift the jaw and tongue up and away from the trachea. Sweep deeply into the victim's mouth from cheek to cheek with the index finger of your free hand.
6. If the object *cannot be removed,* attempt to *ventilate the victim* immediately, using the standard procedure:
   a) Open airway.
   b) Seal mouth and nose.
   c) Attempt to ventilate.
7. If the *airway remains blocked,* immediately implement the *Heimlich manuever:*

a) Straddle the victim's thighs.
b) Position the heel of one hand on the victim's abdomen above the navel and below the sternum.
c) Place the free hand directly over the first hand.
d) Deliver 6 to 10 quick upward thrusts.
e) Each thrust is distinct and delivered with the intent of dislodging the obstruction.
8. Repeat the finger sweep procedure (see step 5).
9. If no foreign object is found, attempt ventilation once again (step 6).
10. If the victim's airway remains blocked, repeat steps 7 through 9 until you are successful in dislodging the foreign body (see Figure 5.6b).

Emergency care for obstructed airway in infants up to approximately 1 year:

1. After determining that an airway obstruction exists and shouting for help, place the infant face down over your forearm, which rests on your thigh. Keeping the infant's head down and supported with your hand, deliver four forceful blows between the victim's shoulder blades with the heel of your free hand.
2. Immediately turn the infant onto his or her back with the head lower than the trunk. Support the head and neck while sandwiching the infant between your hands and forearms. Deliver four thrusts using two or three fingers to the breastbone one finger's width below an imaginary line between the infant's nipples.
3. Repeat steps 1 and 2 until either the foreign body is expelled or the infant loses consciousness.
4. If the infant lapses into unconsciousness, shout for help once again and then check for foreign bodies as discussed in the adult section. If the foreign object is visible, remove it with your fingers. If not, immediately start artificial respiration.

FIGURE 5.6
a, Heimlich maneuver with child standing; b, with child lying.

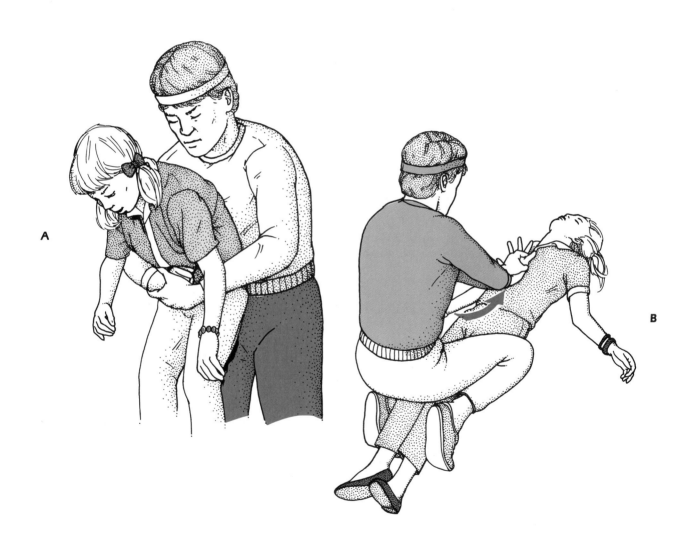

5. If ventilation fails, repeat steps 1 through 4 until successful.

Shock

Shock accompanies all injuries and generally is proportional to the severity of the injury. Treat for shock after any injury.

Shock can be defined simply as a depressed state of bodily functions due to insufficient blood circulation. A person who develops shock and is not properly treated may die. Therefore, it is imperative that emergency treatment for shock be administered to the injured.

Telltale signs of shock:

1. Eyes are vacant and lackluster.
2. Pupils are dilated.
3. Breathing is shallow and irregular, with frequent gasps for air.
4. Pulse is weak or absent.
5. Skin appears pale, cold, and moist.
6. Victim is nauseated.

The treatment for shock is the same for both prevention and care:

1. Keep the victim lying down.
2. If possible, elevate the feet.
3. Cover the victim with a blanket.
4. Administer small sips of water if the victim is conscious and not nauseated.
5. Reassure victim and stay with him or her.
6. Keep onlookers away.
7. If possible, keep the victim from viewing his or her injury.

Common Emergencies

In addition to serious emergencies, other events common to the elementary school will require first aid.

Diabetic Coma

Either not enough insulin or too much insulin can produce some rather startling signs and symptoms. Diabetic coma occurs when the victim has not received enough insulin to carry on bodily processes. The victim's face becomes flushed, with the lips a brilliant red and the skin quite dry. The victim's temperature drops even though he or she appears to have a fever. Acidosis produces an extremely sweet odor on the victim's breath.

Little can be done for the victim of diabetic coma until a doctor arrives. The victim needs insulin quickly. Until the doctor arrives, the teacher should make the child feel as comfortable as possible and offer verbal encouragement.

Insulin Shock

The opposite of diabetic coma, insulin shock is a case of too much insulin in the blood and far too little sugar. The victim of insulin shock exhibits the signs and symptoms of deep shock. The skin becomes quite moist and pallor develops. The pulse is rapid, but breathing is slow and shallow. There is no sweet smell on the breath of the victim. Because the victim is in shock, it would be most beneficial for the teacher to have prior knowledge of the student's condition so that there will be no needless waste of time when and if such a condition might present itself.

A physician should be summoned immediately, but because the victim has too much insulin in his or her system and not enough sugar; there are some immediate measures that can be employed. Giving the victim sugar will in many cases cause a rapid recovery. Even if the child lapses into unconsciousness, a teaspoon or so of granular sugar placed under the tongue will be absorbed into the bloodstream. If the child is conscious, sugar is an excellent choice if available, or a candy bar or orange juice, both good sources of carbohydrates, can be substituted. The teacher who has a diabetic child in class should keep several lumps of sugar in the desk.

Epileptic Seizure

The most common cause of convulsions among school children is epilepsy, and an epileptic seizure is not at all an uncommon occurrence among school children. However, there is a great deal of fear and misconception connected with epilepsy.

The most common forms of epilepsy are grand mal and petit mal. Of the two, grand mal presents more difficulty. The victim of a grand mal seizure has a premonition just prior to the seizure. A child who has had previous seizures may quickly move to a more secluded area and lie down before becoming unconscious. Now the other signs and symptoms of the seizure—foaming at the mouth, violent convulsions, vomiting, loss of bladder control, defecation, and loud, labored breathing—will be apparent. The seizure normally lasts some three to five minutes, but this may seem like an eternity to the attending teacher. Once the seizure subsides, the victim will most likely drop off into a deep sleep for a few minutes and upon awakening may appear to be confused.

To deal effectively with the grand mal seizure requires little skill. *Never* restrain a victim during a seizure. The seizure should be allowed to run its course. It is good practice to clear the area of furniture, etc., so that the victim will not be hurt. A pillow under the victim's head is also a help, especially on a hard floor. Do not concern yourself with the victim's biting his or her tongue; it has been found that such action by an epileptic is an exception to the rule. But if the child is biting his or her tongue, try to slip a hard object between the victim's teeth in an effort to prevent further injury. A wooden ruler, a pencil wrapped with a handkerchief, or the corner of a wallet are readily available items.

When the victim regains consciousness, make him or her feel as comfortable as possible, both mentally and physically. The youngster will also benefit from a rest in an undisturbed environment. Should the child lapse from one seizure into another, trained medical help should be summoned at once. In rare instances, a general anesthetic is required.

Petit mal presents far less of a problem. A petit mal seizure may be unnoticeable to observers. The victim is perfectly normal just prior to and immediately after the seizure, receiving no premonition. The seizure lasts for a very short

FIGURE 5.7
Controlling nosebleed with pressure and packing nostril with sterile cotton.

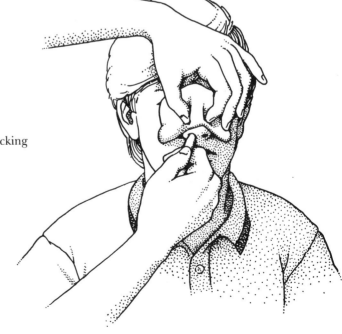

time and consists of little more than minor convulsive movements of the extremities or eyes. At no time does the child lose consciousness.

Fainting

Fainting is not uncommon among young children. Perhaps the most common cause is an unpleasant sight or situation such as the sight of blood. Fainting occurs when the brain is deprived of oxygen, which produces immediate unconsciousness.

The best technique for treating someone who has fainted is to lay the victim flat, with the head lower than the legs if possible. Once in a supine position, the victim will most likely regain consciousness very quickly. If for some reason the victim cannot be stretched out on the floor, the next best thing is to sit the victim down and bend his or her head between the knees. A glass of water with salt is helpful once the victim is fully conscious.

Nosebleed

Nasal bleeding is quite common among elementary school children. A blow to the nose and excessive nose picking are the most common causes. Rupture of the veins very near the surface of the membrane inside the nose is the source.

To treat nosebleeds, keep the victim in an upright position—preferably sitting—to elevate the source of bleeding. Insert a wad of sterile cotton in each nostril and then ask the child to compress his or her nostrils with the thumb and forefinger for *no less* than six minutes (see Figure 5.7). Then have the child gently release the nostrils and check for further bleeding. If bleeding is still present, repeat the process. Once bleeding is controlled, leave the cotton wads in place for as long as possible. When they must be removed, do so gently so as not to remove clots and restart the bleeding.

More information on emergency care is presented in Appendix F.

REFERENCES AND BIBLIOGRAPHY

American National Red Cross. *Advanced First Aid and Emergency Care* (Washington, D.C.: American National Red Cross, 1979).

Brennan, William T., and James Crowe. *Guide to Problems and Practices in First Aid and Emergency Care* (Dubuque, Iowa: Wm. C. Brown, 1981).

Hafen, B. *First Aid for Health Emergencies* (St. Paul, Minn.: West Publishing Co., 1985).

Thygerson, Alton L. *First Aid and Emergency Care Workbook* (Boston: Jones and Bartlett, 1987).

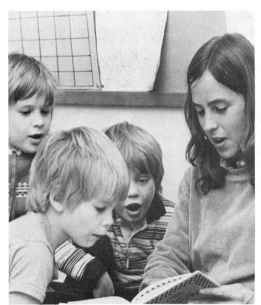

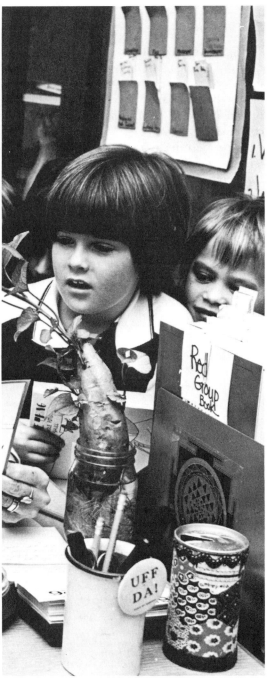

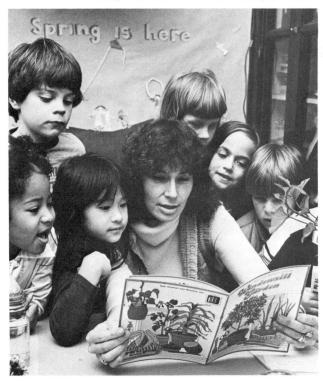

Part Three

Health Education in the Elementary School Curriculum

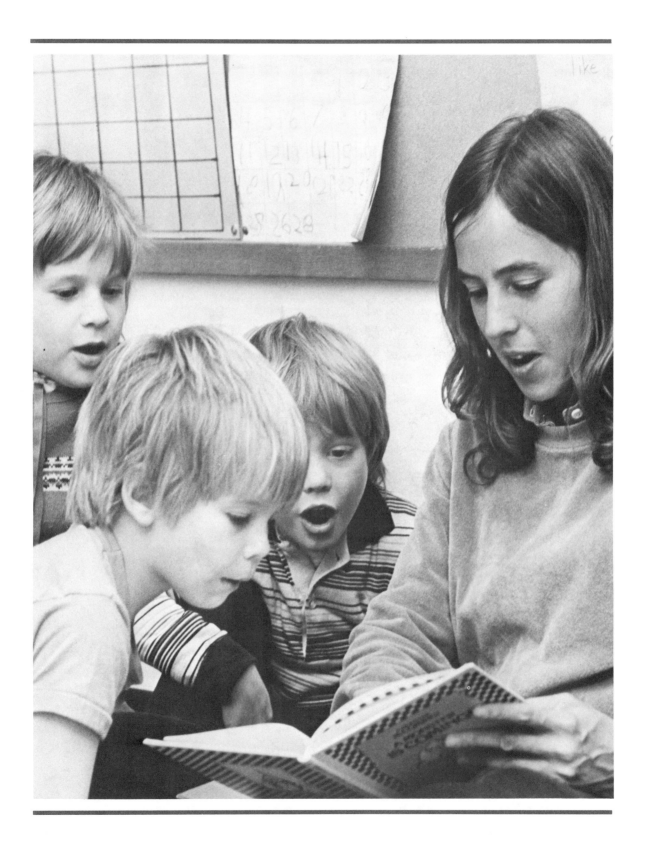

Chapter 6

The Role of the Teacher in the Elementary School Health Program

INTRODUCTION

Teaching at the elementary level is no easy task. The skills required are both complex and demanding. In fact, the elementary school teacher will have at least as much influence on the overall development of the youngster as any of the other immediate forces within the child's environment. Unfortunately, many elementary school teachers do not realize their profound influence on the youngsters they teach.

This premise has implications for elementary health science. The primary responsibility for the health of the elementary school child rests with the parents, and the school's role is to supplement their efforts. However, in all too many instances the role of the school becomes primary. The child may receive very little or perhaps no direct health instruction at home. If this is the case and if the child is deprived of quality health instruction in the school, it is not difficult to forecast the outcome. The unhealthy child's efficiency level is drastically impaired, and in the long run his or her accomplishment will be altered. Failure in itself can be devastating for a child. Failure of a child at any level for unattended health reasons is inexcusable.

The elementary school years are particularly important to one's health. Much of the learned behavior and attitudes about health that will prevail throughout a lifetime are established during the elementary school years. If these habits and attitudes are sound, the child will most likely continue through life exhibiting healthful practices and attitudes.

This theory contributes to the goal of modern health education. The goal underlying all education is the attainment of intelligent self-direction on the part of the student. Elementary health instruction can prepare the youngster to protect, preserve, and promote his or her health.

The vehicle for such preparation is the teacher, who must possess the insight and understanding necessary to teach health via a precise blending of experiences and information that will complement the student's immediate needs and interests.

THE HEALTH EDUCATION PROCESS

The teaching of elementary health science can be thought of as a process of disseminating information in order to influence youngsters' health practices, attitudes, and understanding. In theory, the concept of health education is developed in much the same manner as any of the other traditional subjects found in the elementary curriculum. Perhaps the key difference between health and other subjects is in the realm of expected outcomes. The teaching of health is aimed at assisting the youngster to develop intelligent self-direction in health matters. However, what is easily said is not so easily accomplished. The process of health education is a complex art; many factors ultimately bear on the quantity, quality, and effectiveness of the instruction. The teacher should ponder the following questions:

- Why should I teach health? What can I hope to accomplish by providing health instruction for my students?
- Which topics should I teach about?
- What is the most effective way for me to teach health?
- When should I teach health?
- What materials would enhance the instruction?
- How far can I go with the "difficult" areas of health education?
- How can I evaluate my health instruction?

Education that is motivating, relevant, and timely and that provides for student/teacher involvement requires careful planning and organization. Health education is no exception to this rule. The quantity and quality of the health instruction in your classroom are direct reflections of your motivation, planning, and organizational skills. Haphazard education is often misguided, and it lacks the continuity of well-planned teaching. A teacher who desires to be effective with health instruction should make a conscious effort to fulfill several prerequisites. A thorough understanding of the concept of developmental tasks and their relationship to needs, interests, and maturational stages of youngsters (Chapter 3) is indispensable to curriculum planning. Insight about the basis of health behavior is helpful when planning and implementing the instructional program. The ability to develop concepts (Chapter 8) is most helpful. Sound and attainable expected outcomes are also essential. Teachers' qualifications, motivating learning experiences (Chapter 10), and evaluation (Chapter 11) should be carefully contemplated before formal instruction begins.

Elementary health instruction is most complicated. It should be approached with a great deal of forethought and planning in order to contribute to the development of healthful behavior on the part of students.

THE IDEAL TOTAL SCHOOL HEALTH PROGRAM

To clarify the terminology used throughout the remainder of the text, the following discussion of the ideal school health program is essential. To this point we have referred to elementary health education as a process by which children are exposed to enlightening classroom experiences. This is an integral part of the school health program, but it is only one aspect of the ideal picture.

We can begin by defining the ideal total *school health program* as a combination of the many activities provided by the school in an effort to preserve and promote the health of the school child (see Figure 6.1). It encompasses all of the school functions directed at affecting the

FIGURE 6.1
The ideal total school health program.

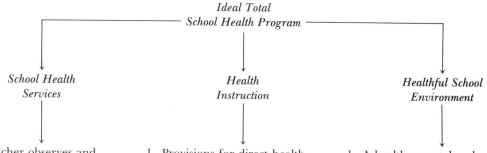

Ideal Total School Health Program

School Health Services

1. The teacher observes and refers students with health problems.
2. Health appraisal through periodic screening tests.
3. Emergency care provisions and procedures.
4. Prevention and control of communicable diseases.
5. Required immunizations.
6. Cumulative health record keeping.
7. Teachers know their students' health status and any special provisions necessary.

Health Instruction

1. Provisions for direct health instruction.
2. Health instruction integrated and correlated with other subjects.
3. Emphasis is placed on the development of sound health knowledge, practices, and attitudes.
4. Instruction is carefully planned, well organized, and sequential in nature. Health curriculum is followed.
5. Prepared teachers.
6. Adequate resource materials.

Healthful School Environment

1. A healthy mental and emotional relationship between teacher and students.
2. School day is arranged in a wholesome fashion.
3. School facilities are safe as possible.
4. Lighting, acoustics, heating, and ventilation are conducive to good health.
5. Proper sanitation is maintained.
6. Nutritious school lunches.
7. Traffic safety program.

health of the child, and it includes *health services, health instruction,* and *healthful school environment.* These activities are not mutually exclusive. For the school health program to operate effectively, the interrelationship among these three traditional aspects of the program should be carefully outlined.

Health services should be designed to appraise, promote, protect, and maintain the health of students. Carried out through a wide variety of activities and procedures, health services require the cooperative efforts of teachers, physicians, nurses, students, parents, and others. School health services are generally considered to include:

1. Health appraisal
2. Counseling appropriate to appraisal findings
3. Assistance with the rectification of remediable defects
4. Assisting in the planning of educational experiences for the handicapped
5. Pupil observation
6. Referral to the proper medical authorities of any student with a suspected medical problem
7. Assistance in the control and prevention of communicable diseases
8. Provisions for emergency care

Health instruction is the planned sequential activities designed to influence students' knowledge, attitudes, and practices. Cognitive lessons emphasize such skills as knowing, analyzing, evaluating, synthesizing, comprehending, and applying gained insight. Teaching of sound attitudes and practices instills behavior that will improve the youngster's health. The health practices of the student while at school are observable and offer an opportunity for evaluation, but just as important are practices and attitudes the student exhibits outside the school. To influence the attitudes and practices that govern the student outside the school is indeed a formidable challenge.

Rounding out the ideal school health program is the *healthful school environment.* The school has a responsibility to provide an environment conducive to the students' good physical, social, and emotional health. This includes safe and healthful water supply and sewage and refuse disposal as well as grounds free from unnecessary hazards. Heating, lighting, and ventilation are important. The food service program is integral to the school environment.

The criteria for the environment we have so far discussed are physical. They are essential to a healthful school environment, but so also are the people. Healthy interpersonal relationships among teachers, students, staff, and administrators are paramount if the school is to be effective in teaching health.

SPECIFIC RESPONSIBILITIES OF THE ELEMENTARY SCHOOL TEACHER

Within the realm of the ideal school health program, the elementary school teacher has many responsibilities. Indeed, the teacher has a responsibility to contribute to *all* aspects of the school health program, being in a unique position of authority. The teacher occupies the key role in the elementary school health program. The student will surely benefit from a teacher who is interested in and motivated to teach health science. If, on the other hand, the teacher cannot find time for health education, the school health program never has a chance to play an influential role.

HEALTH SERVICES

The precise role of the teacher in health services is *observation and referral.* The elementary school teacher sees a child every day over an extended period. Appearance, behavior, and emotions are easily compared from one day to the next. If abnormalities appear, the teacher has an obligation to refer the youngster to the proper authorities.

However, responsibility does not stop there. It is imperative that a serious deviation in the health of the youngster be alleviated. The dedicated and empathic teacher not only refers the afflicted child, but also follows up to ensure that the situation is remedied to the fullest extent possible. The fledgling teacher is encouraged to follow all of the proper channels of authority in referring a youngster. Failure to follow the proper procedures may involve you, the child, and the child's parents in an embarrassing legal entanglement. You may have to persevere longer, but if the child is ultimately helped, the time and effort will have been well spent.

It is safe to assume that rarely will a year pass without a confrontation with at least one, if not more, abnormalities of health among the students. When such an occasion occurs, the teacher has an expressed responsibility to obtain help for the child.

Child Abuse: A Special Area of Concern for Teachers*

One major area of concern of particular importance to the elementary school teacher is child abuse. Many states now define teachers as "mandated reporters," which means that by law you must report any known or suspected cases of child abuse, on penalty of being found liable for negligence. *Child abuse* is physical injury, physical neglect, sexual abuse or emotional maltreatment intentionally inflicted on a child under 18 by any other person.

School personnel play a critical role in the detection of abuse and neglect. Signs—injuries, listlessness, poor nutrition, disruptive behavior, absenteeism or depression—are often first seen by school personnel. Because immediate investigation of suspected abuse may save a child from repeated injuries, even death, school personnel should not hesitate to report suspicious injuries or behavior (Figure 6.2).

---

*The material in this section is adapted from the *Child Abuse Prevention Handbook*, Office of the Attorney General, Sacramento, CA: California Office of State Printing, 1985.

Most school districts have special procedures for reporting suspected child abuse. No administrator should interfere with the classroom teacher's report, nor is the classroom teacher absolved of responsibility by relying on an administrator to file a report.

Unless blatant falsehood in a report can be substantiated, those who file mandated reports of abuse have absolute immunity from civil and criminal liability as a result of providing a required report of suspected child abuse. It is also important to note that the identity of all persons who report suspected child abuse is strictly confidential, as is all the information in the report.

Most jurisdictions investigate child abuse reports via local police or the county child welfare agency or both. If the subsequent investigation does not reveal evidence of child abuse but does indicate other family problems or the potential for child abuse, the investigating agency can attempt to intervene and prevent a crisis.

Child abuse is a crime and the primary consideration is the protection of the child. The police have authority to investigate and arrest, status in the community that induces cooperation, and the ability to respond immediately.

A small percentage of child abuse cases are found to be severe and heinous in nature. Approximately half of reports to child welfare agencies are for neglect. A small percentage of the children in the remaining cases have to be placed in protective custody or foster homes. Very few of the reported cases actually result in prosecution or the termination of parental rights.

As the abused child suffers, the family also suffers in most instances. Child abuse and neglect in a given family are often an intergenerational problem. There is no question that some abuse cases reflect severe mental illness or character disorder. However, it is also a fact that many parents of abused or neglected children were abused themselves.

Child abuse occurs in all cultural, ethnic, occupational, and socioeconomic groups. Although it is often assumed that parents are the only culprits, it is important to understand that children are abused by other relatives, family friends, neighbors, acquaintances, and strang-

SUSPECTED CHILD ABUSE REPORT

TO BE COMPLETED BY INVESTIGATING CPA

VICTIM NAME: _____

REPORT NO./CASE NAME: _____

DATE OF REPORT: _____

TO BE COMPLETED BY REPORTING PARTY

A REPORTING PARTY

NAME/TITLE _____

ADDRESS _____

( )

PHONE   DATE OF REPORT   SIGNATURE OF REPORTING PARTY

B REPORT SENT TO

○ POLICE DEPARTMENT   ○ SHERIFF'S OFFICE   ○ COUNTY WELFARE   ○ COUNTY PROBATION

AGENCY   ADDRESS

( )

OFFICIAL CONTACTED   PHONE   DATE/TIME

C VICTIM

NAME (LAST, FIRST, MIDDLE)   ADDRESS   BIRTHDATE SEX RACE
( )

PRESENT LOCATION OF CHILD   PHONE

SIBLINGS

1. _____   4. _____
2. _____   5. _____
3. _____   6. _____
NAME   BIRTHDATE SEX RACE   NAME   BIRTHDATE SEX RACE

D PARENTS

NAME (LAST, FIRST, MIDDLE)   BIRTHDATE SEX RACE   NAME (LAST, FIRST, MIDDLE)   BIRTHDATE SEX RACE

ADDRESS   ADDRESS
( )   ( )

HOME PHONE   BUSINESS PHONE   HOME PHONE   BUSINESS PHONE

E INCIDENT INFORMATION

IF NECESSARY, ATTACH EXTRA SHEET OR OTHER FORM AND CHECK THIS CIRCLE. ○

1. _____   _____   *(CHECK ONE)* ○ OCCURRED ○ OBSERVED
DATE/TIME OF INCIDENT   PLACE OF INCIDENT

IF CHILD WAS IN OUT-OF-HOME CARE AT TIME OF INCIDENT, CHECK TYPE OF CARE:
○ GROUP HOME OR INSTITUTION   ○ FOSTER CARE   ○ OTHER PLACEMENT (SPECIFY _____)

2. TYPE OF ABUSE: *(CHECK ONE OR MORE)*   ○ PHYSICAL   ○ MENTAL   ○ SEXUAL ASSAULT   ○ NEGLECT   ○ OTHER

3. NARRATIVE DESCRIPTION: _____

4. SUMMARIZE WHAT THE ABUSED CHILD OR PERSON ACCOMPANYING THE CHILD SAID HAPPENED: _____

5. EXPLAIN KNOWN HISTORY OF SIMILAR INCIDENT(S) FOR THIS CHILD: _____

FIGURE 6.2
Suspected Child Abuse Report form. (Adapted from material from the Office of the Attorney General, Department of Justice, State of California.)

**THIS FORM, AS ADOPTED BY DEPARTMENT OF JUSTICE, IS REQUIRED
UNDER PENAL CODE SECTIONS 11166 AND 11168**

REPORTING RESPONSIBILITIES

- No child care custodian, medical practitioner or nonmedical practitioner reporting a suspected instance of child abuse shall be civilly or criminally liable for any report required or authorized by this article (California Penal Code Article 2.5). Any other person reporting a suspected instance of child abuse shall not incur civil or criminal liability as a result of any report authorized by this section unless it can be proved that a false report was made and the person knew or should have known that the report was false.

- Any child care custodian, medical practitioner, nonmedical practitioner, or employee of a child protective agency (CPA) who has knowledge of or observes a child in his or her professional capacity or within the scope of his or her employment whom he or she reasonably suspects has been the victim of child abuse shall report such suspected instance of child abuse to a child protective agency immediately or as soon as practically possible by telephone and shall prepare and send a written report thereof *within 36 hours* of receiving the information concerning the incident.

- Any child care custodian, medical practitioner, nonmedical practitioner, or employee of a child protective agency who has knowledge of or who reasonably suspects that mental suffering has been inflicted on a child or its emotional well-being is endangered in any other way, may report such suspected instance of child abuse to a child protective agency. Infliction of willful and unjustifiable mental suffering must be reported.

REPORTING PARTY DEFINITIONS

- ''Child care custodian'' means a teacher, administrative officer, supervisor of child welfare and attendance, or certificated pupil personnel employee of any public or private school; an administrator of a public or private day camp; a licensed day care worker; an administrator of a community care facility licensed to care for children; headstart teacher; public assistance worker; employee of a child care institution including, but not limited to, foster parents, group home personnel and personnel of residential care facilities; a social worker or a probation officer.

- ''Medical practitioner'' means a physician and surgeon, psychiatrist, psychologist, dentist, resident, intern, podiatrist, chiropractor, licensed nurse, dental hygienist, or any other person who is currently licensed under Division 2 (commencing with Section 500) of the Business and Professions Code.

- ''Nonmedical practitioner'' means a state or county public health employee who treats a minor for venereal disease or any other condition; a coroner; a paramedic; a marriage, family, or child counselor; or a religious practitioner who diagnoses, examines, or treats children.

- ''Child protective agency'' means a police or sheriff's department, a county probation department, or a county welfare department.

INSTRUCTIONS

I. CASE IDENTIFICATION (Upper Box)—*To Be Completed by Investigating Child Protective Agency.*

   Case Identification: Enter the victim name, report number or case name, and the date of report.

II. SUSPECTED CHILD ABUSE REPORT (11166 PC)—*To Be Completed by Reporting Party.*

   A. Reporting Party: Enter name/title, address, phone number, and the date of report, and sign.

   B. Report Sent To: 1) Check the appropriate child protective agency to whom this report is being sent; 2) Enter the name and address of the child protective agency to whom this report is being sent; 3) Enter the name of the official contacted at the child protective agency, phone number, and the date/time contacted.

   C. Victim: Enter the name, address, physical data, present location, and phone number where victim is located (attach additional sheets if multiple victims).

   Siblings: Enter the name and physical data of siblings living in the same household as the victim.

   D. Parents: Enter the names, physical data, addresses, and phone numbers of father/stepfather and mother/stepmother.

   E. Incident Information: 1) Enter the date, time, and place the incident occured or was observed, and check the appropriate circles; 2) Check the type of abuse; 3) Describe injury or sexual assault (where appropriate, attach form DOJ 900, Medical Report—Suspected Child Abuse or any other form desired); 4) Summarize what the child or person accompanying the child said happened; 5) Explain any known prior incidents involving the victim.

III. DISTRIBUTION

   A. Reporting Party: Complete form SS 8572, Suspected Child Abuse Report (11166 PC). Retain yellow copy for your records and submit top four copies to a child protective agency.

   B. Investigating Child Protective Agency: Upon receipt of form SS 8572, Suspected Child Abuse Report (11166 PC), send white copy to police or sheriff, blue copy to county welfare or probation, and green copy to district attorney *within 36 hours*. Complete form SS 8573, Suspected Child Abuse Preliminary Investigation Report (11169 PC), attach pink copy to pink copy of SS 8572, and forward to DOJ *immediately*.

ers. Abusers are sometimes teachers, child care providers, or foster parents. Abusers can be male or female and they may be adults, adolescents, or other children.

Early identification, reporting, and intervention are very important in the effort to protect the victim, because the abuser typically will repeat the abuse and may even escalate it.

Many factors are associated with child abuse; it is rarely the result of any single one. One or more of the following factors could trigger an abusive act:

1. Emotional stress such as marital or employment problems
2. A predisposition to maltreatment, perhaps as a result of having been abused or neglected as a child
3. A lack of constructive outlets for tension
4. Anger or aggression
5. Poor impulse control

Indicators for Suspicion of Child Abuse

The following indicators are to assist the prospective teacher who is expected to report all known or suspected cases of child abuse.

One of the most important grounds for suspecting child abuse is the child's telling you that he or she is abused. If a child tells you that he or she is being abused, it is imperative that you report that fact exactly according to your district's procedures. Most states do not consider communication between a teacher and a child as privileged, and the teacher must report suspected or known child abuse. This requirement normally applies to physical abuse, severe emotional maltreatment constituting willful cruelty or unjustifiable punishment, neglect, and sexual abuse.

Physical Abuse

Physical abuse is any act that results in a non-accidental physical injury. Physical injury most often is the result of unreasonably severe or unjustifiable punishment. This usually happens when the parent is frustrated or angry and strikes, shakes, or throws the child.

Deliberate assault, such as burning, biting, cutting, poking, twisting limbs or otherwise torturing a child, is also included.

The primary zone of injuries is the back of the body from the neck to the knees. Such injuries constitute the largest percentage of identified abuse. Injuries from abuse are not typically located on shins, elbows, or knees.

The known history includes all facts about the child and the injury:

- Whether the child states that the injury was caused by abuse
- Injury that is unusual for the age group (any fracture in an infant)
- History of injuries
- Injuries to the child that the parent is unable to explain; discrepancies in explanation; blame placed on a third party; explanations inconsistent with medical diagnosis

The following behaviors may result from child abuse:

- Parent or caretaker delays seeking care for a child or fails to seek appropriate care.
- Child is excessively passive, compliant, or fearful; or excessively aggressive or physically violent.
- Child or parent or caretaker attempts to hide injuries; child wears excessive layers of clothing, especially in hot weather; child is frequently absent from school or physical education classes.

Bruises

Bruises resulting from abuse are found particularly on the buttocks, back, genitals, and face. They may appear in the outline of a hand, paired bruises from pinching, or an impression of an item of jewelry (such as a ring) or a disciplinary imprint (such as a paddle, switch, or coat hanger). Linear bruise marks, strap marks, and loop marks going around a curved body surface are almost always evidence of abuse.

Multiple bruises may all be the same color, or different colors if the injuries were sustained at different times. Red, red-blue, violaceous, black-purple, green tint, pale green, and yellow color as well as crisp or fading margins reflect various stages of healing. When bruises differ in color, it is useful to take color photographs of them for evidence.

Where bruises may be bite marks, investigators should be prepared to seek the expertise of forensic odontologists.

Blows from a heavy object (such as a baseball bat or fist) on soft tissue result in deep muscular bruises or hemorrhage. These are rarely discolored but in time may be seen on x-rays.

Burns

The location of a burn and its characteristics (shape, depth, margins) may indicate abuse. It is important to keep in mind that children instinctively withdraw from pain. Burns without some evidence of withdrawal are highly suspect because a child will usually try to escape—which will result in splashes, uneven burns, and sometimes burns on the hands.

Scalding with hot liquid is the most common abusive burn. Young infants are scalded by immersion and older children by having liquids thrown or poured on them.

When children are forcibly held in hot water, there are often sharply demarcated burns. If held in water in a jackknife position, only the buttocks and genitalia may be burned. If held down forcibly in a sitting position, the center part of the buttocks (if pressed tightly against the tub) is spared from burning, resulting in a doughnut-shaped burn. If the extremities are forcibly immersed in hot water, glove or sock burns result. The burns are often symmetric and an immersion line is readily evident.

"Zebra" burns also indicate abuse. Such burns result when a child is held by his or her hands and legs under a running hot faucet. The tissue on the child's abdomen and upper legs folds up, preventing burning in the creases. The resulting "zebra stripes" from scalding of exposed tissue are clearly evident.

Abuse may also be suspected when burns are pointed or deeper in the middle. This indicates that hot liquid was poured on, or a hot object (poker, utensil) pressed into the skin.

Another burn characteristic of abuse has the shape of a recognizable object evenly burned into the victim's skin. Such burns indicate forced contact or "branding" with, for example, the grill of an electric heater, the element of an electric stove, or an iron.

Cigarette burns are difficult to diagnose, but they are often multiple and are often found on the palms or soles. There is a searing effect, perhaps with charring around the wound.

Rope burns appear around wrists or ankles when children are tied up.

Bite marks

Bite marks, which may be found on any part of the body, are doughnut-shaped or double horseshoe-shaped. In some bites, tooth impressions may be seen and used to identify the biter. The uniqueness of human dentition allows bite-mark evidence to be admissible in the courts of California and many other states, as well as in United States military cases.

Time is of the essence in recording bite marks. They should be photographed by law enforcement officers daily for as long as a week. Impressions should be made, and salivary swabbings may also provide evidence.

Abrasions, lacerations

Again, the number and location of wounds should be considered. Lacerations under the tongue or in the small piece of tissue connecting the gum to the lip could be caused by falling with an object in the mouth or by the use of excessive force during feedings. Both are suspicious injuries when the victim is an infant who is still unable to stand.

Whipping a child with a belt buckle may cause lacerations resembling a "C" or "U" shape or other distinctive shape.

Head injuries

Whenever abuse or neglect is suspected, a careful examination of the child's eyes and nervous system should be performed, looking for signs of intracranial injury. A skull x-ray may be an important part of the examination. Serious intracranial injury may occur without visible evidence on the face or scalp but may cause brain damage or death if untreated.

Head injuries are the most common cause of death from child abuse and an important cause of chronic neurological disabilities.

Shaken infant syndrome

This syndrome is intracranial and intraocular hemorrhage in the absence of signs of external injury to the head. Shaking, using excessive force, may produce not only these injuries, but also lesions of the long bones.

The only early indicators of shaking may be vomiting, rapidly enlarging head, and subtle neurological signs, including learning problems; the injury may go undiagnosed for years. More severe damage, such as blindness, deafness, and paralysis, may appear, especially if early signs are not heeded.

Shaking can kill. A careful post-mortem examination of every child who dies in infancy is required to detect the cause of death and to avoid erroneous diagnoses.

Internal injuries

Blunt blows to the body may cause serious internal injuries to the liver, spleen, pancreas, kidneys, and other vital organs and occasionally cause shock and result in death. This is the second leading cause of death for victims of child abuse.

Surface evidence of such trauma is present only about half the time. Physical indicators of serious internal injuries include distension of the abdomen, blood in urine, vomiting, and abdominal pain.

Fractures

Any unexplained fracture in an infant or toddler is cause for inquiry. Spiral fractures of the long bones, which result from twisting forces, are almost always caused by abuse when they occur before a child begins walking.

Other fractures that raise suspicion are chip fractures at the end of long bones; multiple rib fractures, especially on the back; unexplained healing or healed fractures revealed by x-rays. X-ray bone surveys are important tools for diagnosing physical abuse. Radioisotope bone scans may pick up healing fractures, subperiosteal hematomas, and so on.

Physical Neglect

Neglect is the failure to provide care and protection to a child by a parent or caretaker under circumstances indicating harm or threatened harm to the child. The term includes both acts and omissions and can be severe as well as general in nature.

Severe neglect is the failure of a parent or caretaker to protect the child from physical injury as a result of severe malnutrition or failure to thrive that is not attributable to physical conditions. It includes allowing the person or health of the child to be endangered and the intentional failure to provide adequate food, clothing, shelter, or medical care.

General neglect is the failure to provide adequate food, clothing, shelter, medical care, or supervision where no physical injury to the child has occurred.

Children may be neglected because their working parents are unable to arrange child care. The shortage of affordable child care has created the latchkey children. They are left unsupervised when they are out of school and their parents are working. Parents of latchkey children may be unable to locate affordable child care or may consider their children old enough to be left on their own. Although these parents may not regard themselves as child abusers, leaving young children without supervision constitutes general neglect. Children left in these circumstances are particularly vulnerable to accidents, injuries, and crime.

Neglect may be suspected if the following conditions exist:

- The child lacks adequate medical or dental care.
- The child is always sleepy or hungry.
- The child is always dirty, demonstrates poor personal hygiene or is inadequately dressed for the weather.

- There is evidence of poor supervision (repeated falls downstairs; repeated ingestions of harmful substances; a child cared for by another child); the child is left alone at home or unsupervised under any circumstances (in car, street).
- The conditions in the home are unsanitary (garbage, animal or human excretion).
- The home lacks heating or plumbing.
- There are fire hazards or other unsafe conditions.
- The sleeping arrangements are cold, dirty, or otherwise inadequate.
- Nutrition is poor.
- Meals are not prepared (children snack when hungry).
- There is spoiled food in refrigerator or cupboards.

While some of these conditions may exist in any home, the *extreme* or *persistent* presence of these factors indicates some degree of neglect.

Extreme conditions resulting in an unfit home constitute severe neglect and may justify protective custody and dependency proceedings as well as criminal neglect charges. Disarray and an untidy home do not necessarily mean the home is unfit.

Psychosocial failure to thrive

Infants or young children who are very small for their age can be a difficult diagnostic problem for physicians. After excluding infants who are small because they were small at birth, there remains a large group of infants with low weight (and perhaps shortness and small head circumference). Most of these children are small because of a failure to meet their nutritional and/or emotional needs. These children may also demonstrate delayed development and abnormal behavior. Some small children have hidden medical problems. Hospitalization may be required to screen for significant illness and to see if the child responds to adequate nutrition and nurturing with a rapid weight gain and more appropriate behavior. Evaluation consists of more than weighing and measuring the baby. The behavior of the child and the parent should

be observed, ideally during feeding, and the child's response to feeding should be noted.

If left untreated, the health or person of the child may be endangered, and emotional disorders, school problems, retardation, and other forms of dysfunction may result.

Sexual Abuse

Sexual abuse is defined as sexual assault on or sexual exploitation of minors. Sexual abuse encompasses a broad spectrum of behavior. It may consist of many acts over a long period (chronic molestation), or a single incident. Victims range in age from less than one year through adolescence. Sexual assault includes rape, rape in concert, incest, sodomy, lewd or lascivious acts upon a child under 14 years of age, oral copulation, penetration of a genital or anal opening by a foreign object, and child molestation. Sexual exploitation includes conduct or activities related to pornography depicting minors, and promoting prostitution by minors.

The nature of sexual abuse, the shame of the victim, and the possible guilt of parent, stepparent, friend, or other caretaker, make it extremely difficult for children to report sexual abuse. Yet reports of sexual abuse continue to increase. This increase is usually attributed to the passage of the Child Abuse Reporting Law, the public's increased concern for the child victim, and the detection and reporting by professionals.

Sometimes a child who seeks help is accused of making up stories, since many people cannot believe that the person involved could be capable of sexual abuse. When the matter does come to the attention of authorities, the child may give in to pressure from the family and deny that any sexual abuse has occurred. Even if protective attention is gained, the child may feel guilty about turning in the abuser or breaking up the family and so withdraw the complaint. This process leads many to be skeptical of a child's complaint of sexual abuse and leaves the child feeling helpless and guilty.

The sad reality of sexual abuse is that without third-party reporting, the child often remains trapped in secrecy by shame, fear, and the threats of the abuser or the family.

Sexual abuse of a child may surface through a broad range of physical, behavioral, and social symptoms. Some of these indicators, taken separately, may not be symptomatic of sexual abuse. They are listed below as a guide and should be examined in the context of other factors.

History
- Child reports sexual activities to a friend, classmate, teacher, friend's mother, or other trusted adult. The disclosure may be direct or indirect: "I know someone"; "What would you do if?"; "I heard something about somebody." (It is not uncommon for disclosure by children experiencing sexual abuse to be delayed.)
- Child wears torn, stained, or bloody underclothing.
- A child's injury or disease is unusual for the age.
- Child has a history of recurrent injuries or diseases.
- Child has injuries or diseases the parent is unable to explain; there are discrepancies in explanation; blame is placed on a third party; explanations are inconsistent with medical diagnosis.
- A young girl is pregnant and has a sexually transmitted disease.

Behavioral indicators
- Detailed and age-inappropriate understanding of sexual behavior, especially by younger children
- Inappropriate, unusual, or aggressive sexual behavior with peers or toys
- Compulsive masturbation
- Excessive curiosity about sexual matters or genitalia of self or others
- Unusually seductive with classmates, teachers, and other adults
- Prostitution or excessive promiscuity
- Excessive concern about homosexuality, especially by boys

Behavioral indicators in younger children
- Enuresis
- Fecal soiling

- Eating disturbances (overeating, undereating)
- Fears, phobias, compulsive behavior
- School problems or significant change in school performance (attitude and grades)
- Age-inappropriate behavior (pseudomaturity or regressive behavior such as bedwetting or thumb sucking)
- Inability to concentrate
- Sleeping disturbances, e.g., nightmares, fearful about falling asleep, fretful sleep pattern, sleeping long hours

Behavioral indicators in older children and adolescents
- Withdrawal
- Clinical depression
- Overcompliant behavior
- Poor hygiene or excessive bathing
- Poor peer relations and social skills; inability to make friends
- Acting out, running away, aggressive or delinquent behavior
- Alcohol or drug abuse
- School problems, frequent absences, sudden drop in school performance
- Refusal to dress for physical education
- Nonparticipation in sports and social activities
- Fear of showers or restrooms
- Fear of home life demonstrated by arriving at school early or leaving late
- Sudden fear of familiar people, places, or activities
- Extraordinary fear of males (in cases of male perpetrator and female victim)
- Self-consciousness of body beyond that expected for age
- Sudden acquisition of money, new clothes or gifts with no reasonable explanation
- Suicide attempt or other self-destructive behavior
- Crying without provocation
- Setting fires

Physical symptoms
- Sexually transmitted diseases
- Genital discharge or infection

- Physical trauma or irritations to the anal or genital area (pain, itching, swelling, bruising, bleeding, lacerations, abrasions, especially if unexplained or inconsistent)
- Pain on urination or defecation
- Difficulty in walking or sitting due to genital or anal pain
- Stomachaches, headaches, other psychosomatic symptoms

Incestuous and Intrafamilial Sexual Abuse

Sexual abuse of children within the family is the most hidden, least publicized form of child abuse. In spite of the taboos against it and the difficulty of detection, some researchers believe such abuse may be more common than physical abuse.

Incest is sexual activity between persons who are blood-related; *intrafamilial* refers to sexual activity between family members not related by blood (stepparents, boyfriends).

In most reported cases the father or another man acting as the parent is the initiator, with girls as the most frequent victims. However, boys are victims much more often than previously believed. The embarrassment and shame used to deter girls from reporting such abuse has an even greater effect on boys, since the abuse is most often homosexual.

The initial sexual abuse may occur at any age from infancy through adolescence. However, the largest number of cases involves girls under the age of 11. Sexual abuse is followed by shame-provoking demands for secrecy and threats of terrible consequences if the secret is revealed. The child fears disgrace, hatred, or blame for breaking up the family if the secret is revealed. Regardless of how gentle or forceful or how trivial or coincidental the first approach may have been, sexual coercion tends to be repeated and to escalate over years. Often the child eventually accepts the blame for tempting and provoking the abuser.

The mother may purposely stay isolated from sexual abuse. Sometimes she is distant and uncommunicative or so disapproving of sexual matters that children are afraid to speak up. Sometimes she is insecure and the fear of loss of her husband or partner or of scandal is so threatening that she cannot allow herself to believe that her child is at risk. She may have been a victim of child abuse and may not trust her judgment or her right to challenge male authority. Some mothers know of sexual abuse but look the other way. Until the victim is old enough to realize that incest is not a common occurrence, and/or he or she is strong enough to obtain help outside the family, there is no escape.

Child Molestation

Children are sometimes manipulated into becoming consenting or noncomplaining victims by adults who receive sexual gratification from them.

This does not fit with society's image of an unsuspecting child being lured into a car with a candy bar. A child molester often uses pornographic literature to steer a normal conversation with a juvenile toward a sexual theme. The materials are used to stimulate both the perpetrator and the victim and to assist in breaking down the inhibitions of the victim. The nature of the literature usually will correspond with the molester's particular sexual inclinations, and the models used are usually of the age he or she prefers. This is evidenced by the ever-increasing volume of pornographic material seized in investigations of sexual exploitation cases. Pamphlets seized by police provide suggestions for child molesters and pedophiles about what to do, where to go, and come-ons. They include cartoons depicting sexual activity to which a child can relate.

Child sexual abuse usually involves an adult known or related to the child, although offenders have been as young as 10. The offender typically uses implicit or direct coercion to involve the child in sexual activity and to secure compliance. Coercion may take the form of psychological pressure, exertion of adult authority, misrepresentation of moral standards, gifts or rewards, and sometimes force or threats. Children may cooperate because of needs for love, affection, and attention or a sense of loyalty to the adult.

Child Rape

Rape is most commonly associated with adolescent victims, although forcible sexual assaults involving young children are also reported. The assault is usually forced oral, vaginal, or anal penetration. Injuries may result either from the act or the force used to subdue the victim. Although child rape can occur within the family, the offender is usually not known to the victim. Typically, enticement or abduction is used to separate the child from family and friends.

Exploitation/Child Pornography

Although it is impossible to determine the exact number of children who have been the victims of pornographic exploitation, it is clear that by even the most conservative estimate, the number is alarmingly high.

The difficulty in assessing the number of children involved in pornography is compounded by a number of factors. First, the evidence indicates that in the vast majority of cases, this kind of sexual exploitation goes unknown even to the parents of the children. The ever-increasing number of juvenile runaways in recent years, together with the growing problem of child prostitution, also contributes to the difficulty in making this assessment; the runaway juvenile, alone in a strange city, is a particularly attractive target for pornography or prostitution. Finally, some parents use their own children to produce pornographic material. Therefore, the only reasonable conclusion is that the number of children involved is substantial. Moreover, the number appears to be growing.

In recent years, police have increased the number of arrests of persons suspected of producing and disseminating child pornography. These arrests have resulted in seizure of thousands of films, magazines, and still photographs that depict children (some as young as 4) in sexual activity. However, the problem outweighs the arrests by a large margin.

Emotional Maltreatment

Just as physical injuries can scar and incapacitate a child, emotional maltreatment can cripple and handicap a child emotionally, behaviorally and intellectually. Severe psychological disorders have been traced to excessively distorted parental attitudes and acts. Emotional and behavioral problems in varying degrees are very common among children whose parents abuse them emotionally.

Excessive verbal assaults (belittling, screaming, threats, blaming, sarcasm), unpredictable responses (inconsistency), continual negative moods, constant family discord, and double messages are ways parents may subject their children to emotional abuse.

Behavioral indicators shown by children
Emotional abuse may be suspected if the child:

- Is withdrawn, depressed and apathetic
- Acts out and is considered a behavior problem
- Is too rigid in conforming to instructions of teachers, doctors and other adults
- Displays other signs of emotional turmoil (repetitive, rhythmic movements; inordinate attention to details; no verbal or physical communication with others)
- Says things like "Mommy always tells me I'm bad."

This behavior may have other causes, but the suspicion of abuse should not be precluded.

Behavioral indicators shown by parent or caretaker
A child may become emotionally distressed when:

- Parents or caretakers place demands on the child that are unreasonable or impossible or without consideration of the child's developmental capacity
- The child is used as a battleground for marital conflicts

- The child is used to satisfy the parent's or caretaker's own ego needs, especially if the child does not understand
- The child victim is referred to as "it" by the perpetrator

Emotional abuse can be seen as proving a self-fulfilling prophecy. If a child is degraded enough, the child will begin to live up to the image communicated by the abusing parent or caretaker.

Emotional abuse is extremely difficult to prove, and *cumulative documentation by witnesses is imperative.* Such cases should be referred for treatment as soon as possible.

Only suspicion of severe emotional abuse that constitutes willful cruelty or unjustifiable punishment of a child is required to be reported. However, mandated reporters *may* report any degree of emotional abuse.

Deprivation

Emotional deprivation is the deprivation suffered by children when their parents do not provide the normal experiences producing feelings of being loved, wanted, secure and worthy.

Emotional deprivation should be suspected if the child

- Refuses to eat enough and is very frail
- Is unable to perform normal functions for a given age, e.g., walking, talking
- Displays antisocial behavior (aggression, disruption) or obvious delinquent behavior (drug abuse, vandalism) or is abnormally unresponsive, sad or withdrawn
- Constantly seeks out and pesters adults such as teachers and neighbors for attention and affection
- Displays exaggerated fears

When parents ignore their children, whether because of drugs or alcohol, psychiatric disturbances, personal problems, or other preoccupations such as outside activities, serious consequences may occur. However, these situations are not reportable unless they constitute abuse, as it is legally defined.

Recognizing a Child's Drug Problem

An adult's drug abuse problem can often be traced to behavior learned early in childhood. Unfortunately, with each passing school year we find the onset of drug use among school children occurring at an earlier age. Youngsters in grades four, five, and six are especially susceptible to the many influences that lead to experimentation with drugs.

It is important that teachers refer a student exhibiting signs of drug use. The following signs, especially in combination, may indicate a drug problem:

1. Sudden mood swings, irritability, depression
2. Neglect of personal appearance
3. Sudden deterioration in school attendance, discipline, and quality of work
4. Unusual and pronounced change in degree of activity
5. Inappropriate weight loss or gain
6. Slow and slurred speech
7. Diminished alertness
8. Deterioration in relationships or radical change of friends
9. Theft of items that can be converted to cash
10. Sudden display of more money than normal
11. Possession of drugs or drug paraphernalia

Dealing with the Problem

Misuse and abuse of drugs are insidious. Drug problems tend to progress slowly, and in most cases destructive behavior and harmful effects are seen only after a child has been misusing drugs for some time; by the time a youngster's drug problem is discovered, it is likely to be serious. Faced with a child who is using drugs, resist the urge to act precipitously; instead, attempt to deal with the situation rationally and objectively. Like an adult alcoholic, the youngster confronted with drug abuse will probably resort to denial. Once parents are involved, there is likely to be family conflict. Some parents will believe the denial, at least for a time, hoping there is not a problem. Other parents will over-react and worsen the problem. Most parents eventually face the truth, but not until after much anguish.

School health personnel should work with the child, classroom teacher, and parents to gather as much information about the youngster's situation as possible. It is important to know what substances are being used, how, and why. Proper diagnosis and careful evaluation are essential to selecting an appropriate treatment.

Many young chronic drug abusers are depressed and have serious emotional, psychological, or physical problems. These problems, in addition to a family history and the youngster's social functioning, are all considered when developing a treatment plan. The diagnosis and treatment should also consider the possibility that the youngster has a learning disability.

Depending on the severity and complexity of the problem, treatment may be confined to individual counseling combined with small group interaction. More complex and advanced cases may involve inpatient hospital treatment and follow-up outpatient day care or residential program. Aftercare for the young drug abuser is extremely important. Many drug abusers find it difficult to remain drug free if they return to the peer group, family, or school situation that prevailed prior to intervention.

Good aftercare does not cease abruptly. It is important that support personnel be readily available when problems arise, anxieties build, and peer pressure or temptation to use drugs surfaces. Some aftercare programs use peer group support to meet this need. These groups of youngsters in recovery are organized and conducted by professional and peer counselors. Often youngsters respond more openly to peers than to professionals about their problems. They are also more receptive to feedback from their peers.

Parents' participation is very important. Most parents' love and understanding will be tested. It is important that the parents be prepared to respond with their love, time, understanding, patience, and ongoing support.

Why Do Some Youngsters Abuse Drugs?

Drug use among the young is probably best attributed to social interaction and experimentation. Young people are egocentric, and this often contributes to a false sense of invulnerability. The idea "I can stop whenever I so desire" often clouds young people's thinking. Part of growing up is the desire to make decisions, and warnings of impending danger from parents and teachers often go unheeded.

Factors believed to increase the likelihood of a youngster taking drugs:

1. Coming from a home whose members smoke, drink, or use drugs.
2. Living with a family that is tolerant of drug use or believes it is harmless or an expected aspect of growing up.
3. Associating with friends who use drugs.
4. Experimentation, often traced to the glamorous portrayal of drug use in the media.
5. The thrill of taking a risk.
6. Biological vulnerability to drug abuse (a distinct possibility, as research on alcoholism is indicating).
7. Disciplinary tactics of adults; research indicates that children of authoritative parents are less likely to abuse drugs than are children of authoritarian or permissive parents.
8. Differences in the values and aspirations of youngsters. A strong desire for independence based on achievement is one of the most important protective factors for prevention and cessation of drug abuse.
9. Young people who know the consequences of drug abuse and who care about their health and future are less likely to experiment with drugs.

School-age drug abusers behave differently from nonusers. Nonusers are more likely to be involved with extracurricular activities such as a sport, club, or job. Those on drugs tend to be involved in sexual activity, truancy, and delinquency; hyperaggressive and rebellious behavior as well as poor relationships are common. One important question is which problem precedes the other.

School-based Intervention

The drug education programs of the 1970's were primarily based on information and fear arousal. Often lacking in credibility, the programs of that era were in some cases actually responsible for raising the level of drug use by participants. The programs failed to provide students with specific skills to resist pressures to use drugs.

Contemporary drug education is more psychosocial. It provides for a more rational framework to assist students in dealing with the recurrent decision whether or not to use a drug. Present-day school-based drug education and intervention differ from previous approaches in who delivers the message (classmates, older peer, teacher, or a combination), teaching techniques for resisting social pressures (role playing, sociodrama, modeling), and the use of social contracts (written commitment not to use drugs).

The AIDS Epidemic: Its Effect on the Educational Community

The AIDS epidemic is a health issue of major proportions. Acquired immune deficiency syndrome (AIDS) is a transmittable viral disease characterized by a severe breakdown in the body's immune system, resulting in increased susceptibility to infection that is eventually fatal to the AIDS victim.

Heterosexual contact is an efficient mode of transmission of AIDS. Therefore, the epidemic is sure to become more widespread. It has been reliably estimated that 1 in 30 males between the ages 20 and 50 are infected. By 1991, AIDS will be second only to accidents as a cause of premature death among American men. As of this writing, no successful treatment is available. The only FDA-approved treatment so far—for patients infected by the virus but not yet ill—is the drug azidothymidine (AZT). AZT has been shown to suppress reproduction of the AIDS-causing virus, called human T-lymphotropic virus (HTLV-III). Appendix C contains a more detailed explanation of AIDS.

An infected mother can pass the AIDS virus to an infant before or during birth, so it is inevitable that AIDS-infected school-age children will become more common. Also, a small number of AIDS victims have been infected via contaminated blood and blood products from AIDS-infected donors. The infected child presents a unique problem for the affected school district. Just as controversial is the AIDS-infected teacher. While it is easy to intellectualize about hypothetical dilemmas, the reality is that such a situation will be emotionally loaded for all involved.

While the AIDS virus has been isolated in infected patients' blood, seminal fluid, saliva, tears, cerebrospinal fluid and breast milk, documentation to date indicates that the actual transmission of the disease is via blood, vaginal secretions, and semen only. Consequently, many school districts have developed policy and procedures that treat AIDS as a communicable disease and closely monitor the child or employee for any change in health that could affect school attendance.

HEALTHFUL SCHOOL ENVIRONMENT

The teacher has direct control over the environment in the classroom. The physical characteristics of the classroom can do much to enhance or hinder learning. A student who is in a cheery, bright, and comfortable room is likely to feel good about her or his surroundings. Atmosphere in the classroom bears on the behavior of students.

The classroom environment can also contribute to long-range social betterment. Children in whose homes the basic practices of good hygiene are not followed can gain valuable insight and experience from a classroom that adheres to a higher standard of living. Ideally, through such an experience the deprived student will develop the incentive to establish more healthful living at home. The student who comes from a home that already has a high standard of health will receive reinforcement for present practices.

There is little the elementary school teacher can do about the architectural surroundings the school provides. However, the teacher can contribute tremendously to the efficiency of the structure. For example, it is most important that the teacher have burned-out lights replaced in the classroom. An improperly lighted classroom will contribute greatly to eye fatigue.

Room temperature is another flagrantly disregarded aspect of the classroom environment. The room that is too hot or too cold is a strong deterrent to the learning process. Teachers should be careful not to impose their wishes on students. Because of their activity level, youngsters generally like a cooler room than adults do. The teacher who has difficulty adjusting to the temperature preferred by the students should make a special effort to offset such a discrepancy, perhaps dressing more warmly.

Ventilation is also important. Whenever possible in the room lacking air conditioning, the windows should be adjusted so as to provide sufficient air transference. When ventilation is poor and the heat is up, the students are likely to suffer drowsiness, headaches, depression, and a general loss of vigor.

The teacher should strive for a classroom temperature between 66° F and 71° F. Humidity can also affect the comfort of a classroom. Relative humidity of 50 percent is ideal at 70° F. However, without central air conditioning, the teacher stands little chance of having any control over the humidity of a classroom.

Perhaps the most important component of a healthful school environment is the people themselves. Even if all of the considerations above were at the epitome, the social environment would be dependent on the people who occupy it. Certainly, the teacher is the most important of these people. Without his or her guidance, empathy, and love for children, the physical structure of the school lacks life itself. Students will only be as enthusiastic, vibrant, and full of love for life as their teacher.

Teacher-Student Involvement

Glasser (1969) has much to say about involvement between teachers and students. His premise is that when students become involved at an affective level with responsible teachers, they are better able to make responsible choices and to behave constructively.

All too often, teachers stand aloof from their students and do not become involved. Many avoid being warm, personal, and sincerely interested in their students. This is indeed unfortunate, especially for the youngster who is lonely and desperately in need of warmth and recognition from an adult.

The involvement concept deals directly with the students' mental health. There is perhaps no nonacademic aspect of elementary education more important than the development and maintenance of the students' emotional well-being. Much can be done for the child with little effort by the teacher. However, "involvement" is difficult to teach. Prospective teachers can be told to involve themselves with their students, but unless they are naturally inclined to do so, it is indeed difficult. Involvement is important at every level of education, but perhaps most so at the elementary level.

Many young students have no opportunity to identify with an adult who is responsible and successful in coming to grips with life. Some youngsters' attempts to grow up are thwarted; they have no adult who will assist them in this process.

Ideally a youngster establishes meaningful relationships with adults other than the teacher. Adult models may be parents, older brothers and sisters, clergy, responsible peers, a relative. However, many children are never given the opportunity to get involved with a responsible person. Many young persons readily admit that their quality of life can be attributed to an understanding teacher who took an interest in them as individuals.

You cannot please and meet the needs of every student. This does not mean that you need not strive to meet every student's needs. Indeed, you should make a pronounced effort, although there will invariably be some students with whom you will have difficulty establishing rapport. There will be many others who will benefit tremendously from your concern and interest in them.

Several simple techniques foster involvement. Some guidelines:

1. Get to know the youngsters' first names as soon as possible. A youngster who is not called by name in and out of school knows that you have no interest in him or her.
2. Make an effort to know the student's background—home life, interests, hobbies, anxieties. However, you should not pry personal information from the student. By being a good listener, you can gather insight into the child's personal life. The ability to see from the child's point of view is extremely helpful to both you and the student.

   Becoming a good listener is difficult for most. All too often, the teacher wants to do the talking, give advice, and offer constructive alternatives—more than likely just what the student does not need. The youngster may need little more than a responsible adult who will listen.
3. Deal with misconduct in a caring way. A child misbehaves for a reason. The teacher must realize that students are responsible for their behavior. By expecting or demanding anything less than responsible behavior, the teacher adds to the deviant child's troubles. Children's behavior is directed mainly by emotion. Successful behavior produces pleasant emotion, and the converse holds true for unsuccessful or unacceptable behavior. Ideally, the teacher should make an effort to deal with the deviant child's behavior if any success is expected in dealing with the child's emotional well-being.

   By developing warm involvement with students and working with their behavior, the teacher may improve their emotional health. Keep in mind that emotion is a result of behavior, but it is the behavior, and the behavior alone, that can be con-

trolled. When we affect the child's behavior, we instill feelings of worth, which produce better behavior in every aspect of the child's life.

Assuming that you are willing to become personally involved with a child who has a behavior problem, you must assist that child in changing his or her behavior if you are to help. Essentially, the youngster must be induced to make a value judgment about the behavior. If the child doesn't believe that there is anything wrong with the behavior, there is little you can do to help. The child must suffer the consequences of refusing to change the behavior.

However, you should never give up on a child. No matter how many times a child misbehaves or fails, he or she should again and again be asked to make an honest value judgment about the situation. Sooner or later, the youngster will doubt that what he or she has been defending is best.

After the child perceives the problem, the teacher and student together pursue a more reasonable and constructive course of behavior. If the child doesn't know a better course, the teacher must suggest some alternatives and help the child set goals. Once the child becomes committed to a new course of action, there is no acceptable excuse for not following through. The teacher who really cares accepts no excuses. This is discipline at its best. Every child needs discipline and guidance.

In another respect, Glasser's approach to dealing with pupil behavior also accentuates the concept of commitment. It is not enough to get the child to evaluate his or her behavior. The child must be persuaded to choose a better way to behave and then make a commitment to that choice. Commitment of this nature develops maturity and feelings of worth in a youngster that ideally will carry through a lifetime.

Glasser is careful to differentiate between discipline and punishment. Schools and society use punishment mainly to deal with misbehavior. The advantages of punishment are questionable. The system of discipline discussed above allows the child to suffer the painful consequences of misbehavior, but no attempt is made to induce excess pain or to be punitive. The child should be excluded from class activities, or school if necessary, for blatant misbehavior. However, the child is excused for an arbitrary time that is completely up to him or her. After proposing an acceptable behavior plan and making a commitment to that plan, the child should be allowed to return to class.

If this system of involvement is to succeed, the teacher cannot accept any excuse for a commitment going unfulfilled. If a teacher does accept an excuse for the breaking of a commitment by the student, involvement too begins to break down. The sensitive student knows that the teacher who really cares will not let him or her get hurt. Involvement ceases when the person who makes the commitment is allowed to excuse himself or herself for breaking the commitment.

There is no question that involvement and commitment are well within the province of mental health. Properly employed, this kind of classroom management can do much to ensure a healthful classroom environment.

HEALTH INSTRUCTION

Ineffective health instruction at the elementary level continues to plague our schools. This is especially important because sociological and psychological health problems are increasing tremendously in both magnitude and complexity. The need for sound health practices and attitudes has never been more important.

The elementary school years are crucial for health education. Some basic knowledge will be acquired by the child; the foundation for the attitudes that will guide the youngster throughout life is laid; and many of the habits that will affect the pupil's health are formed. The implications for elementary health education become obvious when one critically perceives the many public health problems that we are faced with today.

Elementary health education is consistent with the national trend toward promotion of healthful habits, risk reduction, and disease prevention (USPHS, 1979). Elementary health education can make an important contribution to healthful knowledge, attitudes, and practices.

Our goal is to intervene with our students as early as possible to assist them in resisting unhealthful behavior, which leads to premature illness, disability, disease, and death. While improvements in health behavior are an admirable goal, one must question whether the elementary school provides a worthy setting for such a complex endeavor. Healthful behavior is influenced by many diverse factors.

The school is a relatively weak influence on a youngster's behavior when compared with the pressure exerted by peers, family, the community, and its attendant forces (Chapter 1). Even under optimal conditions (the ideal total school health program), the time devoted to formal health instruction is quite limited.

Therefore, the school is best suited to reinforce healthful behavior via the dissemination of knowledge and the fostering of healthful attitudes and practices. In essence, we are promoters of good health. We strive to support behavior that will enhance the youngster's ability to practice healthful behavior.

For example, elementary teachers should be more concerned with teaching about factors that influence the decision to smoke or not than with teaching about smoking-cessation strategies (Green, 1980).

Developing Healthful Attitudes, Practices, and Knowledge

The emphasis placed on the development of healthful attitudes, practices, and knowledge varies at different educational levels (Figure 6.3). Research suggests that at certain stages, children are more inclined to establish healthful practices, at other stages are more likely to develop attitudes, and at still other periods in their lives will seek to procure knowledge.

FIGURE 6.3

Changing emphasis to be placed on imparting health knowledge, evolving attitudes, or developing habits at various grade levels.

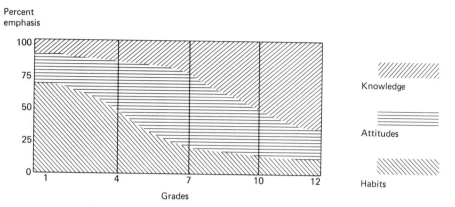

Piaget has described the process by which children develop the capacity for grasping concepts (Pulaski & Pulaski 1971). His theory, applied to elementary health science, is helpful in evolving a pattern of instructional emphasis. The best results are attained by assigning primary emphasis to the development of health practices during the early years of school life. Theoretically, health attitudes will also be developed as by-products through installation of sound health habits at the primary level.

The middle elementary grades provide the most opportune time for the development of healthful attitudes. This does not mean that practices and knowledge are disregarded during the intermediate grades. It simply means that the development of attitudes is given top priority at that time because the child is most ready for the cultivation of attitudes in this period. At this age the youngster is highly impressionable. Desirable attitudes toward health reinforce established health practices.

Knowledge to sustain, support, and reinforce practices and attitudes then becomes important. The upper elementary grades or junior high school is the level at which health knowledge becomes increasingly important. Such knowledge is necessary to reinforce practices and attitudes. Junior high youngsters rapidly become interested in the how and why of health matters. Furthermore, they are capable of digesting and assimilating such cognitive in-

formation. They have reached the level at which factual information is meaningful and relevant to their world.

Keep in mind that the junior high years are highly experimental for the youngster. Peer pressure is intense, and many youngsters' first real value conflicts are occurring. Young people are in dire need of objective health information at this time. Ideally, such information, combined with previously established practices and attitudes, will assist the child in making an informed decision regarding his or her health behavior.

REFERENCES AND BIBLIOGRAPHY

Anderson, C. L. *School Health Practice* (St. Louis: C. V. Mosby, 1980).

Cornacchia, Harold J., Larry Olsen, and Carl Nickerson. *Health in Elementary Schools* (St. Louis: Times Mirror/ Mosby, 1984).

Green, L.W., et al. *Health Education Planning: A Diagnostic Approach* (Palo Alto, CA: Mayfield, 1980):15.

Glasser, William. *Schools Without Failure* (New York: Harper & Row, 1969).

Office of the Attorney General. *Child Abuse Prevention Handbook* (Sacramento, CA: California Office of State Printing, 1985).

Pulaski, Mary, and Spencer Pulaski. *Understanding Piaget* (New York: Harper & Row, 1971).

U.S. Public Health Service. *Healthy People: The Surgeon General's Report on Health Promotion and Disease Prevention* (Washington, DC: Government Printing Office, 1979).

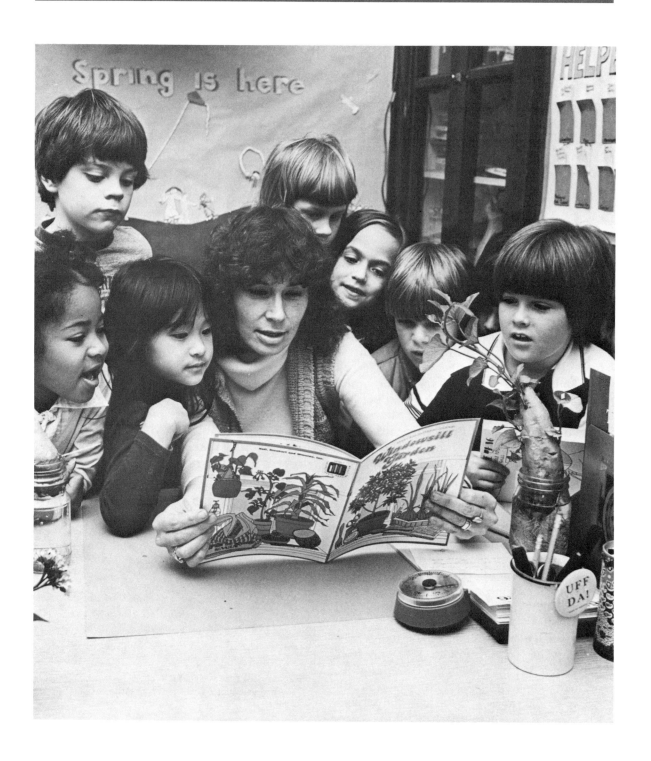

Chapter 7

The Elementary Health Education Curriculum

WHY INCLUDE HEALTH IN THE ELEMENTARY CURRICULUM?

Never have children been more acutely aware of what is taking place around them. They are the television generation, and this fact is responsible for their being exposed to more spectacles in a year than their parents could have been expected to perceive in a decade. Without question, today's elementary school youngsters are brighter, more sensitive, and more provocative than in any preceding generation. The child of today matures quite quickly and very often exhibits as much insight as a person twice as old.

It is generally agreed that values and attitudes have a strong relationship to emotional, physical, social, and spiritual well-being. The earlier in life one develops a positive outlook on health behavior, the greater the chances of living a wholesome, happy, and productive life. It follows that the logical place to initiate health education is the elementary classroom. Ideally the health education that takes place in the classroom will supplement the health education the child receives at home and in the community.

It seems logical that if our socially aware elementary school youngsters received formal health education, they would be more inclined to develop a healthy and wholesome outlook toward optimal well-being. Unfortunately, many children never get formal health education during their developmental years. It is indeed regrettable when a youngster's knowledge, attitudes, and practices of health are unsound simply because he or she was never taught sound health principles. If we expect young people to seek a meaningful and rewarding life, we must help them to establish a firm foundation of health knowledge, attitudes, and practices early in life. Failure to assist the child with this may very well deprive him or her of the ability to reach maximum potential and enjoy a wholesome life.

The responsible and sensitive elementary school teacher is concerned about the health and welfare of students. Actually, the teacher has a legal as well as moral responsibility for the promotion and development of good health behavior in pupils. This is no easy task. The development of optimal well-being is one of the most challenging undertakings in life. The informed and concerned elementary school teacher can significantly contribute to this worthy goal.

In addition to this philosophical rationale in support of the inclusion of health education at the elementary level, there are also other, more objective reasons:

1. It is common knowledge that Americans follow poor health practices. Our diet, activity level, dental habits, weight control, and techniques for dealing with stress border on atrocious at times. For many of us, such poor health practices are a direct reflection of our failure to develop proper health habits at an early age.

2. Many Americans have difficulty in establishing proper health practices because they lack the information necessary to make intelligent decisions about health matters. A well-planned and coordinated elementary health science program can contribute immensely to public health education.

3. The general attitude of the average American toward well-being is not good and appears to be getting worse. Perhaps "future shock" is the best term to describe the state of affairs that confronts most of us. Change is so rapid that only the hardiest can adjust and keep his or her wits. Technology has done many wonderful things for us, but not without trauma. Reality can become too much to bear, and all too often the occasional escape to a world of illusion becomes habitual. The drug problem, divorce rate, incidence of sexually transmitted disease, and ecological problems are just a few of the indicators of future shock in the United States. If we are to survive, we must effectively deal with the way of life we have created. Health education at an early age can assist young people to cope with a complex and demanding way of life.

4. The most pressing health issues that this nation faces today are in most instances sociological. Such topics as mental health,

114

mood-modifying substances, family life, sex education, and ecology are monumental social health issues. In addition, they are all highly attitudinal. Education about these topics will be helpful in developing a socially aware young adult who will be likely to contribute significantly to the solution of these problems.

5. Health is one of the cardinal objectives of education. Every national policy-forming body in the United States for the past five generations has indicated that one of the major objectives of education is good physical and mental health. In addition, most state laws require a teacher to do certain health teaching, to recognize illnesses in pupils, and to prevent accidents. The recommendations in the *School Health Education Study* (1964) not only included health instruction among priorities for the school, but also recognized it as a distinctive responsibility of the school. Implicit in this recommendation was the belief that health instruction belongs in the school curriculum because such knowledge is necessary to direct behavior, is most effectively learned in school, and is not available from other public agencies.

6. The landmark report of the Surgeon General of the United States entitled *Healthy People* (U.S. Department of Health, Education and Welfare, 1979) emphasized the fact that the overall health of Americans is directly affected by four major factors: (1) unhealthful approach to lifestyle, (2) an inadequate health care system, (3) existing environmental hazards, and (4) human biology. The report further identified fifteen areas targeted for intervention:

1. High blood pressure
2. Family planning
3. Pregnancy and infant health
4. Immunization
5. Sexually transmitted disease
6. Toxic agent control
7. Occupational health and safety
8. Injury control and accident prevention
9. Dental health and fluoridation
10. Control of infectious disease
11. Smoking
12. Drug misuse and abuse
13. Nutrition
14. Physical fitness
15. Controlling stress and violent behavior

A companion report entitled *Objectives for the Nation* (U.S. Department of Health and Human Services, 1980) developed specific objectives for each area. Results are expected by 1990. As might be expected, the schools are considered one of the richest potential sources for behavior change and achievement of the *objectives for the nation*.

APPROACHES TO TEACHING ELEMENTARY HEALTH SCIENCE

There are three distinct theories of health education. Health science as a discipline can be taught through correlation, integration, and/or direct instruction. Authorities disagree as to which approach is best for elementary school children. The following discussion is intended to help you form your own opinion.

Correlation

Correlation is the incorporation of health education into another appropriate subject area. This requires a strong relationship between health and the subject with which it is being correlated. Proponents argue that correlation allows the teacher more latitude. It helps remove the traditional barriers of the curriculum and offers a new avenue for teaching old topics. In addition, correlation is purported to enrich the content by broadening and adding relevance to subject matter.

Actually, elementary health science can be incorporated into any subject normally taught in elementary school. Language arts, reading, mathematics, art, geography, music, science, history, and physical education all provide opportunities for teaching health. For example, a chart of students' height and weight for the year can demonstrate mathematical principles, and a discussion of the relationship among growth, development, and health can be prompted.

Teaching health through correlation requires an expert teacher. Assuming that health objectives for the year are established, the teacher must determine which activities are best suited to the health curriculum.

The pitfalls are obvious. It would be easy to force the correlation of health education. When sound planning is lacking, it is not at all difficult to become irrelevant, waste the students' time, and duplicate someone else's efforts. When there is no significant relationship among the ideas being correlated, students can easily miss the point or ignore what may be very important information. On the other hand, correlation properly implemented does much to help children see the importance of health in everyday living.

Integration

Integration organizes learning around a central objective, theme, or area of living. It best lends itself to elementary school because the lessons usually cross subject-matter lines and are centered on life's activities. The integrated curriculum can be thought of as a core surrounded with broad fields. For it to be effective, the teacher must skillfully draw on the various school subjects and programs for those that can best contribute to the lesson.

It is easy to understand why correlation and integration are often confused and used synonymously. One thing is certain: Where there is an integrated plan, there must be correlation in the subjects in the integrated curriculum. On the other hand, there can be correlation of health education with another subject or two without integrating such instruction into an overall instructional plan.

The following discussion by Rash (1974) clarifies the distinction:

As has been suggested, integration is sometimes erroneously confused with correlation. The confusion results from the complete misuse of the word integration, not from any close similarity in meaning. In reality integration has two meanings. The first, and original, meaning is related to integrate, "to make whole." In this connotation integration is the process of making whole. *The second meaning, resulting from attempts to describe a plan of organization of a school curriculum is defined in the* Dictionary of Education *as: "a curriculum in which subject matter boundaries are ignored, all offerings of the school being taught in relation to broad areas of study and in relation to one another as mutually associated in some genuine life relation."*

The concept of correlation in which one subject field is related to another subject field is in direct conflict with the concept of integration, in which subject matter boundaries are ignored. Correlation relates to method while integration relates to plan of organization.

In summary, the elementary classroom does lend itself to these approaches to education. The fact that the classroom is self-contained offers flexibility the teacher can use to decided advantage. The skillful elementary school teacher can go from teaching by correlation to direct instruction or vice versa. When the same teacher is responsible for providing all of the students' instruction, the teacher has a degree of freedom that can be found only in the self-contained classroom. However, such freedom is not without its pitfalls. For example, it would be easy to slight health instruction because the teacher felt that students' health needs were being met entirely through correlation.

The most important point is that we try to meet the students' health needs. Correlation can be most effective for this. Combined with direct instruction, it becomes even more effective.

Direct Instruction

Direct health instruction is scheduled, planned, and directed toward the fulfillment of pupils' health needs and interests.

We have already established that the primary school youngster is held responsible for very little specific knowledge in regard to health. However, children's natural curiosity demands more specific information as their capacity for understanding advances. It is especially desirable to provide information about health from the third grade on. There is no single perfect approach, but the primary grades best lend themselves to development of sound health practices; the intermediate grades to the establishment of positive health attitudes; and the junior high level to the building of new positive attitudes and indepth health knowledge. Direct health instruction becomes the vehicle for such an approach.

Perhaps you have now developed your own opinion as to what is the best approach to health education. Keep in mind that no matter what the choice, it is the teacher on whom responsibility for success rests. Perhaps the best approach to health instruction centers on direct instruction, implementing correlation where possible. That way, health instruction is afforded the same amount of emphasis as the other traditional subjects taught at the elementary school level.

THE ELEMENTARY HEALTH CURRICULUM

To speak of the elementary health education curriculum is a much more difficult task than one might imagine. First and foremost, it is the aspect of health education that you, the prospective elementary school teacher, will probably be able to affect the least. Perhaps Fenton's (1967) discussion of textbook writing and course of study development will clarify these statements.

In the past, university professors and public school teachers wrote the textbooks used in the schools. Usually the most qualified experts, busy at research, refused to turn their hands to writing. Moreover, publishers feared to risk their stockholders' money on radical new approaches which might fail on the market. As a result, one text looked pretty much like another, and almost all lagged behind the latest research.

Typically, a board of education, accepting the recommendations of a small committee of teachers, authorized the use of one text in preference to others. Starting with the text, a committee of teachers developed a course of study during summer vacation. It often turned out to be an expanded table of contents followed by an extensive bibliography. No teacher can develop an imaginative curriculum in a month. Then the textbooks, along with the course of study, passed into the hands of classroom teachers. The curriculum reformers recognized that conventional texts and courses of study were built-in obstacles to chance.

Curriculum can be thought of as the "what" to teach. In most school districts, the elementary health curriculum has been established by a group of so-called experts supposedly well qualified and willing to extend themselves in a more imaginative manner than those cited by Fenton. Ideally, the elementary health curriculum should be designed to meet the needs and interests of the students and should be flexible enough to provide for individual differences from school to school and class to class. Such an undertaking, if it is properly approached, is a monumental project and requires much time, skill, and insight.

In recent years all disciplines have undergone curricular changes. Some have enjoyed more success than others. Over a decade ago, for example, the new mathematics created a fever among students, teachers, and parents alike. The repercussions of the new math are still being felt today. About the same time came the increased emphasis on science. Spurred by Sputnik and financed generously by private foundations and the government, these reforms have spread throughout American schools. However, the books and articles that attempt to explain the new math and science to bewildered parents so they can help their children testifies to the failure of many curricular reforms. Perhaps even more interesting is that already a newer math, designed to consolidate and improve on the work of the original reformers, is on the drawing boards. The problem in health science—that of identifying a new and relevant curriculum, initiating it, and having it accepted by the teachers and public at large—is similar to that of mathematics and science. However, radical curriculum revision is not without dangers.

THE SCHOOL HEALTH EDUCATION STUDY

Health education curricula have not been immune to investigation and revision. About the same time most other subjects were receiving critical evaluation, so was health. It was obvious around 1960 that the health curriculum was out of date compared with that of the other subjects. Following Sputnik I's appearance in orbit, many schools quickly moved to bolster their math and science curricula, often at the expense of health instruction.

This prompted one of the most important national studies in the field of education. The School Health Education Study (SHES) was born in the fall of 1960. Financed by the Samuel Bronfman Foundation, the study was designed to determine the national status of health education and to provide the data necessary for the creation of a sound school health instruction program. Initially, the study was funded for only one year. Later the scope was expanded, and the Bronfman Foundation continued its support through 1965. Approximately one third of a million dollars was allocated for the study.

In its early stages, the study consisted of two surveys. One survey was designed to determine the status of and practices common to health instruction in the public schools. Particular attention was paid to the time devoted to such instruction; whether it was required or not; the course content by grade level; organizational patterns; student groups; course titles; by whom taught; teacher qualifications; credit value, if any; special facilities; textbooks; in-service teacher training; problems peculiar to health instruction; and recommendations. The second survey was designed to determine the behavior of the students in terms of knowledge, attitudes, and practices of health.

In 1961 the SHES team selected a valid statistical sample of the 35,000 or so public school systems in the United States. They randomly selected 135 school systems in 38 states. The survey forms dealing with the status of instruction were completed by the chief administrative office of the school system. The student health behavior instrument was administered to students in one sixth, one ninth, and one twelfth grade in each school system. The gathering of data continued through 1962. After a great deal of analyzing and refining, the SHES staff published a summary report of its findings (1964).

The report confirmed the worst suspicions of the SHES staff. Health education at all levels was in dire difficulty. The subsequent publication *School Health Education: A Call for Action* (1968) more vividly depicted the status and quality of health education in the nation's schools. Among the most important conclusions:

The response by school administrators and teachers . . . revealed a marked deficiency in the quantity and quality of health education in both the elementary and secondary schools. The problems confronting school personnel included: failure of parents to encourage health habits learned at school; ineffectiveness of instruction methods; parental and community resistance to discussions of sex, venereal disease and other controversial topics; insufficient time in the school day for health instruction; inadequate professional preparation of the staff; indifference toward and lack of support for health education on the part of some teachers, parents, administrators, health officers and other members of the community; inadequate facilities and instructional materials; student indifference to health education; lack of specialized supervisory and consultative services. . . .

Regarding the health behavior, knowledge, attitudes, and practices of the surveyed students, there were equally appalling findings. For example:

The health behavior—knowledge, attitudes and practices—of students was likewise appalling. The sixth graders surveyed could answer correctly—on the average—just over 20 of their 40 test questions.

Ninth and 12th graders, on the average, could answer about 50 of 75 questions correctly. Girls, consistently, did somewhat better than boys. Consistently, too, the students were not practicing many of the things they did know—but one sixth grader in five regularly brushed his or her teeth after meals; three out of four ninth grade boys (and half the girls) said a parent or counselor would be their last resort on a question concerning sex.

Equally appalling were the misconceptions held by a great many students. Up to 70 percent of the seniors surveyed, for example, firmly believed that: fluoridation purifies drinking water, legislation guarantees the reliability of all advertised medicines, popular toothpastes kill germs in the mouth and prevent cavities, chronic diseases are contagious, pedestrians are safe under all circumstances in marked crosswalks, venereal diseases can be inherited, venereal diseases have never been a social problem, public funds support the voluntary health agencies, the best man to see for a persistent cough is a pharmacist.

As appalling as these findings may appear, it is not at all surprising that such conditions and beliefs existed, in view of the general quality and quantity of health instruction in 1962.

After the summary report was published in 1964, the SHES Advisory Committee charted a course of action designed to combat the poor status of health education. The original scope of the project was expanded to include the designing of a school health education curriculum for grades K through 12. Eight health education specialists from five states were selected to develop the curriculum, and four sites were selected to test the curriculum once it was completed. The four tryout centers represented the major geographical subdivisions of the United States.

The writing team began work in 1964. After a great deal of research and discussion, it was determined that a concept approach appeared to be the most realistic, potentially effective, and economical way to develop a sound health curriculum. The rationale was that health is not a fact but a comprehensive, generalized, and unified concept. Health is physical, mental, social, and spiritual in nature. It is also a matter of

knowledge, attitudes, and practices into which must be incorporated the interaction among the individual, his or her family, and the total community. Hence many interdependent components combine to influence one's health. Helping young people to recognize and understand this interaction was the challenge for the SHES writing team.

The writing team developed a comprehensive K through 12 health curriculum that is an excellent model for health education. While the SHES project is somewhat dated today, it still reflects the turning point in contemporary health education.

Since the completion of the SHES project, other curricula have been developed and may well serve as the basis for the health education in your school district. Among the more renowned are the Health Activities Project (HAP) developed at the University of California at Berkeley; Health Skills for Life; Growing Healthy; You, Me and Others, developed by the March of Dimes; and The Heart Treasure Chest from the American Heart Association.

CONTENT AREAS OF HEALTH EDUCATION: WHAT AND WHEN SHOULD WE TEACH FOR HEALTH?

Anspaugh, Ezell and Goodman (1987) list 12 content areas. Pollock and Middleton (1984) cite 10; Cornacchia, Olsen and Nickerson (1984) illustrate 14; Haag (1965) mentions 13; Kilander (1968) lists 11; Fodor and Dalis (1966) describe 11; and Willgoose (1974) defines 12. At first glance, there appears to be little agreement among the authorities as to just what should be taught. Further analysis, however, reveals much more agreement. Some authors combine content areas; others prefer to subdivide them.

While the scope of elementary health education does vary among states and school districts, the following list illustrates a typical elementary health curriculum:

1. Consumer health
2. Mental and emotional health

TABLE 7.1
Cycle Plan for Elementary Health Education Content Areas

| | GRADE LEVEL | | | | | | | | |
| | Primary | | | | Intermediate | | | Junior High | |
Content Area	K	1	2	3	4	5	6	7	8
1. Consumer Health							X	X	X
2. Mental and Emotional Health		X			X	X	X		X
3. Drug Use and Misuse			X		X	X	X		X
4. Family Life and Sex Education			X		X	X	X	X	
5. Body Systems and the Senses		X	X	X	X				
6. Nutrition		X		X			X		X
7. Personal Health	X	X	X		X			X	
8. Disease and Disorders			X			X			X
9. Environmental Health						X		X	X
10. Safety and Accident Prevention	X	X			X			X	

3. Drug use and misuse
4. Family life and sex education
5. Body systems and the senses
6. Nutrition
7. Personal health
8. Disease and disorders
9. Environmental health
10. Safety and accident prevention

Ordering the content is another major consideration. A strong program provides for the direct instruction about selected content areas during each year of elementary school in order to ensure that appropriate content is timed to satisfy pupils' needs, interests, and ability to comprehend. This is often termed a cycle plan (see Table 7.1).

PHILOSOPHY OF ELEMENTARY HEALTH SCIENCE

In summary, elementary health science should be an integral part of the elementary curriculum. After all, what is more important than our young people's health? Without health, life can never offer the true zest that accompanies optimal well-being.

Through elementary health education, we can actively assist young people in becoming capable of making intelligent and informed decisions about their health behavior. Behavior is the most influential factor in determining the health of the student. Heredity and environment are also important, but behavior is generally the crucial constituent.

Based on the premise above, we attempt to influence youngsters' behavior by improving their knowledge, attitudes, and practices. Health as a concept is highly value-oriented and attitudinal in nature. The school health program should provide the example and guidance necessary to influence and assist young people in attaining optimum health.

REFERENCES AND BIBLIOGRAPHY

Anderson, C. L. and W. H. Creswell. *School Health Practice* (St. Louis: C. V. Mosby, 1985).

Anspaugh, David, et al. *Teaching Today's Health* (Columbus, Ohio: Merrill, Co., 1987):58.

Cornacchia, Harold J., and others. *Health in Elementary Schools* (St. Louis: Times Mirror/Mosby, 1984):170.

Fenton, Edwin. *The New Social Studies* (New York: Holt, Rinehart and Winston, 1967):2.

Fodor, John T., and Gus T. Dalis. *Health Instruction: Theory and Application* (Philadelphia: Lea and Febiger, 1981).

Framework for Health Instruction in California Public Schools (Sacramento: California State Department of Education, 1970).

Green, Lawrence, et al. *Health Education Planning: A Diagnostic Approach* (Palo Alto, CA: Mayfield, 1980).

Haag, Jessie Helen. *School Health Program* (New York: Holt, Rinehart and Winston, 1965):246.

Kilander, H. Frederick. *School Health Education* (New York: Macmillan, 1968):278.

Michaelis, John U., Ruth H. Grossman, and Floyd F. Scott. *New Designs for the Elementary School Curriculum* (New York: McGraw-Hill, 1967).

NEA-AMA. *Healthful School Living* (Washington, D.C.: National Education Association of the United States, 1957).

————.*Health Education* (Washington, D.C.: National Education Association of the United States, 1961).

————.*School Health Services* (Washington, D.C.: National Education Association of the United States, 1964).

Oberteuffer, Delbert, Orvis A. Harrelson, and Marion B. Pollock. *School Health Education* (New York: Harper & Row, 1972).

Pollock, Marion and Kathleen Middleton. *Elementary School Health Instruction* (St. Louis: C. V. Mosby, 1984).

Rash, J. Keogh. *The Health Education Curriculum,* 2nd ed. (Bloomington: Indiana University Press, 1974):134.

School Health Education Study: A Summary Report. (Washington, D.C.: School Health Education Study, 1964).

School Health Education Study. *Health Education: A Conceptual Approach to Curriculum Design* (St. Paul, Minn.: 3M Education Press, 1967).

School Health Education Study. *A Call for Action* (St. Paul, Minn.: 3M Education Press, January-February, 1968).

Sorochan, Walter D. "Health Instruction—Why Do We Need It in the 70's?" *Journal of School Health* (April 1971):209-214.

U.S. Department of Health, Education and Welfare. *Healthy People: The Surgeon General's Report on Health Promotion and Disease Prevention.* (Washington, D.C.: U.S. Government Printing Office, 1979).

U.S. Department of Health and Human Services. *Objectives for the Nation* (Washington, D.C.: U.S. Government Printing Office, 1980).

Willgoose, Carl E. *Health Education in the Elementary School* (Philadelphia: W.B. Saunders, 1974).

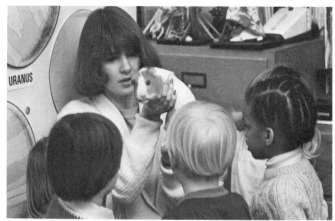

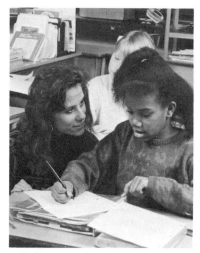

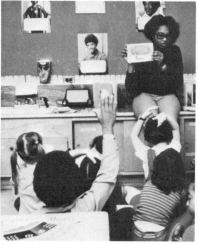

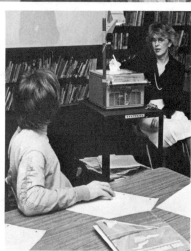

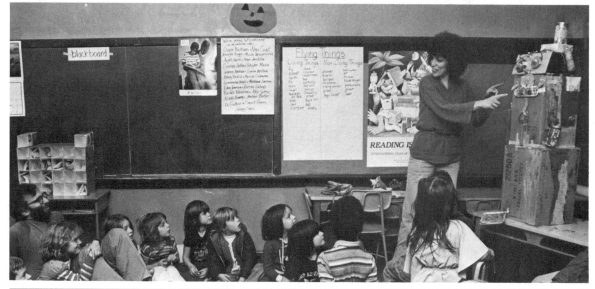

Part Four

Developing the Instructional Program

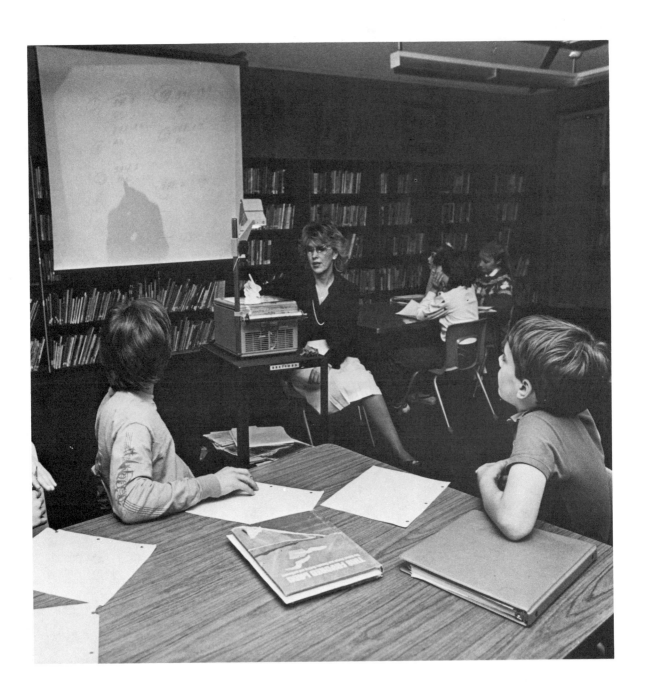

Chapter 8

A Conceptual Approach to Elementary Health Instruction

INTRODUCTION

Like the gills of a trout, the sensory organs extract from the flow of daily experience the mental "oxygen" from which the brain can make its concepts and create the intellectual life. The brain, however, cannot think without sensory data. Conversely, the senses cannot receive preconstructed concepts; they can only accept sensory impressions from the actual referent of our concepts. There is no way into the brain except through the senses. Hence, the teacher must feed sensory impressions to the students, and then coach them through discussion as the students (not the teacher) turn the sensory data into concepts through their own mental processes. (Woodruff, 1951)

Traditional teaching of the past consisted of presenting facts to be memorized. Often these facts were unrelated to one another or to the child's personal well-being. Teachers emphasized information, assuming that once in possession of the necessary facts, children would take intelligent action. Unfortunately, the assumption is not valid. Misuse of drugs and nutritional malpractice demonstrate that the mere provision of facts has not resulted in better health.

Only since 1960 have health educators turned to the concept approach to structure or modify personal health habits and public health practices. Among the programs are the School Health Education Study-3M project *Health Education: A Conceptual Approach to Curriculum Design* (1967); the American Association for Health, Physical Education and Recreation publication *Health Concepts: Guides for Health Instruction* (1967); the National Dairy Council's *Big Ideas in Nutrition Education and How to Teach Them—Grades K-6* (1970); the American Home Economics Association's national project *Concepts and Generalizations* (1970); and numerous state curriculum guides such as the *Framework for Health Instruction in California Public Schools* (1970).

Under such a program the child should arrive at his or her own health concepts by thinking. As the concepts are internalized, the child restructures his or her thinking, feelings and values, and habits and modifies his or her behavior. The foundation for the conceptual approach to health instruction has been devised in part from the content and the beliefs of the preceding chapters. The concept of well-being presented in Chapter 1 structures the basic values and meanings of health for the child as well as adult. Chapter 3 makes us aware that maturation provides a state of readiness to understand. Before understanding can develop, the child's brain and nervous system must develop, and the sense organs must become functional. Physical growth and development set the pace for socioemotional maturity, which in turn paces the intellectual and conceptual development of the whole child.

Definition of Concept

Just what is a concept? There is little agreement, although there is general agreement that concept formation is desirable in transmitting health information to children and in providing the means for understanding such information. More important, concepts may be used to reinforce desirable habits and behaviors.

One problem is the confusion surrounding use of the term "concept." In literature dealing with teaching in general, one can find the terms concept, conceptual scheme, theme, organizational thread, major generalization, major concept, minor concepts, subconcepts, fundamental or key idea, big ideas, and major principles used synonymously. "Concept" provokes further anguish when the elementary teacher discovers that each learner evolves his or her own concepts. It is with these ambiguities in mind that we move toward further clarification.

A concept is a person's mental image of an object or event. Woodruff (1951) defines concept as "some amount of meaning more or less organized in an individual mind as a result of sensory perception of external objects or events and the cognitive interpretation of the perceived data. *It is a relatively complete and meaningful idea in the mind of a person.* It is an understanding of something. It is his own subjective product of his way of making meaning of things he has seen or otherwise perceived in his experience." The School Health Education Study (1967) reinforces this definition by viewing concepts as "the summarizers of experience; they are inventions of the mind to explain or group certain categories of perception. Concepts are mental configurations invented to impose order on an endlessly variable environment and to make adequate responses to events a possibility." Concepts result when the learner relates the facts and information to himself or herself and makes them meaningful. An effort to illustrate such a process is presented in Figures 8.1 and 8.2. This implies that there are different levels of concepts, with each level relevant to a specific maturational (age) stage. The meaning of "concept" will become clearer when you understand the process of concept formation.

Value of Concepts

Concepts result when a child understands. Health behavior is influenced by the child's concepts of well-being. Adjustment to life is greatly influenced by understanding of the environment, other people, and self. For example, the child who understands the danger of automobiles will be more cautious in crossing a street than a child who does not. One of the greatest values of understanding well-being is that it enables a child to adapt to changes, both personal and environmental, and to control the developing body. The child who understands body changes and why they occur will react with less fear, anxiety, or resentment than the child who does not understand.

The child's own concepts are important because she or he is better able to think about self and others, as well as to control his or her feelings. The child's concepts are important because they determine to a large extent what he or she does. The more sound health concepts a child has, the better developed and the more accurate they will be, and the greater the child's understanding will become.

The conceptual approach to health instruc-

FIGURE 8.1

A simple behavioral process, showing the linkage among stimuli, concept, and behavior.

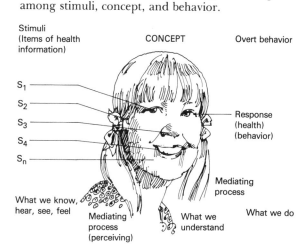

tion is intended to allow children to relate health information to themselves and to their environment, making such information more meaningful. Once information becomes meaningful, it may be used by children to guide them in everyday life experiences.

Concepts as Mediators of Behavior

Concepts are mediators of what we do. Consider Figures 8.1 and 8.2 as a way of understanding this idea (Bourne, 1966). The child interprets the numerous items of health information or stimuli (S_1-S_n) by synthesizing, organizing, and classifying the information. Eventually the interrelationships of all the stimuli are perceived, and a big idea, or concept, emerges. The revelation provides the motivation for a new behavioral response. The concept is the mediator of subsequent behavior, just as the stimuli were mediators of the concept itself. It is the link between the desired behavior and the fragmented information and observations. Concepts as mediators are building blocks from which higher abstract concepts evolve and which in turn affect behavior. The teacher's task is to provide lessons so that the child will perceive the concept for himself or herself.

FIGURE 8.2
A big idea, or concept, evolves from perceived stimuli.

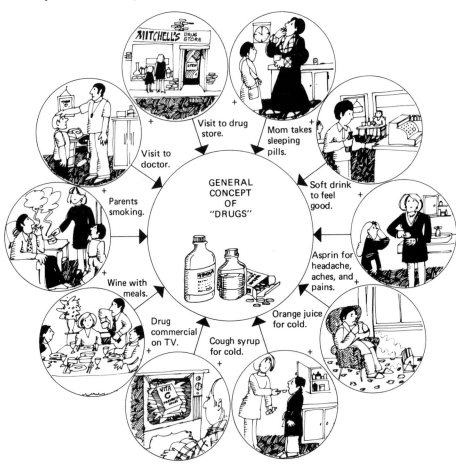

FORMING CONCEPTS

Concepts may be formulated from the way human beings behave. Facts may be grouped to suggest at least three ways of forming new concepts: (1) perceiving a common characteristic from numerous variable phenomena; (2) combining old concepts or grafting new ones onto

old ones; and (3) inferring underlying states or constructs from observations and experiences (Brookbeck, 1965). Analysis of what is involved in each case may throw some light on the subtle and devious process by which concepts are formed.

When the numerous variable phenomena have similar structures, or interpret similar behavior among individuals, or relate a unique relationship between individuals, or have a similarity of function or organization, a common characteristic may be perceived. The newly derived concept is more abstract than the data suggesting it. For example, the functions of the pituitary gland are summarized by the concept "The pituitary gland is the master gland in the body" (see Figure 8.3).

New concepts may also be formed by combining concepts already at hand. By speculating that two or more variables act jointly, a child forms a new concept out of them. For example, a concept on nutrition, "Eating a balanced diet regularly keeps us healthy," and a concept on stress, "Emotional stress causes many disorders," may be used as cues and synthesized to evolve a new concept, "Well-being is enhanced by right style of living." The new concept is valid, since it operates according to sociocultural and physiological laws, has universal application, and is significant for well-being. However, most children will need more than two concepts, or big ideas, as cues to evolve a new or major concept.

The third way of evolving new concepts is to infer underlying states or constructs. From our observations we frequently make inferences about something not observed (see Figure 8.4). In order to help explain certain behavior, the teacher or child may formulate concepts that name unobserved states of an organism. For example, children might rush into the classroom from recess. The teacher forms a concept by remarking, "You behaved like a herd of buffalo."

FIGURE 8.3
Illustration showing how a major concept may be evolved from supporting information.

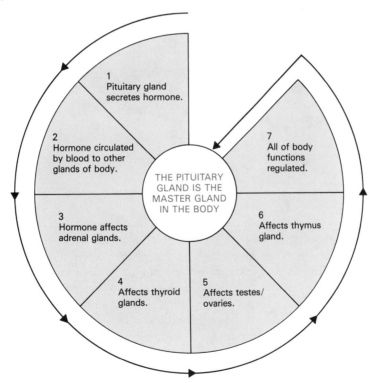

1
Pituitary gland secretes hormone.

2
Hormone circulated by blood to other glands of body.

3
Hormone affects adrenal glands.

4
Affects thyroid glands.

5
Affects testes/ovaries.

6
Affects thymus gland.

7
All of body functions regulated.

THE PITUITARY GLAND IS THE MASTER GLAND IN THE BODY

FIGURE 8.4

A series of experiences may contribute to the building of a key concept. At each step of the sensory experiences (planned and incidental), the child evolves emotional responses, which in turn help him or her to generalize more and more about air pollution.

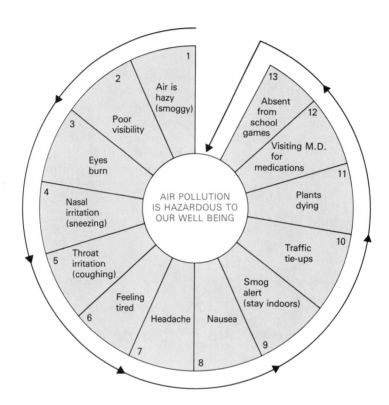

The children's behavior is inferred from an indirect movie or television experience, with which everyone in this culture is familiar, but which no one has directly observed. Such a concept is referred to as a construct.

There are other theories (Bourne, 1965; Pulaski and Pulaski, 1971; Selberg, Neal, and Vessel, 1970; Woodruff, 1951) of how concepts are formed and categorized. Most of these suggest a developmental sequence, arguing that conceptual behavior is based on a sequential decision-making activity in which later decisions are contingent on earlier ones. The diversity of theories suggests that more research is needed in this area.

The application of concepts as mediators of behavior seems a rational approach to exploring concept formation. This approach has merit for elementary school teachers in that the main emphasis is to evolve constructive sociohygienic habits. New concepts evolved by teachers and children may be formed by one or more of the suggested ways.

Criteria of Good Concepts

Related to the general definition of concept are criteria for identifying a good concept. Brookbeck (1965), Gage (1965), and Phenix (1964) suggest that a good concept may be identified as:

1. A generalized summary statement about items of concept or information
2. An abstract idea of what the detailed and specific content is all about
3. Representing meanings of an object or an event
4. Representing a class (body systems), a process (well-being), or a property (height) expressed by a symbol (inches)
5. Reflecting or supporting a basic theory or law (that explains behavior, cause, and effect)
6. Defined in terms of observable individuals
7. Specifying what is the same in different individuals
8. Generalizing about time
9. Valid if it yields successful predictions or outcomes
10. Implicating desirable behavior, ability, or skill
11. Reworded or organized at various levels of complexity (complexity of concepts increases with age and experience)
12. Always symbolized and easily evolved from pictorial material
13. Moving from specific to general, from simple to complex, and from concrete to abstract

The criteria above are abstract. They help to clarify what good concepts should represent and how such concepts should be structured. Unfortunately, many of the concepts evolved by children are too simple and may not meet these criteria. Teachers should keep in mind that children's concepts differ from those of adults more in degree than in kind. For example, children's concepts are more personalized; change with age; and move from simple to complex, from concrete to abstract, from discrete to organized, from egocentric to more "social." Concepts are cumulative for children. In addition, children's concepts are emotionally weighted. Teachers' concepts may have similar characteristics to those of children, but will be on a higher abstract

level. Elementary teachers should regard the criteria as general guides to help them in evolving lesson plans. The application of such guides is presented in the next section.

Steps in Forming Concepts

Prospective teachers are no different from their pupils in evolving concepts. The secret of this process of concept formation lies in understanding the definition of the term "concept." Since a concept is a big idea, or generalization, it may be thought of as a summary about a number of facts. Everyone can form concepts, but not everyone can form good concepts. Children and adults at different stages of development and maturity will vary in the kinds of concepts they evolve about a topic. Teachers should have some expertise in this process if they are going to be able to develop and teach a concept lesson plan.

Teachers need to develop an awareness of the following essentials of forming worthwhile concepts:

1. A basic belief in the fact that optimal well-being is a vehicle to accomplish and therefore is a prerequisite to more abundant living
2. Familiarity with the criteria for identifying good concepts
3. Familiarity with the different kinds of concepts
4. Familiarity with the purpose and function of concepts
5. Familiarity with the subject matter about which concepts are to be formed
6. Familiarity with the semantic structural components of a good concept

The criteria for identifying good concepts, the different kinds of concepts, and the purpose of concepts have already been discussed. Having a rich knowledge of the content is a prerequisite to forming good concepts. A teacher cannot teach something she or he knows nothing about, much less evolve concepts. The more the teacher knows, the easier it will be to evolve concepts. Lack of familiarity with subject matter tends to stifle the formation of concepts. Often an alert teacher will discover a concept from the readings on the topic. Good writers often begin a paragraph with an introductory statement that provides clues for the reader about the remainder of the paragraph. Likewise, writers often end the paragraph with a statement summarizing the contents of the paragraph. Teachers should become aware of paragraph structure and be "looking" for concepts at the beginning and end of a paragraph. This has limitations, however, because someone else's concept may not be meaningful for the teacher. Therefore, teachers should be receptive to rephrasing someone else's concepts. The secret to evolving relevant concepts is possessing a large body of knowledge as background. Although concepts may be stated by someone else, they need to be discovered by the teacher as a learner. Concepts learned from books tend to be superficial. On the other hand, concepts discovered through experience tend to be more meaningful and self-directing. These observations also hold true for children.

The remaining prerequisite to forming sound concepts is familiarity with the semantic structural components of a concept. A good concept has at least three identifiable parts:

1. A *main theme,* such as air pollution or cigarette smoking
2. A phrase suggesting, specifying, or implying a certain kind of behavior or *consequence*
3. A statement of *future ramifications* made by stating the expected outcome and/or by designating persons or things

For example, consider the following concept: Cigarette smoking is hazardous to one's well-being. We can divide this concept as follows:

1. *Main theme*—"cigarette smoking"
2. *Consequence*—"is hazardous"
3. *Future ramifications*—to one's well-being

The three semantic parts of a concept should be stated simply and in as few words as possible. The fewer the words in a concept, the better. As a rule of thumb, a concept sentence should not be longer than 10 to 12 words. Concepts longer than this tend to be confusing for the elementary school child. Both a child and a teacher may forget the main theme when they get to the end of a long-winded concept. If the concept is to communicate understanding and act as a mediator of health behavior, it must be short, concise, abstract, and simple. Only then do words, as concepts, begin to have power as mediators.

Competence in forming sound, relevant, and worthwhile concepts accrues from practice. The mastery of this skill may be reinforced by college professors providing opportunities for prospective teachers to evolve concepts. Such competence is essential to planning lessons.

REFERENCES AND BIBLIOGRAPHY

Big Ideas in Nutrition Education and How to Teach Them: Grades K-6 (Los Angeles: Dairy Council of California, 1970).

Bourne, Lyle E., Jr. *Human Conceptual Behavior* (Boston: Allyn and Bacon, 1966).

Brookbeck, May. "Logic and Scientific Method in Teaching," in *Handbook of Research on Teaching,* ed. N. L. Gage. (Chicago: Rand McNally, 1965), 44-93.

Concepts and Generalizations: Their Place in High School Home Economics Curriculum Development (Washington, D.C.: American Home Economics Association, 1970).

Framework for Health Instruction in California Public Schools (Sacramento: California State Department of Education, 1970).

Gage, N. L. *Handbook of Research on Teaching* (Chicago: Rand McNally, 1965) 48-72, 884-887.

Health Concepts: Guides for Health Instruction (Washington, D.C.: American Association for Health, Physical Education and Recreation, 1967).

Inhelder, Barbel, and Jean Piaget. *The Growth of Logical Thinking* (New York: Basic Books, 1959).

Klausmeier, Herbert J., and Chester W. Harris, eds. *Analyses of Concept Learning* (New York: Academic Press, 1966).

Komisar, Paul B., and C. J. B. MacMillan. *Psychological Concepts in Education* (Chicago: Rand McNally, 1967).

Perry, C.L. "A Conceptual Approach to School-Based Health Promotion," *Journal of School Health* (1984):54(6).

Phenix, Philip H. *Realms of Meaning* (New York: McGraw-Hill, 1964).

Phillips, John L., Jr. *The Origins of Intellect: Piaget's Theory* (San Francisco: Freeman, 1969).

Pulaski, Mary, and Spencer Pulaski. *Understanding Piaget* (New York: Harper & Row, 1971).

School Health Education Study. *Health Education: A Conceptual Approach to Curriculum Design* (St. Paul, Minn.: 3M Education Press, 1967):6.

Selberg, Edith M., Louise A. Neal, and Mathew F. Vessel. *Discovering Science in the Elementary School* (Reading, Mass.: Addison-Wesley, 1970).

Woodruff, Asahel D. *The Psychology of Teaching* (New York: Longmans, Green, 1951):69, 84.

———. "The Use of Concepts in Teaching and Learning," *Journal of Teacher Education* (March 1964):81-89.

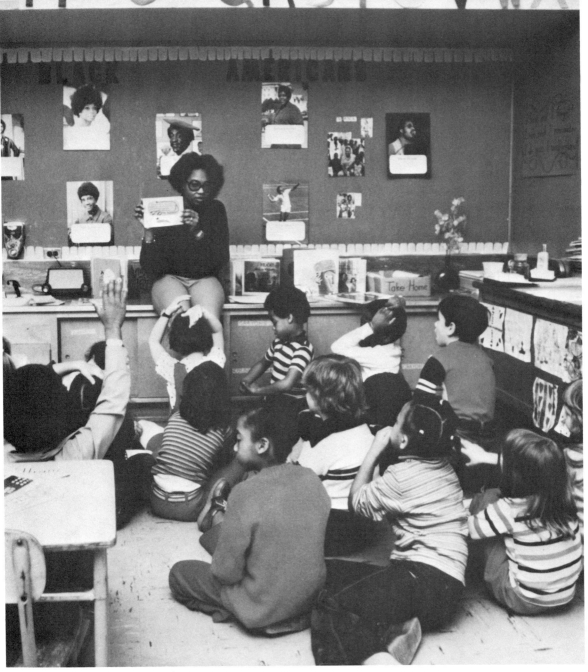

Chapter 9

Stating Behavioral Objectives

INTRODUCTION

Behavioral objectives describe what students will be able to do after completing a prescribed unit of instruction (Kibler, 1970). Other terms used for behavioral objectives are objectives, outcomes, goals, competencies. In this text, the term will be *expected student outcomes*.

In essence, expected student outcomes further the instructional process once concepts have been developed. Like concepts, they provide direction to both the instructor and the student in terms of what should be taught, how it should be taught, and whether or not that which is taught is learned.

Properly stated behavioral objectives are not only useful but also essential to high-quality health education. Failure to prepare behavioral objectives leaves the instructor and the student with no direction in terms of lesson design, goals, and evaluation procedures. On the other hand, properly stated outcomes serve to communicate the goals of the lesson to all interested parties. They identify the specific content to be covered, the expected changes in student behavior, and the form of evaluation necessary to ensure accountability.

LEVELS OF SPECIFICITY

Instructional objectives can be written in degrees of specificity. They can be very general ("to promote healthful behavior"), or they can be highly specific ("in a half-hour essay examination at the end of the unit, the student will describe the physical effects in the body from the time tobacco smoke is first inhaled into the respiratory system. The student's response must be complete and sequential and correspond with the description found in the textbook.") Most objec-

<hr>

The material in this chapter is adapted from Walter D. Sorochan and Stephen J. Bender, *Teaching Secondary Health Science*, New York: Wiley, 1978.

FIGURE 9.1
Continuum of objectives.

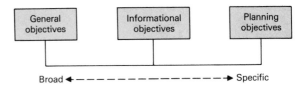

tives fall between these extremes, for example, "The student will be able to describe in sequence the physiological effects of inhaling tobacco smoke."

Kibler (1970) defines these categories of objectives as general, informational, and planning. Figure 9.1 depicts the three different types of objectives on the continuum. Some objectives do not fit neatly into any of the three categories. However, to simplify, we have elected to focus on informational and planning instructional objectives in this text.

VALUE OF PLANNING AND INFORMATIONAL OBJECTIVES

Planning objectives, which are very specific, are for the planning and evaluating of instruction. They are teacher-oriented objectives, most helpful for guiding the curricular process. Kibler (1970) perceives teachers and instruction designers benefiting in several ways from defining planning objectives:

1. *Given clearly defined goals to work toward, teachers can design instructional experiences to achieve them and can evaluate the effectiveness of such experiences according to whether the goals are achieved.*
2. *Students can be examined prior to beginning instruction to determine whether they have already mastered any of the objectives.*

Information regarding their preparedness for the instruction to follow can also be obtained.

3. *Each student can be evaluated on mastery of the unit's objectives. In this way every student can be required to master all objectives. This is in contrast to grading students on how well they performed in comparison with the rest of the class (grading on the curve) or in achievement of a certain percentage of the objectives of the unit.*

Informational objectives, by contrast, are designed to inform others of what the teacher hopes to accomplish in a given lesson. Informational objectives are more or less abbreviations of planning objectives, developed by the teacher after the planning objectives have been established. Kibler (1970) perceives students, curriculum planners, student advisers, teachers, and administrators as benefiting in the following ways from the use of informational objectives:

1. *Research indicates that students can be more efficient learners if they are provided with objectives. Perhaps one of the reasons students do better when given copies of the objectives of a unit of instruction is that they are spared the frustrations and time-consuming effort of trying to guess what the teacher expects of them.*
2. *Given such clearly specified objectives, curriculum planners are better able to arrange sequences of courses or units of instruction. Knowing what students (hopefully, all students) are able to do at the end of courses and what students are able to do at the beginning of courses (prerequisites), it should be possible to eliminate unnecessary overlap of courses and to identify and fill in gaps between courses.*
3. *Students and their advisers are able to plan their course programs better when they can read course descriptions which include informational objectives.*

4. *Through clear behavioral objectives, teachers are able to tell other teachers what they teach. Stating that "students learn to name each state and its capital in the United States" tells considerably more than stating "United States geography is taught."*
5. *Teachers and administrators can determine the level of objectives students will be able to achieve in terms of the three taxonomic classifications to be discussed in Chapter III [Kibler, 1970]. For example, in the cognitive domain, objectives can be classified as knowledge, comprehension, application, analysis, synthesis, and evaluation, thereby avoiding undue emphasis on a certain level of objectives.*

STATING EXPECTED STUDENT OUTCOMES

For the purposes of this text, we will focus on the developmental procedures surrounding planning and informational objectives.

Planning Objectives

As previously stated, planning objectives are most helpful to teachers in preparing a lesson. They are more precise and include more specific details than do informational objectives. Recall that the example of a planning objective describes quite specifically the *behavior* (the student will be able to *describe*) the student will be expected to exhibit to be deemed competent with reference to the objective. In addition, the *content* or result of the student's behavior *(physiological effects in the body from the time tobacco smoke is first inhaled into the respiratory system)*, plus the *conditions* under which the behavior is to be performed *(half-hour written essay examination at the end of the unit)*, and the *standard* to be used in determining whether or not the performance is satisfactory *(the student's response must be complete and sequential and correspond with the description found in the textbook)* must all be included for the objective to be termed a planning objective.

In an effort to simplify the foregoing analysis of the component parts of a planning objective, the following list of elements is provided (Kibler, 1970):

1. *WHO is expected to perform the required behavior. For our purposes this will almost always be "the student," "learner," "pupils," etc.*
2. *The BEHAVIOR to be exhibited by the student to demonstrate his competency. Verbs like "write," "speak," "demonstrate," etc., describe this component. There is a need to use sound action verbs for clarity's sake.*
3. *The CONTENT or result of the student's behavior which will be evaluated to determine the student's level of competency. With cognitive oriented planning objectives, it is merely what the student will be able to discuss, define, identify, etc.*
4. *The CONDITIONS under which the student is expected to perform the behavior. Examples might be a "one-hour examination," "in front of class," etc.*
5. *The STANDARDS which will be employed to determine whether or not the student is minimally competent. Statements such as, "Ninety percent" or "three out of five satisfactory responses," are indicative.*

Now let us view another planning objective that exhibits all of the elements described above: "In a 15-minute quiz the day following instruction, the student will be able to describe the physiological process by which an individual becomes intoxicated due to alcohol abuse. The student's answer must be in complete agreement with the lecture outline presented in class." Note that all of the listed elements are present:

1. *Who*—"the student."
2. *Behavior*—"to describe."

3. *Content*—"physiological process by which an individual becomes intoxicated due to alcohol abuse."
4. *Conditions*—"15-minute quiz the day following instruction."
5. *Standard*—"the student's answer must be in complete agreement with the lecture outline presented in class."

Informational Objectives

Whereas planning objectives guide the instructor in the instructional process, informational objectives are designed to convey instructional intent to others. The informational objective is less specific than the planning objective, but by no means is it less important.

It is sound educational practice to provide students with a copy of the informational objectives for each lesson. It will help them become more efficient learners by providing directions to their learning activities. It also helps the student to understand better his or her own competency level once the unit of instruction is complete and the evaluation procedures have been implemented.

In that informational objectives are abbreviations of planning objectives, it is wise to develop informational objectives after the planning objectives have been established. This means that the informational objective contains all of the elements of a planning objective except the conditions and standards, for example, "The student will be able to describe the physiological process by which an individual becomes intoxicated due to alcohol abuse." Note that the conditions ("in a 15-minute quiz the day following instruction") and standard ("the student's answer must be in complete agreement with the lecture outline presented in class") have been omitted. However, other teachers, administrators, and students are still well informed as to what is to be taught in a given class and what the students are expected to grasp.

In conclusion, the three key elements of an

informational objective are the who, the desired observable behavior, and the content, or result the student is expected to produce. The greater the clarity of these elements, the greater the probability that the objective will clearly communicate to the recipient what he or she is to learn.

A WORD ABOUT PRECISENESS

It is always good practice to make planning and informational objectives as precise as possible. For example, "the student realizes that immunization is one way of controlling communicable disease" and "the student knows about communicable disease" both possess the essential elements (who, behavior, content) of objectives, but they are far too vague. In the first objective, the term "realizes" has many interpretations. What evidence would be required to determine if the pupil does indeed "realize"? In the second objective, both behavior ("knows") and the content ("communicable diseases") are too broad. Does "knows" mean simple recall, being able to tell in one's own words, or explaining relationships? The words "communicable disease" could conceivably mean anything from a single communicable disease to a complete understanding of the infectious-disease cycle.

Imprecise terms such as "understand," "know," and "realize" are open to broad interpretation. In the construction of objectives they serve only to contribute to ambiguity and confusion. It is much more advantageous to employ terms that better describe or define the behaviors sought. The use of more precise terms strengthens the educational process by providing better direction to both the student and the teacher. The student will know better what is expected of him or her, the teacher will be better able to provide learning opportunities that will enable the student to attain the objective, and there will be a better opportunity for more precise evaluation. The following list (Fodor and Davis, 1981) provides a contrast between behavioral terms that are vague and open to many interpretations and those that are more precise in describing behavior:

Less precise terms — many interpretations	*More precise terms — few interpretations*	
Know	*Define*	*Interpret*
Realize	*Distinguish*	*Describe*
Enjoy	*Recall*	*Name*
Believe	*Recognize*	*Construct*
Understand	*Demonstrate*	*Compare*
Appreciate	*Apply*	*Translate*
Value	*Organize*	*State*
Comprehend	*Discuss*	*Illustrate*
Desire	*Identify*	*Summarize*
Feel	*List*	*Classify*
Respect	*Diagram*	*Select*
	Acquire	*Order*

CLASSIFYING BEHAVIORAL OBJECTIVES

We have established that behavioral objectives should be stated in terms of changes in student behavior—thinking, feeling, and doing. By using such terms, we can begin to determine the classes of behavior reflected in the objectives we prepare. Classification can be helpful because it can:

1. Assist with avoiding overconcentration in any one area when formulating instructional objectives
2. Provide insight into the appropriate instruments for evaluation

For instructional purposes, objectives can be classified into one or more of the following domains:

1. *Cognitive:* range from recall or recognition of knowledge to the development of intellectual skills and abilities

2. *Affective:* emphasize a feeling, an emotion, or a degree of acceptance or rejection. Objectives in this domain are often vaguely described as appreciation, attitude, interest, or value and are difficult to measure.
3. *Action:* emphasize some muscular or motor skill, manipulation of material and object, or act that requires neuromuscular coordination.

It is possible to classify behavioral objectives into progressive labels of development. Bloom (1956) and Krathwohl (1964) conducted a systematic survey of the educational objectives in the cognitive and affective domains and prepared taxonomies for the two classes of behavior. To date, there has not been any effort to develop a taxonomy for the psychomotor domain.

Bloom's three domains provide an analysis of 16 terms that may be used in more closely described behavior. Note the progressive levels of development for each domain:

1. Cognitive domain (intellectual processes of the learner)
   a) Low level
      (1) Knowledge—recognition and recall of information, terms, classes, procedures, theories, structures
      (2) Comprehension—interpretation of what has been learned
   b) High level
      (1) Application—use of knowledge in *new* situations
      (2) Analysis—breaking whole units into related parts (deduction)
      (3) Synthesis—combining elements into new wholes (induction)
      (4) Evaluation—judging materials and methods, using standards of criteria
2. Affective domain (emphasis on emotional processes, e.g., feelings, interests, values, and adjustments)
   a) Low level
      (1) Receiving—passive attention to stimuli (sensory inputs)
      (2) Responding—reacting to stimuli (complying, volunteering, and so forth)
   b) High level
      (1) Valuing—actions consistent with a belief or value
      (2) Organization—commitment to a set of values (discussion, formulating values)
      (3) Characterization—all behavior conforming to internalized values (philosophy)
3. Action domain (emphasis on motor behavior involving neuromuscular coordination)
   a) Low level
      (1) Perception—sensitivity to stimulus normally leading to action (cue sensing and so on)
      (2) Preparation—involves readiness to perform (possesses knowledge, bodily stance, willingness)
      (3) Orientation—knowing and/or deciding an appropriate response to be made
   b) High level
      (1) Pattern—a learned response that is habitual, smooth, and confident (a skill pattern or low error response)
      (2) Performance—response that is a complex motor action involving a high degree of skill (polished behavior, complicated responses made with ease and control)

REFERENCES AND BIBLIOGRAPHY

Bloom, B. S., *et al.*, ed. *Taxonomy of Educational Objectives: Domain* (New York: David McKay, 1956).

Fodor, John T., and Gus T. Davis. *Health Instruction: Theory and Application* (Philadelphia: Lea and Febiger, 1981).

Gronhund, Norman E. *Stating Behavioral Objectives for Classroom Instruction* (New York: Macmillan, 1970).

Kibler, Robert J., *et al. Behavioral Objectives and Instruction* (Boston: Allyn and Bacon, 1970):20, 22, 23, 33.

Krathwohl, D. R., *et al. Taxonomy of Educational Objectives: Affective Domain* (New York: David McKay, 1964).

Mager, R. F. *Preparing Instructional Objectives* (San Francisco: Fearon, 1962).

Sorochan, Walter D., and Stephen J. Bender. *Teaching Secondary Health Science* (New York: Wiley, 1978).

Woodruff, Asahel D. *The Psychology of Teaching* (New York: Longmans, Green, 1951):69.

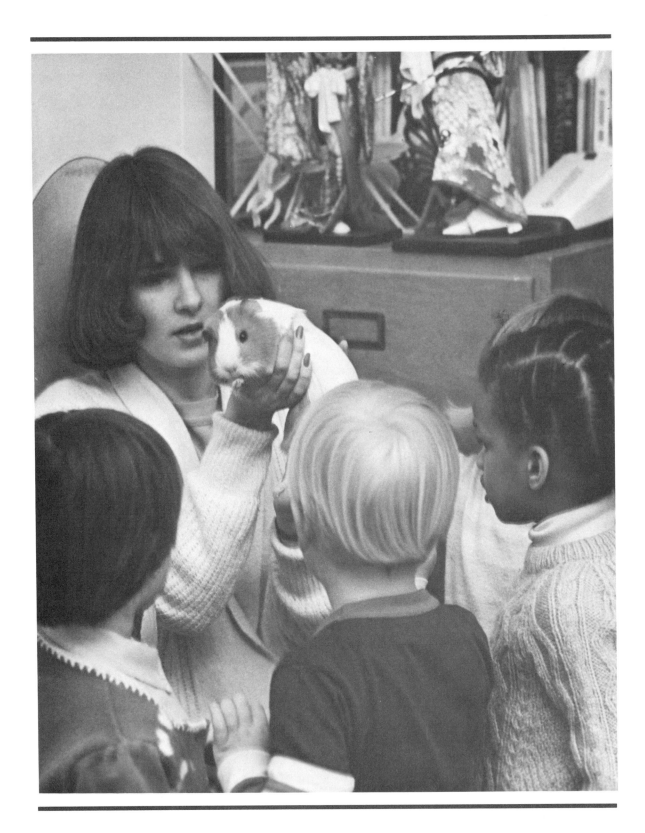

Chapter 10

Appropriate Elementary Health Learning Experiences

INTRODUCTION

To see
To hear
To touch
To feel
To wonder?
  To do
  To discover
  To understand
  To learn. . . .
    To be
    To feel good
    To be well
    To live
    To be happy!

This poem suggests the nature and purpose of this chapter. The first part of the poem has to do with the natural ability of children to learn and the body senses children use to receive messages from the teacher. The middle part of the poem suggests how the message (information) is internalized through learning experiences. What does the latter part suggest? All three are involved in the learning process.

Teaching is both a science and an art. Teachers apply science in selecting relevant content, materials, and methods and in projecting expected behavioral objectives. The effective blending of these into an educational recipe to ensure continuing progress of children toward optimal well-being and more abundant living is an art. This chapter provides suggestions on how elementary school teachers may develop greater skill in the art of teaching for health. The value of suggested methods depends on the way they are used. Methods should motivate children to discover understandings and feelings and to evolve their own concepts. Some methods work better than others, but methods alone are not enough. The message they pass along needs to be reinforced by materials and visual aids. Thus the medium of the method is enriched by the materials and becomes a message. The teacher blends methods and materials so that children may internalize the message. Out of such learn-ing experiences should emerge constructive sociohygienic behavior.

The first part of this chapter explores the nature of methods and how methods may be used. The second part explores methods relevant to elementary health science instruction. Teaching aids and materials and their relationship to methods are discussed in the final section. The chapter content is summarized in Figure 10.1.

Examples of the methods are not included in this chapter. Instead, numerous examples of how methods and materials may be used are included in later chapters dealing with lesson plans.

DEFINITION

There was a time when teaching was accepted as the act of delivering priceless pearls of wisdom to a captive audience of learners. It was also assumed that the mere telling of things to be learned fulfilled the obligation of the teacher. Today this misconception of teaching is seldom found among elementary school teachers. The emphasis in teaching for health today is on behavior rather than on the imparting of facts and information.

Teaching has been recognized as a process of stimulating and directing learning. Although teaching and learning take place at the same time, learning is what happens to the pupils, whereas teaching is what the teacher does. Rash (1965) defines health teaching as fostering an environment favorable to learning. The word "method" is defined in *Webster's New Collegiate Dictionary* as "orderly procedure or process . . . orderly arrangement." Obviously this is not adequate for the teaching context, where it not only covers strategy and tactics of teaching, but also involves what is to be taught at any given time, identification of the expected pupil outcomes, the means by which content is to be taught, the order in which the content is to be taught, and evaluative procedures. All of these aspects of the teaching act should be considered

FIGURE 10.1
Conceptualization of this chapter.

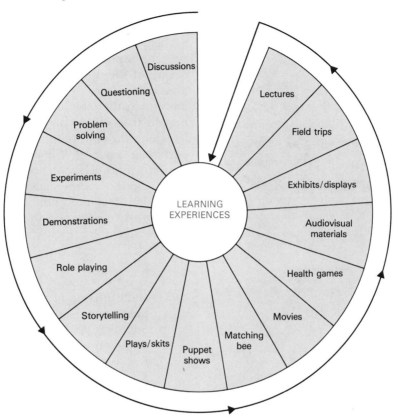

when selecting or using a method. The term "method" covers the how of teaching. In this chapter we are most concerned with that phase of the teaching act that the teacher chooses and uses in designing teaching/learning strategies. The teacher reaches into his or her "bag of tools" for the most appropriate technique or activity to help children to discover for themselves the concept, feeling, or habit. Such learning experiences include role playing, plays, demonstrations, experiments, and discussions. Activities of this nature may be referred to as strategies. The teacher manipulates the classroom activity so as to help each child have a specific experience which allows the child to progress toward or achieve proficiency in specific behavioral or sociohygienic skills or tasks.

Beginning teachers are often mesmerized by teaching strategies. We have found that prospective teachers are more concerned about how to teach than about what or where to teach. This is a good example of putting the cart before the horse. Before the horse is harnessed to the cart, we must have a load for it to pull, and we must also know where the barn is. The analogy between this illustration and teaching is illustrated in Figure 10.2. The load of hay may be thought of as the subject matter to be taught, the horse as the vehicle or technique of moving the hay, and the barn as expected pupil outcomes. Methods are like the horse; they help the teacher to communicate the information to the pupils. All three—what, how, and where—are interrelated aspects of the teaching/learning process.

FIGURE 10.2
Conceptualization of the relationships among content, method, and expected pupil outcomes. Which should be considered first in teaching for optimal well-being? Method is simply a way of communicating the ideas and information from teacher to pupil.

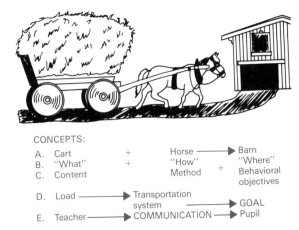

CONCEPTS:

A. Cart   +   Horse ⟶ Barn
B. "What" +   "How"   "Where"
C. Content   Method + Behavioral objectives

D. Load ⟶ Transportation system ⟶ GOAL

E. Teacher ⟶ COMMUNICATION ⟶ Pupil

NATURE OF METHOD

Although method consists of many elements, it is more than a collection of tricks, artifices, and ruses; it is a pattern of knowledge, purpose, skill, respect for others, and the basic means of communication. The core of content—the facts and knowledge—must be presented to the pupils so that they can assimilate, relate to, and internalize the material.

Communication requires sharing and participating. The teacher, as a speaker, only starts the process; the student, as a hearer, must complete it. The teacher has information, an idea, an attitude, a feeling, or an undertaking to share with the pupils. The process of transmitting these elements and receiving responses constitutes communication, which may be verbal, nonverbal, or both. The teacher should continually adapt the teaching method on the basis of feedback from the pupils.

Selecting the best way to communicate with children is most important. Perhaps the first thing the teacher should be aware of is how children receive information. Weaver and Cenci (1960) point out that we learn through our senses. Table 10.1 summarizes the importance of body senses in learning. Most health and living experiences are sociological in nature, so the reactions of others play a significant role in how we behave hygienically.

The implications for teaching are many. The nature of the topic and the behavior expected may call on one of the lesser-rated senses far more than the table indicates. This may be especially true where children are unable to read. Teaching through the senses becomes very important at this level. When peer-group pressure to conform in behavior becomes important, especially in the intermediate grades, the sense of feeling becomes important. Educators in general have failed to recognize the potentiality of this sensory area. The teacher must be always conscious to:

1. Use those senses most important to the child in relation to the specific lesson at hand
2. Stimulate senses as often as possible for retention of learning
3. Use as many senses as possible

We have all heard a sentence or word that recalled a song; a phrase that made us recall a poem; a familiar scene, an event; an exercise, our good physical feeling; a smell, a process; a

TABLE 10.1
Importance of body senses to learning.

Sense	Importance (in education) (Victor, 1970, p. 6)	Estimated importance in health science instruction
1. Sight	75%	52%
2. Hearing	13	13
3. Touch	6	6
4. Smell	3	3
5. Taste	3	3
6. Balance	—	3
7. Kinesthetic	—	—
8. Feeling (emotions)	—	20

touch, a material; a social occasion, a wonderful feeling of belonging and happiness; or a taste, a good or a poor product. Stimulating a special sense or more than one sense gives the student an additional dimension to learning and recalling. Senses are the receivers of communication.

The goal of all methodology is to facilitate communication so that children internalize the information presented.

FACTORS AFFECTING METHODOLOGY

There is no one best way to teach effectively. "One man's meat is another's poison." However, some approaches may be more appropriate than others. There are many variables affecting the selection and use of methods (Broudy and Palmer, 1965; Gage, 1965; Phenix, 1964; Veneker, 1964). These include:

1. Teacher behavior such as personality, dress, deportment, mannerisms, use of voice and diction, movement and tics, mastery of subject matter, communicative skill, exemplar model, and so on
2. Pupil receptivity and motivational behavior (closed or open mind, desire to learn)
3. Media of teaching (methods, materials, instruments, audio-visual aids)
4. Socioemotional environment of the classroom and school
5. Sociocultural traditions and influences of community (the tendency to teach as we were taught)
6. Pupil maturity (physical, emotional, social, intellectual)
7. Expected pupil outcomes (teacher objectives) for the lesson
8. Content or subject matter

All of these variables affect the learning process. Much research has been conducted to provide evidence that one method is superior to another. Because early researchers overlooked these variables in their research designs or ignored controlling them during the research, the conclusions they reached were biased and inconclusive. Gage, in his *Handbook of Research on Teaching* (1965), reviewed research on teaching methodology up to 1964. His conclusions are noteworthy:

1. Methods of teaching reflect teacher effectiveness and consistency in communicating and affecting students.
2. Until 1950, most research attempted to discuss and describe patterns of teachers' behavior or roles. Considerable research was conducted from 1950 to 1964 on the effectiveness of various teaching methods. For example, is the lecture method better than the discussion or TV? Reviewers have found that these studies were weak in design; did not specify, and hence did not control, variables; and did not specify teachers' roles or behavior. Hence the conclusion about research on effectiveness of teaching up to 1964 was that different teaching procedures produced little or no difference in the amount of knowledge gained by students. There is little evidence to favor one method over another.
3. Effectiveness of teaching method and teaching aid depends on the specific instructional objectives or pupil outcomes. There is a need to base methods on goals. Any procedure that achieves the goals is a good one.
4. There is a need to base teaching methods and their use on a learning model stemming from psychological research and developmental task theory.
5. Teaching methods emphasize certain principles and neglect others.
6. There is a great need to design teaching methods that make as much use as possible of a wide range of learning principles.
7. Effective use of teaching methods and the success of those methods are dependent on the teacher's (a) personality; (b) motivation and interest in the subject; (c) interest in pupils; (d) mastery of subject matter; (e) behavior or perception of his

or her role as a teacher; (f) aspirations for ideal teaching; (g) acquaintance with various methods of teaching; and (h) understanding of pupil's developmental tasks and learning processes.

There have been many studies on teaching methodology since 1964. Most of these have been unable to incorporate Gage's recommendations for controlling the variables. The general conclusions of Gage and his reviewers are still valid today. Thus selecting and using appropriate learning experience is an art—a prescriptive judgmental phase of teaching much like the physician's approach to selecting and prescribing a course of treatment for a patient.

APPLICATION OF METHODS

Learning experiences are the means by which children learn both the content and the process of health science. Children acquire understanding, attitudes, and habits that help them to attain, maintain, and conserve their well-being at an optimal level and to live more abundantly. The teacher should use a wide variety of learning experiences to help children realize these goals.

Many teachers use more learning activities than are necessary. This tends to prolong the unit unnecessarily, slow down learning, and dull pupils' interest. The experienced teacher employs learning activities wisely and economically, realizing that sometimes one activity is enough. Occasionally one good activity will provide an understanding of more than one concept. Other times, when a concept is difficult or abstract, more than one activity may be necessary. Slow learners usually learn better when more than one activity is used.

The grade level may also influence the number of learning experiences needed. In the lower grades, the children's attention span is short, and their ability to think abstractly is not well developed; therefore, more than one activity is often necessary to obtain satisfactory understanding. The teaching strategy may have to be repeated several times, or another strategy may have to be introduced. However, in the upper grades one well-chosen activity is usually sufficient. In all cases the best procedure is for the teacher to use as many—but *only* as many—activities as are necessary to ensure satisfactory learning. Teachers should choose and modify methods in light of specific situations. In practice, no method can or should remain static; all of them yield to the purposes and procedures of particular classes. Method is a process, not a predetermined formula. The effective teacher does not select a method, but instead develops a flexible procedure that is applicable to a particular situation. Effective teaching and learning do not come as a result of merely using the visual method, or a field trip, or a discussion. Progress in social learning is the result of the blending of the elements that constitute growth and development. Chapter 2 set the stage for making the elementary teacher sensitive to developmental concepts and learning principles. Chapter 8 suggests that certain methods or learning experiences help children to internalize facts and evolve desirable sociohygienic habits. Chapter 9 suggests the need for the teacher to be concerned about selecting learning experiences that help pupils to attain expected outcomes (behavioral objectives in a lesson plan). Prospective teachers would do well to review these chapters before reading the remainder of this chapter. They should reflect on the major concepts of these earlier chapters when selecting and using learning experiences.

LEARNING EXPERIENCES FOR HEALTH INSTRUCTION

Because of the nature of elementary school children, the subject matter with which they deal, and the educational goals established for them, some learning experiences are more appropriate than others. Appropriate experiences for primary children include storytelling, puppet shows, skits and plays, simulation or acting out, demonstrations, problem solving, and discussions. Others include exhibits and displays, health fairs, field trips, surveys, guest speakers, debates, panels, lectures, programmed instruction, and contract teaching. Learning experiences at the intermediate level may include all of the primary experiences, as well as cardboard games, experiments, role playing, computer-assisted health education, and matching bees.

The learning experiences to be discussed are appropriate for elementary school children. Because they have great potential for helping children to discover concepts and to apply them to everyday living, they will be explored in some depth.

The following criteria can be used to determine whether a particular learning experience is appropriate:

1. Does the learning experience contribute to pupils' attaining the *expected behavioral objectives* or *outcomes?*

2. Does it help children to evolve and discover the *topic concept?* (This discovery occurs only through the learning experience!)

3. Is it *action-oriented* instead of listening-oriented? That is, learning experiences that contribute to developing affective behaviors should take precedence over those focusing primarily on cognitive behaviors. Likewise, learning experiences that evolve or modify health habits and behavior should take precedence over those that focus on cognitive and/or affective behavior.

4. Does it *teach through two or more sense organs?* A learning experience that communicates through two or more body sense organs—eyes, ears, nose (smell), tongue (taste), skin (touch), glands (emotions), muscles (neuromuscular)—is more effective, clearer, and more enduring than one that communicates through just one sensory organ. The information picked up by one sense organ should be reinforced by another. Thus the ears are complemented by the eyes. If a third sensory organ is added, the effect on the student is stronger and more enduring. More important, it helps the student more readily discover the health concept. Keep in mind that the only way a person can receive information is through the

sense organs. The more sense organs involved in recording and decoding the information, the more meaningful the information.

5. Is it economical in terms of time and cost (the materials and visual aids)?

6. Is it appropriate for the subject matter as well as for the expected pupil outcome?

Discussion and Questioning

These two approaches to effective learning take place in all classrooms. Both are used as follow-up to other learning experiences. Questioning the students as a means of treating the topic at hand is the teacher's chief means of directing discourse. The students question the teacher and one another about the topic. Questions prompt thinking about specific subjects. In a discussion topics are formulated as questions because a question sets the mind working. According to research, questions constitute about one third of a classroom discourse, and teachers ask about 86 percent of the questions (Hyman, 1970). Because questioning is essential in the classroom, special attention is given to it here.

A discussion involves the verbal interaction of a number of individuals who perceive one another as participants in a common activity. It is designed to use cooperative participation toward the resolution of a particular problem or question. Discussion usually requires some degree of moderation to guide group thinking. It provides children with an opportunity to review facts and to synthesize them into generalizations with practical applications to health problems.

A good classroom discussion requires (1) an emotionally favorable classroom environment that permits students the appropriate freedom of expression, and (2) participants with sufficient information to discuss the topic sensibly. The first condition results from the teacher's general spirit or attitude. He or she should avoid ridicule and generally regard any sincere response as a useful contribution to the discussion. The second condition, adequate knowledge, is important to avoid the rambling and unproductive "pooling of ignorance." Therefore, discussions are usually more successful after the students have done some reading or viewed a film, a puppet show, skit, role play, demonstration, or experiment.

Discussion usually centers on the teacher— with the teacher directing the questioning. Often the teacher may want more participation from the pupils and can get this from small-group discussions, or *buzz sessions*. Three to five children may be organized into a group. A leader and a recorder may be appointed. The theme or goal of the group is written down. After 10 to 20 minutes of buzzing—researching for ideas, sharing feelings, suggesting alternative solutions, and so on—the recorder from each group should make a brief oral report. The teacher, as mediator, should entertain questions from the class, allow the pupils to answer, and in the end summarize the discussion. Buzz sessions sensitize students to the feelings of their peers as well as to health issues.

Questioning facilitates a good discussion. Questions should lead students to think, to reason, to clarify, and to classify information. Questions may also be asked in order to:

1. *Get a particular student to participate.*
2. *Check on the student's comprehension.*
3. *Attract a student's attention.*
4. *Test a student's knowledge of the topic.*
5. *Diagnose a student's weaknesses.*
6. *Break the ice and get a discussion going.*
7. *Allow a student to shine before his classmates.*
8. *Establish an explanation for a problem.*
9. *Review work for yesterday's absentees.*
10. *Build up a student's security when the teacher is quite sure the student will respond correctly.*
11. *Learn about a student's personal activities (which affect his classroom performance).*
12. *Attack issue A rather than B.* (Hyman, 1974)

In order to use questions to direct discussion, the teacher must phrase the questions appropriately to the context of the discourse and the level of the students. The teacher's role as a discussion leader is to facilitate participation. He or she does more than ask questions. The teacher

summarizes and sharpens the responses and reactions by rephrasing them. He or she plays "traffic cop," acknowledging students who wish to speak and requesting others to comment on previous remarks.

The teacher should not expect correct answers to all of the questions. To act as mediator, the teacher should formulate key questions in advance and include them as part of the lesson planning. Written questions will serve as a guide. However, the teacher needs to be responsive to the spontaneity of the classroom discussion.

Perhaps the greatest task facing the teacher in questioning is to encourage the students to question both the teacher and one another. Students' questions should arise from a desire to understand both the topic at hand and the position taken by the other participants.

Problem Solving

Exercises in problem solving have great relevance to everyday living. They can help children to develop their thinking, creative expression, critical analysis, and reasoning. Perhaps the greatest appeal of problem solving lies in helping children to learn how to cope with their day-to-day problems. Problem solving, like discussion and questioning, has the potential of permeating all learning experiences. Its format and nature change with the topic, the students, and the learning experience.

Problems occur when children are unable to find personal, socially acceptable, and worthwhile solutions to sociohygienic situations. Problems, small and big, arise every day, and meeting them head on and resolving them contributes to successful living. Problem solving provides an opportunity for children to apply what they learn in the classroom to the solution of everyday problems. It helps to counter wasteful trial-and-error approaches to solving problems and to avoid the feeling of failure in living.

The process of problem solving is a natural one. The teacher and pupils identify real or hypothetical problems and proceed to solve them. There are two basic ways to use this technique. In the first, the problem may be posed in paper-

and-pencil form, with suggested alternatives, or pupils may be asked to supply the alternatives. They select the best or most appropriate alternative and justify their choice. A discussion may be useful as a follow-up to help children understand why one answer is better than another. The immediate and long-range consequences of each alternative should be brought out during the follow-up. In the other approach to problem solving, children identify a sociohygienic problem in the community as a field project and then proceed to solve it. The procedure is the same, except that the latter is a long-lasting field experience, whereas the former is theoretical in nature and short in duration. Both approaches should be used.

Children may solve problems by working individually or in teams. If a health problem has social overtones, the peer-group process will be more effective not only in solving the problem, but also in demonstrating to the students that the problem exists.

The steps of problem solving may be identified as follows:

1. Recognize the problem.
2. Gather information about the problem.
3. Apply facts to analyze the problem.
4. List trial solutions or alternatives.
5. Apply personal and social values to the alternatives and indicate immediate and long-range consequences for each of the alternatives.
6. Select the best alternative as a solution to the problem.
7. Try out the alternative. If it fails to work, select another alternative.

Almost all problems of living may be solved by following the steps suggested above. The only way children will be able to solve problems is by applying the guidelines.

Experiments

Experiments are procedures undertaken to discover suspected truths or to prove or disprove a specific point. Experimentation generally attempts to demonstrate how things are done, how they work, or what the truth is by employing precise controls so as to validate results. The purpose of an experiment is to illustrate the content or concept under consideration. Experiments can help children to internalize, investigate health phenomena, and weigh and sift evidence. This process enables them to evolve their own concepts.

The following steps are helpful in conducting experiments:

1. Define the problem to be solved.
2. Select methods or procedure to be used.
3. Identify and assemble necessary materials and apparatus needed.
4. Conduct the experiment.
5. Collect and record data.
6. Select, organize, and interpret data.
7. Prepare conclusions.
8. Discuss the outcomes of the experiment and what was learned. Identify key concepts and relate to everyday living.

Experiments may be demonstrated by the teacher or a pupil or conducted individually by each pupil. They are an excellent way of arousing interest in a health topic and solving problems. Along with demonstrations, experiments provide an excellent opportunity to help the slow learner while challenging the rapid learner. The elementary school teacher should continually involve the children when doing the experiments. However, if the procedure involves a hazard or a risk of accident, the teacher should perform the experiment or avoid it altogether. The wise teacher keeps the experiment simple and stimulating enough to encourage children to think, uses it to help children answer a question or understand an idea.

Demonstrations

A demonstration, similar to an experiment, illustrates what is already known, whereas an experiment is a way of finding a fact. A demonstration is a process of graphic explanation of a selected idea, fact, relationship, or phenomenon.

Demonstration provides a visual explanation. Children like to be entertained; they like to see things done before their eyes, especially if there is an element of the mysterious. The teacher who describes some body function through skillful demonstration encourages the class to want to do it themselves. Demonstrations may be conducted by the teacher, the pupil, or the group. Any demonstration requires planning to be effective.

Sociodramas

Children like to play. They like to pretend, to imagine, and to imitate others. It is part of growing up socially. To the child, play is real. Through it learning takes place, and life takes on social meaning. By use of sociodrama and simulation games, children learn about living. Children play house, school, doctor and nurse, cowboys and Indians, cops and robbers, and other life roles. Pretending at play is part of being young. Pretending is an interesting learning experience—trying out various real or fantasy characters. By pretending to be a firefighter, the child sees or dreams about what it is like to be a firefighter. Dramatic play of this sort may be used by elementary school teachers to gain insight about their pupils and to help the children discover the art of living for themselves. Sociodramas having a natural appeal to children are simulation, let's pretend, role playing, puppets, plays and skits, storytelling, and health games.

Most sociodramas may be used effectively through the following procedures:

1. *Selecting the situation.* The situation should be a fairly simple one, involving one main idea or issue. It should also involve personalities. The issues should be those that arise because people have different desires, beliefs, hopes, and aspirations or ones that arise from the inability of people to understand the point of view of others.
2. *Choosing participants.* When first trying out role playing, the teacher should select students who are fairly well informed about the issue to be presented and who are imaginative, articulate, and self-assured. After the students have become familiar with the technique, the teacher should ask for volunteers.
3. *Preparing the audience.* Just before the sociodrama, the teacher should direct the class to observe for certain feelings, behaviors, and events.
4. *Acting out the situation.* The teacher should allow children to be as actively involved as possible. As a cross between director and audience, the teacher should, when necessary, remind the students of their role in the sociodrama and then withdraw into the audience. The sociodrama should be challenging, mentally stimulating, and fun for everyone.
5. *Following up.* A good sociodrama will generate interest and arouse comments and questions. Follow-up has to do with effective completion of the learning process. The valuable concepts conveyed through sociodramas need to be nailed down by means of reviews, discussions, and question-and-answer sessions. This kind of follow-up is a part of all good learning experiences.

The teacher should express pleasure at how well the players performed. He or she should have thought out a series of questions to guide the ensuing discussion. An attempt should be made to identify main ideas and emotional reactions and to stimulate class involvement through questions, comments, and observations. At the end, the key points should be summarized. Ideally, the students will be able to internalize the main idea of the sociodrama and to evolve their own life-mediating concept. With slow learners and especially primary children, follow-up activities might include creative writing, drawing, and construction work.

Role Playing

Role playing is the unrehearsed acting out of a situation or a problem. It is a form of improvisation in which the participants assume the identity of other persons and imitate the role model's behavior in a particular set of circumstances. On the spot acting out can portray a concept or dramatize problem solving. Two or more people may participate, and ordinarily a short time is allowed for planning. This learning experience has great potential to increase awareness or to modify attitudes. It may also be used to introduce a health topic, to give students an opportunity to use what they have learned by applying some principle to the solution of a problem, or to illustrate the influence of tradition, values, or social pressure on individual behavior. Role playing differs from the usual type of drama in that no script, memorization, and rehearsal are needed. In fact, the value of role playing as a teaching device lies in the spontaneity of presentation. The action comes directly from the individual's creative use of his or her own experience.

The problem should be relevant to the health topic under study and should deal with a significant idea or issue involving personalities in a real-life situation. The problem should encourage the involvement of feelings and attitudes rather than straight factual information. A certain amount of planning is necessary. The problem and the roles to be acted out need to be identified. The specific roles and a limited background regarding the personalities and attitudes to be projected should be briefly described on slips of paper. The duration of the play should be short—one to three minutes. Two to five players are usually needed for a single episode. The roles assigned to students may be either congruent to or opposite from their real-life feelings. In either case the roles should be portrayed as the children perceive them and as the plot develops. The role playing should be stopped at the end of a specified time, when the idea or point has been reached, or when the dramatization begins to lag. The teacher should thank the participants for their performances and allow them to discuss the play. The teacher should follow up the role playing by pointing out the main ideas and emotional reactions presented.

Plays and Skits

A play is a carefully rehearsed dramatization that involves a script, props, and scenery. It can be extremely useful in portraying important so-cial concepts. Play scripts may be obtained in professional form or developed as a class project. The latter has the advantage of student involvement and the discovery and application of knowledge to individual and group problems.

The skit or playlet is a relatively brief dramatic presentation. It too may be a planned satirical or comic story, but it requires little rehearsal. It has great appeal to primary school children, for it is short and may be used to help children explore problems in human relations. It may be presented in the classroom by simply providing scripts to students and asking them to act out as they read the script.

The emphasis in both examples should be on attaining and maintaining healthful living and not on dramatization. Humor and mild ridicule in the script may be used to influence student behavior. The play, probably more appropriate for the intermediate grades, should last five to ten minutes, whereas the skit may last from three to five minutes and be used at both the primary and intermediate levels. Intermediate-grade pupils should be encouraged to write a skit or play and present it to primary-grade children or to their own class. After the presentation, the class can analyze the skit or play and its relationship to them, their needs, and their lives.

Puppets

Puppets are small figures. Marionettes are manipulated by attached strings or wire. Hand puppets, made from cloth or paper, are worn on the hand. Movement of the hand gives the puppet movement and expression.

Puppets are fascinating to most children. Puppets can make statements that will be remembered longer than those made by the teacher. Interest may be maintained at an even higher level when the puppets are made by the class and spontaneous dialogue added. Puppets have great attitudinal effect on primary children, as well as allowing for creativity.

A puppet show may be presented very effectively by the pupils. The teacher merely facilitates the process. A health theme or situation should be selected by the class and teacher for dramatization. A variety of methods may be used in the actual construction; consider, for example, hand puppets, stick puppets, paper-bag puppets, sock puppets, *papier-mâché* figures, and one- and two-string puppets. The characters assumed by the puppets may be taken from *Sesame Street* or other familiar television shows as well as favorite storybook situations. The stage may be a sheet or blanket stretched out as a curtain with the puppet manipulators behind the curtain, the puppets above it, and the audience on the other side, or a large cardboard box with a curtain as a stage. The extended sheet as a curtain has appeal because it is quick and easy to rig up and adds to a relaxed and informal setting. An added advantage is that it provides space for mass participation of the pupils. One group can manipulate the puppets, another can hold the curtain, and the third group can provide the dialog. Puppets provide an ideal opportunity for creativity and subject correlation with art, English, drama, and health science. As with all sociodramatic techniques, a follow-up is necessary.

Storytelling

Storytelling has been used by the world's greatest teachers. Jesus used it, as did Plato, Confucius, and other great philosophers and teachers. It has great appeal to primary school children because it lets them hear living language—language that communicates at a level above and beyond that of everyday usage. Storytelling is defined by Means (1968) as the narration to a class of incidents or events, true or fictitious, read, told, or presented through various forms of expression. Its general aim is to present a message, interpret literature, or inspire reading and expression. Anderson (1970), Chambers (1970), and Means (1968) point out that one tells stories to children to:

1. Entertain and charm them. Life is made rich by sharing the adventures of others, finding new solutions to old problems, and seeing the familiar in a new way.
2. Explain about human nature. As the child identifies with characters, he learns to recognize his own feelings about health topics.

3. Give reassurance that life is good. With news of today stressing violence and the exceptional, children especially need reassurance that most people are kind and thoughtful, that most persons have only good intentions, or that most people feel the same about work, play, and well-being.
4. Give meaning to the big ideas of life. The good, the true, and the beautiful are learned concepts. Storytelling creates a concrete situation in which ideas and judgments can be tested and applied to personal experiences.
5. Give children a sense of competence to face each day, an appreciation of our environment, or an understanding of self.
6. Encourage the development of good listening skills and provide aesthetic enjoyment.
7. Stimulate the imagination and provide opportunities for creative expression.

The storyteller should be honest and relaxed and tell the story in a sincere manner. The story should possess substance and involve content related to the topic under study. The beginning storyteller should explore the children's collection in the library for suitable stories and should review the story in detail so as to know it well but should avoid rote memorization. The storyteller uses his or her own personality as a teller— that is, his or her own choice of words, voice, pace, gestures, facial expressions, and so on— sending it to the ears and imagination of the listeners. When desirable, visual aids should be used to stimulate imagination, but not so that they distract from or interfere with the story. There is a need to create a visual picture of the story, to project into its character, and to consider ways in which effectiveness might be enhanced. The teller selects and arranges supplementary materials. Pictures are an important aid in helping primary children to understand stories. The storyteller should also arrange the seating so that there is closeness and a relaxed atmosphere. Visual aids and materials should be set up so that they communicate at the children's eye level.

The class needs to be motivated to listen attentively to the story. One way of doing this is to use an eye-catching or ear-catching technique to ensure initial attention and a warm emotional climate (see Figure 10.3). The teller then unfolds the story by dramatizing it enthusiastically. The teller avoids interrupting the story unnecessarily but allows for some student reaction and response. As with other learning experiences, there is a need to provide for follow-up activities.

Health Games

These are board games, similar to Monopoly, Concentration, checkers, ludo, fox and geese, and other commercial games for adults and children. The format and process of playing these board games may be adapted to the health area. Health games should be designed to help children become more knowledgeable, clarify misconceptions, reinforce positive attitudes, and develop constructive health habits (see Figure 10.4). A good health game has a main theme, such as drug misuse, ecology, water or air pollution, or disease control. Tokens, symbols, or colors may represent the players on the board. The players take turns, throwing dice, spinning an arrow, moving marked staves, or using some other chance technique. The game should provide for risk taking and acknowledge the consequences of good and bad decisions. Good decisions are rewarded with success; bad decisions are penalized by loss of reward or disaster. The progress of the game should be based on emotional and psychological factors, cultural values, and the benefits of maintaining optimal well-

FIGURE 10.3
Children should be encouraged to tell health stories.

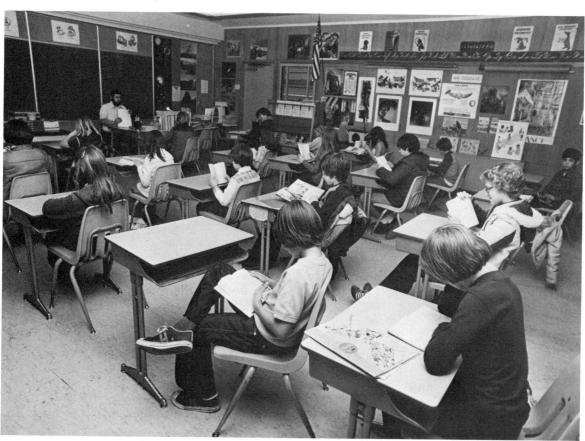

FIGURE 10.4

Teacher/pupil–made health games allow for pupil participation. They may be used as bulletin boards or adapted for groups of four to five students.

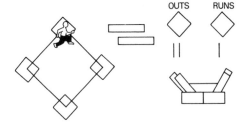

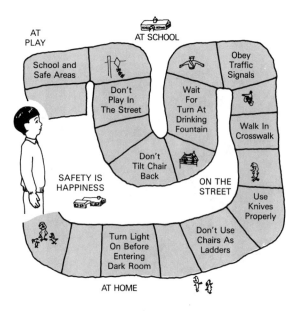

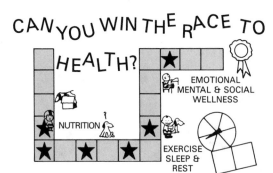

being. The game should allow for victory, success, or reward; attempt to solve problems; provide for varying degrees of skill and chance; and be bound by simple rules that allow the game to be completed in a short time. Children in the intermediate grades are mature enough to play and to learn from such games. In playing the games, children act out their feelings and wishes and project their understanding of social and health issues.

Teachers and pupils should create their own games. The quality of a game will depend on the psychology of the teacher and his or her creativity, knowledge of the subject matter, acquaintance with gamesmanship, and interest in games. For more on this teaching technique, see Sleet and Stadsklev (1977).

Computer-Assisted Health Education

Computers have been employed in teaching for over a quarter of a century. Early on, computers were used almost exclusively in a programmed instructional format. However, early computer-assisted education was not met with a great deal of enthusiasm by the educational community. Both hardware and the limited amount of commercially available software were prohibitively expensive and too new to be widely accepted.

My, how times have changed! The 1980's have seen the computer assume a major role in education. Without question, we will see the computer play an even more active role in the 1990's. The microcomputer has led to the classroom use of computers in many schools throughout the nation. Also, many students now come from homes where a microcomputer has been used for everything from word processing to playing games. Computer literacy will soon be as much a part of a good education as reading, writing, and mathematics.

Like other disciplines, health education has grown rapidly with respect to available software. Computer-assisted health education may be classified on the basis of how pupils use the software and computer. Available software can provide learning experiences that:

a) provide information

b) analyze data, behaviors, and habits

c) predict high risks because of health habits; appraise risks

d) simulate real-life situations with many choices

e) develop skills for managing time, stress, and so forth

f) keep records, monitor progress

g) perform math functions and statistical analysis

Health education software can enhance a health lesson. It can be fun to use and mentally challenging, help with problem solving, and increase the attention span of children through use of color, graphics, animation, and sound. Computers can facilitate learning and promote better health by providing immediate feedback. They allow pupils to learn at their own pace and provide reinforcement for attitude or behavior modification.

Health education programs often request that the student respond with a choice provided by the computer, or provide personal information used by the program to analyze individual behavior and make recommendations for change.

As with other learning resources, teachers who have at least one computer available for their pupils to use should clearly identify their lesson objectives first and then select the appropriate software. If software is to provide a positive learning experience, it must be used correctly. This requires good management by the teacher. Computer-assisted health education provides the teacher with an advantage over other learning resources when it performs better than the teacher could do without the computer.

More and more health education software is being made available. While it is impossible in a text of this nature to provide a comprehensive up-to-date list of software, a good sampling of packages is provided in the appendices.

Matching Bees

Matching bees motivate cognitive learning. There are two ways to set up matching bees—teacher and pupil. In the teacher matching bee

FIGURE 10.5
A matching bee on parts of the ear. All of the parts, their names, and the functions are mobile. The three sequences illustrate the progression of the matching bee.

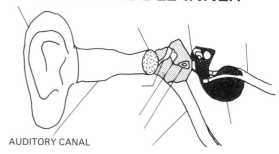

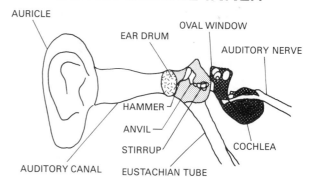

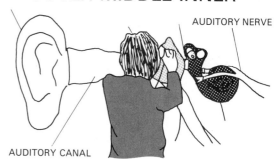

the teacher uses the bee as a visual aid to supplement a lecture. For example, the teacher may use the bee to explain how the digestive system works. A life-size outline drawing of the body is made on a large piece of cardboard. Each part of the digestive system is of a different color, life size, and mobile. The name of each part may be printed on 3″ × 12″ mobile cards. The function of each part, described in one to three words, is also printed on a separate mobile card (see Figure 10.5). As the teacher comes to a part of the digestive system, she or he matches the colored part with the proper location on the body, places the name of the part adjacent to it, and finally places the function of the part alongside the

name. This procedure, repeated for each of the parts, should not last more than three to four minutes. In this way the audible explanation is visually reinforced.

The pupil matching bee is similar in technique to the teacher bee. One pupil matches a part, another the name, a third the function, a fourth spells the word, and so on until all of the parts have been matched and all the pupils have had a chance to participate. Pupil matching bees may be run off as competitions, with the class organized into two teams. Rules for playing the matching bee as an educational game may be structured by the class and teacher. It is important that competition not be allowed to destroy the matching bee as an educational game. Winning should be deemphasized.

Matching bees are educational in that children can be motivated to acquire cognitive health skills on their own initiative. They may be adapted to teach about body organs and systems, food groups and dieting, and most health topics (see Figure 10.6). As a learning process, the matching bee surpasses the lecture, for pupils are actively involved in the matching bee.

FIGURE 10.6
Adapting the matching bee to teach about diseases.

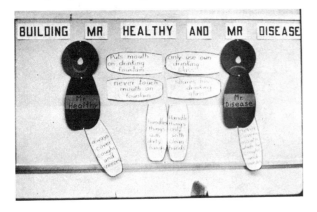

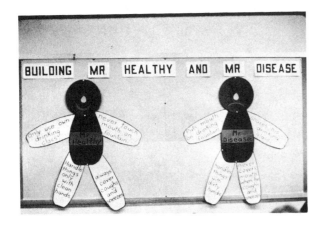

RELATIONSHIP BETWEEN METHODS AND MATERIALS

Materials and teaching aids are part of methodology. It is often difficult to distinguish between the two. A film by itself is a teaching aid. It becomes a part of methodology when children discuss what they saw and heard. Likewise, cut-out pictures of foods may be used with a flannel board or bulletin board as teaching aids. When these items are used to demonstrate a balanced daily diet, they structure an organized teaching method. Materials may facilitate a method. They should make the method more meaningful. Good teachers use a variety of materials and methods. Perhaps it is wise to think of both methods and materials as contributing to more effective learning. Use of both helps children to make well-being a dynamic and valued force in their lives.

TEACHING AIDS AND MATERIALS

Teaching aids and materials should be used to enrich and to supplement learning experiences. However, they do not replace the teacher. They are sensory aids and constitute a medium of communication (see Figure 10.7).

Various terms have been used in reference to teaching materials: supplementary materials, audiovisual aids, multisensory materials, perceptual aids to learning, and instructional materials. Perhaps the safest way of categorizing materials is this: (1) *printed materials,* such as textbooks and pamphlets, overhead transparencies, workbooks, songs and poems, graphs, flip charts, flash cards, and cartoons; and (2) *audiovisual aids,* including films, filmstrips, projectors, videotape, records, cassette tapes and recorders, photographs, slides, mobiles, models, posters, specimens, bulletin boards, flannel boards, and so on. Printed materials are like a second teacher, for

they may temporarily remove the burden from the teacher. The latter aids are used by the teacher while actively engaged in teaching.

Materials and aids enrich learning experiences by facilitating communication. They should give the spoken word and printed symbols meaning and life and help children to discover and to extend understanding. They should help to crystallize sociohygienic concepts, thereby motivating the children toward positive attitudes and habits.

Materials and aids should be varied from time to time. Such change avoids boredom, adds excitement to the learning process, and brings forth new freshness and interest. The elementary teacher should also remember that some aids are better than others at various grade levels. For example, to children who cannot read, a photograph may be more effective than a cluttered poster.

To this point, we have implied that children will be presented only with learning experiences,

FIGURE 10.7
Teaching about the symptoms of rheumatic fever, using Charlie Brown and his facial expressions as the communicatory technique between teacher and class.

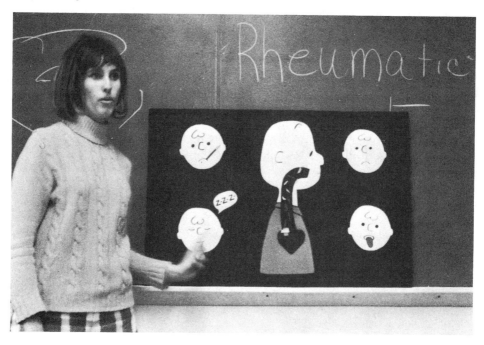

teaching materials, and aids in the classroom. Obviously, nothing could be further from reality. The current generation is more media-oriented than ever before. The contemporary classroom extends well beyond the school. To a large degree television has been responsible for this expansion of extracurricular learning. Often children can be counted upon to learn more about health topics from watching commercial television than from formal classroom education. Of course, this can be destructive as well as constructive in terms of molding positive health knowledge, attitudes, and behavior.

The video cassette recorder, another innovation, has evolved to the point where 4 out of 10 American households and 6 out of 7 of the nation's public schools possess one. The VCR has proven to be a stimulus without equal in instructional television's quarter-century quest to secure and expand its influence on public education. Improved video materials and more versatile distribution has served to kindle a new interest in instructional television. Just as important is that the VCR is simple to operate, especially when compared with the threading and rewinding that film requires. VCRs also eliminate scheduling problems, making it possible for the teacher to tape off-air programs for classroom use at a more convenient time.

Many elementary health education videotapes are readily available. Two excellent sources are the Public Broadcasting Service (PBS) and National Educational Television (NET). On occasion the commercial networks produce programs suitable for classroom use. A growing list of commercial health videotapes are also available for purchase. The innovative teacher also has the option of producing his or her own videotape if the time, motivation, and equipment are available.

REFERENCES AND BIBLIOGRAPHY

Anderson, Paul S. *Story Telling with the Flannel Board*, Book Two (Minneapolis, Minn.: T. S. Denison, 1970).

Berelson, Bernard, and Gary A. Steiner. *Human Behavior:* *An Inventory of Scientific Findings* (New York: Harcourt, Brace and World, 1964).

Beyrer, M. K., A. E. Nolte, and M. K. Sollender. *A Directory of Selected References and Resources in Health Instruction* (Atlanta: U.S. Department of Health and Human Services, 1983).

Blough, Glenn O., and Julius Schwartz. *Elementary School Science and How to Teach It* (New York: Holt, Rinehart and Winston, 1969).

Broudy, Harry S., and John R. Palmer. *Exemplars of Teaching Method* (Chicago: Rand McNally, 1965).

Chambers, Dewey W. *Storytelling and Creative Drama* (Dubuque, Iowa: W. C. Brown, 1970): 14-43.

Davis, Morton D. *Game Theory* (New York: Basic Books, 1970).

Gage, N. L. *Handbook of Research on Teaching* (Chicago: Rand McNally, 1965).

Gold, S. and D. Duncan. "Computers and Health Education," *Journal of Health Education* 50 (1980): 455-458.

Goodwin, Arthur B. *Handbook of Audio-Visual Aids and Techniques for Teaching Elementary School Subjects* (West Nyack, N.Y.: Parker, 1969).

Hilgard, Ernest R., and Gordon H. Bower. *Theories of Learning* (New York: Appleton-Century-Crofts, 1966).

Hoyman, Howard S. *Teacher's Manual: Your Health and Safety* (New York: Harcourt, Brace and World, 1963).

Huey, J. Frances. *Teaching Primary Children* (New York: Holt, Rinehart and Winston, 1965).

Humphrey, James H., Warren R. Johnson, and Virginia D. Moore. *Elementary School Health Education* (New York: Harper and Brothers, 1962).

Hyman, Ronald T. *Ways of Teaching* (Philadelphia: Lippincott, 1970): 217.

Hyman, Ronald T. *Ways of Teaching*, 2d ed. (Philadelphia: J. B. Lippincott, 1974): 290-296.

Irwin, Leslie W., Harold J. Cornacchia, and Wesley M. Staton. *Health in Elementary Schools* (St. Louis: C. V. Mosby, 1966).

Klausmeier, H. J., and K. Dresden. *Teaching in the Elementary School* (New York: Harper and Brothers, 1962).

Means, Richard K. *Methodology in Education* (Columbus, Ohio: Charles E. Merrill, 1968): 35.

Oberteuffer, Delbert, Orvis A. Harrelson, and Marion B. Pollock. *School Health Education* (New York: Harper & Row, 1972).

Phenix, Philip H. *Realms of Meaning* (New York: McGraw-Hill, 1964).

Platt, Ellen S., Ellen Krassen, and Bernard Mausner. "Individual Variation in Behavioral Change Following Role Playing," *Psychological Reports* 24 (1969): 155-170.

Rash, Keogh J. *The Health Education Curriculum* (Bloomington: Indiana University Press, 1965): 44.

Selberg, Edith M., Louise A. Neal, and Mathew F. Vessel. *Discovering Science in the Elementary School* (Reading, Mass.: Addison-Wesley, 1970).

Sleet, David A., and Ron Stadsklev. "Annotated Bibliography of Simulations and Games in Health Education," *Health Education Monographs* 5 (1977): 75-90.

Timmreck, T. "Creative Health Education through Puppetry," *Health Education* (Jan/Feb 1978).

Veneker, Harold, ed. *Synthesis of Research in Health Education* (Washington, D.C.: School Health Education Association, and National Education Association, 1964).

Victor, Edward. *Science for the Elementary School* (Toronto: Macmillan, 1970).

Weaver, Gilbert G., and Louis Cenci. *Applied Teaching Techniques* (New York: Pitman, 1960): 6.

Willgoose, Carl E. *Health Education in the Elementary School* (Philadelphia: Saunders, 1969).

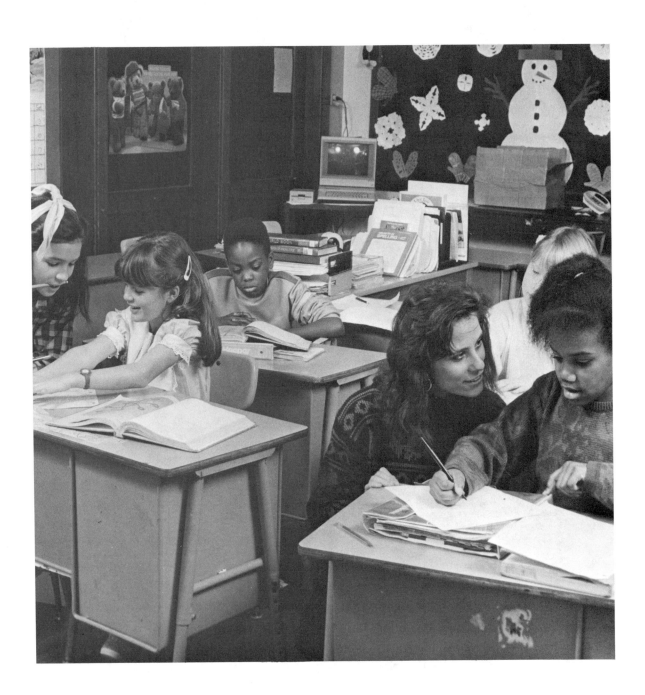

Chapter 11　Instructional Accountability

INTRODUCTION

Assessment of teachers is one of the most controversial topics in American education. The average tax-paying parent, already overburdened, is more than ever concerned about the quality and quantity of the education his or her child receives. Administrators are continually under pressure to prove the effectiveness of their programs. Institutions of higher learning are taking a harder line than ever on admission requirements, much to the dismay of open-admission advocates. Younger and younger students are rebelling against the traditional grading system and avidly advocating such alternatives as a credit/no credit system of grading, which removes the pressure of grades and allows the student to explore those learning experiences most appropriate to his or her needs and interests. One thing is for sure: As a prospective teacher, you are destined to be confronted with your share of difficulties directly related to evaluation. It is our opinion that you will change your personal philosophy relative to evaluation numerous times as you progress through your neophyte years of teaching.

To explore this issue, we must first come to grips with some basic questions relative to the concept of evaluation. Thus we will attempt to determine what evaluation is, why it is important, and how it is implemented.

EVALUATION DEFINED

Unfortunately, the term "evaluation" is misused by many educators. What is often referred to as evaluation is little more than test scoring. For clarity, we need to differentiate among the terms testing, measurement, and evaluation (see Table 11.1).

Testing

Testing is the process of using tests. Emphasis is placed on the instrument used in the process. Such tools as observation, checklists, inventories, questionnaires, rating scales, and interviews are used. The administration of a 25-question multiple-choice test about nutrition to a fifth-grade class is a typical example of testing.

Measurement

Measurement answers the question "How much?" Essentially, we are assigning numerals to a criterion according to a preconceived set of rules. Functions such as ranking, classification, comparison, description of status or change, and prediction are all included. A multitude of tech-

TABLE 11.1
Interrelationship of Testing, Measurement, and Education.

Term	Definition	Concept	Point of Reference
Testing	Procedure of systematizing observations, e.g., a 25-question multiple-choice nutrition examination for fifth graders.	Instrument (tool)	Tests, check lists, rating scales, observation, etc.
Measurement	Assigning symbolic significance, e.g., a score of 95 percent.	Score (quantity)	Rank, status, classification comparison, etc.
Evaluation	Determining the worth of measurement, e.g., the number of scores above 95, the mean score for the test.	Value (quantity)	Goals, objectives, expected outcomes

niques and instruments may be employed to fulfill these functions. Consider the use of several kinds of tests such as rating scales and score cards as well as systematic observation to measure achievement. When all is said and done, measurement is probably best referred to as a condition of quantity. For example, a score of 95 percent on the multiple-choice nutrition test is a measurement.

Evaluation

Evaluation is far more complex than either testing or measurement. Compared with measurement, evaluation refers more to value and quality. Evaluation deals with questions and judgments of worth rather than amount. Evaluation should be thought of as a much more inclusive process whereby quantitive statements are incorporated en route to ultimate value judgments.

The evaluation of public schools is an age-old process. Right or wrong, good or bad, evaluation finally is taking place around us. Most people find it quite easy to discuss the drawbacks and merits of American education. The average person on the corner can tell you exactly how he or she thinks schools ought to be run and will most likely add, "it ain't like it used to be in the good old days." There never has been, and surely never will be, a lack of both good and bad evaluation in education.

PURPOSES OF EVALUATION

Education is frequently conceptualized as a process comprising three major elements: the determination of objectives, the planning and organization of learning experiences and materials for fulfilling these objectives, and the evaluation of the educational program. Figure 11.1 shows the interplay among these elements and their relationship to the process of elementary health education.

FIGURE 11.1

Interplay of the three major elements of the educational process and their relationship to elementary health education.

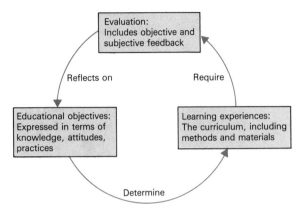

This premise raises many evaluative questions about elementary health education. For example, what is happening as a result of our instruction? Are we accomplishing what we set out to achieve? Is what we are doing helpful to students? Most authorities agree that effective evaluation can answer these questions. However, there has been a great deal of controversy and mixed emotion as to just what is the best, most productive technique for assessment. More on approaches to evaluation later.

These are some of the reasons why we evaluate health instruction:

1. Perhaps one of the most important purposes of evaluation is to assist in the *diagnosis* and/or *classification* of pupils who are in need of special help. In addition to indicating a need for help, evaluation might also determine the specific kind of help needed by the youngster.

   The health services of the school health program provide an excellent reference point. The youngster failing to meet the minimum standards for the Snellan Eye Test (most often administered by the school nurse as a screening device) is referred for a more comprehensive eye examination. Let's say that the youngster is found to be nearsighted and needs glasses. The conscientious teacher would take advantage of this information and seat the child in the front of the classroom so the youngster can see the chalkboard.

Diagnosis can be viewed in another way. The teacher may want to use an examination to introduce a unit of study in an effort to determine just what the class already knows and does not know about a particular topic. Data of this nature can be helpful in determining where the greatest amount of instructional emphasis should be placed. Periodic evaluation of this nature can also be helpful with updating a course of study.

2. Evaluation can be thought of as *accountability*. Without some form of accountability, we can never be sure whether or not our objectives have been attained. With reference to health education, we are concerned with whether our students are improving their health behavior, attitudes, and knowledge. The dedicated teacher wants to know if his or her teaching has been effective. Meaningful evaluation of instruction can be helpful in providing a valid indication of the effectiveness of the teacher's effort.

   The task is assessing pupils' progress. True appraisal of changes in health knowledge, attitudes, and practices resulting from organized classroom learning experiences is no easy task. Building on the concept of evaluation as diagnosis, the teacher could administer the same test at both the beginning and end of the unit and compare the results. There is no question that such an approach lends itself in a more realistic fashion to the cognitive domain. Objective measurement of change in attitudes and behavior is quite difficult. We will address this subject later.

3. For those still operating within a traditional numerical grading system, sound tests of knowledge provide *objective information on which to base grades*. This partic-

ular approach to evaluation has come under the greatest criticism of late at the elementary school level. Today, there appears to be a strong trend away from the categorical approach to grading at the elementary level. Instead, more and more emphasis is being placed on the descriptive analysis of each child's academic progress, thus eliminating the traditional grading approach. However, it is still necessary to measure cognitive progress if any meaningful descriptive evaluation is to be employed. So although letter grades may be eliminated, testing may very well still play a large role in the evaluation process.

4. Some educators steadfastly assert that evaluation devices (tests) are excellent *motivational devices* for students. Certainly tests can be challenging and educationally rewarding for many students—perhaps all students under the right conditions. However, wrongly used tests can be a most deadening influence. Needless to say, then, this purpose of evaluation is highly controversial. All too often our opinion is influenced by our own success with educational measurement. It is indeed sad to see the teacher who attempts to use testing as a prime motivating force for his or her students. If tests were taken away from this type of teacher, what control would she or he have over the class? Misguided rationale such as this on the part of the teacher is most unprofessional.

Summary

Evaluation should be thought of as a means to an end, not an end in itself. The greatest value of evaluation lies in the use to which it is put. Properly implemented evaluation in health education can be diagnostic, provide for accountability, be used as a basis for letter-grade assignment if necessary, and perhaps even be motivational if realistically approached. Keep in mind that evaluation in health education is far more than *how much* the child knows.

Just as important is how the child feels and what she or he does about health matters. This is what makes meaningful evaluation of health education such a difficult task. Although most teachers easily develop the ability to measure students' health knowledge, much skill is required to develop effective techniques that can validly measure their health practices and attitudes.

Knowledge of good health practices has long been considered a basis for health behavior. Proponents of this theory have argued that what the child knows will have a strong bearing on how she or he feels and will act in health matters. No doubt a person adhering to such a philosophy would place a great deal of emphasis on how much the child knows about health. However, there is little evidence to support such a theory. Knowledge is just one of the many influential factors affecting health behavior, and given the multitude of avoidable health problems clearly evident in our enlightened American culture today, one wonders how important it is. Just as important are how the youngster feels and behaves. Ideally, we should strive to evaluate students' health practices and attitudes as conscientiously as we do their health knowledge.

PRINCIPLES OF EVALUATION

It is impossible to list a standard set of evaluation procedures that can be applied to health education. The variety of conditions and situations unique to each health teaching assignment precludes the establishment of a step-by-step format to evaluation. However, it is possible to discuss the generally accepted principles of evaluation. The neophyte teacher would do well to ponder the following considerations before endeavoring to assess any aspect of the school health program. Ask yourself:

1. Have I familiarized myself with the instructional objectives or expected outcomes of the lesson, unit, or course I am attempting to evaluate?
2. In light of my response to question 1, have I precisely defined what it is I want to measure and eventually evaluate?
3. Do I have the insight and ability to select the most appropriate form of measurement?
4. Do I possess the skill to develop reliable and valid assessment tools?
5. Am I capable of analyzing, interpreting, and eventually evaluating the results of my measurements?
6. Am I dedicated enough to apply my findings and conclusions in the future?

Failure to consider the principles above will more than likely yield faulty evaluation. This is unfortunate, given the importance of evaluation in terms of the time it consumes and the ultimate influence it has on the student. Indeed, poor and misguided evaluation is probably worse than no evaluation at all.

Although we cannot here present the fine points of sound tests and measurement, we are in no way minimizing the importance of educational assessment. To the contrary, we encourage every prospective teacher to develop competencies in the area of measurement along the lines of the principles listed above. Should your teacher-education program not require a measurement course as a prerequisite to your degree, we encourage you to take one as an elective.

METHODS OF APPRAISING HEALTH ATTITUDES AND PRACTICES

If you were asked to list the most popular form of evaluation used by teachers today, what would your answer be? If it is paper-and-pencil knowledge tests, you are right. In many instances this is the only form of evaluation used by the teacher. Such an inflexible approach is unacceptable in health education. Health is a way of life, and knowledge is only one aspect of the health-educated person. To do the topic justice, it is necessary to assess student health practices and attitudes as well as knowledge. Following are several suggested approaches to the evaluation of health education at the elementary level.

Observation

One of the easiest and most meaningful forms of evaluation is observation. Actions do speak louder than words, and the observant teacher can perceive a great deal about a youngster's health practices and attitudes. The creative teacher can foster situations that will provide the opportunity to observe students' health behavior. By critically observing typical situations, we can determine if our instruction has had any significant impact on our students' health behavior.

The implications for such an approach are far-reaching. Whenever beginning a health unit, the teacher decides what he or she will regard as a satisfactory change in student health behavior after the unit has been completed. Since the expected outcomes for each lesson plan are for the most part behaviorally stated, they offer the direction needed to determine the observable behavior for which the teacher might watch.

From a more practical standpoint, let us consider the following example. You are undertaking a unit of study in nutrition with your fourth-grade class. One of the expected outcomes of the day's lesson is "Is capable of selecting a balanced meal." Once the instruction is complete, the teacher merely observes the quality of the eating practices exhibited by the students in the lunchroom. Due to the fact that cafeteria lunches purchased by the child are already balanced, it would be advantageous to reserve evaluation for the days when the youngster brings his or her own lunch.

The possibilities for evaluation of this sort are unlimited. Every content area of elementary health education offers an opportunity for ob-

servation and evaluation. Perhaps the only drawback of observation is that it is subjective and prone to error and bias. However, every effort can be made to clarify and define observation by knowing precisely what one is looking for. By adhering to the principles of evaluation and maintaining a critical and precise attitude about what is being observed, the elementary school teacher can ascertain a great deal about the health practices of his or her students.

Conferences

A one-to-one conference can be most effective for learning about a youngster's health attitudes and practices. In keeping with Glasser's comments relative to "involvement" (1969), the warm, empathic teacher is capable of establishing a rapport with students, becoming both friend and confidant. Such a relationship is conducive to learning about a student's health behavior. It also provides an excellent opportunity to determine if there are any hidden problems. Often the student will refrain from discussing his or her feelings or behavior in front of the class for fear of being embarrassed. By the same token, the teacher should be careful not to raise any question about a student's health behavior in front of the class if it might prove embarrassing for the youngster. Such inquiries are better left to individual conferences. The teacher's job is to assist young people in developing their maximum health potential. If individual conferences can contribute to this goal, they are worthy of implementation. Based on the results of such a conference, the teacher will, ideally, be able to evaluate any problems and proceed accordingly.

Self-Evaluation

Student input is becoming more of an issue with each passing day, and rightfully so. A student who is allowed to be a part of the evaluation process cannot help getting involved. When the measurement is developed by the student or as a result of a group endeavor, it is likely to be much more meaningful to the student.

Primary-grade children are entirely capable of developing simple checklists or rating scales for evaluating individual or group health behavior. The teacher simply acts as the class facilitator for developing the instrument of self-evaluation. Once the instrument is developed, the students introduce it and rate their own health behavior.

Intermediate and junior high school students find it more challenging to develop their own expected outcomes, learning experiences, and accountability techniques. Much to the amazement of many teachers, students are often tougher on themselves than the teacher would have been. Motivation can also be greatly enhanced. Care should be taken when such an approach is pursued to be sure that students build in feasible and attainable accountability factors. It is easy for students to become overzealous and set their sights too high. The teacher's role is one of mediator and guide.

Even so, do not be surprised if your first attempt at introducing self-evaluation falls far short of your expectations. This will be true especially if the students have never attempted it before. Keep in mind that students are trained to expect direction from the teacher. When the roles are reversed, most students are overwhelmed at first and respond rather erratically.

However, the more that students are subjected to such an approach, the more proficient they become in dealing with self-evaluation. In the long run, the benefits in terms of motivation and personal satisfaction will far outweigh the detriments of any initial confusion and uncertainty. Modern psychology and democratic social values both hold that important educational strides can be achieved by eliciting student participation in evaluation. The present trend in education will continue to place more and more responsibility on students themselves for evaluating their own achievement. If such an endeavor is taken seriously by both the teacher and student and every effort is made to make it as valid as possible, there is no question that self-evaluation can be most desirable.

Checklists and Rating Scales

Checklists and rating scales are excellent tools of evaluation, especially when used to supplement self-evaluation. In essence, they serve as self-administered inventories and can easily be developed to assist in the evaluation of health practices. Use of a checklist or rating scale makes assessment more objective. Hence order and continuity are added to the evaluation process.

Health checklists and rating scales are similar in nature. Both are designed to seek an indication of the quality and quantity of the student's health behavior. The main difference lies in degrees of measurement. More precisely, the checklist requires only a simple yes or no answer. The respondent either is or is not performing a particular health practice.

We can turn our attention to the charts and checklists presented in this text for examples. In Chapter 19 the chart entitled "Are My Meals Balanced?" asks the child to judge the degree to which his or her diet is well balanced. The picture quizzes on bicycle safety in Chapter 21 and the picture quiz on how to avoid a cold (Chapter 22) provide examples in which a variation on the theme has been developed.

Rating scales differ from checklists in that more latitude in responding is provided. The factor of degrees is introduced. Often a straight yes or no response does not completely or correctly answer the question. Rating scales attempt to offset such a possibility by adding more response categories. The traffic safety education rating scale for the primary grades shown in Figure 11.2 is an example.

If all of the statements are expressed positively, numerical values can be assigned to the response alternatives. This quantitative aspect can be helpful to the evaluation process. The category "always" can be assigned three points; "usually," two points; "seldom," one point; and "never," a zero. A total score can be determined

FIGURE 11.2
Example of rating scale for traffic safety education.

	Always	Usually	Seldom	Never
1. I cross streets only at marked crosswalks and refrain from jay-walking.	_____	_____	_____	_____
2. When I do cross at a marked intersection, I am sure that all traffic is stopped and that I can make the entire crossing safely.	_____	_____	_____	_____
3. I obey "walk" and "don't walk" signals.	_____	_____	_____	_____
4. I obey the safety patrol and traffic officers.	_____	_____	_____	_____
5. I walk my bicycle across intersections.	_____	_____	_____	_____
6. I do not play in the street.	_____	_____	_____	_____
7. I enter and get out of cars on the curb side.	_____	_____	_____	_____
8. If I must walk in the road, I do so facing traffic.	_____	_____	_____	_____
9. If I am out at night and near traffic, I wear white or carry a light.	_____	_____	_____	_____

by simply adding the values for each response. With "always" being the most desirable response, the best possible score is 27 points. The teacher and students can establish ranges for evaluation purposes. It might look something like this:

1. A perfect score of 27: Excellent traffic safety practices.
2. 22 to 26 points: Good traffic safety practices, but room for improvement.
3. 21 and below: You are an excellent candidate for an accident, and you will probably have one unless you quickly improve your traffic safety practices.

In conclusion, the uses of checklists and rating scales are most important. Only the most naive teacher would ask students to engage in such an activity and then use the results for grading purposes. Such an approach would only encourage students to be dishonest in their responses, and both the students' and the teacher's time would be wasted. To the contrary, students should be made well aware of the fact that such an undertaking will not be graded and that it is designed so they can assess their personal health practices and benefit from recognition of their level of well-being. The teacher should derive some input in terms of secondary evaluation by viewing the responses of the students. The results do reflect on the effect of the teaching that has preceded the checklist or rating scale.

Any evaluation should be twofold. On the one hand the teacher can ascertain the status of certain of the student's health practices. In light of these findings, future instruction can be altered if necessary. On the other hand, the child is afforded an opportunity to evaluate his or her own health practices and ideally, make adjustments where necessary.

Summary

It is no secret that health attitudes and practices are exceedingly difficult to measure and evaluate. Nevertheless, the importance of positive health attitudes and practices requires assessment, if only to assist in the evaluation of the instruction. This is based on the premise that health practices reflect attitudes and understanding. As the child grows older, this statement takes on added meaning. The concept of developmental tasks (see Chapter 2) can be considered the key to successful teaching for healthful attitudes and practices. The most successful instruction is timely. By introducing the exercises that are most appropriate to the youngsters' developmental level, there is an excellent chance of fostering positive health habits that may last a lifetime.

Evaluating this is another story. All one can do is attempt to evaluate the immediate behavioral results of health instruction. From a practical standpoint, the best the teacher can do is to evaluate the change in student health behavior over the span of the academic year. But this can be deceiving, because health behavior hardly begins or ends in the classroom, and worse yet, some health behavior cannot be evaluated during the school years. The outcome of some health instruction may not be measurable for years to come and consequently never is evaluated. Besides, health behavior is greatly influenced by elements outside the classroom. Peer-group pressure, advertising, parental influence, the church, and all other environmental forces have an effect on health behavior. The direct instruction that takes place in the classroom is only one of the many factors influencing students' health behavior. Ideally, the other factors influencing the child's health practices and attitudes will supplement and reinforce the school's activities.

In conclusion, carefully planned, systematic, and ongoing evaluation of students' health practices and attitudes can provide guidance and direction for classroom learning experiences. Use of the preceding methods of appraisal should prove helpful to the teacher.

METHODS OF APPRAISING HEALTH KNOWLEDGE

The assessment of health knowledge presents far less of a problem than does the challenge of evaluating health attitudes and practices. It is in the cognitive domain that the teacher can be most effective in evaluating. However, the basic philosophical question is How useful and meaningful is evaluation in this area? We have already discussed the argument that knowledge alone does not necessarily compel the student to practice wise health behavior. Then again, no one has yet proved that knowledge is not a prerequisite to an intelligent decision regarding health behavior. For example, it is logical to assume that if a person does not know about a vaccine for polio, he or she may never be immunized or see that his or her children are. This outcome is as unfortunate as the one for the person who knows better but fails to act. Keeping in mind the ultimate goal of health education (intelligent self-direction in health matters), it follows that students should acquire certain basic knowledge that will influence the health behavior favorably. This acquisition of knowledge is an objective of health education and should be subjected to evaluation as are the other areas.

In substance, the point of importance is that the evaluation of health knowledge is only one aspect of health education evaluation. Actually, it can be thought of as sharing equal billing with the evaluation of health practices and attitudes.

Constructing Teacher-Made Tests

Teacher-made paper-and-pencil tests are the most common approach to evaluating pupil health knowledge. Examinations developed on the basis of recognized principles of test construction can be an effective means of evaluating both knowledge and understanding. The teacher-made paper-and-pencil test has two forms, which can be combined if desired. We refer to the *short answer* test and the *essay* examination.

Both types of examinations have their merits, as pointed out by Table 11.2 found in Remmers, Gage, and Rummel (1965).

The following discussion examines essay and short-answer tests, with the express purpose of exploring the philosophy underlying each.

Essay Examinations

A good essay examination requires the student to organize his or her thoughts in a logical sequence and to support that position. It requires the student to reveal his or her general grasp of the subject matter being tested and to organize and express facts and documented opinion forthrightly.

In an effort to explore the type of essay questions that can be used for evaluation purposes, Monroe and Carter's (Remmers, 1965) list of the types of essay questions was modified to apply to health education and is presented below:

1. *Selective recall—basis given:* How can heart disease interfere with a normal lifestyle?
2. *Evaluative recall—basis given:* What do you consider are the five most important dental health practices in helping to prevent caries?
3. *Comparison of two things—on a single designated basis:* Compare the effects of stimulants and depressants on the central nervous system.
4. *Comparison of two things—in general:* Compare the definitions of chronic and communicable diseases.
5. *Decision—for or against:* Should illicit drugs be legalized? Support your opinion.
6. *Causes or effects:* How can cigarette smoking cause lung cancer?
7. *Explanation of the use or exact meaning of some phase in a passage:* Explain how digestion takes place.
8. *Summary of a unit of the text or of an article read:* Explain briefly the definition of mental health as stated by the National Association for Mental Health.
9. *Analysis:* Analyze the tobacco-smoking controversy. How did a health practice that is so harmful become so popular?
10. *Statement of relationship:* Why is health behavior important to lifestyle?
11. *Illustration or examples of principles:* Illustrate the correct procedure for mouth-to-mouth resuscitation.
12. *Classification (usually the converse of number 11):* Classify the following drugs according to category and cite their effects: heroin, amphetamine, barbiturate, cocaine, etc.
13. *Application of rules or principles:* If one is

TABLE 11.2
Summary of the Advantages of Essay and Short-Answer Tests. A Plus Sign Indicates the Type Judged to Be Superior as Far as the Factors Listed Are Concerned.

Factor	Essay	Short-Answer
Reliability of scoring		+
Adequacy of sampling student achievement		+
Labor required to prepare	+	
Labor required to score		+
Providing opportunity for student to select, organize, and integrate	+	
Providing opportunity to test effective writing	+	
Possibility for bluffing, "writing around the topic"		+
Opportunity for guessing	+	
Freedom from distortion of grading by skill in expression and quality of handwriting	+	

From *A Practical Introduction to Measurement and Evaluation,* 2nd Edition, by H. H. Remmers, N. L. Gage, and J. F. Rummel. (New York: Harper & Row, 1965):223.

attempting to lose weight, what principles of caloric intake must be applied?

14. *Discussion:* Discuss the functions of the skeletal system.

15. *Statement of aim:* Why is it important to understand how to select a proper diet?

16. *Criticism:* What is wrong with the following meal, and what would you add or delete to improve it?

17. *Outline:* Outline the four food groups and list two examples of each.

18. *Reorganization of facts:* After gleaning the following list of factual type statements about nutrition (some are not true), select the most appropriate and organize them into a paragraph.

19. *Formulation of new questions:* Based on your response to question 13, what other factors could theoretically influence weight control?

20. *New methods of procedure:* How would you approach the problem of drug abuse in the United States?

Note that several of these essay questions can also be easily converted to short-answer questions in the form of completion or simple recall.

Once the essay examination has been formulated and administered, the teacher must grade it. To make the process as objective as possible, the teacher should consider:

1. Grading the papers on an anonymous basis. That way the factor of teacher-student relationship is reduced, and the papers are graded on merit. The object is to eliminate as much prejudice as possible. If the students sign their examinations on the back, the teacher does not know whose paper is whose unless he or she recognizes the style or penmanship.

2. By grading only one question at a time, the teacher can more precisely compare one student's answer to a given question with all other answers to that question.

3. It is important that standards for sentence structure, paragraphing, spelling, and writing ability be set before the test.

Before we consider such criteria in an evaluation, we must decide whether it would be consistent with our educational objectives or expected outcomes. If not, these variables should not be considered in the grading process. In any event, the teacher should make a decision on this point prior to administration of the examination and tell the students of the decision.

Matching type tests are efficient in terms of space and time. They are also particularly useful for making a rapid survey of a specific aspect of a field of subject matter. The disadvantage of matching questions is that great care must be taken to prepare them. Much forethought is necessary if the exercise is to be challenging and free of irrelevant clues, poor alternatives, and awkward arrangement.

Conclusion

When comparing and contrasting essay examinations with short-answer examinations, it is apparent that the short-answer approach does offer some advantages. More material can be covered, there is greater reliability and objectivity than with essay examinations, they are easier to score, and they tend to eliminate bluffing. However, the nature of short-answer examinations limits them to the province of testing factual material and excludes their application to appraising important problem-solving skills.

To be effective, short-answer examinations must be carefully prepared, properly administered, and humanely interpreted. Just how accurately the answers can be evaluated depends largely on the skill and insight exercised by the teacher in preparing the test questions. It is one matter to reward rote recall and another to penalize creative thinking when only *one* answer is considered correct because it is associated with a statement in the required text. Is it not possible that several responses could be correct, depending on the frame of reference of the student?

Teachers should also strive to avoid overemphasizing trivial information. Instead, the teacher should provide positive learning experiences (and tests can be just that) if only major concepts are tested.

APPROACHES TO GRADING

Based on this discussion of assessment and its many procedures, the next question is "What do we do with our findings?" How do we evaluate the health attitudes, practices, and knowledge of our students? The answer is not simple. There are as many opinions as there are educational authorities. Although the information that follows is intended to relate to health education, it can be applied just as well to every other content area found in the elementary curriculum.

We do not pretend to have a catchall answer; instead, we offer several points of view regarding evaluation. We hope that this information will stimulate discussion among your class members as to the merits and drawbacks of each approach mentioned. From the elementary school to the graduate level, grading is one of the most controversial topics in American education. Some school systems have changed from the A-B-C system to other systems. The question at hand: "Is the traditional system of grading the most educationally useful system of evaluation?"

Claims and Counterclaims

More than 70 years ago, E. L. Thorndike (1918) asserted that "whatever exists at all, exists in some amount." Ever since that time (and surely before), educators have been trying to measure that all-important amount.

Since Thorndike's time, many other specialists in educational measurement have added strong support to the process of systematic evaluation in education. Their influence over the years is quite apparent today. Grades; grade-point averages; standardized tests of achievement, intelligence, and personality; proficiency tests; programed instruction; and measurement courses for prospective teachers all attest to the influence of their point of view.

To the testing enthusiast, the achieved score forms the basis for the definition of learning. The test score is the direct and complete evidence of learning. Validity is often considered in the narrowest context, and statistical reliability is substituted for evidence of relevance. The entire process at best must be considered within an extremely pragmatic and data-centered frame of reference. Keep in mind that we are discussing one of the most cherished and widely practiced aspects of American education. Without the fear of grades to hang over students' heads, many a teacher would be lost. How else would it be possible to coerce students into doing what the teacher wants them to do?

Through the years, several renowned educational authorities have argued that the entire process of measurement and evaluation is useless and damaging to students. Hoffmann (1962) charges that bright and creative students are penalized by contemporary test practices. Wernick (1956) suggests that the whole basis for employing tests is so shaky that tactics such as cheating and physical refusal to be tested are justifiable on the part of those subjected to the tests. Holt (1969) considers testing unnecessary, of no value, and inexcusable. He further states that testing does more harm than good and at its worst hinders, distorts, and corrupts the learning process. He believes that our chief concern should not be to improve testing but to find ways to eliminate it. Glaser (1969) sees grading as being the most influential factor in producing failure among students. He points out that grades do not motivate students at both ends of the scale. He feels that grades have become a substitute for real learning, a symbolic replacement for knowledge. One's transcript status becomes more important than his or her education.

So there you have it, a philosophical discussion of the merits of grading. Do you still think it is necessary to grade health education or for that matter any other subject in the elementary education curriculum? Is it possible to motivate students to learn without the fear of a grade hanging over their heads? Can we make health education as well as other subjects interesting and relevant enough to turn kids on to learning without the threat of grades? Is it possible to evaluate our teaching without testing?

Alternatives to Traditional Grading

Just in case you are not befuddled enough at this juncture, the following alternatives to the traditional grading system, which were compiled by Kirschenbaum, Simon, and Napier (1971), are offered as food for thought. Many of you will teach in a school district that has adopted an alternative approach. That alternative approach will more than likely resemble one of the following.

A. *Written Evaluations**
  1. *Description*
     The teacher uses all *the letters of the alphabet to evaluate to parents, kept on file in the school and eventually sent to colleges and employers.*

     Frequently, teachers are provided with a form to guide them in their written evaluations. Such a form might have spaces for the teacher to discuss "strengths," "weaknesses" and "recommendations for improvement." Or it might have a more detailed breakdown of various aspects of a subject, e.g., reading, writing, discussion skills, etc.

     Teachers' written evaluations are sometimes combined with the student's written self-evaluation, and both become part of the student's record and are sent to colleges and employers. When a checklist *form of grading is used, there is often room for the teacher's additional comments. This would be a form of written evaluation.*

     One school has teachers send out evalua-

     tions throughout the year, rather than at specific marking periods. They also provide equal space for the parents' written response.
  2. *Advantages*
     a) *These evaluations are much more helpful to the students than letter or number grades. They have an educational value.*
     b) *Written evaluations are much more meaningful to parents and admissions officers.*
     c) *They encourage the teacher to think more about each student as an individual, rather than as a set of numbers in the grade book.*
     d) *The school with ongoing evaluation and parent response says their system encourages ongoing attention to student needs, better school-community relations, and parental responses which help the teachers write more meaningful evaluations.*
  3. *Disadvantages*
     a) *Written evaluations allow teachers to be even more subjective than usual in evaluating students. Teachers might unconsciously minimize the strengths and focus on the weaknesses of students they dislike. Test scores averaged out into a letter grade, in some ways, prevent this kind of subjectivity.*
     b) *Not all teachers know how to write meaningful, helpful individualized evaluations. Some teachers will rely on vague terms like "excellent," "fair," "poor," "needs improvement," "good worker" and so on; their evaluations will be no more meaningful than letter grades.*
     c) *This is a much more time-consuming method of evaluation for teachers.*
     d) *Written evaluations create extra work for the school's records office.*

B. *Self-Evaluation*
  1. *Description*
     There is a need to distinguish between self-evaluation and self-grading. In a formal system of self-evaluation, the student evaluates his own progress, either in writing or in a conference with the teacher. In a system of self-grading, the student determines his own grade. Presumably self-grading cannot take place without prior self-evaluation. On the other hand, some

---

*From Wad-Ja-Get? The Grading Game in American Education *by Howard Kirschenbaum, Rodney W. Napier, and Sidney B. Simon, copyright © 1971 by Hart Publishing Company, Inc., New York. Reprinted by permission.*

schools have self-evaluation, but no self-grading.

An English department in a Michigan high school has its students write out their own evaluations each quarter. These evaluations then go to the teacher who writes his own comments and reactions to the self-evaluation, if he desires. These evaluations are then sent to the parents and included in the student's permanent records. There are no grades.

The student's self-grade can be combined with the teacher's grade for him and the two averaged out to determine the recorded grade. Peer evaluations can be included. Sometimes forms for self-evaluations are devised to guide the student's self-appraisal.

In some settings, students are given freedom to determine many of their educational goals and the means to achieve them. In these cases, students evaluate their progress toward their own goals. Where educational goals and activities are determined by the teacher, self-evaluation implies that students evaluate their progress toward the teacher's goals. Even here, students can help establish the criteria for evaluation, so they can more meaningfully evaluate themselves according to agreed upon criteria.

2. *Advantages*
   a) It is an important learning experience for students to evaluate their own strengths and weaknesses.
   b) Most teachers who use self-evaluation and self-grading report that students are very fair and objective and often harder on themselves than the teacher would be.
   c) Self-evaluation might tend to encourage students to want and teachers to allow students more responsibility for setting educational goals and means of achieving them.
3. *Disadvantages*
   a) Initially, students may take the "experiment" of self-evaluation and self-grading very seriously, but once the novelty wears off, they may give less thought to their self-evaluation and grade. There is some research to show that, over time, students' self-grades become less accurate.

b) When students respect their teachers they want to grade and evaluate themselves fairly, so the teachers will respect them. When students do not respect or when they dislike their teachers, they might tend to abuse the opportunity of grading themselves.
   c) Because of the enormous pressure on students these days to get high grades, self-grading makes honest self-evaluation extremely difficult.

C. *Give Grades But Don't Tell The Students*
   1. *Description*
      Students receive grades as usual, but they are not told what their grades are. A strong, personalized advising system keeps students apprised of their progress, informs them when they are in danger of failing, and gives them a clear perspective of how they stand in relation to their peers when they are ready to apply to college. At some schools students can find out their grades a certain number of years after they have left the institution.
   2. *Advantages*
      a) Once the students get used to the idea, tension over grades decreases.
      b) Without grades, students stop comparing themselves to one another and begin to shift their focus away from grades and toward learning. Reed College has had this system for over 50 years, and periodic polls show that its alumni are in favor of keeping this system.
   3. *Disadvantages*
      a) Initially, it might increase tension. For some students, the tension always remains.
      b) Although it may reduce tension and help the focus shift away from grades somewhat, many of the problems of traditional grades remain. Even at Reed, there is a movement to introduce pass/fail courses.

D. *The Contract System*
   1. *Description*
      There is a need to distinguish between contract grading applied to a whole class and contract grading applied separately to the students.

      When applied to a whole class, the contract system means that if the student does a certain type, quantity, *and, ideally,* quality *of work, he will automatically receive a given grade. For example, one teacher made the following contract with his class:*

Anyone who neither comes to class (type) regularly (quantity) nor turns in all (quantity) the required work (type) will receive an F.

Anyone who only comes to class regularly or only turns in all the required work will receive a D.

Anyone who both comes to class regularly and turns in the required work will receive a C.

Anyone who comes to class regularly, turns in the required work, and the work meets the following criteria (quality) will receive a B.

Anyone who comes to class regularly, turns in the required work that meets the following criteria and does the following extra report will receive an A.

Sometimes the teacher alone states the terms of the contract. Sometimes they are reached by a group decision. In either case, the same contract applies to the whole class.

Another practice is to have each student *design his own contract to which the teacher must agree. This use of the contract system implies that students are setting their own goals and ways of reaching those goals, and therefore, different grading procedures will be appropriate for different students. For example, in one social studies class,*

Student X might contract to read three books on the United States' political system and write a report on the three books.

Student Y might contract to study the process of how a bill becomes a law and to lead the class in a simulated exercise that would help the class to understand this process better. Student Z might contract to work two afternoons a week in the campaign headquarters of a local political candidate.

Since each contract calls for a very different type of activity than the others, each contract needs to include its own agreement as to how the student's grade will be determined. One of *the grading variables in this situation will be* who *will do the evaluating. In the case of student X, the teacher might be the sole judge of the grade. For student Y, the class feedback on the simulated exercise might play a part in the grade. And the local candidate might evaluate the work of student Z. But in all cases, the method of evaluation is decided upon jointly by student and teacher and stated clearly in the original, written contract.*

In some classes, the type *and* quantity *of work are the only components of the contract. Ideally, a contract should also include a statement of how the* quality *of the work will be judged, what criteria will be used and what levels of proficiency are necessary to earn a given grade. To do this adequately requires use of the "mastery approach" toward grading, which is discussed in the next section.*

2. *Advantages*

   a) *Much of the anxiety is eliminated from the grading process because the student knows, from the beginning of the year, exactly what he has to do to get the grade he wants.*

   b) *To the extent the teacher specifies the quantity and quality required for each grade, some of the subjectivity is eliminated from the grading process, and students have a clearer idea of what is expected of them.*

   c) *The contract system, when applied to students individually, encourages diversity in the classroom, encourages students to set and follow their own learning goals, and decreases unhealthy competition.*

3. *Disadvantages*

   a) *The* quantity *of work is easily overemphasized in contracts and tends to become the sole basis for a grade. To use an extreme example, one English teacher stipulated that five-page compositions would receive an A, four-page compositions would receive a B, and so on. When the quantity of work becomes the sole criterion for the grade, the grade loses its meaning.*

   b) *It is difficult to find creative ways to measure the* quality *of the different types of work students may contract to do.*

c) *There is a danger that teachers will be too ambiguous in attempting to state the qualitative distinctions between grades. To say that work of "excellent" quality will receive an A, work of "good" quality will receive a B, and so on, is no different than the ambiguous and subjective criteria we presently employ.*

E. *The Mastery Approach or Performance Curriculum (Five-Point System)*

1. *Description*

The mastery approach is not only a different method of grading, but an entirely different approach toward teaching and learning. It may be practiced by one class or by an entire department or subject area. In a sense, it is not an alternative to traditional grading; rather, it is the traditional grading system, done effectively.

The mastery approach begins with the teacher deciding what his operational or behavioral objectives are for his students, that is, what exactly he wants them to be able to do as a result of their learnings. He then organizes these learnings into units of study and arranges the units in a logical sequence, each unit serving as a necessary or logical building block to the unit succeeding it. Then the teacher determines how he will measure the extent to which his students have mastered the body of knowledge and skills in each of the units.

For each unit, the teacher designates levels of mastery or proficiency. Thus, if a math teacher wants his students to be able to solve a quadratic equation, he stipulates what the student must do to demonstrate a C level of proficiency, what he must do to demonstrate a B level of proficiency, and so on.

At the very beginning of the course, the teacher provides the students with all this information—what they are expected to learn, how their learnings will be tested, what the criteria are for the different levels of proficiency and what level of proficiency is required before they can move on to the next part of the course. In addition, he explains to the students what resources are available to help them achieve the levels of mastery they desire.

Students are then free to master the course content in their own fashion. Some students will attend class lectures and discussions. Others will work independently. Many students will utilize the various resources the teacher has provided—learning packages, programmed tests, films, tapes, speakers, field trips, etc.

Each student proceeds at his own pace. One student may take a semester to accomplish what is normally done in a year. Another student may take a year to do a semester's work in a particular subject. Under this system the course is oriented much more to the individual student, and the professor spends most of his time in review seminars and in individual tutoring, rather than in large group lectures.

Students ask to be examined when they think they are ready to move on. Usually, when a student has achieved a C level of mastery in one unit of a course, he can choose to go on to the next unit. However, students who want to earn B and A grades will stay with each unit until they have achieved that level of proficiency. A student may take an exam (a different form each time, of course) over again until he is satisfied with his grade.

Using the mastery approach, several teachers or an entire department can get together and plan their courses sequentially—one course building upon the next. This is sometimes called a performance curriculum, since course credits are no longer determined by the length of time a student spends with a given subject ("I had three years of French.") but by the level of performance he has achieved in a given area.

Bucknell's Continuous Progress Program is one example of the mastery approach and performance curriculum. Courses as different as biology, philosophy, psychology, physics, religion and education are all involved.

2. *Advantages*

a) *A student's grade becomes more meaningful to him because it is tied to a performance level. In the performance curriculum, grades become more meaningful because, in several different classes, the same grade now means the same thing.*

b) *Much of the teacher's subjectivity in grading is eliminated.*

c) *When students know where they are heading, they are likely to get there faster.*

d) *The focus of this system is on success, not failure.*

e) *The student has freedom to pursue his own path in mastering the course content.*

f) *The teacher is held accountable for stating his objectives, providing many resources, and helping his students achieve mastery. Sloppy organization and ill-prepared teachers are readily noticeable.*

g) *In the performance curriculum, the cooperation among teachers can generate better morale and the sharing of resources.*

3. *Disadvantages*

a) *To utilize the mastery approach properly requires considerable skill on the part of teachers and administrators. Most educators were not trained in this method and a great deal of retraining will be necessary. The funds are not easily made available.*

b) *The performance curriculum somewhat limits a teacher's freedom to run his classes in just his own way. In some cases this might be desirable; in other cases some creative teachers might be hampered.*

c) *It is possible for teachers to use the mastery approach without allowing students to pursue their own ways of achieving the levels of proficiency. When this happens students might feel, more than many do now, that all their education means is jumping over a series of prescribed hurdles.*

d) *Even when students have freedom to choose* how *they will achieve the teacher's goals, the mastery approach discourages them from setting and working toward their* own *goals.*

e) *The total faculty must be involved in setting up a performance curriculum. The teachers in each subject area would have to carefully study goals and methods and explore new approaches to the subject matter. This could take a very long time and might normally be impossible, since most teachers teach 5 classes, have supervisory duties, and are in-*volved in one or more student activities. A long-term grant might be needed to hire additional personnel to free teachers to do the necessary research and curriculum development.*

F. *Pass / Fail Grading (P / F)*

1. *Description*

At the beginning of the course, the teacher states his criteria for a passing grade, or else the teacher and students together decide on the criteria for a passing grade. Any student who meets these criteria passes; any student who does not meet these criteria fails. Students have the opportunity to redo failing work to bring it up to passing quality.

Pass / fail is a form of blanket grading, with the blanket grade being a P. P / F is also a form of the contract system, since the students know that if they meet the teacher's stated criteria for passing, they will automatically receive a P. Finally, it is also a form of the mastery approach, since the teacher designates the level of mastery needed to pass the course.

2. *Advantages*

a) *Students are more relaxed, less anxious, and less competitive.*

b) *There is a better learning atmosphere. Students feel freer to take risks, disagree with the teacher, and explore the subject in their own way.*

c) *There is no point to cheating or apple-polishing (except for students in danger of failing).*

d) *Students still have to meet the teacher's requirements to get the blanket grade, so plenty of work gets done. Freed from the pressures of traditional grading, some students do even more work than usual.*

3. *Disadvantages*

a) *Some teachers will use blanket grading as an excuse to avoid all evaluation. This deprives the student of potentially helpful feedback.*

b) *The blanket grade does not distinguish between students of different abilities. Therefore, the grade is meaningless except to connote passing work.*

c) *Freed from the pressures of traditional grad-*

ing, some students do less work than usual.

d) *Just as it is difficult for teachers to distinguish between the different levels of mastery in the performance curriculum, it will be difficult to clearly state and measure the level of mastery needed to earn the blanket grade.*

e) *The student in danger of failing still labors under all the pressures normally associated with traditional grading. P/F is no help to our poorer students.*

4. *Note*
   The system of pass/fail grading has two kinds of variations:
   a) *Modified Pass/Fail which adds one category to denote outstanding work. This is called Honors/Pass/Fail (H/P/F).*
   b) *Limited Pass/Fail in which the student may take only some of his courses on a pass/fail basis.*

G. *Credit/No Credit Grading (CR/NC)*
   1. *Description*
      This system works precisely the same way as pass/fail grading, except the two categories are "credit" and "no credit" instead of pass and fail. CR/NC also can be practiced on a modified or limited basis. It is important for systems using CR/NC to note right in their transcripts that NC does not *connote failing work.*
   2. *Advantages*
      Same as those for pass/fail but with one additional advantage: "No Credit" does not connote failure; students simply do not get credit for the course. With this fear of an E removed from those students on the borderline, they, too, can feel freer from the need to cheat and con their way to a passing grade. It is a small difference, but significant for those on the borderline.
   3. *Disadvantages*
      Same as those for pass/fail, except for "e."

H. *Blanket Grading*
   1. *Description*
      The teacher announces at the beginning of the year that anyone in the class who does the required amount of work will receive the blanket grade. Usually, the grade is B. Sometimes classes use the blanket A to make a protest state-ment to the school. Sometimes a blanket C is used, as a way of saying to the school, "See, this is how little we care about grades. The focus in this class will be on learning."

   If a student's work is of such poor quality that the teacher does not feel justified in giving him the blanket grade, he allows the student to keep trying until the quality improves.

   This is a form of contract grading. It is also a form of the mastery approach, since the teacher is saying, "Anyone who achieves this minimum level of mastery will receive the blanket grade."

   Blanket grading is used in individual classrooms only; it is never used by a whole school.

   2. *Advantages*
      Same as those for Pass/Fail Grading.
   3. *Disadvantages*
      a) *Same as those for Pass/Fail Grading.*
      b) *Although teachers frequently use blanket grading without any repercussions, this system would violate most school's written or unwritten grading policies and, therefore, be a risk for the teacher. Same of those for blanket grading.*

REFERENCES AND BIBLIOGRAPHY

Brooks, C. H. and D. J. Howard. "Evaluation of an Activity-Centered Health Curriculum: Assessment of Cognitive Knowledge," *Journal of School Health* (Nov 1982):52.

Dizney, Henry. *Classroom Evaluation for Teachers* (Dubuque, Iowa: Wm. C. Brown, 1971).

Dobbin, J. E. and Henry Chauncey. *Testing: Its Place in Education Today* (New York: Harper & Row, 1963).

Ebel, R. L. *Measuring Educational Achievement* (Englewood Cliffs, N.J.: Prentice-Hall, 1965).

Glasser, William. *Schools Without Failure* (New York: Harper & Row, 1969).

Green, J. A. *Teacher-Made Tests* (New York: Harper & Row, 1963).

Green, L. and F. Lewis. *Measurement and Evaluation in Health Education and Health Promotion* (Palo Alto, CA: Mayfield Publishing Co., 1986).

Gunn, W. J., D. C. Iverson, and M. Katz. "Design of School Health Education," *Journal of School Health* (Sept/Oct 1983):15.

Hoffmann, Banesh. *The Tyranny of Testing* (New York: Crowell, Collier & Macmillan, 1962).

Holt, John. *The Under-Achieving School* (New York: Pitman, 1969).

Kung, K. M. Taylor and M. Dignan. "Health Education Evaluation," *Health Education* (Sept/Oct 1982):13.

Kirschenbaum, Howard, S. B. Simon, and R. W. Napier. *Wad-Ja-Get? The Grading Game in American Education* (New York: Hart, 1971).

Marshall, Max. *Teaching without Grades* (Portland: Oregon State University Press, 1969).

Remmers, H. H., N. L. Gage, and J. F. Rummer. *A Practical Introduction To Measurement and Evaluation* (New York: Harper & Row, 1965):225-226.

Thorndike, E. L. "The Nature, Purposes and General Methods of Measurements of Educational Products," *The Measurement of Educational Products*—17th Yearbook of the National Society For the Study of Education, 1918, Part II.

Wernick, Robert. *They've Got Your Number* (New York: Norton, 1956).

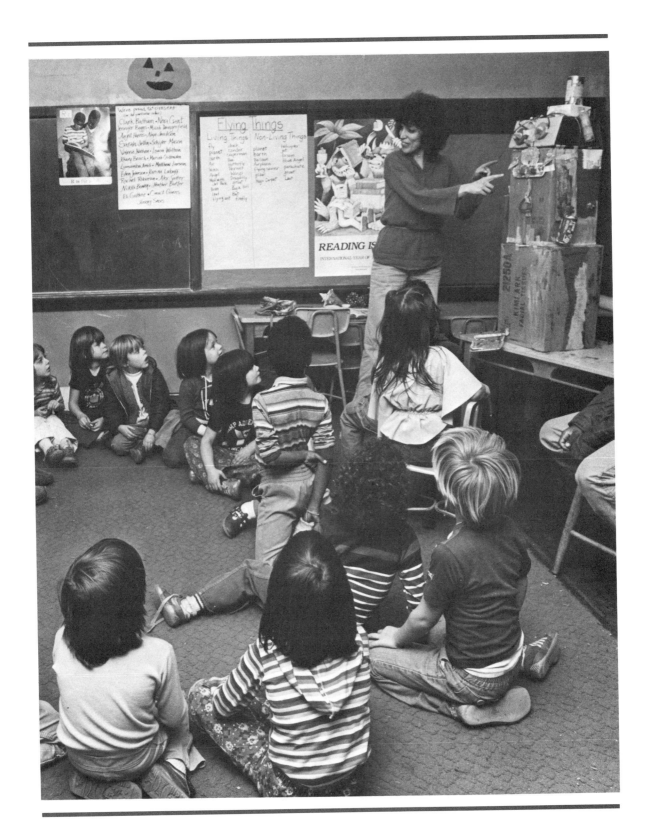

Chapter 12

Organizing for Health Instruction

INTRODUCTION

Among the elements of health instruction are concept formation, objectives instruction, content cognition, method and technique selection, evaluation skills, and unit and lesson plan organization. Failure to master these skills leaves the instructor without the tools so vital to effective health instruction.

This chapter is concerned with organizing material dealing with concepts, objectives, methods, and techniques into a blueprint for learning—the unit and daily lesson plan. This approach is a theoretical model to be used as a guide. Under no circumstances does the effort required to develop such a plan ensure that learning will take place. On the contrary, unit and lesson plans serve only to assist in the organizational process that normally accompanies effective health instruction.

CONCEPT UNIT PLANNING

Modern education has fostered the change from memory-centered education to problem-solving learning. Elementary health education is no exception to this rule. Effective elementary health education is designed to provide a systematic organization of activities, experiences, and situations that contribute to the optimal health development of the youngster.

To accomplish this task, it is necessary to have a well-perceived plan of educational experiences. Such a plan begins with a unit plan. The health education unit plan consists of a number of interrelated concepts, objectives, learning experiences, content, evaluation procedures, and references. Although the literature yields various forms for presenting the unit plan,

This material in this chapter is adapted from Walter D. Sorochan and Stephen J. Bender, *Teaching Secondary Health Science*, New York: Wiley, 1978.

we have found that the parallel-column form possesses considerable merit (see Fig. 12.1).

Unit Title

The title of the unit should be short, clear, and concise. Every effort should be made to convey clearly to the reader the nature of the topic to be discussed. The title should also be so stated that it stimulates the interest of the reader. It is not necessary to spend an inordinate amount of time developing a catchy unit title; however, an effort should be made to write a title that clearly informs and motivates the reader about the topic.

Concepts

The concepts serve as the framework for the unit plan. Concepts are the big ideas that will be emphasized in the unit. They serve as focal points for the development of the remainder of the unit and the entire instructional process. The concepts act as guides to the competencies that are to be demonstrated by the learner.

Concept formation is invaluable. Careful concept formation forms the basis for formal health education.

Expected Pupil Outcomes (Behavioral Objectives)

The unit plan should comprise statements that clearly describe what students will know, feel, and be able to do after completing the unit of instruction. Theoretically, the objectives add further direction to the instructional process once the concepts for a unit have been developed. The objectives suggest what should be taught and how.

Behavioral objectives can be stated in various ways: as objectives, expected outcomes, goals, aims, and/or competencies. Behavioral objectives are referred to in this text as *expected pupil outcomes*. They are skills children are expected to

FIGURE 12.1
Suggested format for a unit plan.

Unit Title _____
Grade Level _____
Instructor _____
Time Period _____

Concepts	Expected Pupil Outcomes	Content	Learning Experiences	Evaluation Procedures	Teaching Aids

attain. Expected pupil outcomes may be any of three types:

1. *Cognitive:* pertaining to knowledge and intellectual skills, such as recall and recognition
2. *Affective:* pertaining to feelings, emotions, interests, values, and the development of appreciation and adequate adjustment or attitudes
3. *Action:* relevant to acting, manipulating, or motor skills or acts of overt behavior.

The elementary teacher should develop appropriate outcomes in all three domains (see Chapter 9).

Content

The content section of the unit plan outlines the subject matter to be taught. More often than not, several content items will be required to achieve each objective. The content should be carefully selected to enhance the development of the desired objectives.

Without content, there is no concept development. Specific details of a topic make up content. Content is a collection of facts and information. Such facts should be relevant to a concept and expected outcomes. It may be difficult for the child to assimilate and categorize numerous facts. Indeed, the child may forget the details of the content in a few minutes. When this happens, the details are overwhelming, and the child will not be able to analyze and categorize the information. The content cannot be internalized.

Teachers make the content meaningful to children by providing the proper learning experiences. The learning experiences should help the child to internalize the content and to evolve his or her own concept. Although most of the details of content will be forgotten in 24 hours, the big idea, or concept, structured by the details will be retained. There are no concepts without content. Content provides the fuel for the discovery of concepts. The spark for igniting such a discovery comes from the learning experience.

In selecting content, the teacher should start out at the pupil's level, then select and present the content in a progressive manner. This sustains pupil interest and provides intrinsic motivation to learning.

Learning Experiences

Once the concepts have been developed, the expected pupil outcomes established, and the content for each outcome determined, suitable instructional methods and techniques must be selected. The learning experiences selected for each content item should be carefully developed to ensure that individual factors such as class differences, strengths, weaknesses, and time allotment are all considered. It may be necessary to develop more than one learning experience to choose from.

Teachers are the facilitators of these learning experiences. Teachers help children to make information meaningful and to evolve concepts. Concepts can be mediators of behaviors. Whether such an internalized process in the child occurs depends to a large degree on the kinds of learning experiences that teachers provide. Learning experiences should help children to discover for themselves the big ideas, or concepts.

Teachers should keep in mind that concepts gradually arise from precepts, experiences, and images of observations. The child perceives by acquiring an awareness of self, the environment, and that which he or she is trying to relate to sensually. Through experience, the child synthesizes information and gives meaning to the information. For example, a kindergarten child watching guppies swimming in an aquarium eventually sees small dark spots in the mother guppies' transparent stomachs and later locates baby guppies; the child synthesizes impressions of color, shape, content and structure, and growth characteristics derived through the light receptors of his eyes. The child perceives an answer to the question, "Where do babies come from?" Learners see, touch, and hear about fish, babies, and other objects to formulate an image of an understanding of their nature. Crucial to learning for elementary school children, then, is the selection of basic experiences appropriate to the concept to be developed.

Some learning experiences are more appropriate than others in evolving specific concepts. Although good research is still lacking in this area, the basis for this is suggested in Table 12.1. The four basic aims of health science instruction are to (1) impart facts and knowledge; (2) develop thinking skills; (3) evolve positive attitudes; and (4) develop positive behaviors. Table 12.1 also summarizes the expected outcomes and suggests learning experiences that may help to attain the outcomes.

Learning experiences are very much how you get where you are going. How do you want to travel to your destination (expected outcome)? Do you travel by car, train, ship, or airplane? Each is a different mode of transportation and places a different priority on time and experience. And so it is with learning experiences, vehicles for attaining expected outcomes and helping children to evolve desirable concepts.

Evaluation Procedures

It is important to implement some form of measurement and evaluation to determine whether or not the established objectives have been attained.

Accountability can take on many forms: knowledge tests, attitude scales, practice inven-

TABLE 12.1
Relationships Among Behavioral Domains, Health Instructional Aims, Expected Outcomes, Behavior, and Learning Experiences.

Domain (Behavioral)	Aims (Health Instruction)	Typical Outcomes (Expected)	Behavior (Overt/Covert)	Typical Learning Experiences
Cognitive	Impart facts	Define, name, state, recall, list	Think	Lecture, discussion, question-answer (Q-A), group reports
	Develop thinking skills	Distinguish, apply, recognize, analyze, identify		Discussion, Q-A, demonstration, field trip, experiment
Affective	Evolve positive attitudes	Aware, sensitive, accept, like, believe, value, appreciate, feel	Feel	Role play, debate, sociodramas, panel-group reports, discussion
Action	Develop positive behaviors	Perform, practice, demonstrate, apply, acquire, participate	Act (does)	Teacher demonstration and pupils practice habit or skill

tories, checklists, rating scales, observations, oral and written reports, and so on. It is important that each objective be measured with an appropriate technique (see Chapter 11).

Teaching Aids

It is important to list any materials, essential supplies, and aids necessary to the instructional process. Films, projectors, screens, models, specimens, transparencies, overhead projectors, videotape, VCR, computer software, slides, and slide projectors are all teaching aids. The list provides the instructor with a quick inventory of the items necessary for the lesson.

References

It is helpful to have one list of references for the instructor and another for the student. The student list can provide exact page numbers if necessary. In some instances it might be more valuable to provide students with general references and leave isolating the relevant material to them.

In any event, it is important that reference lists be kept current.

CONCEPT LESSON PLANNING

Once the unit plan has been established, the *daily lesson* plans must be made. The daily lesson plans provide the day-by-day progression toward the established objectives of the unit. Effective lesson planning requires that the instructor have a clear understanding of the total learning package presented in the unit. With that understanding in mind, the instructor carefully separates the unit into the separate daily lesson plans.

A lesson plan may extend into more than one class period. It may also be designed for completion in one class period but have to be extended into another class period due to the instructor's miscalculation of the time allotment. A most important consideration surrounding the daily lesson plan is that a sense of continuation be observable from one class period to the next and that ultimately the objectives of the unit are met and the concepts realized. Table 12.2 shows the suggested format for the daily lesson plan.

TABLE 12.2

Suggested Format for a Daily Concept Lesson Plan

Topic: _____   Grade Level: _____

Concept(s): _____   Instructor: _____

_____   Date: _____

_____

Expected Pupil Outcome(s): _____

_____

_____

Content	Time Allotted	Learning Experiences	Teaching Aids
1. (*NOTE:* Record "WHAT" it is you are going to disseminate to the students.)		1. (*NOTE:* Record "HOW" you are going to convey the content. Learning experience number 1 should be correlated to content number 1, etc.)	1. (*NOTE:* Record all essential materials, supplies and aids necessary to carry out the instructional process.)
2.		2.	2.
3.		3.	3.
4.		4.	
etc.		(*NOTE:* "Key words & key questions" can be listed under the learning experience where appropriate.)	etc.
		Evaluation Procedures	
		1. (*NOTE:* Some form of measurement and evaluation is important to determine whether established objectives have been attained.)	
		2.	
		etc.	
		References	
		(*NOTE:* List sources that substantiate the validity of your content.)	

The daily lesson plan should be structured so that each component reinforces the other components. For example, the content should reinforce the concept, which in turn should reinforce the outcome. The exercises should specify how each part of the content may be internalized into a concept. Indirectly, the learning experience contributes to the outcome by helping children to discover the concept.

The theme topic and expected outcome for the lesson plan should be accompanied by a developmental task. The specific information relevant to the outcome should be selected next. Third, a concept should be evolved from the content so that it helps to mediate for the outcome. Finally, the learning experience should be plugged into the lesson plan.

In addition to these four major components of a lesson plan, the following may be added:

1. *Key questions* (for review to help children to internalize the content and structure the concept)
2. *Key words* (terms important to developing the concept)
3. References for pupils and the teacher
4. Teaching aids
5. Evaluations, such as quizzes before and after the lesson, observations of behavior
6. Time allotted to each learning experience

Inclusion of these elements in the lesson plan is left to the discretion of the critic and prospective teachers. Examples of lesson plans for various topics on well-being are given in Chapters 13 through 23.

Health instruction, like the practice of medicine, is both an art and a science. It is a science in that it has interdisciplinary content and relies on the principles of educational and developmental psychology. In terms of the knowledge, techniques, and methods employed, it is similar to medicine. Which techniques to use and how to use them is an art in medicine, as in teaching.

Medicine is the art of diagnosing, prescribing, and treating. Selecting appropriate learning experiences to attain expected outcomes is a process of decision making as well as manipulating human behavior. Teaching is an art because the teacher is a social engineer, having pupils evolve new health habits and behaviors and accept public health practices. Dealing with children to attain these outcomes is an art. Thus the conceptual lesson plan is a scientific approach, and its execution is an art.

REFERENCES AND BIBLIOGRAPHY

Bloom, Benjamin S., ed. *Taxonomy of Educational Objectives,* Handbook 1, Cognitive Domain (New York: McKay, 1968).

Bourne, Lyle E. *Human Conceptual Behavior* (Boston: Allyn and Bacon, 1966).

Broadbeck, May. "Logic and Scientific Method on Teaching," in N. L. Gage, ed. *Handbook of Research on Teaching* (Chicago: Rand McNally, 1965), pp. 44-93.

Gage, N. L., ed. *Handbook of Research on Teaching* (Chicago: Rand McNally, 1965), pp. 48-72, 884-887.

Hurlock, Elizabeth B. *Child Development* (New York: McGraw-Hill, 1964).

Kibler, Robert J., Larry L. Barker, and David T. Miles. *Behavioral Objectives and Instruction* (Boston: Allyn and Bacon, 1970).

Klausmeier, Herbert J., and Chester W. Harris. *Analyses of Concept Learning* (New York: Academic Press, 1966).

Mager, Robert F. *Preparing Instructional Objectives* (Palo Alto, Calif.: Fearon, 1963).

Middleton, K. "Back to Some Basics in Health Lesson Planning," Health Education (Mar/April 1976):7.

Phenix, Philip H. *Realms of Meaning* (New York: McGraw-Hill, 1964).

Rash, J. K. *The Health Education Curriculum* (Bloomington: Indiana University Press, 1970).

Sorochan, Walter D., and Stephen J. Bender. *Teaching Secondary Health Science* (New York: Wiley, 1978).

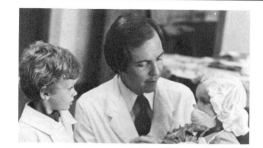
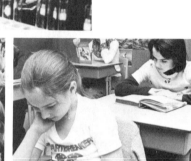
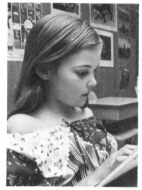
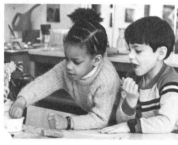
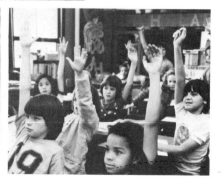
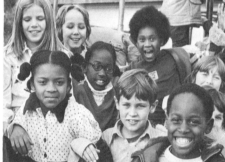
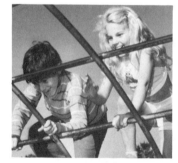
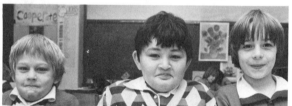
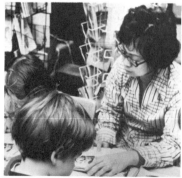
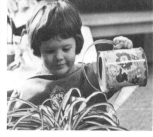

Part Five

Suggested Learning Experiences

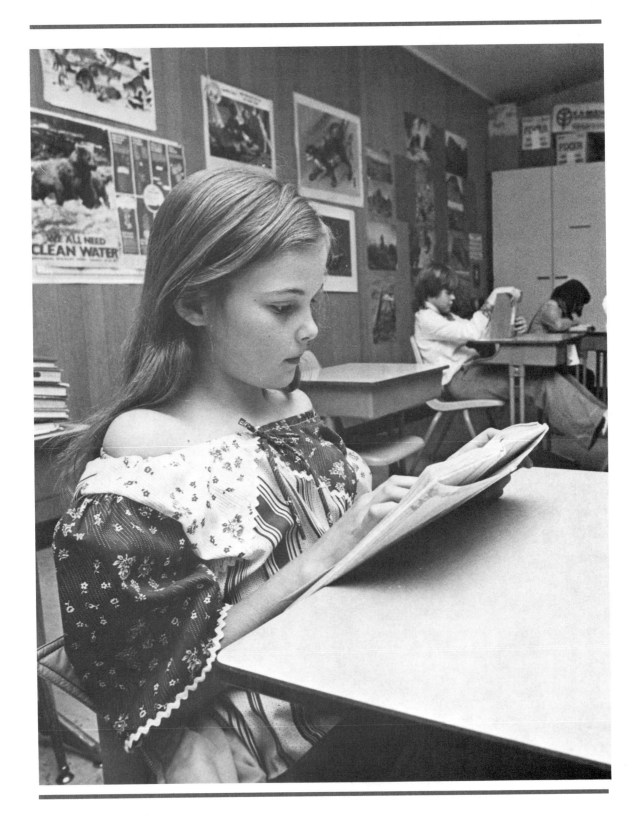

Chapter 13

Teaching About the Human Body

INTRODUCTION

The human body is a marvel of nature. The human machine consists of ten systems and their organs. The skeletal system gives us appearance and protection; the muscular system allows for locomotion; the nervous system and sensory mechanisms facilitate communication; the glandular system regulates body functions and provides a stress-defense mechanism; the cardiovascular system transports blood and other substances; the digestive system processes fuel; the excretory system removes wastes; the respiratory system allows for gaseous exchange; the lymphatic system protects the body; and the reproductive system (see Chapter 23) procreates the species. Collectively, these systems make the human body a complex living organism. Its different parts act and react on one another in ways quite impossible of any other machine. This machine requires a balanced blending of nutrition, exercise, rest, sleep, affection, spiritual purpose, and social interaction to function optimally.

SKELETAL SYSTEM

The skeleton, the bony supporting structure of the body, is made up of 206 bones of different shapes and sizes (Figure 13.1). In vertebrates, the skeleton is covered by soft tissues, such as muscle and fat, and is called an *endoskeleton*. Many invertebrate animals (for example, lobsters, crayfish, and clams) are protected by an *exoskeleton*, which is on the outside of the soft tissues.

The endoskeleton has five principal functions:

1. *Protection.* The hard bony tissue provides internal soft tissues with a defense against trauma. The skull protects the brain; the vertebral column protects the spinal cord.

---

*The first part of this chapter is from Paul D. Anderson, *Basic Human Anatomy and Physiology: Clinical Implications for Health Professions*, Monterey, CA: Wadsworth Health Sciences, 1984.

The rib cage and the bones of the pelvis protect the organs in the thorax and the lower part of the abdomen.

2. *Support.* Most of the body's structures are soft, pliable, and delicate. The skeleton's rigid framework provides a means of suspension for body systems.

3. *Muscle attachment.* Muscles are attached to bone by tendons. The rigidity of bone, combined with the elasticity and contractility of muscle, makes the arms and legs strong levers, tools, or weapons.

4. *Reservoir for minerals.* The *osseous* (bony) tissues of all parts of the skeletal system provide the body with a vast depot of mineral salts such as calcium and phosphates.

5. *Hematopoiesis.* During late fetal life and continuing in some bones through adult life, the red marrow of long bones, the ribs, the sternum, and the pelvic bones produce blood cells—a process called *hematopoiesis.*

It is important to remember that the skeleton is composed of living tissues. Its materials are constantly being dissolved and passed into the bloodstream and replenished by other tissues and from food.

Gross Structure

A typical long bone consists of a shaft (the diaphysis) and two heads (epiphyses). The diaphysis is made up principally of compact bone in which lamellae are arranged to form a hard, solid mass. In the core of the diaphysis is the medullary cavity, a large space filled with yellow bone marrow, a hematopoietic tissue.

Adult bone has two types of marrow: red and yellow. Red marrow is found in the vertebrae, sternum, ribs, and proximal epiphyses of long bones. Its major function is the production of blood cells and platelets. Yellow marrow, found in the cavities of long bones, is mostly adipose tissue (fat cells). Under normal conditions, yellow marrow takes no part in red blood cell production in adulthood, but in certain abnormal circumstances, it may replace red mar-

FIGURE 13.1
Human skeleton, anterior aspect.

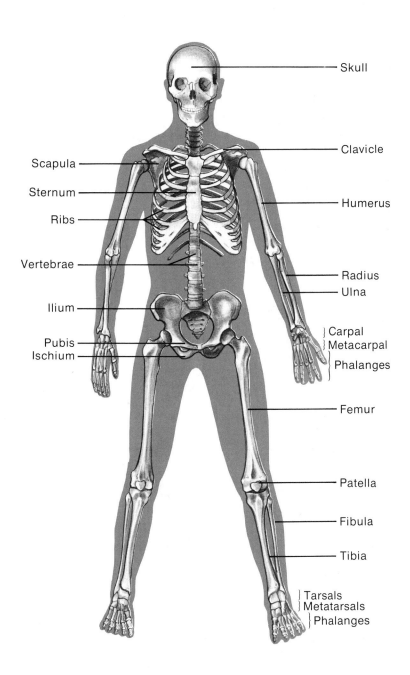

Skull

Clavicle

Scapula

Sternum

Humerus

Ribs

Vertebrae

Radius

Ulna

Ilium

Carpal
Metacarpal

Pubis
Ischium

Phalanges

Femur

Patella

Fibula

Tibia

Tarsals
Metatarsals
Phalanges

row when the supply of the latter becomes depleted.

The bone is covered with periosteum. Nutrients and osteoid components are supplied to the bone by the large nutrient artery as well as by many small blood vessels in the periosteum. These vessels permeate the compact bone and reach the medullary cavity through haversian and Volkmann's canals.

The marrow cavities of bone are lined with a membrane, the *endosteum,* which is a single layer of either osteoblasts or osteogenic cells.

Types of Bones

Each bone is a distinct structural unit. However, all osteoid tissue has the same basic composition. Its pattern varies according to its functions, which are represented by the four basic types of bones:

1. *Long bones.* Long bones are the largest in the body. Included in this group are the prominent bones of the arms and legs. Each has a shaft and two ends. The general function of long bones is to act as levers. Examples are the femur of the leg and the humerus of the upper arm.
2. *Short bones.* These differ from long bones in that they are smaller and have less prominent ends. They are cuboid and are composed of cancellous bone enclosed within a thin shell of compact bone. Their principal function is to provide strength. Examples are the carpals of the wrist and the tarsals of the ankle.
3. *Flat bones.* These are platelike and usually have two broad surfaces (tables) and narrow edges by which one flat bone articulates with another. Each flat bone is thin and is made up of two plates of compact bone that enclose a layer of cancellous bone. The general function of these bones is protection. Examples are the ribs, the scapula at the back of the shoulder, and the cranium.
4. *Irregular bones.* These are so named because of their shapes. Several surfaces may articulate with several other bones. Some of the bones of the skull are irregular, as are the vertebrae and the hip bones. The thinner parts of irregular bones consist of two thin plates of compact bone with cancellous bone between them. The general function of irregular bone is articulation.

MUSCULAR SYSTEM
Skeletal Muscles

Skeletal muscles' principal function is to produce movement. To accomplish this, they must have two attachments (Figure 13.2 a): one to the bone that is fixed, called the *origin* of the muscle; the other to the bone to be moved, called the *insertion* of the muscle. This does not mean that muscles attach only to bones. Some attach to other muscles as well.

Muscles are attached to bones by tendons, cords or bands of white fibrous connective tissue. *Aponeuroses* are sheets of connective or membranous tissue that connect muscle and the part it moves.

Muscles are named for various traits as follows:

- *Location:* intercostal (between the ribs), brachii (arm), occipitalis (head)
- *Action:* adductor, flexor, extensor
- *Shape or size:* trapezius (trapezoid), maximus (largest), minimus (smallest), longus (long), brevis (short)
- *Direction of fibers:* rectus (straight), transversus (across)
- *Number of heads of origin:* biceps (two heads), triceps (three heads), quadriceps (four heads)
- *Points of attachment:* sternocleidomastoid (sternum, clavicle, and mastoid process of the temporal bone)

The motions produced by muscle contraction are described with reference to the standard anatomical position of the body—standing erect

FIGURE 13.2

a, Skeletal muscle attachments. The origin is attached to the less movable bone, whereas the insertion is attached to the more movable bone. **b,** Two examples of muscle action.

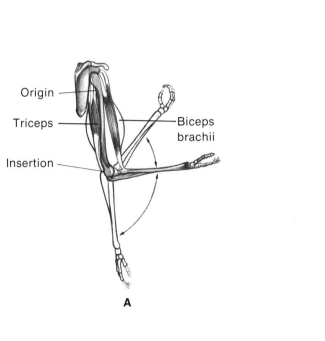

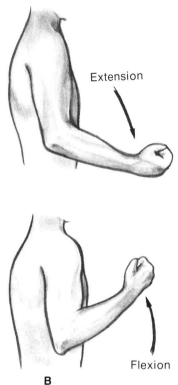

with arms straight down and palms directed forward (Figure 13.3). Movements parallel to the longitudinal axis are flexion, or folding together, and extension, an unfolding movement in the opposite direction (Figure 13.2 b). Abduction refers to movement away from the axis; adduction means toward the axis of the body.

Muscles that produce movement in directions opposite to one another are *antagonists*. Muscles that work together to accomplish a particular movement are *synergists*. Two muscles that bend an arm at the elbow are synergists with one another (for example, the biceps and brachialis flex the lower arm), but both are antagonistic to a muscle that straightens the arm (the triceps extend the lower arm).

NERVOUS SYSTEM

No body system is capable of functioning alone. All must work together so that homeostasis may be maintained. The mechanism that ensures that the organs and systems operate in smooth coordination is the nervous system. Conditions within and outside the body are constantly changing, and one purpose of the nervous system is to respond to these internal and external changes so that the body may adapt itself.

The nervous system is divided into two parts: the central nervous system (CNS) and the peripheral nervous system (PNS). The CNS consists of the brain *and* the spinal cord, which runs up inside the vertebral column and expands into

FIGURE 13.3
Muscles of the body, anterior aspect.

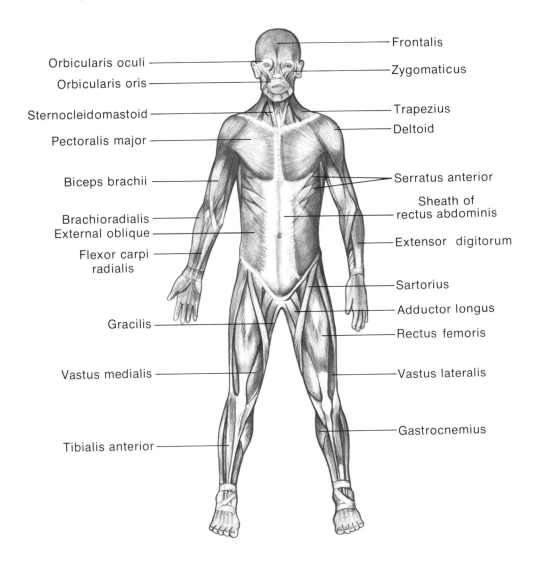

Orbicularis oculi

Orbicularis oris

Sternocleidomastoid

Pectoralis major

Biceps brachii

Brachioradialis

External oblique

Flexor carpi radialis

Gracilis

Vastus medialis

Tibialis anterior

Frontalis

Zygomaticus

Trapezius

Deltoid

Serratus anterior

Sheath of rectus abdominis

Extensor digitorum

Sartorius

Adductor longus

Rectus femoris

Vastus lateralis

Gastrocnemius

the brain. Communicating centers within the CNS and various nerve tracts make possible the appropriate response to sensory stimulus. The PNS is a network of nerves and sense organs that gathers information from the rest of the body and feeds it into the brain. For convenience, peripheral efferent nerve fibers distributed to smooth muscle, cardiac muscle, and glands are referred to as the autonomic nervous system (ANS).

The Neuron

The basic unit of nervous tissue is the nerve cell or *neuron* (Figure 13.4). Neurons are composed of a cell body containing a large nucleus with one or more nucleoli, mitochondria, Golgi apparatus, Nissl bodies (associated with the conduction of a nerve impulse), and numerous ribosomes. Extending from this cell body are two types of threadlike projections of cytoplasm, the

FIGURE 13.4

The structure of a neuron. **a,** Monopolar sensory neuron. **b,** Bipolar retinal neuron in the eye. **c,** Multipolar motor neuron, showing a muscle-nerve synapse. **d,** Structure of a typical nerve. **e,** An enlarged extension of an axon, showing its protective myelin sheath and neurilemma.

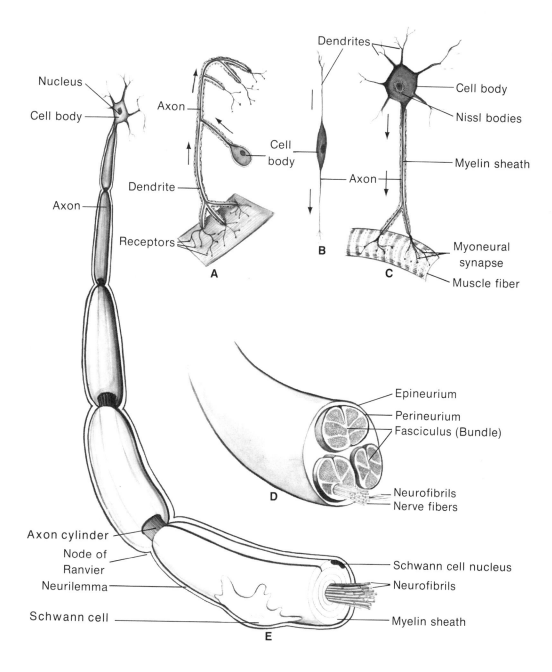

nerve fibers: dendrites, which conduct impulses to the cell body, and *axons,* which conduct impulses away from the cell body.

Types of Neurons

Neurons are classified according to their function as follows:

1. *Motor neurons.* These pass messages from centers in the brain and spinal cord to effector organs such as muscles and glands.
2. *Association (interneuron) neurons.* Also called *internuncial* or *intercalated neurons,* these relay messages between neurons within the brain and spinal cord.
3. *Sensory neurons.* These receive messages from the environment and pass them to centers in the brain and spinal cord.

The Brain

Divisions of the Brain

From a developmental standpoint the brain can be divided into three large areas: the forebrain, the midbrain, and the hindbrain. These areas can be further subdivided as shown in the following outline:

   I. Forebrain (prosencephalon)
     A. Telencephalon (cerebrum)
       1. Cerebral cortex (gray matter) ·
       2. White matter (core)
     B. Diencephalon
       1. Thalamus
       2. Hypothalamus
  II. Midbrain (mesencephalon)
     A. Corpora quadrigemina
     B. Cerebral peduncles
 III. Hindbrain (rhombencephalon)
     A. Pons
     B. Medulla
     C. Cerebellum

The largest part of the brain is the cerebrum, which is divided into the right and left cerebral hemispheres. The brain stem is the lower stem-like portion of the brain connecting the cerebral hemispheres with the spinal cord. It comprises, from the top down, the diencephalon, midbrain, pons, and medulla. The midbrain contains a massive number of cerebral nerve fibers. Below, it is connected with the pons, which is connected with the medulla. Finally, the medulla connects with the spinal cord through a large opening in the base of the skull (Figure 13.5).

Next in size to the cerebral hemisphere is the cerebellum, which is behind the brain stem. It is connected with the pons, medulla, and midbrain by the three *cerebellar preduncles.* Collectively, the cerebellum, pons, and medulla make up the major parts of the hindbrain.

The cerebrum

The cerebrum, the largest part of the human brain, accounts for up to four fifths of the brain's total mass and weight (see Figure 13.5). It fills the entire upper portion of the cranial cavity and contains billions of neurons and synapses. These form a network of pathways. The outer nerve tissue of the cerebral hemispheres is gray matter and is called the *cerebral cortex.* This gray matter is arranged in folds or convolutions *(gyri),* separated by depressions *(sulci)* or deep grooves called *fissures.* The cerebral hemispheres are largely white matter with a few areas of gray matter.

Thalamus

The thalamus is a large oval structure of gray matter; it bounds the third ventricle. It receives all sensory impulses, either directly or indirectly, from all parts of the body. Some of the impulses are associated, some are sorted out, and others are relayed to specific areas of the cerebral cortex. The thalamus is a sensory integrating center where malaise, crude touch, pain, and temperature are interpreted. For this reason it is believed to be a center for primitive, crude sensation. In addition, the thalamus is connected with the motor system and can expedite or inhibit motor impulses from the cerebral cortex.

Hypothalamus

The hypothalamus is the principal center integrating the autonomic or peripheral functions.

FIGURE 13.5

Left side of the brain, showing the cerebrum, cerebellum, pons, medulla, and spinal cord.

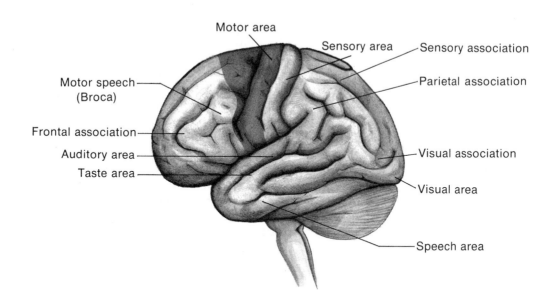

It is directly below the thalamus and forms the floor of the third ventricle.

The hypothalamus is part of an extensive system that regulates food and water intake. Research on animals shows that the hypothalamus's drinking center is lateral and its appetite center is medial.

Research supports the belief that the hypothalamus has two sets of centers: medial centers that are inhibitory and lateral centers that are stimulatory of food intake. Theories for faulty appetite regulation and obesity propose the following causes: (1) a hypothalamic center that does not respond normally to normal impulses; (2) a normal hypothalamic center subjected to abnormal stimuli from other parts of the brain; (3) metabolic abnormalities resulting in a disturbance of factors participating in the homeostatic regulation of appetite.

The neurotransmitters epinephrine, norepinephrine, serotonin, and dopamine, which are found in the hypothalamus, have all been implicated in the control of appetite. Several researchers have reported that norepinephrine in-jected directly into animals' brains causes animals to overeat and serotonin injections cause the animals to undereat.

Cerebellum

The cerebellum occupies the lower and posterior part of the skull cavity (see Figure 13.5). It lies below the posterior portion of the cerebrum and behind the pons and the upper part of the medulla. The cerebellum is oval and constricted in the center. When cut in two, it resembles a tree, and thus sometimes has been called the *arbor vitae*, the tree of life. Like the cerebrum, it has a cortex of gray matter and an interior of gray and white matter.

The cerebellum is made up mainly of masses of nerve tissue called *peduncles*. These are pathways between the cerebellum and the rest of the central nervous system. The cerebellum is a reflex center through which coordination and refinement of muscular movement are brought about. Coordination of impulses from sensory organs and muscle contractions facilitates equilibrium. It is believed that motion sickness is partly due to a disorganization of the part of the cerebellum that coordinates posture and balance through the medulla. Damage to the cerebellum leads to jerkiness of voluntary movements and poor balance.

Medulla

The medulla (sometimes incorrectly called the "spinal bulb") is continuous with the spinal cord and together with the pons is a major component of the reticular formation of nerves that constitutes the upper part of the extrapyramidal pathway (see Figure 13.5).

Reflex activities such as sneezing, coughing, vomiting, and alimentary tract movements, as well as the major system reflex controls, make the medulla the vital reflex center of the body.

The Involuntary Nervous System

The organism becomes aware of changes in its external environment through external receptors such as the eyes and ears, and it uses its skeletal muscles to adapt to these changes. In like manner, internal receptors signal information about the state of the internal environment.

Although the internal organs, such as the heart, lungs, and stomach, contain sensory nerve endings and nerve fibers for conducting sensory messages to the brain and spinal cord, most of these impulses do not reach the consciousness. Sensory neurons from the organs are grouped with those that come from the skin and voluntary muscles. On the other hand, the efferent motor neurons that supply the glands and the involuntary, or smooth, muscles are arranged very differently from those that supply the voluntary muscles. This variation in location and arrangement of the visceral efferent neurons has led to their being classified as part of a separate division—the *autonomic nervous system*.

Functions of the Autonomic Nervous System

The sympathetic and parasympathetic nervous systems are *antagonistic*. This means that the nerves from the two divisions can produce op-

posite effects. However, they also provide a correlated adjustment to meet any physiological demand. Generally, the effects of parasympathetic stimulation are most obvious during calm and rest. For example, fibers in the oculomotor nerve stimulate the smooth circular muscle of the iris, protecting the eye from excess light; fibers in the facial nerve stimulate the secretion of saliva, aiding digestion. Digestion is most suitably carried out during rest, and it is aided further by the vagus parasympathetic fibers, which stimulate secretion of digestive juices and increase the activity of the smooth muscle of the digestive tract. Other vagus nerve fibers decrease the rate and force of the heart beat during rest—a reasonable adjustment inasmuch as the skeletal muscles are inactive and the body's requirement for blood is lower at that time.

In summary, the functions of the *parasympathetic* division are conservative. Narrowing the pupil to protect the eye from excessive light; promoting the digestive processes in a restful environment; slowing the heartbeat to allow the heart muscle and the skeletal muscles to recover their tone; and emptying the bowel and bladder to remove the body's waste materials: these are a few of the many ways the parasympathetic division contributes to the maintenance of the constant internal environment.

The *sympathetic* division is greatly influenced by changes in the environment. It acts to prepare the body for stressful situations and has effects mainly opposite to those of the parasympathetic division. These are commonly referred to as "fight or flight." Fear, pain, anger, and other forms of emotion are a strong influence on the sympathetic system. This effect is made even more general because sympathetic preganglionic fibers innervate the adrenal gland, which secretes the hormone epinephrine into the circulation. Epinephrine and norepinephrine have a stimulating effect. For this reason, the sympathetic division might be called the emergency system, since it prepares us to remain and fight or to take flight.

To prepare the body for stress the sympathetic division produces effects primarily opposite to those noted for the parasympathetic chain. Sympathetic fibers innervate the smooth muscles of the eye that contract and increase the size of the pupil, thus increasing its sensitivity in dim light. Muscular exertions require an increased blood supply, and this is accomplished by sympathetic impulses that stimulate the smooth muscles of tiny blood vessels within the digestive tract, cutting down the flow of blood to the stomach and intestine and increasing the blood flow to skeletal muscle. This augmented blood supply is also aided by cervical sympathetic impulses that cause an increase in the rate and force of the heartbeat.

Whether you are standing, sitting, sleeping, eating, digesting food, or eliminating wastes, your nervous system activates the organs required for the activity. Suppose you have just finished eating and are doing nothing more than sitting on the beach watching the surf crash on the beach. Messages flow along parasympathetic nerves, stimulating into action all body parts that function in digestion. At this time, sympathetic nerves of the digestive system are relatively inactive. Blood vessels supplying your digestive tract are wide open, but those supplying limb muscles and kidney tissue are constricted. Suppose you decide to go swimming before giving your system enough time to digest the food. The strong stimulus triggers chemical messages that race through your body, inhibit parasympathetic nerves, and excite sympathetic nerves. Digestion stops; your skeletal muscles quiver with the excitement of fresh forced blood, and you race into the water. As you exert your skeletal muscles while swimming, your smooth muscles lining the digestive tract remain inactive, allowing the partially digested food to remain stationary causing cramps. Only when you stop swimming and begin resting again do the antagonistic pathways shift priorities, so that digestion resumes and the cramp goes away.

The ANS is under the influence of the CNS at all times, especially certain higher centers of the cerebral cortex, thalamus, hypothalamus, medulla, and spinal cord. Afferent impulses keep these centers informed as to the physiological state of the body and its parts, and efferent impulses are sent from them to the autonomic system to make adjustments as required to maintain the homeostatic state.

Sensory Mechanisms

A *sense organ*, or receptor, is a specialized nervous tissue situated at the peripheral endings of the dendrites of afferent neurons. The receptor's primary function is to provide the body with information, both conscious and unconscious, about degrees of change in the organisms's external and internal environments.

Classification of sense organs

Many have tried to classify the senses into groups, but no one has been entirely successful. Traditionally, the special senses are smell, vision, hearing, equilibrium, and taste; the cutaneous senses are those associated with receptors in the skin; and the visceral senses perceive the body's internal condition.

Different sensations are evoked by stimulation of various specialized sensory receptors. Some of these may be grouped according to the nature of the stimulus:

- *Chemoreceptors:* sensitive to chemical stimuli (necessary for taste and smell)
- *Pressoreceptors:* sensitive to mechanical stimuli (necessary for touch, pain, temperature, pressure, sound, and motion)
- *Photoreceptors:* sensitive to visible light (necessary for sight)

Another classification of the receptors categorizes them according to their somatic or visceral locations:

- *Teleceptors:* detect environmental changes occurring some distance from the body (for example, light rays, sound waves, and odors are detected by teleceptors of the eye, ear, and nose)
- *Exteroceptors:* detect the environmental changes that directly affect the skin (temperature, touch, pressure, or pain)
- *Proprioceptors:* provide the body with information about its position in space (muscles, tendons, and joints)
- *Interoceptors:* maintain the environment within the organs (smooth muscle contraction, peristalsis, visceral contractions)

FIGURE 13.6

Cutaneous senses. Various types of exteroceptors and their sensations found in the skin.

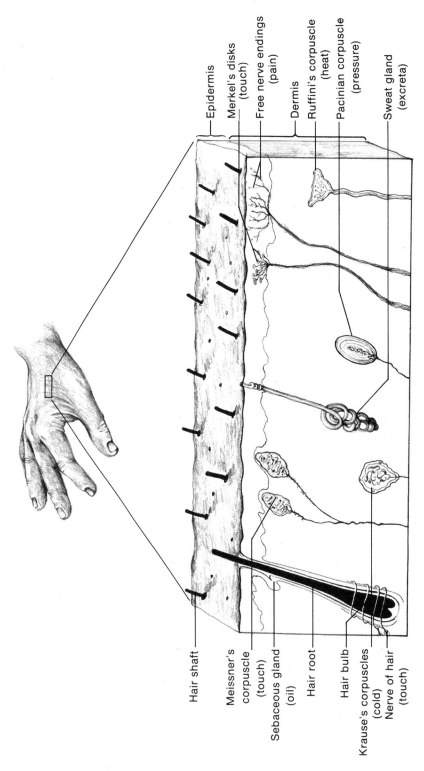

Cutaneous Senses

Touch, pressure, heat, cold, and pain are the cutaneous senses.

Touch and pressure

At least four kinds of receptors—free nerve endings, Meissner's tactile corpuscles, Pacinian corpuscles, and nerve fibers at the base of each hair—give rise to touch sensations (Figure 13.6). The hair nerve ending is stimulated by a change of position of the hair; Meissner's and Pacinian corpuscles sense a quick touch or deformation of tissue, but not a sustained touch. Free nerve endings adapt slowly to continuous stimulation.

Position Sense

Receptors in muscles, tendons, and joints relay impulses that help us judge the position and changes in location of body parts in relation to one another (Figure 13.7). They also inform the brain of the extent of muscle contraction and tendon tension. These widely spread end-organs—proprioceptors—are aided in their function by the semicircular canals of the inner ear.

This sense of position, also called the *kinesthetic sense,* enables us to know the positions of various body parts without actually seeing them. Information from the proprioceptors is needed for the coordination of muscles and is important in everyday activities, such as walking and running, and in more complex skilled movements, such as playing a musical instrument. These muscle sense end-organs (Ruffini's end-organ and Golgi's tendon organ) also play an important part in maintaining muscle tone and posture.

Hunger and Thirst

Hunger and thirst are organic sensations that follow the law of projection. The feeling of hunger is projected to the stomach; the feeling of thirst is projected primarily to the throat (pharynx).

Hunger

The feeling commonly called hunger occurs normally before meals and presumably is due to contractions of the empty stomach that stimulate receptors distributed throughout the organ's

FIGURE 13.7
Proprioceptors in skeletal muscle.

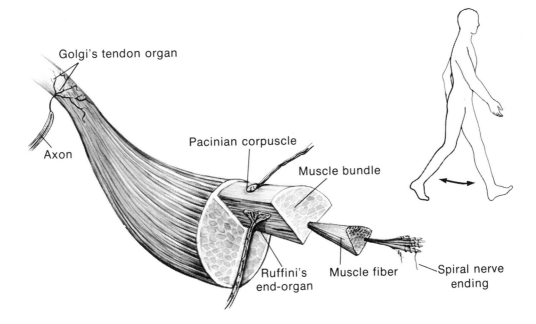

Golgi's tendon organ

Axon

Pacinian corpuscle

Muscle bundle

Ruffini's end-organ

Muscle fiber

Spiral nerve ending

mucous membrane. If food is not taken, hunger increases in intensity for a time and is likely to cause headaches, nausea, and overall weakness. The cliche "never make a decision on an empty stomach" is based on the fact that a hungry individual can become quite excitable.

Appetite differs from hunger. Although it is a desire for food, it often has no relationship to a need for food. Appetite is also a pleasant sensation; conversely, hunger is disagreeable. A loss of appetite is known as *anorexia* and may arise from a great variety of physical and mental disorders.

Thirst

Although thirst may reflect a generalized lack of water in the tissues, the sense of thirst is largely in the mouth, tongue, and pharynx. It is very unpleasant and is continuous until relieved or until death. An excessive excretion of water, as in diabetes, may provoke excessive thirst, called *polydipsia*. The condition in which the tissues lack water is dehydration.

Visceral afferent impulses concerned with the organic sensations of hunger and thirst are conducted to the hypothalamus, where appetite is regulated. The location of the nerve receptors that transmit hunger and thirst impulses is still unknown. They are probably in the muscles lining each respective organ.

Taste and Smell

Taste and smell are considered to be chemical sensations because the taste buds and olfactory receptors respond to substances dissolved in fluids secreted by the oral and nasal epithelial tissues.

Taste

The sense of taste (*gustation*) involves receptors in the tongue and three different nerves that carry taste impulses to the brain. The taste receptors, called *taste buds,* are along the edges of small depressed fissures separating the papillae of the tongue (Figure 13.8). These papillae vary in shape: pointed at the front of the tongue and fat at its base. The papillae give the tongue its characteristic rough appearance. All papillae contain taste buds.

There are essentially four kinds of taste (Figure 13.9):

- *Sweet:* acutely experienced at the tip of the tongue
- *Sour:* detected at the sides of the tongue
- *Salty:* felt at the tip of the tongue and along its sides
- *Bitter:* detected at the back of the tongue

To be tasted, substances must be in solution. At the top of each bud an opening called the taste pore admits materials dissolved in saliva, which stimulate the receptors.

Although the taste buds are structurally alike, they are physiologically different in sensitivity. Bitterness can be detected in a dilution of $1:2,000,000$; sweetness, $1:250$; sourness, $1:135,000$; and saltiness, $1:500$. Sourness is a response to acids and is the most specific of the four taste sensations. Taste sensations other than the basic four are a result of a blending of the fundamental sensations with one another and with odors.

Smell

The olfactory receptors lie in the mucous membrane lining the upper part of the nasal cavity. A layer of mucus secreted by the surrounding supporting cells covers the epithelium and dissolves and absorbs gaseous particles in inspired air (Figure 13.9). Only volatile substances in solution can stimulate the receptors of smell. The amount of air reaching the olfactory region is greatly increased by sniffing, a semireflexive response that usually occurs when a new odor attracts attention.

The human sense of taste depends a great deal on their sense of smell. If you block your nose or have a severe cold, your food is tasteless. This phenomenon is due to the gustatory nerve, which blends sensations of smell and taste. It also creates the strange feeling that you are able to taste something you actually are smelling. For example, if you enter a room that has been perfumed, you can taste sweetness by breathing in the odor. The smell of cooked cabbage can almost be tasted. A principal characteristic of smell is that only a minute quantity of the stimulating

FIGURE 13.8

Taste. **a,** Regions of the tongue that are most sensitive to the various tastes. The tongue appears rough owing to the three types of papillae **b,** that contain the taste (gustatory) cells or buds **c,** embedded deep within each furrow.

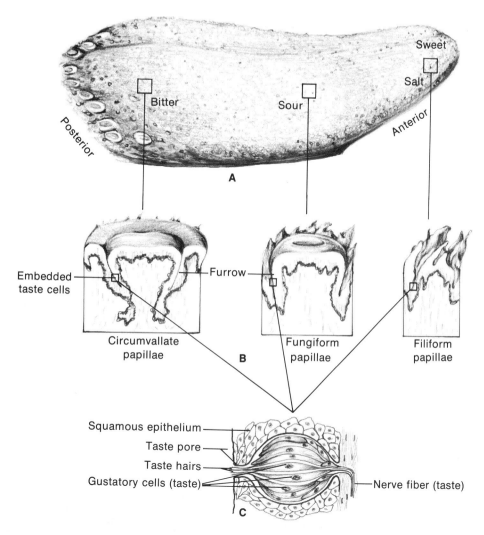

agent in the air is required to evoke the sensation.

Vision

Vision is usually considered the most important of all the senses. Blind people learn to depend on their other senses to a remarkable degree, but nothing approaches complete compensation for loss of vision. Fundamentally, the sense of vision is similar to all the other senses in that there are receptors (sensitive to light), an afferent pathway (optic nerve) that conveys the impulses to the cerebral cortex, and an area (occipital lobe) of the cerebrum necessary for interpretation of these impulses. But vision is far more complex than such senses as hunger and thirst, and therefore it is necessary to consider

FIGURE 13.9

Smell. **a,** Olfactory receptive area in the roof of the nasal cavity, showing the gross relationship of the olfactory nerves to the mucous membrane. **b,** A microscopic sketch of a supporting mucous cell surrounded by olfactory cells that collectively form the olfactory nerve.

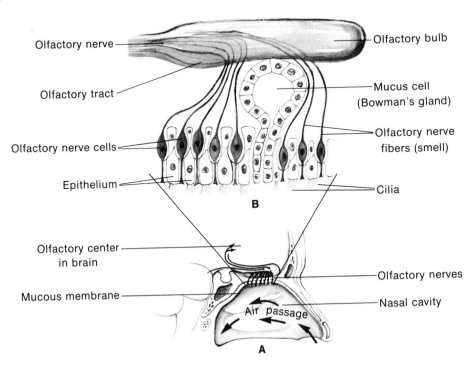

the physics, anatomy, physiology, and biochemistry of sight.

Accessory organs of the eye

The accessory organs of the eye include the eyebrows, eyelids, conjunctiva, lacrimal apparatus, and muscles of the eyeball.

The *eyebrows* are thickened ridges of skin covered with short hairs. They are positioned on the upper border of the orbit of the eye and protect the eye from strong light, foreign materials, perspiration, and so forth.

The *eyelids* are movable folds of skin in front of the eyeball that can cover it. They are lined internally with a mucous membrane, the *conjunctiva*, which begins at the lower edge of the upper lid, progresses down over the eyeball, and ends at the upper edge of the lower lid (see Figure 13.10). A small muscle is attached to the upper lid and elevates it. The orbicularis oculi is a sphincter muscle that lies around both lids and opens and closes them. Eyelids protect the eye and spread its lubricating secretions (tears) over the surface of the eyeball.

The conjunctiva, which lines the eyelids and is reflected onto the surface of the eyeball, is kept moist by tears flowing across the eye. Inflammation of this membrane is called *conjunctivitis* and may be acute or chronic.

The eyelids bear rows of short, thick hairs, the eyelashes. The follicles of these hairs receive a lubricating fluid from sebaceous glands that open into them. The glandular secretions lubricate the edges of the eyelid and prevent adhesion of the two lids. If the glands become infected, a

FIGURE 13.10
Structure of the eye, transverse section.

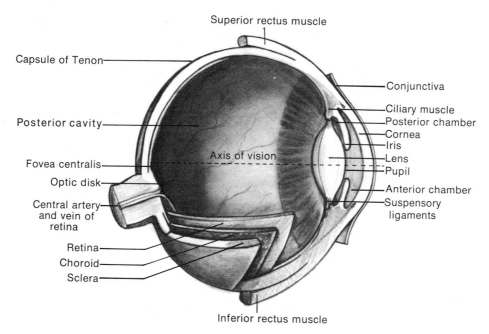

Superior rectus muscle

Capsule of Tenon

Conjunctiva
Ciliary muscle
Posterior chamber
Cornea
Iris

Posterior cavity

Axis of vision

Lens
Pupil

Fovea centralis

Optic disk

Anterior chamber
Suspensory ligaments

Central artery and vein of retina

Retina
Choroid
Sclera

Inferior rectus muscle

stye results. Distention of a sebaceous gland is called a *chalazion*.

Anatomy of the eyeball

The eyeball has three layers of tissue (Figure 13.10): sclera, choroid, and retina. The *sclera*, the opaque white outer layer of tough, fibrous tissue, gives shape to the eyeball and protects its delicate inner layers. The most anterior or forward continuation of the sclera is the transparent *cornea*. The sclera and cornea are fibrous connective tissue and lack blood vessels and nerves—a fact essential for transplants.

The transparent and colorless cornea is referred to as the "window" of the eye. It bulges forward slightly and is the eye's most important refracting structure. Injuries caused by foreign objects or infection may result in scar formation and a slight opacity through which light rays cannot pass. Because the cornea is free of blood and nerves, it is one of the parts of the eyeball that can be transplanted (keratoplasty). Eye banks arrange for cornea transplants from do-

nors to recipients who are blind because of a corneal defect. The transplant should be performed within 72 hours after the death of the donor. The operation has been remarkably successful.

The middle layer of the eye contains primarily the choroid, which is highly vascular and resembles skin. Its principal function is to supply blood to the other layers of the eyeball, especially the innermost retina. The forward extension of the choroid is a thin muscular layer, the *iris* (Figure 13.10), or colored part of the eyeball; an opening at its center allows light to pass. This circular opening is the *pupil*.

The function of the *iris* is to regulate the amount of light entering the eye. This is accomplished by its smooth muscles, which contract or dilate, causing the pupil to become larger or smaller. The larger the pupil, the more light reaches the inner eye. This mechanism is a reflex that allows the eye to adjust to changes in light intensity, a property called *adaptation* (light reflex). When in a dimly lit room, the pupils dilate to permit as much light as possible to reach the retina. When a light is turned on in the room, the pupils automatically contract to protect the retina against damage from too much light.

Homatropine, a drug used in eye examinations, epinephrine, atropine, and cocaine all make the pupil larger. Such drugs are called *mydriatics*. Pilocarpine and morphine cause the pupil to contract; such agents are *miotics*.

The *ciliary muscles,* which support and modify the shape of the lens, are another anterior modification of the choroid layer. The *lens,* a flexible, transparent, colorless body, consists of a more or less semisolid substance enveloped by a thin capsule. It is biconvex (thicker in the middle), and this property serves to converge light rays and focus them on the retina. During youth the lens is elastic and plays an important role in the eye's ability to focus on near objects. With aging, the lens loses its elasticity and therefore its ability to adjust by thickening, resulting in a condition known as *presbyopia.*

The third and innermost layer of the eyeball is the all-important *retina.* The word retina means net, and that accurately describes the network of highly specialized nerve cells, called *rods* and *cones* and their processes. Each eye has approximately 110,000,000 such photoreceptors. The image is focused on this layer, the receptors are activated, and the impulses are transmitted via the optic (second cranial) nerve to the occipital lobe of the cortex.

Figure 13.10 shows two spaces, one between the cornea and lens and another between the lens and retina. The more anterior cavity is the *anterior chamber,* which contains a watery fluid, the *aqueous humor.* Aqueous humor fills much of the eyeball in front of the lens and is continually produced by the ciliary body in the anterior and posterior chambers behind the iris and absorbed by the choroid blood capillaries in the anterior chamber through the canals of Schlemm. This is a matter of physiological importance because blockage of these canals can result in a buildup of fluid in the anterior chamber, producing increased pressure on both the cornea and lens. Continued high pressure on the lens can cause premature hardening and opacity of the lens, a disorder called *glaucoma.*

Hearing and Equilibrium

The ear contains receptors for two sensations, hearing and equilibrium. The external ear, middle ear, and cochlea of the inner ear are concerned with hearing (Figure 13.11). The semicircular canals, utricle, and saccule of the inner ear are concerned with equilibrium (Figure 13.12).

External ear

The external ear, which receives sound waves, consists of an expanded portion, the *pinna,* and the external auditory canal. The *pinna* (or *auricle*) projects from the side of the head as a framework of cartilage covered with skin and joined to the surrounding parts by ligaments and muscles (see Figure 13.11). It is irregular in shape and serves to collect sound waves and direct them toward the external auditory meatus. Although considered cosmetically unattractive, a projected or flapping ear is actually much more effective in trapping sound waves than is an ear set very close to the head.

The *external auditory meatus* is the opening of the auditory canal, a tubular passage about 1.5 inches long. It leads from the pinna to the inner eardrum, forming an S-curve as it progresses inward. Lifting the pinna upward and backward tends to straighten the canal during an examination with an otoscope. The external portion of the auditory canal consists of cartilage; the inner portion is hollowed out of the temporal bone. The canal is lined with skin bearing hairs and with ceruminous glands that secrete the yellow, pasty *cerumen* commonly called earwax. Cerumen acts as protective agent, but excessive amounts may block the ear canal and exert undue pressure on the eardrum, causing earaches. The hairs of the canal protect the ear from foreign substances.

Middle ear

The *tympanic membrane* (eardrum) separates the auditory canal from the tympanic cavity of the middle ear (see Figure 13.11). The eardrum is a thin layer of fibrous tissue covered externally with skin and internally with mucous membrane. The eardrum is attached so that it can vibrate freely when sound waves enter the auditory canal.

FIGURE 13.11

Frontal diagram of the outer ear, middle ear, and internal ear. A section of the cochlear duct has been cut away to show the position of the organ of Corti.

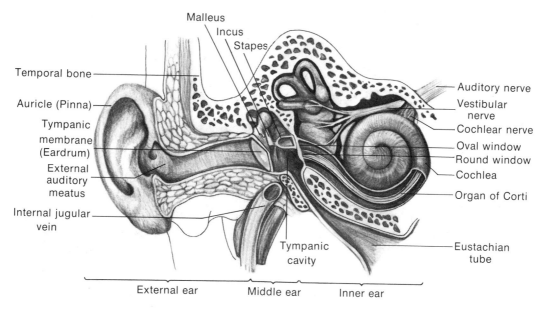

FIGURE 13.12

Cross section through the cochlea showing the relationship between the membranous and bony labyrinths and the structures concerned with balance.

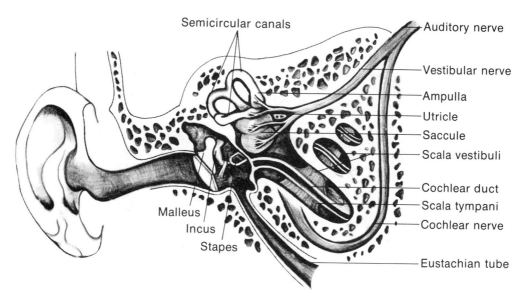

The tympanic cavity is a small, irregular bony cavity in the temporal bone. It is separated from the auditory canal by the eardrum and from the inner ear by two small openings, the *oval window* and the *round window*. In the round window there is an opening into the mastoid process; through this, an infection of the middle ear may extend into the mastoid cells, causing *mastoiditis*.

The middle ear cavity is filled with air that reaches it from the upper part of the throat (nasopharynx) by way of the *Eustachian tube*. The walls of the cavity are lined with a mucous membrane continuous with that of the nasopharynx. Thus it is possible for infection to spread from the nose or throat to the middle ear *(otitis media)*. Accumulations of pus in the middle ear can cause increased pressure on the eardrum. In this case, the membrane should be lanced (myringotomy) to drain the ear and to prevent further problems.

The Eustachian tube equalizes the air pressure of the middle ear with atmospheric pressure. If inflamed, the tube may become blocked and prevent this equalization; hearing is impaired, and permanent damage may result if the inflammation is not relieved. The pharyngeal opening of the tube is closed except during swallowing, yawning, and sneezing. It tends to remain closed when the external pressure is greater. Sudden changes in pressure exerted on the tympanic membrane by loud explosions or rapid falling, as in an airplane's descent, may rupture the membrane. This often may be prevented by swallowing or yawning, which will open the Eustachian tube and balance the pressure. Divers must be examined regularly to prevent ear damage that may result from prolonged intervals spent deep under the water; a diver with a blocked Eustachian tube due to a cold, for example, may easily suffer ruptured eardrums.

Stretching across the cavity of the middle ear from the *tympanic membrane* to the oval window are three tiny, movable bones or *ossicles* named according to their shapes—the *malleus* (hammer); the *incus* (anvil); and the *stapes* (stirrup) (see Figure 13.12). The handle of the malleus is attached to the tympanic membrane; its head is attached to the incus. The long process of the incus is attached to the stapes, and the footpiece of the stapes fits into the oval window. These bones transmit sound waves from the outer ear to the inner ear. They are attached freely to one another by ligaments and are set in motion by any movement of the tympanic membrane. The bones of the middle ear form a series of levers, the effect of which magnifies the force of sound vibrations to about ten times that at the oval window.

Inflammation of the joints between the ossicles may prevent normal vibration and amplification of sound waves. *Otosclerosis* is a type of deafness found in adults, more frequently in women. Bone changes (fusion of the joints) prevent normal vibration of the third ossicle (stapes). An operation to release the stapes so that it will move again has had considerable success.

Inner ear

The inner ear contains receptors for hearing and for position sense. It consists of a bony labyrinth enclosing a membranous labyrinth. The *bony labyrinth* is a series of channels in the temporal bone filled with a fluid called *perilymph*. The inner *membranous labyrinth* more or less duplicates the shape of the bone channels and is filled with a fluid called *endolymph*. There is no communication between the spaces filled with perilymph and endolymph.

The cochlea, a portion of the labyrinth about 1.5 inches long, is a coiled tube resembling a snail shell. The cochlea is divided into three spiral membranous channels that run the full length of the organ.

The actual receptors for hearing are in the cochlear duct. They are several rows of specialized *hair cells,* approximately 20,000 in number. These bear cilia that project into the endolymph from the free end of each cell. The hair cells, supporting cells, and nerves constitute the organ of Corti, which rests on the basilar membrane within the cochlear duct.

Physiology of hearing

Hearing depends on a succession of events. The first is entry of sound waves into the external auditory canal, which causes the tympanic membrane to vibrate. These vibrations are transmitted mechanically by the malleus, incus, and stapes of the middle ear to the oval window at the entrance to the inner ear. The vibrations of the oval window set up pressure waves in the perilymph of the vestibular and tympanic channels. These pressure waves are transmitted through the basilar membrane to the endolymph of the cochlear duct, where the hair cells of the organ of Corti are stimulated. The resulting stimulation of the hair cells arouses nerve impulses that are transmitted by the cochlear nerve to the hearing center in the temporal lobe of the cerebral cortex. This process suggests that a certain portion of the basilar membrane and certain hair cells are affected by sound waves of one frequency. Waves of a different frequency set up vibrations in another portion of the basilar membrane.

According to the just-described place theory of hearing, age and other factors determine the range of hearing among individuals. The human ear can detect sounds ranging in frequency from 20 to 20,000 cycles per second; sounds below or above this range are not heard. The squeaking of a mouse is higher than 20,000 cycles per second. We do not hear it, but the cat does. A dog whistle can be made to produce sounds higher than our hearing capacity. The dog's hearing range goes as high as 24,000 cycles per second; therefore, when we blow the whistle, the dog hears it and we don't.

Equilibrium

In addition to the cochlea, the inner ear contains three organs—the utricle, saccule, and semicircular canals—that play a major role in the sense of equilibrium or balance (see Figures 13.12 and 13.13).

The *vestibule* is a chamber containing the first two membranous sacs, the *utricle* and the *saccule*, each of which is filled with endolymph and is concerned with static equilibrium. Within the walls of these two sacs are special thickenings, or *maculae*, containing receptor hair cells and nerve endings that project into the overlying endolymph. Enmeshed in the hairs are tiny particles of calcium carbonate called *otoliths* or ear stones (Figure 13.13). Any changes in position of the head or body that cause the otoliths to bend in the direction of the pull of gravity initiate nerve impulses that travel to the brain via the vestibular nerve (Figures 13.11 and 13.13). The vestibular nerve joins the acoustic nerve to form the eighth cranial nerve.

The three semicircular canals are hollow tubes containing endolymph. These are the organs of dynamic equilibrium. They are arranged at right angles to one another so that all three planes of space are represented (Figures 13.11 and 13.13). One end of each canal is enlarged into a swelling called the *ampulla*. Within each ampulla is a small cluster of hair cells and nerve endings that project into the endolymph. Movement of the hair cells sets up impulses in the vestibular nerve; whenever movement begins or ends, goes faster or slower, or changes direction, impulses are initiated.

A change in position of the head causes impulses from receptors in the semicircular canals and vestibule to initiate the righting reflex. Balance against gravity is thus maintained by the coordinated effective response of the antigravity muscles. The cerebellum links the impulses that arise from stimulation of the sensory nerves of the canals, joints, and so forth, and sends nerve impulses to the motor centers of the cerebrum and spinal cord.

GLANDULAR SYSTEM
Pituitary Gland

The pituitary gland, also known as the *hypophysis*, is about the size of a small marble. It is attached by a stalk to the floor of the third ventricle in the base of the brain.

Thyroid Gland

The thyroid gland is in the anterior aspect of the neck just below the larynx (voice box). It consists of right and left lateral lobes connected by an isthmus that lies upon the upper part of the trachea.

The thyroid glands secretes two types of hor-

FIGURE 13.13

Equilibrium. Diagram of the organization of the maculae and cupula of the inner ear. Both contain receptors covered by a gelatinous mass. **a,** Otoliths move in the maculae, mechanically stimulating the hair processes of the hair cells. **b,** Endolymph movement stimulates the hair cells in the cupula. Each stimulation is carried to the brain, which interprets the movement.

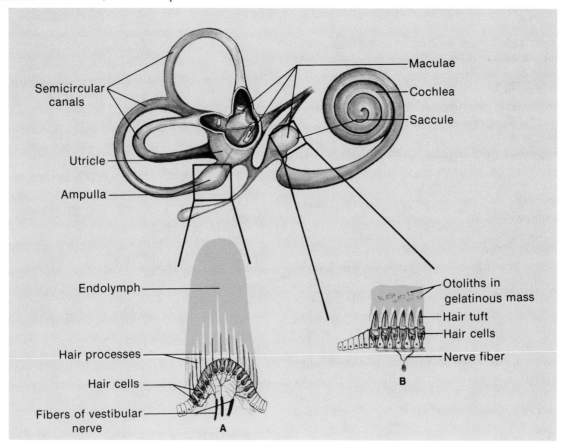

mones: (2) the modified amino acids thyroxin (T_4) and triiodothyronine (T_3), which are involved with iodine metabolism and regulation of the basal metabolic rate (BMR), and (2) calcitonin (thyrocalcitonin), a polypeptide involved in calcium metabolism.

Most of the body's iodine is obtained from the diet and appears in the blood as inorganic iodide. The vast majority of iodide is taken up by the follicles of the thyroid gland and is oxidized to iodine and combined with an amino acid tyrosine to form *thyroxin* (T_4).

The thyroid hormones regulate metabolism of the tissues by mobilizing proteins in adults and increasing protein synthesis, which favors growth in children. They also lower serum cholesterol levels and influence the action of epinephrine with regard to the breakdown of glycogen *(glycogenolysis)* and the subsequent elevation of blood glucose *(hyperglycemia)*. Thyroid hormones are also instrumental in lipid metabolism including synthesis, mobilization, and desaturation of fats. In their absence, tissue oxygen consumption falls to about half its normal resting value; conversely, an excess of hormone speeds up energy production in the cells.

The thyroid gland also produces a hypocalcemic, hypophosphatemic hormone called *calcitonin* or thyrocalcitonin (TCT), which lowers blood calcium and phosphate.

Parathyroid Glands

Two small brownish-yellow parathyroid glands lie on the capsule of the posterior aspect of each thyroid lobe. The four minute glands consist of densely packed secretory cells held in close association with capillaries by a fibrous meshwork. These glands are essential to life, for they regulate the supply, distribution, and metabolism of calcium and phosphorus in the body.

Adrenal Glands

The two adrenal (or suprarenal) glands lie one on each side, just above the kidneys and usually covered by perirenal fat. Each appears to be a compact unit but actually comprises two endocrine glands. The outer part, the *cortex*, secretes several *steroid* hormones synthesized from cholesterol; the core of the gland, the *medulla*, has an entirely separate function, the secretion of epinephrine and norepinephrine.

Adrenal Cortex

The adrenal cortex secretes so many hormones that the classical experiment of removing the glands from animals led to a bewildering series of results. In general, however, the animals showed poor performance and a low tolerance to infection, temperature changes, or any form of stress. They also suffered profound water and electrolyte disturbances. These animals usually died after a few weeks, but their life could be extended for a short time by giving them unlimited access to salt and water.

Histologically, the cortex is subdivided into three zones. The outermost zone, or *zona glomerulosa*, is responsible for the secretion of *mineralocorticoids*, principally aldosterone. The middle zone, or *zona fasciculata*, is the widest of the three zones and secretes the *glucocorticoids*. The inner zone synthesizes sex hormones.

The Adrenal Medulla

The adrenal medulla makes up the pulpy center of the gland in which groups of irregular cells are located amidst veins that collect blood from the sinusoids. This gland produces two very similar hormones, *epinephrine* (80 percent) and *norepinephrine* (20 percent), also known as adrenaline and noradrenaline, respectively. Their molecular structures are relatively simple: both are amines, and they are sometimes referred to as *catecholamines*. Both hormones elevate the blood pressure: epinephrine accelerates the heart rate, and norepinephrine acts as a vasoconstrictor. The two hormones together promote glycogenolysis (glucogenesis), the breakdown of liver glycogen to glucose, causing an increase in blood sugar concentration. Of the two, epinephrine functions most closely as the emergency hormone for the body. Its functions of increasing the blood glucose level (by glycogenolysis) and the blood flow to the skeletal muscles (vasodilation of arterioles), heart, and viscera serve to shunt or direct the circulation of blood where necessary during exertion or increased stress.

The adrenal medulla, unlike the thyroid and other endocrine glands, is not essential for life. It can be removed surgically without causing untreatable damage.

Adrenal Hormones and Stress

When an individual is under severe emotional stress, such as rage or fear, a marked excess of epinephrine is poured into the blood, enabling the person to perform feats of muscular exertion of which he would not ordinarily be capable. This has been called the emergency functions of the adrenals, or the *fight or flight response*.

Pancreas

The pancreas lies close to the posterior abdominal wall behind the stomach (see Figure 13.14). It functions as both an exocrine and endocrine gland. Its exocrine functions involve the secretion of digestive enzymes into the small intestine; this will be discussed in the chapter on metabolism and digestion. The endocrine function of the pancreas is carried on by groups of special tissue scattered throughout the pancreatic tissue called the *islets of Langerhans*. The number of cells

FIGURE 13.14
General location of the major endocrine glands of the body.

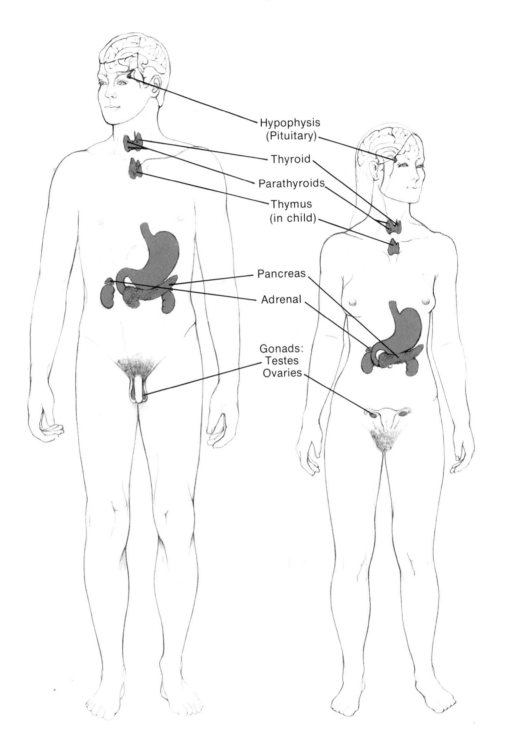

in these islets varies from several hundred thousand to a few million. Each islet consists of several types of cells; those designated as *alpha* and *beta* predominate. The hormone *insulin* is secreted by the beta cells and another hormone, *glucagon,* by the alpha cells. Both are polypeptides and can be synthesized commercially.

The earliest studies on the effect of insulin on carbohydrate metabolism showed four basic effects of the hormone:

1. Increases rate of glucose metabolism.
2. Regulates blood glucose concentration.
3. Increases glycogen storage in the tissues.
4. Promotes a positive nitrogen balance.

Ovaries and Testes

The ovaries and testes are primary sources of the sex hormones that control the maturation and function of the reproductive system (see Chapter 23).

Other Endocrine Glands

The *pineal gland* is a cone-shaped gland in the roof of the third ventricle of the brain. It is very small (5 mm long and 9 mm wide). Covered by a capsule of pia mater, it consists of parenchymal and glial cells. Although the exact function of the gland is still in doubt, some investigators believe it secretes melatonin, a polypeptide hormone that inhibits the secretion of ovarian hormones. It is functional in early childhood and is largely fibrous connective tissue in the adult. Other hormones reportedly secreted by the pineal gland are adrenoglomerulotropin, which stimulates the adrenal cortex to secrete aldosterone, and serotonin, which is a neurotransmitter. The exact nature and function of the pineal gland is still to be determined.

The *thymus gland* is in the upper mediastinum posterior to the sternum and between the lungs. The thymus, like the pineal gland, is functional before and during puberty. After puberty, the lymphocytic thymic tissue atrophies and is replaced by connective tissue. The thymus gland plays an essential role in the immune response of the body. It produces a polypeptide called *thymosin,* which plays an important part in the maturation of T-lymphocytes.

CARDIOVASCULAR SYSTEM

The cardiovascular system comprises: (a) heart, (b) arteries, (c) capillaries, (d) veins, (e) blood.

The Heart

The heart is a hollow, muscular organ that can be thought of as two separate pumps operating in parallel. The right heart receives blood from the tissues and pumps it through the pulmonary arteries to the lungs. There it passes through capillaries, where it is oxygenated and its carbon dioxide removed. The pulmonary veins return the blood to the left heart, which pumps it out again through the aorta to supply the tissues of the body.

Structure

Heart muscle, or *myocardium,* resembles voluntary skeletal muscle (Figure 13.15) in that its fibers are striated. However, in voluntary muscle, the fibers are separate; in heart muscle, which is involuntary, they are joined by side branches, and each fiber has one central nucleus.

The inner lining of the heart is called the *endocardium.* It covers all the heart's projections and irregularities and is modified to form the cardiac valves. The endocardial lining of the heart is continuous with the endothelium that lines all of the arteries, veins, and capillaries of the body. An inflammation of this lining is called *endocarditis.* This may involve the cardiac valves that have been destroyed by rheumatic fever or congenital malfunctions.

Cavities of the heart

The right and left sides of the heart are separated by a muscular partition, the *septum.* Each half is divided into an upper compartment, the

FIGURE 13.15
Diagram of the heart. Arrows indicate direction of blood flow.

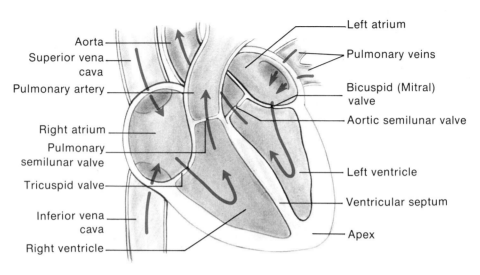

atrium, and a lower compartment, the *ventricle* (Figure 13.15). Before birth there is an opening in the partition between the atria. Soon after birth this closes, so that there is no longer any communication between the right and left sides of the heart. The partition between the atria is called the *interatrial septum;* that between the ventricles is the *interventricular septum.* Each atrium communicates with the ventricle below it on the same side by the atrioventricular orifice of the right and left atrioventricular valves.

The left ventricle ejects blood into the systemic circulatory system under higher pressure than is required of the right ventricle for ejecting blood into the pulmonary (lungs) circulation, which offers less resistance. The thicker muscle is on the left side, where it is needed in this stronger pumping action. The right and left sides of the heart contract and relax almost simultaneously.

Valves of the heart

On the right, the atrioventricular (AV) valve is composed of three irregularly shaped flaps or cusps and is called the *tricuspid valve* (Figure 13.15). The flaps are formed mainly of fibrous

connective tissue covered by endocardium. Their pointed ends project down into the ventricle and are attached to the tips of the papillary muscles by fibrous cords, the *chordae tendineae.* These muscles contract when the ventricular walls contract, preventing the flaps from being pushed back into the atria by the force of blood ejected from the ventricle.

The left AV valve, which bears two flaps or cusps, is called the *bicuspid* or *mitral valve* (Figure 13.15). It is attached in the same manner as the tricuspid valve, which it resembles closely. However, it is much stronger and thicker in all parts. The object of both valves is to allow blood to flow freely from the atria to the ventricles but to prevent its flow in the other direction.

The Cardiac Cycle

The task of the heart is to propel blood to all parts of the body. In doing this, it pumps in definite strokes or beats. In the healthy adult these occur on the average about seventy-two times per minute.

Heartbeats may be felt by placing the hand over the region of the apex of the heart, the *precordium,* in the area just under the left breast about 3½ inches from the sternum. The sensation felt is one of bumping or thrusting, each thrust corresponding to a contraction of the heart.

The series of actions the heart performs is spoken of as its cycle. Starting with any one of the separate actions or movements of the heart, the sequence of events that follows until the original action repeats itself constitutes a complete cardiac cycle. The contraction of the heart is called *systole;* its relaxation is called *diastole.*

For convenience, we can consider the events of the heartbeat starting from diastole, when the heart is relaxed and relatively flaccid. Venous blood from the superior and inferior venae cavae enters the right atrium; at the same time, oxygenated blood from the pulmonary veins returns to the left atrium. Meanwhile, the valves between the atria and the ventricles on each side are open so that the blood can flow through the atria and into the ventricles. The combination of the mild muscular contraction of the atria and the increased pressure of the full atrial chambers ultimately drains the atrial blood into the ventricles.

Shortly thereafter, the ventricles contract. The rising pressure closes the AV valves (see Figure 13.15). As the pressure rises, it forces the pulmonary and aortic valves to open, so that the blood is driven out into the circulation. When contraction is completed, the ventricles relax. The blood in the aorta and pulmonary artery attempts to reflux or flow back into the ventricles. The semilunar valves of the aorta and pulmonary artery close and prevent this reverse flow. During ventricular contraction, the atria once more relax and venous blood starts to fill them. When the ventricles are completely relaxed, the tricuspid and mitral valves open again, blood flows into the ventricles, and the next cycle begins.

Heart sounds

A great deal of information is obtained by carefully listening to the heart with a stethoscope. The first heart sound is associated with the initiation of ventricular systole and the closing of the mitral and tricuspid valves. This first sound is low pitched and longer than the second sound. Both sounds can be heard over the entire area of the heart, but the first sound, "lubb," is heard most clearly in the region of the apex of the heart.

The second sound, "dupp," is sharper, shorter, and lower pitched. It is heard best over the second right rib, since here the aorta is nearest to the chest surface. The second sound is caused mainly by the closing of the semilunar valves during ventricular diastole. The momentum of the moving blood closes the valve cusps, preventing a backflow into the heart. The faint third sound sometimes may be heard following the second in early ventricular diastole. The fourth sound occurs during a trial contraction and immediately precedes the first heart sound.

Defects in the valves can cause excessive turbulence or regurgitation of the blood, resulting in abnormal sounds. Abnormal sounds are called *murmurs.*

General Circulation

The general circulation is shown diagrammatically in Figure 13.16. The heart is a muscular organ that can be thought of as two parallel pumps. The right heart receives blood from the veins draining the tissues and pumps it through the pulmonary arteries to the lungs. Here it passes through capillaries in which it is oxygenated and its carbon dioxide removed. The pulmonary veins return the blood to the left heart, which pumps it out again through the aorta, from which arise the various systemic arteries that distribute blood to the other tissues.

Thus there are two parallel circulations: the pulmonary circulation for gas exchange in the lungs and the systemic circulation for maintaining a constant internal environment in the other tissues. Note that all blood goes through first one system and then the other.

The Blood Vessels

Arteries carry blood away from the heart to the tissues: *veins* return blood from the tissues to the heart. The large arteries nearest the heart divide into smaller vessels. These divide into still

FIGURE 13.16
Diagram of general circulation.

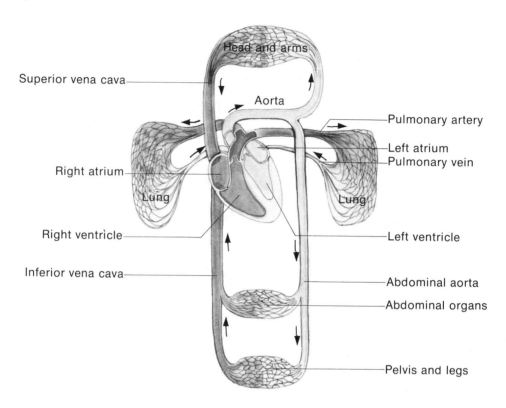

smaller ones, and so on. The smallest arteries are called *arterioles.* These lead into vessels of narrow caliber, the *capillaries.* The capillaries branch and form a network where the exchange of materials between blood and tissue fluid takes place. After passing through the capillary network, the blood is collected into the smallest veins, the *venules.* The venules unite to form small veins; these combine to make ever-larger vessels until eventually the great veins that enter the heart are reached.

The distention of the arteries during systole extends to the periphery and can be detected as a throbbing sensation, known as the *pulse,* in several arteries near the skin.

Capillaries

The walls of the capillaries consist of one layer of endothelial cells continuous with the layer that lines the arteries, veins, and heart (see

Figure 13.17). The capillaries form an interlacing network of variable size.

As noted, it is in the capillary beds that the main work of blood is done—the exchange of materials between cells and blood. A molecule diffuses through the capillary wall into the tissue fluid and from the tissue fluid into the cell, or in the reverse direction as shown in Figure 13.18. In addition to diffusion, some of the fluid part of the blood filtrates through the capillary walls, especially at the arterioles where the blood pressure is high, so that the blood continually contributes to the tissue fluid.

Blood

Functions of blood

Everything required by the tissues for energy or synthesis is carried in the blood, and all waste products derived from the tissues are re-

FIGURE 13.17

Blood vessels. Diagram showing the single-cell endothelium of all the vessels and the layered muscular coats of arteries and veins.

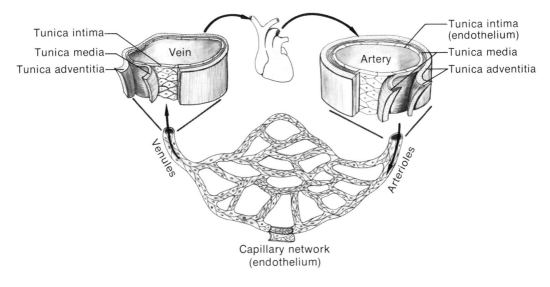

FIGURE 13.18

Diagram illustrating some of the physiological exchanges between capillaries and body cells. RBC, red blood cell.

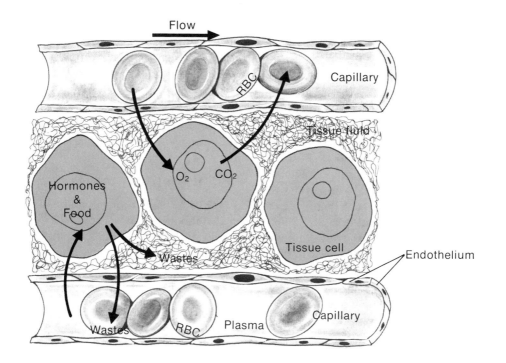

moved by the blood. Following are some of the more evident functions of blood:

1. The blood supplies the cells and tissues with oxygen and nutrients for growth, repair, and other life activities.
2. The blood transports the waste products of cellular metabolism, including carbon dioxide, to the excretory organs for elimination.
3. The white blood cells, antibodies, and other protective substances provide an important defense against damage from injury and disease.
4. The blood helps regulate and equalize body temperature by distributing heat to the body parts.
5. The blood transports hormones, the secretions of the endocrine glands, to the cells and tissues.
6. The blood plays an important role in maintaining the acid or alkaline balance of the tissues.
7. The blood can help to maintain its own volume and composition by forming a clot, reducing bleeding and preventing the escape of body fluids.
8. The blood bathes the various body cells and tissues in fluid, regulating the water and salt content of all tissues. At the same time it maintains the osmotic concentration throughout the body.

Characteristics of blood

Blood is bright red (indicating that it is well oxygenated) in the arteries and dark red (less oxygenated) in the veins. Water flows four to five times faster than blood because blood is four to five times thicker (a property called *viscosity*). Blood's specific gravity (density compared with water) varies between 1.045 and 1.065 (water is 1.0), and its temperature and pH are 38° C (100.4° F) and about 7.38, respectively. The volume of blood in the body has been measured in many ways but can be expected to vary with the size of the body. A useful estimate is that its weight is 8 percent of the body's weight. The blood volume of a man of average size is approximately 6 liters.

Seen with the naked eye, blood appears to be opaque and homogeneous, but microscopic examination reveals that it consists of cell fragments and an intercellular fluid, the plasma (Figure 13.19).

When blood is obtained from a person's vein (by venipuncture) and transferred to a test tube and clotting is prevented by adding certain chemicals called *anticoagulants*, it separates into two distinct layers. The upper layer, yellow and transparent, contains most of the chemical components of the blood in solution; this is the plasma (Figure 13.20). Plasma constitutes about 55 percent of the blood's volume. The lower portion of the blood sample consists of the formed elements: the red blood cells (erythrocytes), the white blood cells (leukocytes), and the platelets (thrombocytes). These are often called *corpuscles*, meaning little body. The percentage of total blood volume contributed by these formed elements is called the *hematocrit*.

Leukocytes

The white blood cells, the leukocytes, are concerned primarily with the body's defense against infection. Leukocytes vary in size and shape. They are less numerous than erythrocytes, numbering 5000 to 9000 per cubic millimeter. They lack hemoglobin, are colorless, contain a nucleus, and are larger than the red cells. White blood cells are extremely active and move under their own power by ameboid motion, often against the flow of the bloodstream. Unlike erythrocytes, white blood cells pass out of the bloodstream and into the intracellular spaces to consume foreign materials (such as bacteria) found between the cells.

Platelets (Thrombocytes)

Only 1 to 2 microns in diameter, the platelet or thrombocyte is not a cell in the strictest sense but a cell fragment. It is made in the bone marrow by the largest cells there, the megakaryocytes (Figure 13.19). As these huge cells mature, their nuclei become smaller and more dense and the cytoplasm becomes increasingly granular. The megakaryocyte then fragments into blood platelets that leave the bone marrow. The cytoplasm's large granules contain chemical substances that

FIGURE 13.19
Microscopic blood smear.

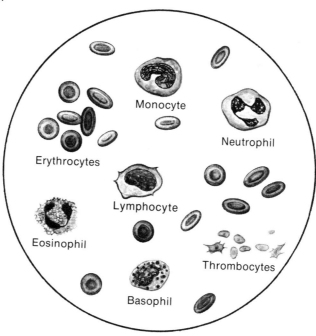

affect blood vessels and the clotting mechanism. After leaving the bone marrow, the platelet survives for about 10 days and then is cleared by the spleen. The normal platelet count is 250,000 per cubic millimeter.

FIGURE 13.20
Centrifuged whole blood, showing the relationship of the fluid portion (plasma) to the formed elements. WBC, white blood cells. RBC, red blood cells.

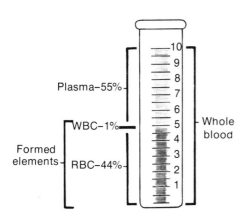

The blood platelet is vital to life. Platelets adhere to other platelets and to the inner surfaces of small blood vessels. When a blood vessel is torn or severed, platelets begin to pile up immediately, adhering to the torn surface of the vessel and to other platelets, forming a plug to slow the loss of blood. As they adhere, they release chemicals of *coagulation,* a clot begins to form behind the platelet plug. The clot ultimately enmeshes more platelets, red cells, and some white cells. A special spiral protein in the platelets contracts much like the proteins in the muscles. When the clot is big enough, the protein contracts and the clot becomes firm. This process is called *clot retraction.* The firm clot forms a bridge over which healing will take place.

Cardiovascular Response to Activity

The heart is one of the most fascinating organs of the body. One of the strongest muscles of the body, it pumps blood through the arteries to all parts of the body. Exercise and stress make the heart beat faster, increasing blood volume per minute by as much as 10 times in trained athletes. During a night's sleep, the heart does work equivalent to carrying a 30-pound pack almost to the top of the Empire State Building—not bad for an organ the size of a clenched fist.

The five quarts of blood in an average adult are replaced once a month. It takes about 23 seconds for the blood to round the circulatory system. During this time, the blood holds enough oxygen for about five minutes during rest; the same amount is used in a fraction of a minute during strenuous exercise. Yet when 10 percent of the blood is lost over a short period, the body goes into shock. Death results when 40 percent is lost.

The average adult male has 100,000 miles or more of blood vessels. It is in the smallest vessels, the capillaries, that the exchange of substances takes place between the blood and the rest of the body. Although the vessels are elastic, the arteries lose their elasticity if the body is not exercised regularly and when the diet is rich in fats. No wonder physiologists say that you are as old as your blood vessels.

The blood supply to the muscles varies in proportion to the amount of muscle work. Active muscle on one side of the body will have 40 to 100 times more capillaries than the inactive muscle on the opposite side of the body. About 750 major muscles are attached to more than 205 bones. After stretching, twisting, and squeezing, muscles return to their original length and shape. In so doing, they oxidize glycogen (body sugar), help with body balance, and generate heat, energy, and minute electrical currents. Muscles have enormous strength. Some, like the biceps in the arm, are capable of lifting a weight 1500 times their own weight. In addition to doing work, muscles support the skeleton and refine body posture and personal appearance. They allow for locomotion. The human being's greatest speed is about 22.2 mph, the equivalent of running 220 yards in 20.3 seconds. People over 70 years of age have diminished work capacities; these are estimated to be only 50 percent of the values of a 17-year-old.

It is little wonder that many doctors and physiologists believe exercise helps to control body weight. Exercise burns food or fat, both measured in calories. To lose one pound of body fat, one must burn off 3500 calories. In so doing, the heat produced, if not checked, would rise and coagulate the protein in muscles. A heat-regulating apparatus keeps body temperature almost constant. This radiator is the skin, which dissipates about 80 percent of the excess heat. This cooling and heating system in the human body is self-regulating.

DIGESTIVE SYSTEM

Before food can be absorbed, it must undergo a number of changes. Some of these are purely mechanical; others are highly complex chemical reactions. Most foodstuffs are constructed of molecules too large to pass through the walls of the intestine, and the purpose of digestion is to convert these into smaller molecules.

During digestion, hydrolysis occurs. Complex molecules are broken down by digestive enzymes, known collectively as the *hydrolases*. These enzymes are present in the secretions of the several digestive glands of the alimentary tract: the salivary glands, the gastric glands, the pancreas, and the intestinal glands.

The alimentary tract or canal extends from the mouth to the anus. Different names have been given to its various parts (Figure 13.21). The greater part of the tract has to do with the actual digestion of food, but it is also concerned with absorption of the nutrient part of food and with the excretion of waste products.

Mouth

When food is taken into the mouth, it is cut and ground by the teeth, mixed with saliva, and finally molded into a semidigestible mass called a *bolus*. Saliva contains a large amount of water, the enzyme salivary amylase (ptyalin), and mucus, which helps to hold the food together and lubricate it for passage down the esophagus.

Salivary amylase hydrolyzes or splits starches into disaccharides, chiefly maltose and dextrin. This chemical process is facilitated by body heat and chemically neutral conditions.

FIGURE 13.21

Human digestive tract. Times indicated along the tract represent how long it takes food to pass through each area during digestion.

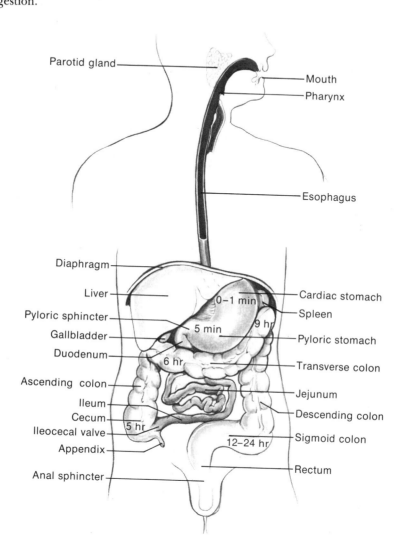

The mechanical breakdown of food *(mastication)* is carried out by the *teeth*.

Stomach

The irregularly shaped, distended stomach lies slightly to the left side in the upper portion of the abdomen, just beneath the ribs and just below the diaphragm, which separates the abdominal and thoracic cavities (Figure 13.22). The stomach has two functions. First, it receives the bolus of swallowed food from the esophagus and begins the digestion of proteins. Second, the stomach delivers food to the intestine.

Small Intestine

The food leaves the stomach through the pyloric sphincter and enters the small intestine, where most digestion and absorption take place. The

FIGURE 13.22

Stomach. **a,** External and internal anatomy of the stomach, showing the layers of muscle, the rugae, and the pyloric valve. **b,** Schematic representation of the gastric mucosa, showing all the layers of the stomach. **c,** Gastric glands from the greater curvature of the stomach. **d,** Detail of the gastric glands.

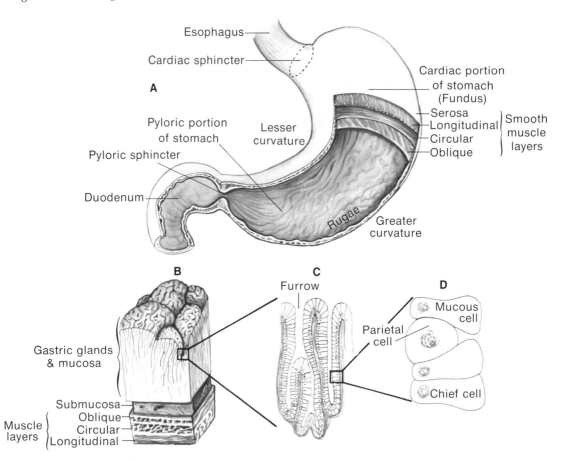

first section of the small intestine is the *duodenum* (Figure 13.21). The duodenum leads into the middle portion, the *jejunum,* and the small intestine terminates in the *ileum* (Figure 13.21). The entire small intestine of an adult male is about 7.5 meters (23 feet) long and 2.5 cm (1 inch) in diameter.

Partially digested food from the stomach passes into the duodenum, where the acidity of the food stimulates the intestine to secrete hormones. These stimulate the pancreas to secrete pancreatic juices and the liver to secrete bile.

Bile salts are produced by the liver and stored in concentrated form in the gallbladder when the intestine is empty. When the chyme, or food, reaches the intestine from the stomach, the bile salts digest and absorb fats. Bile salts

emulsify the fats into minute fat particles, providing a larger surface for the action of pancreatic lipase.

Since the small intestine is where absorption of the end products of digestion occurs, special structural adaptations increase the absorptive surface area.

The innermost lining of the small intestine is not smooth, but has numerous fingerlike projections, the *villi,* which greatly increase the absorptive surface (Figure 13.23). Electron microscopy has shown that this surface is further increased by numerous microvilli so that the total surface of an intestinal lining is estimated to be five times as large as the surface of the exterior of the body.

The muscularis mucosa contracts and re-

FIGURE 13.23

Liver and its relationship with the gallbladder, pancreas, and duodenum. A section has been removed from the liver and the area enlarged to show the arrangement of liver cells, bile ducts, Kupffer cells, and blood sinusoids to one another. Arrows indicate the direction of flow of bile from the gallbladder and liver and of digestive juices from the pancreas into the duodenum.

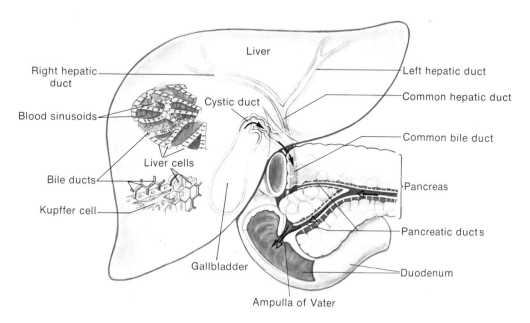

laxes rhythmically (peristalsis) during digestion. This causes corresponding shortening and lengthening movements of the villi that act to stir the intestinal fluids, facilitating absorption of the digestive products.

Within each villus is a network of capillaries and a central lymph vessel or lacteal. Simple sugars, amino acids, vitamins, minerals, and water are absorbed by the capillaries. Fatty acids and glycerol are absorbed by the lacteal, and after absorption they combine to form the triglycerides found in the bloodstream.

Gallbladder

The gallbladder, or *cholecyst,* is a pear-shaped sac lying on the underside of the liver.

Bile passes from the liver, where it is produced by way of the hepatic duct, into the common bile duct and the gallbladder (Figure 3.23). The gallbladder stores the bile as bile salts until

needed for digestion, at which time they are released into the small intestine.

Pancreas

The *pancreas* is the most active and versatile of the digestive organs (Figure 13.23). In the absence of other digestive secretions, its enzymes alone are capable of almost completing the digestion of all foodstuffs. The pancreatic secretion into the duodenum contains all the enzymes needed to break down foodstuffs:

1. *Carbohydrate enzyme,* or *pancreatic amylase* (amylopsin), acts upon starch and glycogen, producing maltose.
2. *Fat enzyme,* or *pancreatic lipase* (steapsin), is the main fat digestive enzyme in humans. Each molecule of fat is broken down into a molecule of glycerol and three molecules of fatty acid.

3. *Protein enzyme,* or *trypsin,* is secreted as an inactive precursor, trypsinogen, which is converted to active trypsin by enterokinase, an enzyme found in the intestinal juices. Trypsin digests proteins and peptides partially digested in the stomach. The products of trypsin digestion are polypeptides and amino acids. A second proteolytic enzyme, chymotrypsin, is secreted by the pancreas as inactive chymotrypsinogen, which is converted to *chymotrypsin* by trypsin. Chymotrypsin acts in a manner similar to that of trypsin.
4. *Nuclease* is an enzyme that splits nucleic acids, producing mononucleotides.

Large Intestine

In humans the junction between the small intestine and the large intestine (colon or large bowel) is usually in the lower right portion of the abdominal cavity. A blind sac, the *cecum,* projects from the large intestine near the point of puncture, the *ileocecal (ileocolic) valve.* Here a small, fingerlike process, the *appendix,* projects from the cecum. The appendix frequently becomes infected and sometimes must be removed surgically (appendectomy).

The cecum and appendix serve no known purpose except as storage centers for microorganisms that aid digestion. Humans cannot digest the complex cellulose found in plant cells without assistance; the stored microbes digest this cellulose for them, but most of the nutritional value of the material is lost. The duodenum, not the cecum, is the principal site of digestion.

The large intestine is about 2 meters (5 to 6 feet) long, and its sections are named according to the directions they travel and the shapes they assume. The cecum leads into the *ascending colon,* which is followed by the *transverse colon, descending colon, sigmoid colon* (shaped like the letter "S"), *rectum,* and *anus.*

The major function of the large intestine is the reabsorption of water into the body. If all the water in which enzymes are secreted into the digestive tract were lost in the waste material

(feces), dehydration would occur.

A second function of the large intestine is the removal of the waste products of digestion by *defecation.* The large bowel is also where excess salts, such as those of calcium and iron, are excreted when their concentration in the blood is higher than normal. The last portion of the large intestine, the rectum, stores the waste materials until defecation occurs. The feces are expelled through the anus.

Occasionally the colon becomes irritated, and peristalsis moves the material through it faster than normal. As a result, not enough water is reabsorbed, and a watery waste material, *diarrhea,* persists until the cause of the irritation is remedied. Conversely, if material moves too slowly, too much water is reabsorbed, and constipation results. Diarrhea may be the result of a bacillary dysentery or of many other causes. *Constipation,* on the other hand, results from an overstimulation of the intestinal muscle, narrowing the canal and preventing passage of fecal material. Nervous tension, excessive amounts of bulky foods in the diet, and use of laxatives contribute to constipation.

Liver

The liver, the largest of the glandular organs of the body, is situated in the upper right quadrant of the abdominal cavity. It lies to a large extent under the shelter of the lower ribs, its upper surface conforming to the lower surface of the diaphragm.

The liver can be thought of as a chemical factory. Besides storing fat-soluble vitamins and maintaining about a 12-hour supply of sugar, the liver synthesizes bile for the small intestine. Perhaps the liver's most important function is to detoxify poisons and complex body chemicals. When these chemicals are broken down into simpler substances, they can be excreted by the kidneys. Many poisons and drugs, such as alcohol, caffeine, and nicotine, are detoxified by the liver. The liver is also capable of making antibiotics, as when it converts the chemical prontosil into sulfanilamide in the fight against bacteria and viruses.

The liver has numerous functions:

1. Production
   a. Blood plasma proteins
   b. Antibodies to fight off diseases
   c. Heparin, a substance that prevents blood clotting
   d. Bile pigments from red blood cells in the form of bilirubin and biliverdin
2. Storage
   a. Vitamins and minerals
   b. Glucose in the form of glycogen
3. Conversion and use
   a. Fats (desaturation)
   b. Carbohydrates (glycogenesis)
   c. Proteins (deamination)
4. Removal
   a. Old blood cells and toxins by phagocytosis (Kupffer cells)
   b. Waste products (urea and ammonia) from amino acids

EXCRETORY SYSTEM

The active life of every cell is accompanied by the production of waste materials. These must be removed quickly if the activities of the tissues are not to be impaired. In the chemistry of the body, some reactions produce starting materials for others, but certain end products may accumulate and disturb the sequence of essential reactions if they are not removed. These materials are the excretory substances, and they are produced in different amounts by all cells.

The process of *excretion* consists of the separation and removal of substances harmful to the body. Excretion is carried out by the salivary glands, skin, lungs, liver, large intestine, and kidneys (Figure 13.24).

The lungs remove carbon dioxide from the blood, and other waste products of metabolism, such as ketone bodies (acetone), are removed by the respiratory system. The salivary glands excrete various salts, particularly sodium chloride. The sweat glands produce water, salts, amino acids, vitamins, and other materials that are carried from the body and deposited on the outer

FIGURE 13.24
Organs of the excretory system.

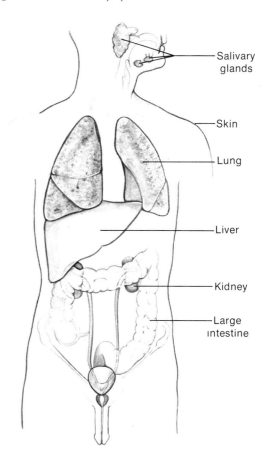

Salivary glands

Skin

Lung

Liver

Kidney

Large intestine

surface of the skin. Excretory functions of the liver include phagocytic action and the removal of bile pigments. The large intestine, following its principal function of water absorption, removes solid waste materials as feces.

Urinary System

The two principal functions of the urinary system are the excretion of wastes and the regulation of the composition of blood. Blood composition must not be allowed to vary beyond tolerable limits, or life will be lost. Regulation of the composition of the blood involves not only the removal of waste products but also the conservation of water and metabolites in the body.

The urinary system consists of two kidneys that secrete urine; the ducts leading from them, the ureters; a urinary reservoir, the bladder; and the tube from it to the surface of the body, the urethra (Figure 13.25).

Kidneys

The *kidneys* are deeply imbedded in the abdominal cavity in the lumbar region (Figure 13.24). They are *retroperitoneal* (behind the peritoneum). Both are protected at the back by the last two pairs of ribs. They are surrounded by a layer of fat, the *perirenal* fat; in front they are covered by renal fascia, the *capsule*.

A kidney is a dark red, bean-shaped organ about 11 cm (4.5 in.) long, 6 cm (2.5 in.) wide, and a little over 2.5 cm (1 in.) thick. An adult kidney weighs about 5 ounces (Figure 13.26).

One of the first organs to receive the oxygenated blood is the *kidney*. The kidneys work in much the same way as a screen does in separating rocks from sand. The waste products of cell and liver metabolism are screened out by the kidneys, stored in the bladder, and excreted as urine. Through filtration, the kidneys control body fluids and maintain a stable fluid environment. Of the 180 quarts of blood filtered by the kidneys each day, only one to two quarts are excreted as urine. Every 20 minutes the entire volume of the blood passes by a set of molecular filters in the two million glomeruli of the kidney. Many vital substances, such as salts, minerals, and vitamins, are retained and recycled by the kidneys.

FIGURE 13.25
Urinary system with blood vessels.

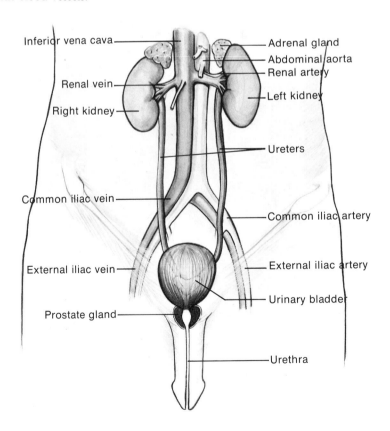

FIGURE 13.26
External **a,** and internal **b,** anatomy of the left kidney.

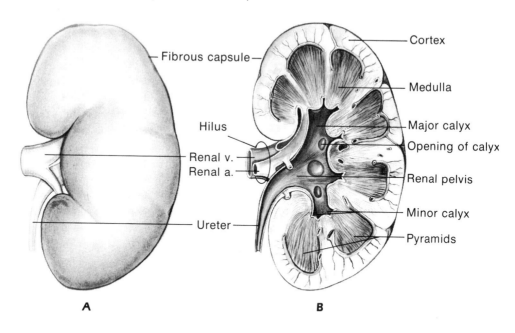

RESPIRATORY SYSTEM

Nature designed the body so that the cardiovascular system is complemented by the respiratory system. Oxygen is necessary for life. The lungs, where exchange of gases take place, contain 700 million to 800 million air sacs, or alveoli. The inner surface of the lungs in an adult is equivalent to the size of a tennis court. Lungs help us to breathe about 12,000 liters of air each day.

The respiratory system comprises:

1. nostrils (nose)
2. trachea
3. bronchus and bronchioles
4. lungs (air sacs)

The trachea divides into two *bronchi* that enter the right and left lung. The right bronchus is shorter, wider, and more vertical than the left. Within the lungs the bronchi subdivide into smaller branches, the bronchial tubes, and finally into bronchioles (see Figure 13.27). Each bronchiole terminates in an elongated sac called the *atrium*; these are lined with numerous pouches, the *alveoli* or air cells (Figure 13.27). Alveolar walls are very thin and highly vascular. They are lined with squamous epithelium, and an exchange of gases occurs through the walls of the capillaries in the alveolus between the blood and the air. The term *intrapulmonary* refers to the spaces within the alveolar sacs.

The two lungs vary in shape and size. The right lung is the larger and has three lobes. It is wider than the left lung but a little shorter. The left lung is divided into two lobes and is somewhat narrower and longer than the right.

The movement of air into and out of the lungs depends on the rhythmical contraction and relaxation of the diaphragm, the intercostal muscles, and other respiratory muscles. Because muscles contract in response to volleys of impulses over the nerves serving them, there must

FIGURE 13.27
Internal structure of the lungs. **a,** Relationship of the lungs to the head and neck. **b,** External and internal appearance of a lung lobule, showing the atrium and alveolar sacs. **c,** Section of a lung, magnified 100 times. **d,** Section of a similar lung with emphysema. Note the decreased number of alveolar sacs and consequent diminishing in the gas exchange area of lung tissue.

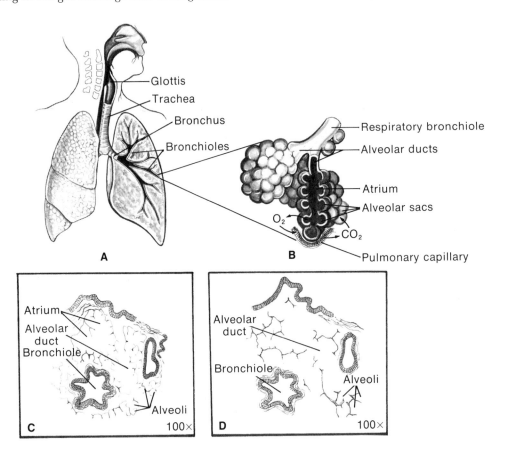

be a control center. This control is performed by the respiratory center in the brain.

LYMPHATIC SYSTEM

Most of the tissues of the body, with the notable exception of the central nervous system, are drained by the lymphatic system.

The lymphatic system gathers and drains filtered fluid and cellular constituents that accumulate in the spaces between the cells. The larger lymphatic vessels drain into veins, which return the lymph to the blood.

Lymphatic Tissues

The following organs containing lymphoid tissue perform somewhat different functions, particularly with respect to the substances that they filter.

Tonsils

These masses are found just beneath the epithelium of the mouth and throat and include the *palatine tonsils* (at each side of the soft palate), the pharyngeal tonsils (behind the nose on the back wall of the upper pharynx, sometimes called the *adenoids*); and the *lingual tonsils* (back of the tongue). Any or all of these tonsils may become so infected with bacteria that their surgical removal is indicated.

Thymus

The thymus gland, usually comprising two lobes, plays a key role in the formation of antibodies in the first few weeks of life and the development of immunity. It is located at the base of the neck and manufactures lymphocytes. Removal of the thymus causes a decrease in lymphocyte production throughout the body and a decrease in size of the spleen and lymph nodes. The thymus is most active during early life; after puberty it undergoes degenerative changes and is replaced by adipose tissue.

Spleen

The spleen is situated in the left abdomen next to the stomach. It is designed to filter blood and to produce lymphocytes that carry on phagocytosis. The spleen has many functions concerned with lymphatic and blood circulation. Prominent structures inside the spleen are round masses of lymphoid tissue, and these justify its classification as a lymphatic organ.

Functions of the Lymphatics

Lymph and the lymphatic system serve the following functions:

1. *Defense mechanism.* Lymphocyte production phagocytizes pathogenic organisms.
2. *Immunity.* Production of antibodies aids in combating disease and infection.
3. *Tissue drainage.* Networks of vessels drain the spaces between the tissue cells and return the metabolites to the system, where they can be reused.
4. *Excretion.* The lymphatic system removes impurities such as carbon particles, waste products, and dead blood cells.
5. *Digestion.* Intestinal lacteals absorb end products of fat digestion and distribute them via the circulatory system.

Lymph Nodes

Lymphatic tissue filters and removes bacteria. Along the course of the lymphatic vessels are small bodies of lymphatic tissue called lymph nodes (Figure 13.28). These usually are oval and are commonly referred to as *microkidneys.*

Research indicates that lymph nodes may afford some protection against infection and disease. Lymphocytes (leukocytes) of the lymph nodes and spleen destroy bacteria and antigens that are introduced into the body. Lymph nodes commonly become swollen and inflamed during severe bacterial infections.

All lymphatic vessels form networks and at certain points carry lymph into the regional lymph nodes. Groups of large nodes are in the neck (cervical), under the arm (axillary), at the elbow (cubital), and in the groin (inguinal).

Lymph Formation

Lymph is the fluid that returns to the circulation from the tissue spaces by way of the lymphatics. Since lymph originates from plasma, its composition is similar to that of plasma.

Lymph is a clear fluid containing a low count of granular leukocytes and a varying number of lymphocytes.

Immunity

The body is continually invaded by microorganisms that enter through the respiratory passages and through small wounds in the skin. In most cases, these invasions are harmless, since they are dealt with immediately by the phagocytic leukocytes and the immune reactions.

Invading organisms and the toxins they produce are composed of proteins. The danger of a foreign protein lies in the reactive chemical groups on its surface, for these can combine with groups in the body and interfere with normal processes. These effects can be avoided if the invading protein is either destroyed or made inactive by combination with another protein.

FIGURE 13.28

The lymphatic system. **a,** Superficial lymphatics of the body. Locations of the major lymph nodes and organs are also shown. Shaded area indicates the segment of the upper right quadrant of the body that drains into the right lymphatic duct. The remaining area of the body is drained by the left lymphatic (thoracic) duct. **b,** Diagram of the lymphatic system, showing its connection with the general circulatory system.

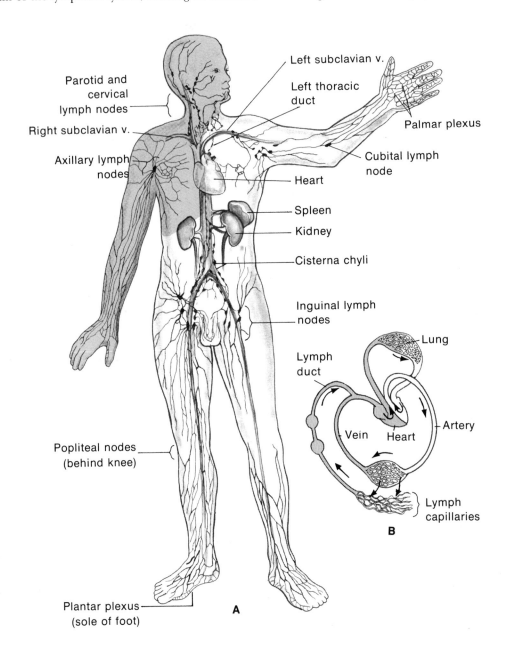

Such a combination or action is, in essence, the *immune reaction*. A foreign protein that will waken the immune reaction is called an *antigen*, and the protein in the individual's system that is produced to react with it is called an *antibody*, or immunoglobulin.

Immunology is concerned with how and why the body reacts against almost anything that is foreign or genetically different from its own substance. The term *immunity* signifies all those properties of the host that confer resistance to a specific foreign agent. This resistance may be of all degrees, from complete insusceptibility. Therefore, resistance and immunity are relative terms implying only that one host is more or less susceptible to a given agent than another host.

Humans have a certain amount of natural immunity, that is, immunity with which they were born, but most immunity is acquired either naturally, by exposure to a foreign agent, or artificially, by immunization.

The capacity to respond to immunological stimuli rests principally in cells of the lymphoid system. During embryonic growth, a stem cell develops in the fetal liver and other organs under differentiating influence of various environments. The stem cell can develop into cells of the red blood cell series or of the granulocyte series. It can also develop into a lymphoid stem cell that may differentiate to form at least two distinct lymphocyte populations. One population, the T lymphocytes, is dependent on the presence of a functioning thymus; the other, theB lymphocytes, is independent of the thymus.

The lymphoid system is composed of small lymphocytes that are present in organized lymphoid tissue (lymph nodes, spleen, and Peyer's patches), in the lymph, and in the blood (see Figure 13.29). The lymphocytes recognize foreign antigens and initiate the immunological response of the animal.

The small lymphocytes belong to two general classes of immunity: B lymphocytes, involved in humoral immunity, and T lymphocytes, with cell-mediated immunity (resistance to infection). Both B and T cells originate from precursors released into the blood from the bone marrow.

B Lymphocytes

B precursors complete their differentiation into mature B lymphocytes, or plasma cells, after passing directly into the lymph nodes, spleen, and Peyer's patches. After the B precursor has become a plasma cell (Figure 13.29), it synthesizes and secretes approximately 2000 antibody molecules per second until it dies, usually within a few days after reaching maturity.

Each B lymphocyte is differentiated by a distinct marker on its surface. This marker is a specific type of immunoglobulin identified as IgM and can be recognized using the fluorescent antibody technique. Characterization of the abnormal lymphocytes by detection of IgM has shown that certain diseases are expressions of one class of B lymphocytes.

T Lymphocytes

These constitute the greater part (65 to 80 percent of the circulating pool of lymphocytes. They are from primitive stem cells that have circulated through the thymus gland and are capable of destroying bacteria, viruses, and fungi and of providing immunological surveillance that can eliminate cancer cells (Figure 13.30).

T lymphocytes divide about three times daily. Once the T cell has entered the bloodstream, it slips between the epithelial cells of the vascular bed or enters special regions of the lymph nodes and spleen. The T cell identifies the intruding antigen and processes its identity so as to allow the B cell to form antibodies. In addition, the T cell can destroy the offending agent outright. The T cell can circulate through the bloodstream via the lymphatic-general circulatory system portal in the thoracic duct and search for foreign substances or malignant cells.

Humoral immunodeficiency can be caused by a lack of either B cells or T cells and is especially prominent in certain malignant states such as multiple myeloma and chronic lymphocytic leukemia. Infectious problems may develop in persons deficient in these lymphocytes and their immune reactions.

Acquired immune deficiency syndrome, or

FIGURE 13.29

Cooperation between T cells and B cells in antibody production. Lymphocytes originate from a stem cell, whose morphology is not clear. This cell migrates through the blood and invades the thymus, dividing many times to form T lymphocytes. In birds, the stem cells are "conditioned" to become B lymphocytes in the bursa of Fabricius, a lymphatic organ of the cloaca. After encountering an antigen, the lymphocyte modulates into a larger cell—the immunoblast—which then proliferates and produces either more T lymphocytes or plasma cells. The so-called thymus-dependent antigens promote the transformation of B lymphocytes into plasma cells only when T lymphocytes are also present. (From L. C. Junqueira and J. Carneiro, *Basic Histology*, 4th Ed. Copyright © 1983 by Lange Medical Publications. Reprinted by permission.)

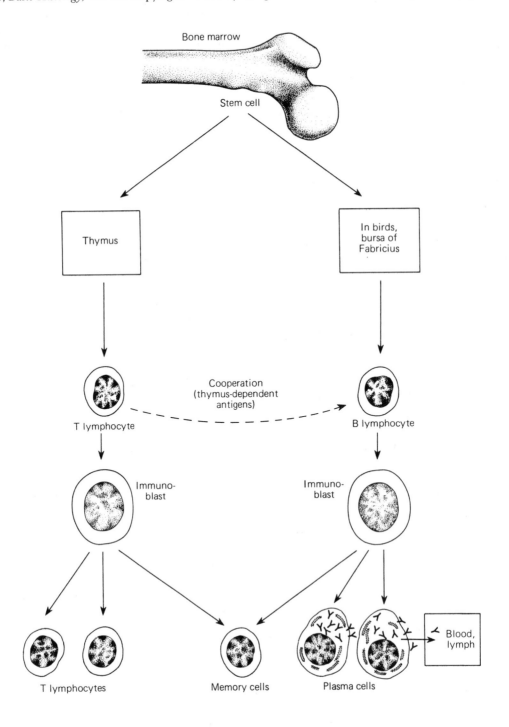

FIGURE 13.30

Bacteria invading bloodstream. Bacteria invade, perhaps through a tiny scratch, and begin to multiply. Some become stuck to monocytes, activating them into more aggressive macrophages. Circulating randomly, T cells adhere to macrophages and to the bacteria. This linkage stimulates T cells to send three messages: (1) Activate and summon more macrophages. (2) Produce more T cells. (3) Signal B cells to proliferate and become plasma cells that produce and release antibodies (Y-shaped molecules). Antibodies latch onto intruder molecules (or antigens) on bacteria and link the yoke of the Y to them. The shaft of the Y attaches to macrophages. They in turn envelop the bacteria, which are consumed by enzymes and become harmless debris.

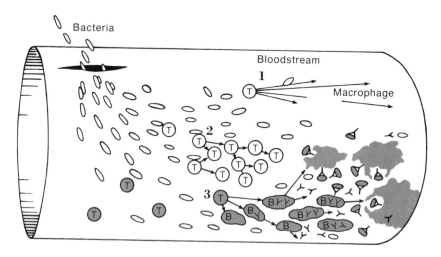

AIDS, has received much public attention recently. Identified just a few years ago, this disease is fatal, and cause and cure are unknown. In AIDS, the immune system is destroyed, leaving victims with no means to fight off infectious agents. Individuals with AIDS suffer recurring infections and often develop Karposi's sarcoma, a rare cancer, and *Pneumocystitis carinii* pneumonia.

The immune system's T lymphocytes appear to be affected by the disease. AIDS victims have a decreased number of these white blood cells, and those that they do have are abnormally shaped and malfunctioning.

Researchers believe that AIDS is caused by a viral agent. The disease is transmitted through certain body fluids, such as blood, semen, and vaginal fluid. AIDS has been diagnosed in homosexuals, intravenous drug users, and persons who have received blood transfusions. The sysmptoms of the disease—fatigue, recurring viral infections, fever, swollen lymph glands, and night sweats—may not appear until months after exposure to the disease.

Antibodies

Antibodies are gamma globulin molecules that circulate in the plasma and are produced by the lymphoid tissues and lymphocytes. Each antigen has a specific antibody that alone can react with it. The particular configuration of the combining sites is seemingly complementary to the determining portions of the antigens that induce their formation—an arrangement comparable to a lock and key. The antigen molecule has many active chemical sites or determining groups protruding from its surface as specific configurations. These determine antigenic specificity and fit into the pocketlike combining sites of the antibody. The number of antibody molecules produced is usually many times greater than the number of antigen molecules present.

A discussion of all immunoglobulins is beyond the scope of this book, but a few are listed below.

- IgG (75%) In maternal/fetal passage allows fetus to fight infection.

- IgM (10%) Responds to antigenic stimulation.
- IgA (12%) Neutralizes viruses and prevents attachment of bacteria to epithelial cells.
- IgO (about 2%) Minimal function found in B lymphocytes in lymphatic leukemia.
- IgE (about 1%) In allergic rections helps to suppress foreign allergen.

Two broad groups of antibodies are recognized: *natural antibodies*, which are formed without apparent antigenic stimulation, and *acquired antibodies*, which appear only after exposure to a known antigen. The anti-A and anti-B blood group antibodies involved in blood reactions are examples of the natural type. Antibodies that are developed during the course of immunization (as for polio, measles, and typhus) are examples of the acquired type.

The thymus has an important role in antibody production. Located in the chest cavity near the lower end of the trachea in children, the thymus is a prominent mass of lymphoid tissue. During early childhood the gland produces lymphoid cells responsible for antibody production during most of the life of the individual. Removal of the thymus in newborn mice has proved fatal; the mice die of infection within a few weeks. Although the thymus is naturally atrophied and inactive in adults, removal of the gland from a child can almost entirely prevent antibody production.

EXEMPLARY LESSON PLANS

In light of the first part of this chapter, peruse the following lesson plans, keeping in mind that they are examples of the types of lesson plans that you will likely be expected to use in your classroom. Remember that they by no means provide a complete unit of instruction. They are offered only as a guide for the formation of a comprehensive unit.

THE GLANDULAR (ENDOCRINE) SYSTEM

Grade Level: Intermediate

Concept: The endocrine glands are essential to normal body function.

Expected Pupil Outcome: The student will be able to name the glands, locations, functions, and products of the endocrine system.

Content: The seven regulatory glands, their location, function, and products:

1. Pituitary: at base of brain; produces master hormones, regulates growth and size. Produces various hormones.
2. Adrenals: top of kidneys; produce stress hormones, or adrenaline.
3. Islets of Langerhans: behind stomach; regulate sugar use, produce insulin.
4. Thyroid: neck region; regulates body use of food (metabolic rate), produces thyroxin.
5. Parathyroid: on thyroid gland; regulates calcium-phosphorus balance, regulates muscle tone.
6. Thymus: lower neck; protects body from early childhood diseases.
7. Gonads: groin and lower pelvic area; produce reproductive hormones, regulate sexual development.

Learning Experiences:
1. Show short film: *The Endocrine Glands.*
2. *Matching bee:* (teacher and pupil play a matching game).
3. Go over work sheet as a final review.

Evaluation Procedures

The final learning experience will serve as the evaluation portion of the lesson. If the students respond favorably to the review worksheet, the stated objective will be deemed attained.

THE LIVER—A CHEMICAL FACTORY

Note: Similar lesson plans may be evolved for other body organs.

Grade Level: Intermediate to Junior High

Concept: The liver works like a chemical factory.

Expected Pupil Outcome: The student will be able to describe how the liver works like a chemical factory.

Content: Ways the liver works as a chemical factory:

1. a) Detoxifies drugs and poisons.
   b) Enzymes in the liver convert poisons (drugs, alcohol) into harmless substances that the kidneys can excrete from the body.
   c) If poisons are continually imbibed, the liver is forced to overwork unnecessarily.
2. Stores vitamins A, D, E, K, B_{12}. Vitamins regulate body processes.
3. Stores sugar (provides quick energy for body).
4. Produces and stores bile. Bile used to break down fats in small intestine.

Learning Experiences:

1. *Experiment/Demonstration* of chemical changes taking place in body. To a test tube of dilute sulphuric acid (colorless), add phenolphthalein (red). Observe the white sodium settling as a precipitate. Phenolphthalein may be conceptualized as the poison and the white precipitate as the detoxified poison. The color change should simulate a chemical factory.
2. *Simulate* vitamins (in capsule form) and adhere on flannel board to picture of liver. Or identify each vitamin with food source and adhere these to picture of liver on flannel board.
3. Stick sugar cubes to picture of liver on flannel board (see Figure 13.31).
4. *Experiment/Demonstration* of the action of soap and water in dissolving butter in a plastic bag. Demonstrate first without soap. Soap could be conceptualized as bile.

Evaluation Procedures

Teacher will develop a short answer paper and pencil quiz covering the content in this lesson. If the class in general scores well, the assumption will be that the expected pupil outcome was accomplished.

FIGURE 13.31
The liver as a chemical factory.

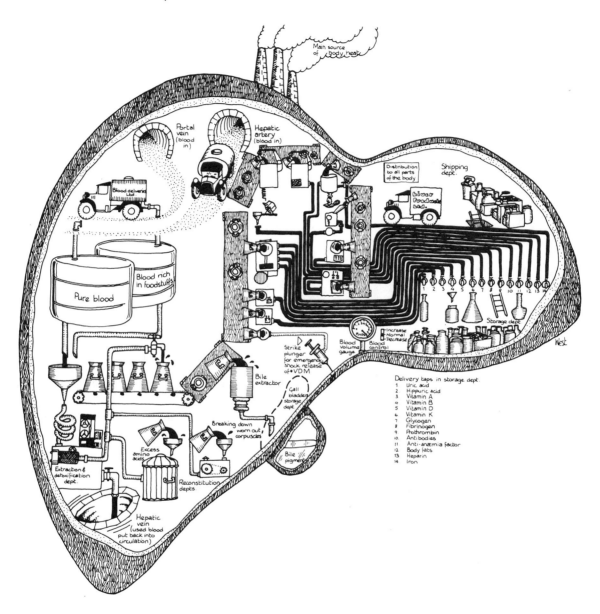

THE EYE AND ITS STRUCTURE AND FUNCTION

Grade Level: Intermediate to Junior High

Concept: The eye functions like a camera.

Expected Pupil Outcome: The student will be able to describe the major components or the eye as well as the function of each.

Content: Parts of the eye and their functions:
1. *Iris* muscles (blue, brown) control amount of light entering lens.
2. *Pupil* is black center of iris through which light passes.
3. *Lens* focuses light rays on retina.
4. *Vitreous humor* helps focus light on retina.
5. *Retina* receives image upside down.

Learning Experiences:
1. *Demonstration:* Obtain beef eyes from a slaughterhouse and dissect one. Then let each pupil dissect one.
   How to dissect an eye.* A bull's or a sheep's eye can be used. Remove the clear front skin, or cornea. This will reveal the iris and behind it the crystalline lens. This lens divides the eye into two parts, the front containing a thin liquid called aqueous humor *and the back a jellylike liquid, the* vitreous humor.

   Removing the lens and vitreous humor, the retina or sensitive surface can be seen. It is more richly served with sensitive cells at a spot opposite the lens called the yellow spot. The nerves carrying the sensations pass out through a hole in the outer sclerotic membrane; this spot is therefore not sensitive to light and is called the blind spot.

   Other body organs, like the lung, heart, and kidney, may be obtained from the local slaughterhouse and dissected for the class.

---

*Excerpted from *700 Science Experiments for Everyone* by UNESCO.

Evaluation Procedures

The teacher will observe each student during the lab portion of the lesson. During the observation session each student will be asked to describe each of the eye parts (both structure/function) they are dissecting. Satisfactory responses will be construed as successful completion of the stated objective.

MAJOR ORGANS OF THE BODY (GENERAL INTRODUCTION)

Note: Body systems may be taught in similar fashion.

Grade Level: Intermediate

Concept: Body organs are necessary to sustain life.

Expected Pupil Outcome: The student will be able to state the names, locations, and functions of the major body organs.

Content: Major body organs:

1. Brain: skull; switchboard of the body, coordinates everything, communication center.
2. Heart: middle chest cavity; pump blood throughout body.
3. Lungs: in upper chest cavity; exchange gases CO_2 and O_2.
4. Kidney: one on each lower side of vertebral column; filters wastes from blood and maintains fluid balance.
5. Liver: right side of abdominal cavity below lung; detoxifies poisons and body wastes, stores body sugar, produces bile.
6. Spleen: behind liver and to left of stomach; although not well understood, it appears that the spleen has much to do with the formation and destruction of blood cells.

Learning Experiences:

1. *Lecture/Discussion* using a *human torso* (Figure 13.32) and/or a *matching bee* (Figure 13.33). Conceptualize function of brain with a film projector.
2. Heart can be compared in size with a clenched fist; function like that of a pump.
3. Lungs: function and appearance conceptualized by balloon.
4. Kidney: physical comparison of kidney shape to bean shape. Conceptualize function by putting chopped carrots through strainer (action of strainer simulates kidney function).
5. Compare liver to sponge.

Evaluation Procedures

Have the students respond to the body organ crossword puzzle (Figure 13.34). If the students perform in a satisfactory fashion, (ie, 90% correct responses), the stated expected pupil outcome will be accomplished.

FIGURE 13.32
A life-size human torso. Parts may be dismantled.

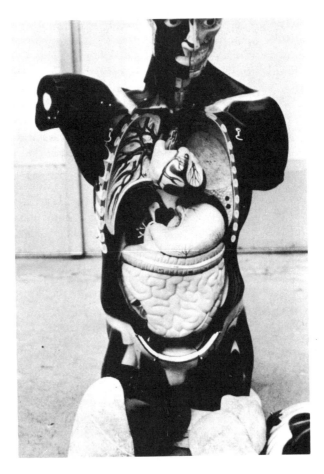

FIGURE 13.33
Organs of the body, locations, and conceptualizations of their functions.

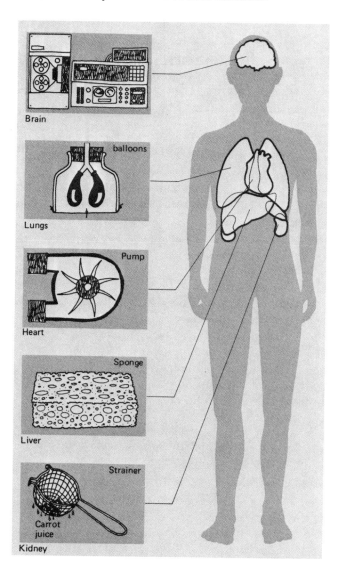

FIGURE 13.34
Crossword puzzle on body organs.

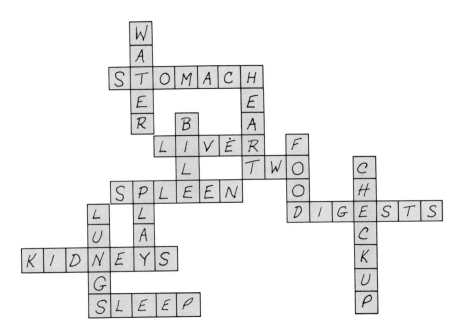

Directions: Each sentence below contains a missing word. Fill in the blank space with the words provided. Then place the word in the crossword puzzle space with the same number, either down or across.

Down:

1. L __ __ __ __ are shaped like balloons.
2. Your body needs 4-5 glasses of W __ __ __ __ daily.
3. You should P __ __ __ outdoors.
4. The liver secretes B __ __ __.
5. The H __ __ __ __ is the size of your fist.
6. The right F __ __ __ is good for your body.
7. You need a health C __ __ __ __ __ __ once a year.

Across:

8. The S __ __ __ __ __ __ can hold one quart of food.
9. The largest glandular organ is the L __ __ __ __.
10. The heart has T __ __ pumps.
11. You can live without your S __ __ __ __ __.
12. The stomach D __ __ __ __ __ __ food.
13. The K __ __ __ __ __ __ are shaped like beans.
14. You need plenty of S __ __ __ __ and rest.

Use these words:

Water	Checkup	Sleep	Liver	Kidneys	Heart	Digests
Food	Play	Bile	Spleen	Two	Stomach	Lungs

REFERENCE

Anderson, Paul D., *Basic Human Anatomy and Physiology: Clinical Implications for the Health Professions*, Monterey, CA: Wadsworth, Health Sciences, 1984.

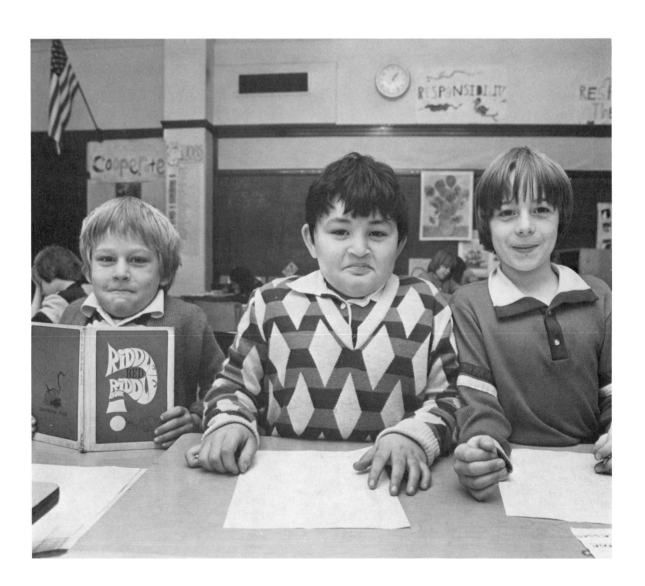

Chapter 14

Teaching About Emotional Well-Being

INTRODUCTION

Emotional well-being is a fascinating topic; it is life itself. Our whole approach to life is dependent on our emotional well-being. Some of us lead happy, wholesome, well-adjusted lives. Others approach each day as sheer drudgery and find life a chore. All too often these unhappy individuals spend a lifetime in misery. Their coping behavior becomes negative, and they enter a downward spiral that may lead to mental disturbance or suicide.

Meeting life's demands is no easy task. One does not inherit good mental health, but rather has to work at it. Life is a series of minor and major developmental tasks (see Chapter 2) requiring mastery. When we fulfill these tasks, our self-esteem receives a boost, and we move closer to full functioning. When we fail, our course— for better or worse—becomes altered.

Emotional well-being is a complex, multifaceted portion of total well-being. Emotional well-being may be interpreted as how one feels, thinks, acts, and behaves. These four are intermeshed and so integrated into the personality that we find it most difficult to recognize them separately. Perhaps for purposes of simplicity, we should think of emotional well-being in terms of the three concepts evolved by the National Association for Mental Health: (1) feeling comfortable about self, (2) feeling right about others, and (3) being able to meet the demands of life. The interpretation of such concepts is culturally determined.

All people have the same fundamental emotional needs. Understanding ourselves and adjusting to others is primarily an emotional task. Stated in another way, if you understand the emotional needs of others, you will not only get along better with them, but come to a greater realization of your own self. Everyone wants to be loved, feel secure, be independent and successful, and be recognized and accepted. To understand that all human beings have precisely these same emotional needs is the first step toward maintenance of good mental health in yourself and fostering sound emotional development in others. In addition to understanding the basic emotional needs, elementary school teachers should make an effort to contribute to the satisfactory fulfillment of these needs in children. Good emotional well-being is based on giving as well as receiving.

Two approaches to teaching emotional well-being have already been implied. The indirect approach is evolving and maintaining a socio-emotional environment that is favorable to learning and the development of emotional well-being. The well-adjusted teacher is part of this environment and becomes involved with his or her students. The direct approach consists of instruction that assists the children in finding their identities, managing their emotions, having positive thoughts about life in general, coping with the problems of living, and behaving in socially acceptable ways.

This kind of instruction has meaning only in a social setting, where behavior arises from coping with others. Direct teaching can help children develop responsibility for self and others. The child should learn to value a synergic social approach, which is predicated on the notion that one becomes a better person by helping others to be better persons—thereby attaining good feelings about self and others. The synergic concept helps us to demonstrate that emotional well-being permeates all avenues of life. That is, emotional well-being is related with a child's attitudes toward school and work, feelings toward sex and family living, behavior in sports and play, and so on. It is for this reason that many educators justify inserting sex education into the mental health unit.

The teacher should structure the learning process as part of the emotional climate of the school. The environment—social, physical, and academic—should ensure more successes than failures for all children. Indeed, every child should succeed in the elementary school, for it is at this level that attitudes toward life are structured and grafted. From this time on, the child's behavior becomes either social or antisocial, he or she either copes or does not cope with life, either withdrawing or mixing with society, either has or does not have identity, either feels comfortable about self and others or does not, and so on. As the child progresses through the secondary school system, the die that was cast in the formative years merely hardens and then comes to direct the child's destiny into adulthood.

It is important that the emotional climate in the elementary school allow the child to try out what he or she learns from direct teaching. It becomes a proving ground for the child, providing opportunities for learning to control emotions, deal with problems and people, and generally acquire ways of becoming adequate and worthwhile—achieving social competence. Social skills arise from physical skills. Both allow the child to be academically successful. The emotional climate in the classroom is essential to reinforcing direct teaching. Teaching for emotional well-being should be so structured that it becomes a humanizing social process.

EMOTIONAL DISTRESS*

We all feel emotional distress. Occasionally feeling angry, anxious, blue, lonely, or depressed is normal.

Most of us would prefer always to feel happy, content, and secure, but that is not possible—or desirable. If nothing ever changed, we might escape emotional distress, but such an existence would be boring.

Besides, humans need certain kinds of stimulation; they do not tolerate long isolation very well. People are creative, curious, interactive beings who induce change in their lives simply by living. Situations that require adjustment arise all the time. Very often the message that it is time for an adjustment in one's thoughts, attitudes, or behavior is communicated by emotional distress, and failure to heed such messages may bring about stress-related illness. Negative emotions signal that something is not right with life, and they motivate individuals to seek ways to feel better. Viewed in this way, emotional distress can

be seen as a stimulus for personal growth and self-improvement.

In this discussion we will consider the dynamics of emotional distress and the ways in which negative feelings can be used to accomplish personal growth. Please remember that the unpleasant feelings, the fears, frustrations, and sadness of everyday life are quite different from the severe distress associated with prolonged periods of abnormal thoughts, feelings, and behavior that seriously disrupt some lives for months or even years. Unfortunately, many conditions that involve feeling bad are often labeled mental illness, and carry with them the stigma of being "neurotic" or "crazy." This is not the case in some parts of the world, where social customs and even employment practices recognize that everyone has occasional blue days and antisocial periods. We prefer to differentiate the emotional distress that accompanies problems of living from the abnormal thoughts, feelings, and behavior that are often the result of severe abnormalities in brain physiology and biochemistry (some of which may be genetically based) or of brain injury.

Motivation, Emotion, and Emotional Distress

Psychologists tell us that much of our behavior is motivated by the desire to fulfill certain basic human needs, of which there are two general kinds: *maintenance needs,* for physical survival, and *growth needs,* sometimes called needs for self-actualization, for emotional stimulation and spiritual growth. This theory, advanced by Maslow (1970), is based on the premise that most people are unable to concentrate on philosophical or spiritual development if they are starving or sick (Figure 14.1).

Although basic needs are intrinsic to all humans, the ways in which people satisfy them are not. Everyone may need to eat, but not everyone obtains food in the same way. Neither does everyone eat the same kind of food. Similarly, people engage in a great variety of living arrangements, jobs, and recreation to find the best

---

*The material in this section is from Gordon Edlin and Eric Golanty, *Health & Wellness: A Holistic Approach,* Third Edition, (Boston: Jones and Bartlett Publishers, 1988).

FIGURE 14.1
Maslow's hierarchy of human needs.

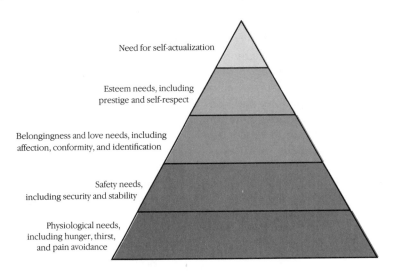

Need for self-actualization

Esteem needs, including prestige and self-respect

Belongingness and love needs, including affection, conformity, and identification

Safety needs, including security and stability

Physiological needs, including hunger, thirst, and pain avoidance

way to fulfill their needs for love, security, and self-esteem. The many different ways in which people fulfill their basic needs are remarkable examples of human creativity.

From childhood, people develop and refine strategies for meeting their basic needs. For infants, the repertoire of need-fulfilling abilities is very limited. A child can cry for food or attention and smile to encourage touching and play, which fulfill needs for love and stimulation. As people grow up, they acquire more tools to fulfill their needs. Among them are a set of values, beliefs, attitudes, and behavior that they expect will help them by producing harmonious interactions with the environment—especially with people with whom they exchange love and trust. When individuals fulfill their needs, they experience joy, happiness, and contentment. When individuals are not successful, however, they experience *emotional distress*. We get hungry when we need food or thirsty when we need water. Hunger and thirst are basic discomforts that motivate us to fulfill those maintenance needs. If we confront an obstacle that prevents us from satisfying a certain need, we can become frustrated and angry (see box). If our security is threatened, we can become fearful or anxious. The loss of love or self-esteem can bring about depression.

Dealing with Emotional Distress

Such is the condition of human life that people never reach complete satisfaction. Even if all your maintenance needs were met, and even if you lived in wonderfully harmonious family relationships and worked at a fulfilling job you would still face frustration and conflict because you would continue to seek new and enriching experiences. There are times, of course, when everything seems to be going really well, and reasonably long periods of great joy are possible. One of the principal goals of holistic health is to maximize the time you are joyous and happy and to minimize emotional distress.

The various ways people devise to solve their life problems are *coping strategies*. Coping is "any response to external life-strains that serves to prevent, avoid, or control emotional distress" (Pearlin and Schooler, 1978). There are three general ways people can cope: (1) they can try to change the situation that is causing the emotional distress, (2) they can try to alter their interpretation of the significance of the situation so it has less importance and therefore is not so distressing, or (3) they can try to alter the negative feeling without trying to change the situation or how they think about it.

DEALING WITH ANGER

Anger is one of the most common expressions of emotional distress. At all stages of life from infancy to old age, people get angry if their needs are not met. They get angry if they are cheated, lied to, hurt, punished, betrayed, or prevented from realizing their desires. People get angry when others whom they care for are hurt. They sometimes get angry at others—as a form of self-defense—when they feel disappointed with themselves or guilty about something they did (or did not) do.

For many people anger is difficult to deal with, usually because it is difficult to express. When it is directed toward an authority figure, anger can be difficult to express for fear of retaliation. Anger at a loved one is sometimes hard to express because of the risk that the other person may become angry in turn and withdraw his or her love. Some people are confused by their anger at loved ones. They see it as inconsistent with love and hence become unable to express it, even if they feel justified in doing so. Another reason anger is hard to deal with is that it is often associated with the desire to inflict physical harm.

Psychologists say that anger is the result of frustration, which is the feeling that comes when you are prevented from attaining a particular goal. Therefore, one good way to handle anger is to assess the merits of the goal you cannot attain and the strategy you have been employing to attain it. We often get angry with other people because we ask them for things that they cannot give, or because they are not providing the help we expect from them. Often, however, we haven't told them what the goal is, or how we expect them to help. So it's no wonder they don't perform the way we want them to.

Before you get angry at someone or something, ask yourself if your goal is attainable.

Have you expected too much of yourself? Have you expected too much of someone else? Have you tried to get what you want in the best possible way? If you have set an unattainable goal for yourself, or your strategy for attaining a goal is not well thought out, then you have no one (or nothing) to blame for your anger but yourself—and this realization usually makes angry feelings evaporate. Remember, most of the time other people don't make you angry. *You* make yourself angry. Being honest with yourself and direct with others is one way to prevent anger, and a reassessment of your goals and strategies is one way to diffuse an anger-provoking situation.

There are times, of course, when feeling anger and expressing it are appropriate. For example, anger is justified when someone knowingly physically or psychologically abuses you or someone or something you care for. Anger is also appropriate if the person abuses himself or herself. Another time is when someone breaks a promise. It's always wise to be very clear about promises. There would be a lot less anger and frustration if people promised to do only things that they knew they could follow through on.

What about dealing with someone who is angry at you? Receiving anger makes you want to protect yourself from physical or psychological harm resulting from hostility. One way to protect yourself is to get angry in return. However, this is rarely a good solution. It is better to realize that the angry person is frustrated, disappointed, and emotionally upset. If the angry person were wounded and bleeding, you would try to help. Think of anger as an emotional wound. Be patient with the angry person and try to offer support. This will help remove the pain of frustration and eventually the anger will subside.

There are many ways of changing a situation that is causing emotional distress. One is to make a rational appraisal of the situation and attack the problem directly by removing or surmounting the obstacle. Another is to withdraw from the situation—either by avoiding it altogether or by deciding to be patient in the belief that circumstances will ultimately change. Still another way to change the situation is to adapt oneself to it. This can be done by changing habitual ways of thinking, feeling, and behaving, by modifying unrealistic assumptions about how people are supposed to act, and by increasing self-knowledge and insight.

Attempts to alter the significance or interpretation of a distressing situation are probably used the most often (Pearlin and Schooler, 1978). One way people do this is to make positive comparisons, which are represented by sayings like "count your blessings," "we're all in the same boat," or "things are bound to get better." Another way is to focus on the good in a situation and try to minimize or ignore the bad. Most everyone can see the flaws in another person, but how often do we notice a person's good qualities?

It is also impossible to devalue a goal that might have been important and to replace it with another. For example, one might come to believe that taking time for meditation and physical relaxation each day is preferable to a day full of tension-producing work. Another way to alter the significance of a situation is to turn awareness for a time to the inner, private, perhaps mystical nature of being rather than on external experience and pressures. This can be done by increasing both body and mental awareness through any number of methods, such as exercise, yoga, dance, and various forms of meditation. Those who take time to expand self-awareness often claim increased self-knowledge and increased mastery over their feelings; they say that they have found a way to personal and emotional peace. In response to the charge that they are simply escaping from their problems, they answer that there is much to gain by "turning off the world" for a brief period each day. "It's still there when you turn it on again, but it usually looks a lot different . . . and better."

People can also cope with a distressing situation by trying to alter their negative feelings about it. Some people release their emotions in ways other than confronting the distressing situation. For example, they can express their anger at their boss or a family member by taking part in competitive sports or by hitting a punching bag. Some people adjust by accepting the bad feelings that accompany difficulties, thinking that perhaps it was "meant to be" or that "you have to take the bad with the good." And some people are like the Biblical Job: they endure their distress in the belief that such behavior is a virtue that will be rewarded in the hereafter. People also try to cope by escaping into books, films, or television or by ingesting alcohol or drugs. Although trying to change how you feel can help reduce the intensity of a negative emotional state, it does not change the situation causing the problem and in some cases may actually delay permanent solution.

Depression

According to the National Institute of Mental Health, each day approximately one person in seven experiences some form of depression, characterized by such feelings as dejection, guilt, hopelessness, and self-recrimination and by some or all of the following depressive symptoms: loss of appetite, insomnia, reduced interest in previously enjoyable activities, withdrawal from social contacts, inability to concentrate and to make decisions, lowered self-esteem, and a focus on negative thoughts and the bad things in life. If asked how they feel, most depressed people respond by saying something like "I've got the blues," or "Life's a drag," or "What's the use of doing anything?"

Most commonly, depression is a reaction to one of two kinds of event: the loss of status in the group; or the loss of love, companionship, and group belonging (Henry and Stephens, 1977). Thus, people become depressed and feel worthless and defeated when they receive criticism or fail at an important task. People also feel depressed when they are lonely.

One of the characteristics of depression is that it feeds on itself, creating what is called the depressive cycle. The depressed person's negative thoughts, social withdrawal, the loss of interest and activity only serve to reinforce feelings of worthlessness, helplessness, gloom, and doom. The fact that depression can make itself worse means that overcoming depression often necessitates a two-pronged strategy: (1) to interrupt the depressive cycle, and (2) to correct the situation that brought on the depression. Sometimes they can be accomplished simultaneously by a particular life change.

Dealing with Depression

The best way to deal with depression is to get life moving again. Little improvement can be expected unless the cycle of withdrawal and inactivity is interrupted. One way to do so is to establish a simple, attainable goal and then to set out to accomplish it. It should be a concrete act or task that can be done in a brief period, and it should involve movement. That way inactivity stops and some sense of mastery over life is restored. Perhaps the reason jogging helps depressed people feel better is that it provides an attainable goal that is "good for you." When people jog, they learn that they are capable of succeeding at something that improves their lives. It may also be that physical exercise alters the chemistry of the brain and the body and produces positive feelings in place of negative ones.

It is also important for depressed people to increase their interaction with other people. Remaining in seclusion reinforces feelings of loss and worthlessness. Depressed people are not necessarily pleasant if they dwell on their troubles during conversations. Thus, it may be preferable for depressed people to begin by going to a movie or playing tennis rather than by discussing what's wrong with them with an acquaintance. By becoming active, they will divert attention from their negative inner dialogue, and this will help break the depressive cycle.

In most cases, depression is a reaction to a particularly disturbing event, such as the loss of a loved one. As such, it is normal. But when the severity and length of a depressive episode are excessive, or when the depression cannot be attributed to any unfortunate life change, the cause may be an imbalance in brain biochemistry. Many authorities support the hypothesis that malfunctions in the normal processes that control the brain levels of certain neurotransmitters can lead to the onset of depressive symptoms (Schildkraut, 1978).

Other biological factors than malfunctions in neurotransmitters may play a role in the onset of certain types of depression. Certain people react to excessive sugar with a surge in insulin secretion that lowers blood sugar and brings about the symptoms of mild depression. People with an unusually high requirement for a certain vitamin or other nutrient may suffer occasional depression if they do not receive sufficient amounts of that nutrient. Treating these people with large doses of nutrients can sometimes completely eliminate their depressive episodes.

Depression and Suicide

One of the most worrisome aspects of depression is the possibility of suicide. The psychological states most commonly associated with suicide are hopelessness, helplessness, and intolerable despair.

During the 1970's, the National Center for Health Statistics reported approximately 27,000 suicides per year in the United States, which ranked suicide among the 10 most frequent causes of death. The number of reported suicides represents only 10 percent to 15 percent of the number of people who attempt suicide (Schneidman, 1979). Among young people, suicide ranks behind only accidents and murder as a leading cause of death. And in recent years the suicide rate among young people has increased (Figure 14.2).

Suicide is not a disease, nor is it a disorder that can be inherited. Suicides are not caused by unusual weather or by a full moon. Most important of all, many people who contemplate suicide are not psychotic. Most people who consider suicide do so because they feel overwhelmed by some unhappy situation and believe suicide to be the only option for dealing with extreme distress. Much of the time, people who seem to attempt suicide do not really want to die but want to express anger or to signal for help. Such suicide gestures are characterized by limited self-destructive acts, such as taking less than a lethal dose of sleeping pills or arranging to be discovered in time to be saved.

Occasionally a person will express thoughts of suicide to a relative or a friend. This can be extremely distressing for the listener, who may react with disbelief ("You've got to be kidding"), panic ("What am I supposed to do about it?"), or avoidance ("Why tell me?"). In attempting to deal with these uncomfortable feelings, a listener might say things like "Cheer up," or "You're better off than I am," or "You can't be serious." These and similar statements deny the distressed person's feelings. According to suicidologist Louis Wekstein (1979), the best approach is to speak directly about the suicidal thoughts ("Tell me more about why you want to kill yourself"), to offer the distressed person nonjudgmental sympathy and concern, and firmly, but patiently

FIGURE 14.2

Suicide rate of white and black males and females ages 15 to 24, 1950-1980. (Data from the U.S. National Center for Health Statistics.)

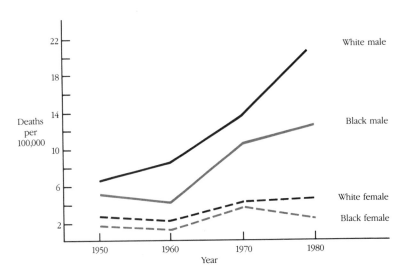

and sympathetically, to direct the distressed person to seek professional help immediately.

A suicidal individual may offer excuses for not seeing a professional and may even try to blackmail a friend into silence with covert threats. But the friend must hold firm and if necessary make an appointment with a counselor, psychiatrist, student health center, hospital emergency room, or suicide prevention center and deliver the distressed person there. If possible, parents or a spouse should be informed. The attempt to help a suicidally distressed person should be shared by as many concerned people as possible.

When a person contemplates suicide, life can seem exceedingly hopeless. But few life problems are beyond solution. Crises do pass and distressing situations improve; time does heal many hurts. The experience gained by working through a distressing time can bring confidence, insight, and understanding. As you acquire experience and understanding, you are better able to cope with life's problems. And you are better able to help others deal with theirs.

The Definition of Stress

Although most people have been what they would call "under stress" or "stressed out," it is important to recognize a significant difference in how the word "stress" is used in these two expressions. The phrase "under stress" refers to the *cause* of the disruption of psychological or physiological balance or both, as in the example, "She was under stress having to take five final exams in two days." "Stressed out," on the other hand, refers to consequences, as in the example, "During final exams she was so stressed out that she suffered from stomach cramps, diarrhea, and insomnia."

Because it is confusing to use the word stress to represent both causes and results of challenging or disruptive experiences, the term *stressor* will refer to circumstances and events that produce disruptions in mind-body harmony. The term *stress* will refer to the symptoms resulting from stressors. More specifically, stress can be defined as "a relationship between the person and the environment that is appraised by the

---

HINTS FOR EMOTIONAL WELLNESS

People Who Have a Positive Self-Image	*People Who Feel Positive About Other People*	*People Who Are Able to Meet Life's Demands*
. . . are not incapacitated by fear, anger, love, jealousy, or guilt.	. . . are able to love and accept others the way they are.	. . . do something about their problems as they arise.
. . . can take disappointments in stride.	. . . have satisfying personal relationships.	. . . accept their responsibilities.
. . . have a tolerant attitude toward themselves and others; they can laugh at their shortcomings and mistakes.	. . . expect to like and trust others and take it for granted that others will like and trust them.	. . . shape their environment whenever possible; otherwise they adjust to it.
. . . respect themselves and have self-confidence.	. . . respect the many differences they see in people.	. . . plan ahead but do not fear the future.
. . . are able to deal with most situations.	. . . do not need to push around or control other people.	. . . welcome new ideas and experiences.
. . . get satisfaction from simple, everyday pleasures.	. . . feel a sense of responsibility to friends and society.	. . . use their natural capacities and talents.
		. . . set realistic goals for themselves.
		. . . get satisfaction from what they accomplish.

---

person as taxing or exceeding his or her resources and endangering his or her well-being."

Defining stress in terms of a person's response focuses attention on an individual's experience rather than on some external factor (the stressor) as being the key element in the relationship between stress and illness. Moreover, this distinction places the avoidance or prevention of stressful experiences under the control of the individual and suggests that stress-related illnesses can be prevented by reducing stressful interactions or by coping with them in ways that do not cause a breakdown of harmony between the mind and the body.

How Stress Contributes to Illness

Although stress can be described as a disruption of harmony between the mind and the body, a more detailed and scientific definition is required in order to understand how stress can contribute to illness (Table 14.1). Stress-related illnesses such as high blood pressure (hypertension),

TABLE 14.1
Some Disorders That Can Be Caused or Aggravated by Stress

Gastrointestinal disorders	Skin disorders	Metabolic disorders
Constipation	Eczema	Hyperthyroidism
Diarrhea	Pruritus	Hypothyroidism
Duodenal ulcer	Urticaria	Diabetes
Anorexia nervosa (severe loss of appetite)	Psoriasis	Cardiovascular disorders
Obesity	Musculoskeletal disorders	Coronary artery disease
Ulcerative colitis	Rheumatoid arthritis	Essential hypertension
Respiratory disorders	Low back pain	Congestive heart
Asthma	Migraine headache	failure
Hay fever	Muscle tension	Menstrual irregularities
Tuberculosis		Cancer
		Accident proneness

asthma, arthritis, ulcers, and skin problems have traditionally been referred to as psychophysiological or psychosomatic disorders. These illnesses are not phantom problems, as the term *psychosomatic* is sometimes thought to mean, but are real physical conditions. They do not, however, necessarily stem from the direct action of some physical agent on the body. Instead, psychophysiological disorders are the result of a physical response to emotionally charged—stressful—situations and events. The physical response is mediated by the nervous, endocrine (hormone), and immune systems, which link the centers of thought and feeling of the brain with the rest of the body.

When a person suffers stress, the feelings associated with that experience activate the nervous and endocrine systems, which produce changes in body physiology (Figure 14.3). These

FIGURE 14.3
Stressful incidents produce hormonal and nervous system reactions that can lead to abnormal changes in body physiology.

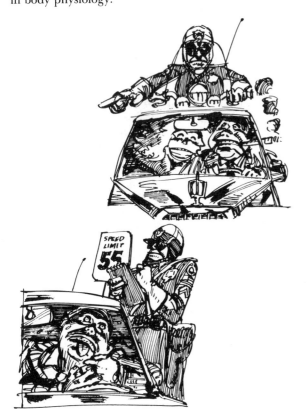

nervous and endocrine responses are a characteristic of normal physiology, meant to deal with immediate and short-term stressful situations. Illness arises when these stress-response mechanisms are continually activated and overstimulated organs begin to wear down or become diseased. Stress can also impair the immune system. Lowered immunity is probably responsible for the increased susceptibility of stressed people to infection and perhaps even cancer (Hales, 1983).

Current theories of stress (Eisdorfer, 1985; Smith, 1985) identify three components of the stress-illness relationship (Figure 14.4): (1) activators, (2) reactions, and (3) consequences. *Activators* are occurrences, situations, or events that are potential stressors. They become actual stressors only when an individual reacts to them in ways that disrupt harmony. Reactions refer to an individual's physiological and psychological responses to the stressor. It is through one's reactions that a given situation becomes stressful; some people react very strongly to an event while others take no notice. For example, if someone we are close to dies, we become emotionally upset; if we read about the death of someone we do not know in the obituary column, we do not become emotionally upset. Consequences are the effects of a reaction. When a reaction is severe or prolonged, a consequence may be unhealthy behavior—increased cigarette smoking, overconsumption of alcohol, or abuse of tranquilizing drugs—to quell the upsetting emotions. Another possible consequence is illness. A study of Detroit-area residents revealed that occupational stress was associated both with health-harming behaviors such as drinking alcohol and various kinds of illnesses (House, 1986).

Activators of Stress

Activators are situations that disrupt a person's emotional or mental state. Activators or stressors can be major external events (war, flood, famine) or unpleasant interactions with people (divorce, job loss), or they may be changes in the body resulting from puberty, accident, or aging. An activator can also be an unmet emotional need or even a happy event such as marriage or winning a lottery.

To identify and measure the potential for certain experiences to be activators, Thomas Holmes and Richard Rahe (1967) devised the Schedule of Recent Experience (SRE). The SRE lists common events and for each event a corresponding number of life change units (LCUs) is assigned that measure the relative stressfulness of the event (Table 14.2). The SRE scores the death of a spouse as requiring the most adjustment (arbitrary numerical LCU of 100); mar-riage carries a value of 50 LCUs, and a vacation has a value of 13 LCUs.

Research using the SRE has shown that the accumulation of more than 150 LCUs in a year correlates with a high probability of negative health change within that year or soon thereafter. The likelihood of negative health changes increases as the number of accumulated LCUs increases. The negative health changes include heart attacks, accidents, infectious diseases, worsening of a previous illness, injuries, and metabolic disease.

TABLE 14.2

The Schedule of Recent Experience (SRE)

Rank	Event	Life change units	Rank	Event	Life change units
1	Death of spouse	100	23	Son or daughter leaving home	29
2	Divorce	73	24	Trouble with in-laws	29
3	Marital separation	65	25	Outstanding personal achieve-ment	28
4	Jail term	63			
5	Death of close family member	63	26	Wife begin or stop work	26
6	Personal injury or illness	53	27	Begin or end school	26
7	Marriage	50	28	Change in living conditions	25
8	Fired from job	47	29	Revision of personal habits	24
9	Marital reconciliation	45	30	Trouble with boss	23
10	Retirement	45	31	Change in work hours or condi-tions	20
11	Change in health of family member	44	32	Change in residence	20
12	Pregnancy	40	33	Change in schools	20
13	Sex difficulties	39	34	Change in recreation	19
14	Gain of new family member	39	35	Change in church activities	19
15	Business adjustment	39	36	Change in social activities	18
16	Change in financial state	38	37	Mortgage or loan less than $10,000	17
17	Death of close friend	37	38	Change in sleeping habits	16
18	Change to different line of work	36	39	Change in number of family get-togethers	15
19	Change in number of argu-ments with spouse	35	40	Change in eating habits	15
20	Mortgage over $10,000	31	41	Vacation	13
21	Foreclosure of mortgage or loan	30	42	Christmas	12
22	Change in responsibilities at work	29	43	Minor violations of the law	11

FIGURE 14.4
The hypothetical stress-illness relationship.

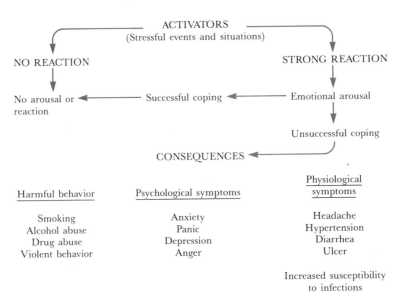

Recognizing that people's reactions to various situations may differ in intensity, Irwin Sarason and his colleagues (1986) developed the Life Experience Survey (LES). The LES lists 47 life events that are potential activators of stress (34 of which appear on the SRE) but does not rate their importance. Each respondent is asked to rate the degree of distress experienced with each event. Results of research with the LES are similar to the results obtained with the SRE.

It is important to remember that surveys such as the SRE and LES are culture-bound; that is, their effectiveness in predicting health problems associated with activators depends on the similarity of the people in the group being surveyed. The potential for health changes depends on the meaning and importance people place on certain events. Because individuals from different social strata or ethnic groups have different values, beliefs, and attitudes, they often respond differently to activators (see Box).

Reactions to Activators

Reactions depend largely on the individual's personality and emotional makeup and not on the activator itself. Everyone interprets the world and events differently. Each of us is born with a capacity for certain behavior, which is greatly modified and shaped by what we learn and experience. Each of us reacts to a particular situation according to individual values, beliefs, and attitudes.

Because of these differences, a situation that may be very stressful to one person may not bother another. According to stress researcher Folkman (1984), experiencing stress requires that an individual interpret a given situation as significant (This situation is important to me) and that he or she decide what to do with the situation (What can I do about it?). For most people situations that are interpreted as stressful include (1) *harm and loss,* (2) *threat,* and (3) *challenge.*

Harm and loss include the death of a loved one, theft or damage to one's home, physical injury or loss of an organ, physical assault, or loss of self-esteem. Harm and loss create stress because an important physical or psychological need is not satisfied. Emotions that signal harm or loss include sadness, depression, and anger. Note that eight of the first ten items on the SRE involve harm and loss.

Threats are perceived and interpreted as

ARE YOU SUSCEPTIBLE TO STRESS?

Some persons are more susceptible to stress than others. The following test, developed at the Boston University Medical Center, can give you some indication of your susceptibility. Score each item from 1 (almost always) to 5 (never) as it applies to you. Any number less than 50 indicates you are not particularly vulnerable to stress. A score of 50 to 80 indicates moderate vulnerability, and over 80, high vulnerability.

___ 1. I eat at least one hot, nutritious meal a day.

___ 2. I get seven to eight hours sleep at least four nights a week.

___ 3. I am affectionate with others regularly.

___ 4. I have at least one relative within 50 miles on whom I can rely.

___ 5. I exercise to the point of sweating at least twice a week.

___ 6. I smoke fewer than ten cigarettes a day.

___ 7. I drink fewer than five alcoholic drinks a week.

___ 8. I am about the proper weight for my height and age.

___ 9. I have enough money to meet basic expenses and needs.

___ 10. I feel strengthened by my religious beliefs.

___ 11. I attend club or social activities on a regular basis.

___ 12. I have several close friends and acquaintances.

___ 13. I have one or more friends to confide in about personal matters.

___ 14. I am basically in good health.

___ 15. I am able to speak openly about my feelings when angry or worried.

___ 16. I discuss problems about chores, money, and daily living issues with the people I live with.

___ 17. I do something just for fun at least once a week.

___ 18. I am able to organize my time and do not feel pressured.

___ 19. I drink fewer than three cups of coffee (or tea or cola drinks) a day.

___ 20. I allow myself quiet time at least once during each day.

TOTAL ___

Adapted from a test developed by L. H. Miller and A. D. Smith.

---

likely to produce harm or loss whether or not any harm or loss actually occurs. The experience is one of continually warding off demands that tax one's abilities to cope with life. Emotions associated with threat include anger, hostility, anxiety, frustration, and depression.

Challenges are perceived and interpreted as opportunities for growth, mastery, and gain. Very often such situations involve major transitions such as leaving one's family to start life on one's own, graduating from college, or getting married. Even though they are interpreted as "good," transitions can nevertheless be stressful because they require considerable psychological and physical adjustment. Often a transition involves both sadness and excitement: sadness for the loss of what is familiar and excitement in anticipation of the new.

Besides interpreting a situation as harmful, threatening, or challenging, reacting to a situation also involves deciding what to do about it. This is *coping*. Coping is effort to manage a situation and is independent of outcome. This definition differs from the popular idea that coping with a problem necessarily includes success.

The ability to cope often depends on a person's belief about how much control he or she has over the situation. Control, in turn, depends on how powerful the situation is perceived to be and resources that the individual can muster to meet the challenge (Table 14.3). People who believe that they can control their environment,

TABLE 14.3
Various Factors Affecting Coping with Stress

PHYSICAL
Genetic predisposition to stress illness
Health status
Nutritional status
Physical strength and endurance

PSYCHOLOGICAL
Beliefs and attitudes about change
Beliefs and attitudes about one's abilities and skills
Motivation to manage challenge and change
Previous history with managing challenge and change
Self-esteem

SOCIAL
Availability of other people who offer care and support
Social climate (absence of prejudice, racism, expectations)
Institutional support and services
Stable social and economic environment

MATERIAL
Income, food, shelter
Access to information
Access to helping services
Access to tools and equipment

who perceive life changes to be opportunities for growth, who hold a personal commitment to respond to challenges, and who are optimistic about success have been shown to feel less stress than those who believe that they lack control, who are helpless in the face of change, who hold little hope for a positive outcome, and who seek permission from others before acting.

Consequences of Reactions

Although it is the mind that interprets a given situation as harmful, threatening, or challenging, it is the nervous and endocrine systems, which link the brain with the rest of the body, that bring about the changes in physiology that lead to harmful behavior or to disease. The feelings associated with stressful experiences (fear, anger, sadness) activate the nervous and endocrine systems, which produce changes in the immune system and in physiology. Illnesses arise when the nervous and endocrine systems are continually activated or overstimulated. As a consequence, organs begin to wear down or become susceptible to disease.

The challenge-response systems activate the *fight or flight* response. All mammals, including humans, are capable of displaying this particular response when confronted with challenges they interpret as frightening or as a threat to survival. The response is characterized by a coordinated discharge of the sympathetic nervous system and portions of the parasympathetic nervous system and by the secretion of a number of hormones, especially epinephrine. When a person (or other animal) perceives a threat, the emotions (usually fear or rage) that rise in the limbic system portion of the brain are translated into the appropriate physiological responses through nervous and hormonal pathways mediated by the hypothalamus.

Some of the more prominent aspects of the fight or flight response are an elevation of the heart rate and blood pressure (to provide more blood to muscles), constriction of the blood vessels of the skin (to limit bleeding if wounded), dilation of the pupil of the eye (to let in more light, improving vision), increased activity in the reticular formation of the brain (to increase the alert, aroused state), and liberation of glucose and free fatty acids from storage depots (to make more stored energy available to the muscles, brain, and other tissues and organs). Figure 14.5 lists the physiological reactions of the fight or flight response.

Everyone is capable of this response; it is part of human biology. Individuals display this reaction to some extent when they narrowly escape from a dangerous mishap or when they get angry or frustrated and lose their temper. The heart rate quickens, the person becomes more alert and tense and feels a rush of excitement from increased epinephrine in the blood. In short, the person becomes ready to act to deal with the situation.

In our society, however, fleeing from a threatening situation or engaging in physical

FIGURE 14.5
The fight or flight response.

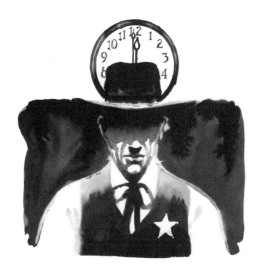

Heart
Increase in heart rate and force of contractions

Blood vessels
Constriction of abdominal viscera and dilitation in skeletal muscles

Eye
Contraction of radial muscle of iris and relaxation of ciliary muscle

Intestines
Decreased motility and relaxation of sphincters

Skin
Contraction of pilomotor muscles and contraction of sweat glands

Spleen
Contraction

Brain
Activation of reticular formation

combat is often inappropriate—and sometimes impossible. Social norms dictate that people handle many difficult situations civilly. Moreover, many threats are symbolic. The fear of losing a job, social status, or a lover is not the same as being confronted by a ferocious animal or thug, but the anxiety can produce similar physiological responses. Thus, one of the consequences of having a highly evolved brain with the ability for symbolic thought and the intellectual capacity to produce a civilized society is social norms that make people unwilling or unable to take direct action when confronted with threats. The fight or flight reaction has outgrown most of its usefulness. However, human biological changes have not kept pace with cultural and social changes. Thus, we are left with a biological response that is inappropriate for most stressful situations.

General Adaptation Syndrome

Hans Selye (1983), a pioneer in researching responses to stress, found that continued physiological responding to stressors led to a characteristic response called the General Adaptation Syndrome (GAS). The GAS is characterized by a three-phase response to any stressor (Figure 14.6). In the first phase, called the *alarm*, a person's ability to withstand any type of stressor is lowered by the need to deal with the stressor, whether it is a burn, a broken arm, the loss of a loved one, or the fear of losing one's job. During the second phase, the *resistance*, the body adapts to the continued presence of the stressor by increasing resistance—for example, by producing more epinephrine, raising the blood pressure, activating the immune system, releasing glucose into the blood, tensing certain muscles. If interaction with the stressor is prolonged, the ability to resist becomes depleted, and the person enters the *stage of exhaustion*. During exhaustion disease may be initiated. Because many months or even years of wear and tear may be required before the body's resistance is exhausted, illness may not appear until long after the initial interaction with the stressor.

Experiments with laboratory animals performed by Selye and others have demonstrated that profound changes in vital body organs—principally the adrenal glands, the thymus gland, the lymph nodes, and the lining of the stomach—can be caused by activation of the GAS. For example, stomach ulcers in humans or other animals can often result from prolonged interaction with a stressor. In a study of air traffic controllers, more than half were found to be suf-

FIGURE 14.6

The three phases of the general adaptation syndrome. In the stage of alarm, the body's normal resistance to stress is lowered from the first interactions with the stressor. In the stage of resistance, the body adapts to the continued presence of the stressor and resistance increases. In the stage of exhaustion, the body loses its ability to resist the stressor and becomes exhausted.

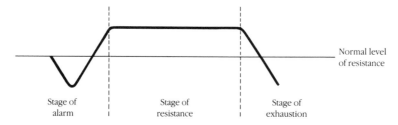

fering from gastrointestinal illness. Among those who were ill, more than half were diagnosed as having peptic ulcers. The constant stress from worrying about airplane crashes and collisions caused ulcers in many of the persons engaged in this kind of job (Cobb, 1973).

Animals receiving an intermittent mild electric shock tend to develop more ulcers than animals that are not shocked. More significantly, animals receiving warning of an impending electric shock develop fewer ulcers than do those not given a warning. Of special relevance to humans is the observation that animals given the opportunity to avoid or delay the shock develop only slightly more ulcers than do animals who receive no shock at all (Weiss, 1972). This implies that if ways are found to avoid persistent stress, or at least to modify its effects, many stress-related illnesses can be avoided.

Type A Behavior and Stress

Physicians Meyer Friedman and Ray Rosenman (1974) proposed that some people respond to stress in a way that predisposes them to heart disease; they dubbed this response the *type A behavior pattern*. They defined type A persons as being "engaged in a relatively chronic struggle to obtain an unlimited number of poorly defined things from their environment in the shortest period of time, and, if necessary, against the opposing efforts of other things or persons in the

same environment." In short, the type A behavior pattern is a "hurry sickness" (see Box).

Friedman and Rosenman suggest that a personality type opposite that of type A—type B—is associated with greater health. The type B person "is rarely harried by desires to obtain a widely increasing number of things or participate in an endlessly growing series of events in an ever-decreasing amount of time." Despite an enormous amount of research, recent evidence does *not* support the idea that type A persons are more susceptible to heart disease and heart attacks.

Stress and the Immune System

Long-term activation of the nervous and endocrine systems is responsible, at least in part, for reduced functioning of the immune system, which produces increased susceptibility to infections. For example, Jemmot (1983) showed that stress associated with taking exams can reduce the level of antibodies (in this study, immunoglobulin A) that are normally present in saliva. Samples of saliva were taken from a group of students at various times during their first year of dental school. Students returning from vacation had the highest levels of antibody, whereas during the exam periods the students' antibody levels were significantly lower. These data may explain the longstanding observation that colds and other infectious diseases increase in student populations during exams. If stress

---

DO YOU HAVE "HURRY SICKNESS"?

	Almost always ·	Only sometimes	Almost never
1. Do you interrupt other people before they have finished speaking?			
2. Are you irritated when you have to wait in line?			
3. Do you eat fast?			
4. Do you try to do more than one thing at a time?			
5. Are you annoyed if you lose at sports or games?			
6. How often do you forget what you were going to say?			
7. Do you tap your fingers or bounce your feet while sitting?			
8. Do you speed up and drive through yellow caution lights at intersections?			
9. Do you race the car engine while waiting for the signal to change?			
10. Do you fall behind in the things you need to accomplish?			

Here's how to determine your score. If you checked almost always, give yourself 3 points; if you checked only sometimes, 2 points; and for almost never, 1 point. Add up all of the points. If you scored 25 to 30, you probably have hurry sickness (don't worry, it's not fatal) and need to work on slowing down or relaxing more. If you scored 16 to 24, you have a potential for hurry syndrome. If you scored less than 16, you are probably pretty laid back.

---

can interfere with immune system responses, then it also can predispose one to infections and other diseases.

Other studies have confirmed that stress can impair the functioning of the immune system. For example, Stein (1985) found lower-than-normal levels of immune system cells in men whose wives had recently died. This may explain the observation that among older people a surviving spouse has an elevated risk of death during the period of bereavement. Unhappily married and recently divorced people also have reduced immune system functions.

Managing Stress

Stress-related illness is the result of a chain of psychological and physiological responses that consists of (1) the appraisal of a situation as per-sonally threatening or disruptive, (2) unsuccessful attempts to deal with the disruption, and (3) persistent activation of the nervous, hormone, and immune systems that eventually results in exhaustion and illness.

Because stress-related disorders depend on mental attitudes and processes, it is possible for people to control the steps that may lead to illness. For example, people can change how they interact with disruptive persons and situations by disengaging from a stressful situation (change jobs, change roommates, change college major).

An individual also can try to alter the response to a situation by changing beliefs and attitudes, and goals. Winning may be an athlete's highest goal, but the fear of losing may bring about an ulcer. The solution need not be to give up sports but to change one's priorities—perhaps by emphasizing one's performance and not the outcome of the competition. Another way to handle stress is to change one's usual way of coping. People who are inclined to act regardless of the situation may find that being patient and postponing action will produce greater rewards. At the other extreme, people who are inclined not to act may find it useful to become more assertive when confronted with a stressful situation.

The key to dealing with stress is to change some aspect of life or to change the way that situations are experienced. There is no stress-reduction pill; neither do alcohol nor tranquilizers offer any real solution to reducing stress. Tranquilizers, although often prescribed by physicians to reduce stress, offer at best only limited short-term relief—and at worst, habituation to and even physiological dependence on a drug. The best way to deal with stress is to replace stressful ways of living with beliefs, attitudes, and behaviors that promote peace, joy, and harmony. That does not mean that you must become reclusive or try to eliminate all sources of conflict, tension, and anxiety. People need a certain degree of tension to overcome challenges in order to be creative and to grow psychologically and spiritually. It may mean, however, that it would be wise to change some habitual ways of being and thinking that are self-destructive.

Another way to deal with stress is to employ a technique that produces a psychophysiological condition opposite to the fight or flight response. This condition has been termed the *relaxation response*, or *hypometabolic state*. Its use is based on the notion that continual discharge of the sympathetic nervous system and excessive secretion of adrenal hormones ultimately lead to ill health and that reducing these psychophysiological reactions to stress can improve health. The techniques that produce the relaxation response include autogenic training, meditation, progressive relaxation, and hypnosis. Apparently the physiology of the relaxation response can be elicited by any of these techniques and is not specific to any one of them. We urge everyone to learn some mental relaxation technique and to use it to reduce the physiological effects of stress.

Nearly all stress-related illnesses are preventable by avoiding or reducing stressors. Although you cannot avoid all potentially stressful situations, you can choose an occupation consistent with a peaceful frame of mind rather than with continual stress. Each person has to be sure that his or her choice of a livelihood is consistent with personal goals. For some, the tensions of (for example) air traffic control are too great and bring on illness. Clearly, these people should not continue as air traffic controllers unless their duties change to become less stressful or they learn to cope with their duties more successfully. For others, the challenge of air traffic control is stimulating and they have no problems with it. The same applies to any kind of work—firefighting, law enforcement, tax accounting, or child care. Good health comes from avoiding situations that are stressful to the point of causing illness.

EXEMPLARY LESSON PLANS

In light of this discussion, peruse the following lesson plan examples, keeping in mind that they are the type you will likely be expected to implement in your classroom. Remember that they by no means encompass a complete unit of instruction. They are simply offered as a guide for the formation of a comprehensive unit.

TOPIC: COPING WITH PROBLEMS

Grade Level: Intermediate

Concept: Most problems can be solved.

Expected Pupil Outcome: The student will be able to describe effective ways to deal with different problems.

Content: Typical problems children face:
1. Getting along with others (fighting)
2. Homework
3. Lying

Learning Experiences
1. *Problem solving:* Teacher prepares a worksheet on problem situations, reads each to the students and then discusses their suggestions for solving each problem. (See problem solving scenarios below.)

Problem Solving **Key Questions**

The following questions are suggested as a follow-up for stimulating and guiding the discussion of each problem. The direction such questioning takes should be based on (1) the teacher's use of each situation to make pupils aware of the steps for solving problems, and (2) the reactions and needs of the pupils.

1. Is there a problem?
2. Who has it?
3. Is it a recurring problem?
4. How would you solve it? Why?
5. Is there a good immediate solution?
6. Is this the best solution for later on?
7. Do you agree with _____ and his solution?
8. How would you solve it differently?
9. Does anyone have a different solution?

Problem 1: Getting Along with Others

Bill and Gary are team captains. Both teams are playing softball. Bill says "out" on a play and Gary disagrees. They begin to argue and Bill hits Gary. What should Gary do?

Alternatives:

1. Hit Bill back.
2. Tell the teacher Bill hit him.
3. Ask Bill if that made him feel better and suggest taking the play over.
4. Call Bill a name.
5. Run away from Bill.

Problem 2: Homework

Sue has just started working on her homework assignment. Lynn calls Sue on the telephone and asks her if she can play after supper. What should Sue do?

Alternatives

1. Close her book, forget about her homework, and go play with Lynn.
2. Copy Sally's homework and then go over to Lynn's house to play.
3. Tell Lynn she has to finish her homework, but if it's not too late, she can play afterwards.
4. Tell Lynn she's busy and will play with her tomorrow after school.
5. Go to Lynn's house to play, and then stay up late to do her homework.

Problem 3: Lying

Jim and some of the other boys are on the playground throwing rocks. Jim's rock hits a classroom window and breaks it. The classroom is empty. No one saw Jim throw the rock. What should Jim do when the teacher asks the class who threw the rock?

Alternatives

1. Admit he broke the window.
2. Say nothing.
3. Blame it on someone else.
4. Say nothing at school, but that evening tell his mother he broke a window at school.

Evaluation Procedures   During the discussion of each problem solving situation the teacher will evaluate the students' ability to select the most effective alternative offered. If the students are generally correct in their choices the objective will be considered attained.

TOPIC: RULES CONTRIBUTING TO GOOD EMOTIONAL WELL-BEING

Grade Level: Intermediate

Concept: A healthy lifestyle contributes to good emotional well-being.

Expected Pupil Outcome: The student will be able to practice the rules contributing to good emotional well-being.

Content: Fifteen rules of good living helping us to have good emotional well-being:

1. Be cheerful.
2. Be calm about things you do.
3. Think before you do things.
4. Be dependable.
5. Be patient.
6. Practice self-control.
7. Respect rights of others.
8. Plan what you do.
9. Be fair.
10. Do your share.
11. Do unto others as you would have them do unto you.
12. Do something for others without any strings attached.
13. Believe in yourself.
14. Develop good skills in the three R's.
15. Develop good social skills.

Learning Experiences

1. *Class discussion:* The teacher uses pictures depicting bad and good lifestyles as they relate to the fifteen rules of good living.

Evaluation Procedures   Teacher will subjectively evaluate the quality of the students' response during the class discussion. If the students display a good attitude in general, the objective will be considered fulfilled.

TOPIC: QUALITIES OF A GOOD FRIEND

Grade level: Primary

Concept: Good friends help us to be happy, better people (good friends help each other).

Expected Pupil Outcome: The student will be able to recognize qualities of a good friend.

Content: Good friends are
1. Honest
2. Kind and considerate
3. Thoughtful and polite
4. Helpful—do things for us
5. Cooperative and share things
6. Clean and neat
7. Cheerful
8. Interested in you
9. Responsible and dependable
10. Fun to be with
11. Good companions and listeners
12. Able to bring out the best in you

Learning Experiences
1. *Role play and dialogue* of poor and good qualities of a friend. Teacher reads off statement, and two to four children act out roles; rest of pupils identify kind of quality projected.

Evaluation Procedures The teacher will evaluate the quality of the dialogue following each role play session. If the students are successful in identifying the "Good Friend" qualities, the objective will be attained.

REFERENCES AND BIBLIOGRAPHY

Cobb, S., and R. M. Rose. "Hypertension, Peptic Ulcer, and Diabetes in Air Traffic Controllers," *Journal of the American Medical Association*, 224 (1973): 489-492.

Edlin, G., and E. Golanty. *Health and Wellness*, Third Edition (Boston: Jones and Bartlett, 1988).

Eisdorfer, C. "The Conceptualization of Stress and a Model for Further Study." In Michael R. Zales (Ed.), *Stress in Health and Disease*. New York: Brunner/Mazel, 1985.

Folkman, S. Personal Control and Stress and Coping Processes: A Theoretical Analysis, *Journal of Personality and Social Psychology*, 46: 839-852, 1984.

Friedman, M., and R. H. Rosenman. *Type A Behavior and Your Heart* (New York: Alfred A. Knopf, 1974).

Hales, D. "Mind over Body: Old Theories, New Proof," *Medical World News* (October 10, 1983):58-72.

Henry, J. P., and P. M. Stephens. *Stress, Health, and the Social Environment* (New York: Springer-Verlag, 1977).

Holmes, T. H., and R. H. Rahe. "The Social Readjustment Rating Scale," *Journal of Psychosomatic Research*, Vol. 11 (1967): 213-218.

House, J. D., V. Strecher, H. L. Metzner, and C. A. Robbins. "Occupational Stress and Health Among Men and Women in the Tecumseh Community Study," *Journal of Health and Social Behavior*, 27 (1986):62-77.

Maslow, A. W. *Motivation and Personality* (New York: Harper & Row, 1970).

Pearlin, L. I., and C. Schooler. "The Structure of Coping," *Journal of Health and Social Behavior*, Vol. 19 (1978): 2-21.

Sarason, I. G., B. R. Sarason, and J. H. Johnson. "Stressful Life Events: Measurement, Moderators, and Adaptation." In Susan R. Burchfield (Ed.), *Stress*. Washington, D. C.: Hemisphere, 1985.

Sarason, T. G., J. G. Johnson, and J. M. Siegel. "Assessing the Impact of Life Changes: Development of the Life Experience Survey," *Journal of Consulting and Clinical Psychology,* 46 (1978): 932-946.

Schildkraut, J. "The Biochemistry of Affective Disorders: A Brief Summary." In A.M. Nicholi, Jr. (Ed.), *The Harvard Guide to Modern Psychiatry* (Cambridge: Harvard University Press, 1978).

Stein, M., R. C. Schiavi, and M. Camerino. "Influence of Brain and Behavior on the Immune System." *Science,* 191 (1976), 435.

Weiss, J. M. "Psychological Factors in Stress and Disease," *Scientific American* (June 1972):104-113.

Wekstein, L. *Handbook of Suicidology* (New York: Brunner/ Mazel, 1979).

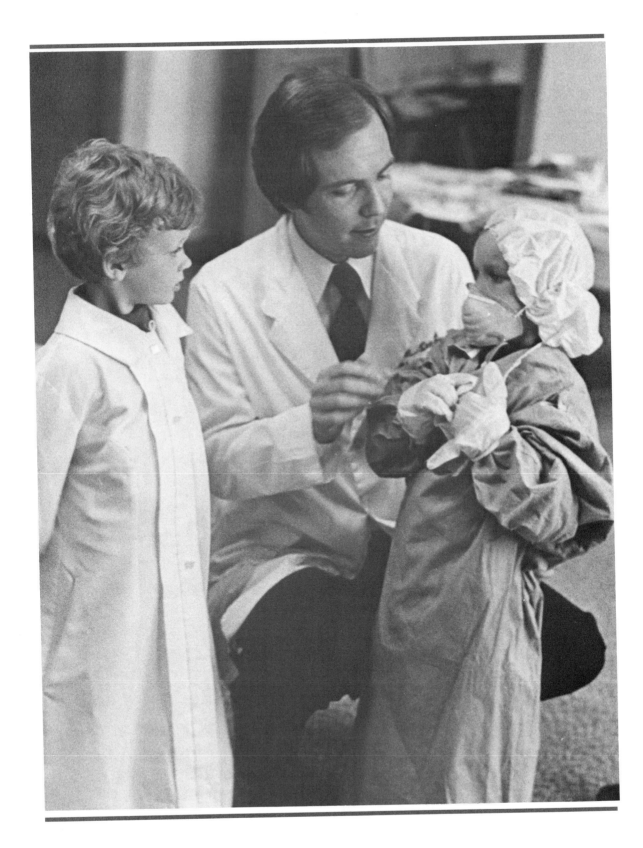

Chapter 15   Teaching About Drugs

INTRODUCTION

Perhaps no other health issue today commands more public attention than drug use and abuse. Nearly every school system has a formal drug education program. However, effectiveness of many of these programs is debatable.

The classic assembly program at which a local narcotics officer lectures on the ill effects of drugs while dragging on a cigarette may satisfy an administrator's ego, but it does little to impress students. The teacher who adamantly denounces the popular hallucinogenic drugs but fails to discuss alcohol and tobacco is not only naive, but possibly hypocritical as well. Inviting a rehabilitated narcotic addict to "tell it like it is" can be impressive but should hardly be considered as either all-encompassing or constituting the appropriate focal point of drug education. The use of inaccurate or outdated teaching aids is also a serious error. Youngsters are far more sophisticated about drug use and abuse than one might believe. Many may be far more experienced than you.

So what do we do? Is there one best way to approach drug education? Probably not. Surely many teachers are doing an effective job of drug education, and chances are that each uses a different technique. However, these underlying principles are basic to effective drug education:

1. Only sound, scientific, up-to-date information has a place in drug education.
2. Scare tactics have little long-lasting value.
3. Drug education includes instruction about *all* mood-modifying substances; alcohol and tobacco are no exception.
4. When biases or moralizing becomes apparent, the objectivity of drug education suffers and instruction loses its impact.
5. Instruction about drug use and abuse should be handled only by a well-informed, empathic, competent teacher.

6. Drug education is ongoing and comprehensive. "One-shot" endeavors are of little value.
7. Drug education encompasses far more than information. Drug education deals with behavior, and this implies that the affective and action domains are explored.

By now it should be obvious that drug use and abuse are not just a passing adolescent fad. The complexities of our culture provide the basis for what in many instances is irresponsible, self-destructive behavior in the form of drug abuse. Drug use is not new. People have abused drugs for centuries. The only new thing many young people have done is to expand the horizon of illusion and experiment with a wider variety of mind-altering drugs.

Surely our most important task at hand is to deal with the sources of drug abuse. We have already discussed the behavioral nature of drug education, and it follows that one of the greatest emphases in instruction should be on exploring the reasons why people chemically escape from reality. Alternatives to drug abuse are also important. Last but not least, we should provide children with the most up-to-date, objective information about the physiological effects of drugs on the body.

HISTORICAL PERSPECTIVE

People have been ingesting substances that alter thoughts, feelings, and behavior for thousands of years—ever since somebody first noticed that eating a particular plant changed the way he or she felt or behaved. That eating a particular mushroom or chewing the leaves of a certain plant could bring about pleasant feelings, relieve pain, produce strange visions, or increase physical vigor was probably an accidental discovery made while trying a new kind of food. Throughout the centuries since that discovery, potions, herbals, elixirs, and extracts have been used to change consciousness, to produce sleep, to heal

Much of the material in this chapter is from Gordon Edlin and Eric Golanty, *Health & Wellness: A Holistic Approach*, Third Edition (Boston: Jones & Bartlett Publishers, 1988).

the sick and wounded, to drive out evil spirits, and even to restore family and tribal harmony. Today drugs and medications continue to be used for many of these same purposes.

Advances in modern chemistry in the nineteenth century and the rise of new technologies produced a revolution in human drug taking. In 1803 a substance was crystallized from opium poppies and named morphine, after Morpheus, the Greek god of dreams, because of its numbing effects on the brain. Since that time thousands of biologically active substances have been prepared, no longer from the "eye of newt and toe of frog, wool of bat and tongue of dog," but isolated in pure form from plants, fungi, bacteria, and animals and synthesized by chemists. While many prescribed drugs are of enormous value in relieving human pain and suffering, in curing disease, and in facilitating healing, indiscriminate use and overuse of drugs—especially tranquilizers—has become a major health problem in our society. This section discusses legal drugs—those that are purchased over the counter or by a doctor's prescription and what are popularly referred to as *recreational* drugs—those that are taken primarily for pleasure or for reasons that have nothing to do with curing sickness or increasing health.

WHAT ARE DRUGS?

A *drug* is a single chemical substance that constitutes the active ingredient in a medicine. A medicine may contain two or more drugs (aspirin and codeine, for example) because the combined effect is greater than that of either drug alone, which is called *synergism.* (Other drug-drug and drug-food interactions are discussed later.) In the scientific sense, no distinction is made between a drug and a medicine—both are substances used to prevent illness, to cure disease, or to aid the healing process in some other way.

There are three principal ways that drugs are used in medical treatment. One is curative, as with antibiotics that destroy pathogenic microorganisms or certain drugs that destroy cancer cells. In one case we are cured of the infection; in the other we are cured of cancer. Another way drugs are used is to suppress symptoms. For example, morphine or codeine can suppress pain, and cortisone can suppress inflammation from allergies or arthritis. Third, drugs are used as preventive measures, such as vaccines that protect against viral infections or oral contraceptives that prevent pregnancy.

The *dose* of a drug is the amount that is administered, whether in the form of a tablet, a liquid, or an injection. Once a drug enters the body, the effects and consequences of its chemical activities can vary widely from person to person and from one administration to the next. The correct dose is the amount that will accomplish the desired therapeutic effect with a minimum of other (undesirable) effects. The effective therapeutic dose is modified by the presence of other drugs or chemicals in the body and by the person's experience with and expectations about the drug. It is important to know the effective therapeutic range for a drug, since too small a dose may provide no relief whereas too large a dose can be dangerous, even lethal.

How Do Drugs Act?

The number of chemicals that can act as drugs is large, and so diverse are their chemical structures that it is impossible to classify drugs into single chemical categories. Therefore, drugs are usually classified according to the physiological system on which they exert a primary effect (central nervous system, gastrointestinal system, and so on) or by the principal physiological effect they produce (lower blood pressure, relieve pain, stop coughing). For instance, all substances that increase urine production, regardless of their chemical structure, are called diuretics; those that inhibit pain, analgesics; those that relieve anxiety, tranquilizers, and so on.

Nor is there any single biochemical mechanism by which drugs alter physiology. Many drugs have been shown to interact directly with molecules inside cells or with receptor sites on the surface of cells (Figure 15.1). Once the drug

FIGURE 15.1

Binding of drugs to cellular receptor sites. The molecular structure of many drugs is similar to that of molecules normally produced in the body. The drugs compete for binding sites on cells and alter the physiological functioning of organs and tissues.

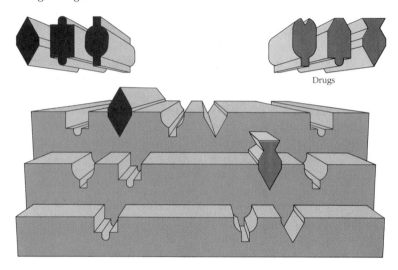

Drugs

molecules bind to or are absorbed into cells and tissues, they can inhibit or activate enzyme functions, stimulate or retard the release and synthesis of hormones and neurotransmitters, and change the flow of chemicals into and out of tissues. Frequently the chemical structures of drugs mimic (closely resemble) the structures of natural body components, such as enzymes, hormones, neurotransmitters, and vitamins. The brain produces molecules called endorphins that block pain by binding to certain pain-receptor sites in brain cells. The drugs morphine and heroin bind to the same cellular receptors as the endorphins, also blocking pain. Another drug, naloxone, inhibits the binding of both morphine and endorphin to receptors and is an *antagonist* of those substances. Recently, brain cell receptor sites for the tranquilizing drug Valium and for the hallucinogenic drug LSD have also been identified.

The discovery of receptor sites on cells allows scientists to understand the mechanisms of drug action and to develop new drugs that can produce specific and desirable changes in physiology. For example, it would be of great benefit to have pain-relieving drugs that are as effective as morphine but that do not cause physical dependence. Solomon Snyder (1980), of the Johns Hopkins Medical School, believes that today's rapid advances in understanding receptor sites for drugs may soon lead to the development of nonaddicting drugs for pain relief.

Many antibiotics recognize receptors that are specific to bacteria but that are not present in human cells. In this way antibiotics inhibit the growth of disease-causing bacteria in our bodies without interfering with our own cells. Most drugs used in the treatment of cancer are *antimetabolites*. That is, they adversely affect biochemical reactions that are vital to the growth of cancer cells as well as to the growth of normal cells. The aim of such treatment (chemotherapy) is to destroy the cancer cells completely, then to allow the normal, healthy cells to recover once the drug treatment is stopped.

Another type of drug mechanism can be seen in magnesium hydroxide, the active component of milk of magnesia. This drug acts outside the cells, in the body's spaces and fluids. It is poorly absorbed into tissues and while present in the gastrointestinal tract it tends to draw water out of the body, producing a laxative effect.

The Effectiveness of Drugs

The effectiveness of a drug depends on many factors, some of which can be controlled and some not. The dose can be controlled; however, once the drug enters the body, its effect will depend on how rapidly it is absorbed into the tissues, how much reaches the target organs or binds to the appropriate receptors, and how rapidly the drug is broken down and eliminated from the body.

Drugs are taken into the body by mouth, by inhalation, by injection into the muscles or skin (from which they diffuse into the surrounding tissues and into the blood), or by injection directly into the bloodstream (intravenous injection). Most drugs remain in the body for a relatively short time, often only a few hours, which is why most drugs are prescribed to be taken every few hours.

Inhalatory anesthetics are eliminated from the body with every breath. Other drugs are filtered out by the kidneys and are excreted in the urine. The liver and to a lesser degree the lungs possess special enzymes that break down drugs so that they become inactive and are excreted. Drug molecules are generally too small to be recognized by the immune system, so drugs usually do not evoke an immune response. An important exception is the allergic response to penicillin, which is discussed in a later section of this chapter.

Interaction of Drugs

The effectiveness of a drug in the body can be markedly altered by interaction with other substances, particularly with alcohol and with certain foods (Table 15.1). For example, antibiotics such as erythromycin and penicillin are destroyed by excess stomach acid. When taking these drugs, a person is usually instructed to avoid acid foods, such as citrus fruits and juices, vinegar, tomatoes, and cola drinks. The action of tetracycline antibiotics is inhibited by calcium-rich foods, such as milk, cheese, and ice cream. Because both are acidic, the frequent use of aspirin with orange juice can damage the stomach lining and even cause ulcers.

Alcohol interacts with many drugs that affect the central nervous system, such as tranquilizers and sedatives, and should *never* be used while taking such medications. Whenever your phy-

TABLE 15.1
Drug and Food Interactions That Should Be Avoided

If you take	Avoid	Because
Erythromycin- or penicillin-type antibiotics	Acidic foods: pickles, tomatoes, vinegar, colas	These antibiotics are destroyed by stomach acids
Tetracycline-type antibiotics	Calcium-rich foods: milk, cheese, yogurt, pizza, almonds	Calcium blocks the action of tetracycline
Antihypertensives (to lower blood pressure)	Natural licorice (artificial is OK)	Natural licorice causes salt and water retention
Anticoagulants (to thin blood)	Vitamin K: green leafy vegetables, beef liver, vegetable oils	Vitamin K promotes blood clotting
Antidepressants (monoamine oxidase inhibitors)	Tyramine-rich foods: colas, chocolate, cheese, coffee, wine, avocados	Tyramine elevates blood pressure
Diuretics	Monosodium glutamate (MSG)	MSG and diuretics both increase water elimination
Thyroid drugs	Cabbage, brussels sprouts, soybeans, cauliflower	Chemicals in these vegetables depress thyroid hormone production

sician prescribes a drug ask him or her whether there are any foods that you should avoid or other precautions you should observe while taking the prescribed drug. When in doubt about any drug, ask a physician or pharmacist.

Dangerous Complications of Drug Use

Even though a drug may be intended to have a single therapeutic effect, this goal is seldom achieved because the chemical reactions in the body are very complex. Drugs may have side effects, may cause allergic reactions, or may be harmful to developing embryos.

Drug Side Effects

Unintended drug actions are called *side effects*. From a biological point of view, they are completely normal. From the patient's point of view, however, the side effects of a drug are undesirable and often dangerous. For example, oral contraceptives are synthetic hormones designed to inhibit ovulation by affecting the hypothalamus, but they are so similar to natural hormones that they also affect other hormone-sensitive organs, such as the breasts and vagina, to produce occasional undesirable side effects.

Virtually all drugs produce some undesirable reactions in some people. One hopes the beneficial effects of the drug will far outweigh the undesirable side effects. For many people, however, this is not the case—which is why it is always wise to inquire about the benefits and risks of any drug and not simply to accept another person's assurances, even if that person is a physician. For example, many physicians prescribe a tranquilizer if a patient seems anxious or stressed, even though it would be much more beneficial to eliminate the cause of the anxiety or stress. Drugs are often prescribed for hypertension or ulcers when the cause of such symptoms is stress that may be reduced by other means.

Side effects are not a drug's only potential dangers. A drug may be harmful if it is taken in large doses or if the taker has some medical condition that will be aggravated by that drug. Such conditions are called *contraindications*. The necessity of controlling dosage and the need to screen for contraindications are two reasons most potent drugs are available by prescription only.

Physicians should, of course, be knowledgeable about the side effects of drugs and what constitutes safe dosages. Yet it is estimated that about *one-third* of hospital stays are needlessly extended because of doctor-induced illness, called *iatrogenic illness,* caused principally by improper medication (Steel, 1981).

Drug Hypersensitivity

Some people exhibit an allergic response to certain drugs. This condition is known as *drug hypersensitivity.* Usually a mild reaction, such as a rash, indigestion, or a stuffy nose, occurs on initial exposure. A second exposure to the drug often produces a more severe reaction. Perhaps the best-known example of drug hypersensitivity is the allergic reaction to penicillin.

Such persons produce antibodies specific to penicillin after they have been exposed to the drug. These antibodies are different from the antibodies for infectious bacteria and viruses. Months or years later another exposure to penicillin can re-stimulate antibody production and produce a severe reaction in a sensitive person.

As much as 5 percent of the population exhibits a penicillin allergy. Often the allergy shows up as a rash or inflammation in some part of the body. However, some people have a more severe reaction known as *anaphylaxis,* which can lead to death within hours or even minutes. For this reason repeated use of penicillin to treat bacterial infections may be unwise for some allergic persons, and use of other antibiotics may be safer. A physician will usually inquire if a person has any allergies before prescribing an antibiotic.

Legal Drug Abuse

People take prescription and over-the-counter (OTC) drugs for many reasons that are unrelated to illness, injury, or therapy. In 1983 the American Medical Association concluded that "The abuse of prescription drugs results in more injuries and deaths to Americans than all illegal drugs combined. . . . Prescription drugs are involved in almost 60 percent of all drug-related deaths." The most abused prescription drugs are the stimulants (amphetamines, anorexiants) and the depressants (opioids, barbiturates, benzodiazepines). OTC drugs that are frequently overused and abused are sleep and cold remedies, analgesics taken for aches and pains, and cough remedies.

People over 65 years of age are the largest consumers of both prescription and OTC drugs, which explains why TV drug ads usually show older persons as sufferers. Older persons often take numerous drugs for a variety of complaints, and these drugs may interact in unforeseen ways to cause additional problems. It is not uncommon to find older people who daily take 10 or more different medications prescribed by different physicians at different times. Older people are physiologically less able to tolerate drugs than younger people and often suffer more serious side effects. Quite often elimination of all drug use for a brief period will cause many symptoms to disappear, which is a clear indication that the combination of drugs is causing problems. Patients need to ask for and use fewer drugs; physicians need to become less willing to prescribe unnecessary drugs.

Teratogenic Drugs

Drugs and other substances that cause defects in developing embryos are called *teratogens.* In the 1960s several thousand babies were born all over the world with an uncommon congenital birth defect characterized by deformation of the arms or legs. A study subsequently revealed that during early pregnancy all the mothers of the affected children had taken the tranquilizer thalidomide, which caused the abnormal limb development (Figure 15.2). The thalidomide incident is a tragic reminder that any drug, no matter how safe it might seem in an adult, may have disastrous effects on a fetus. Many drugs are known or suspected to be teratogenic, including such common substances as antibiotics and alcohol (Table 15.2). The further to complicate matters, drugs that are teratogenic in one species may not be in another. Aspirin, for example, is

FIGURE 15.2
Many pregnant women who took the tranquilizer thalidomide gave birth to children whose arms did not develop normally. These individuals are normal in all other respects, including intelligence and the capacity to have normal children when they grow up. Butch Lumpkin was able to overcome the birth defect to become a professional tennis instructor. (Photo by UPI/Bettman Newsphotos).

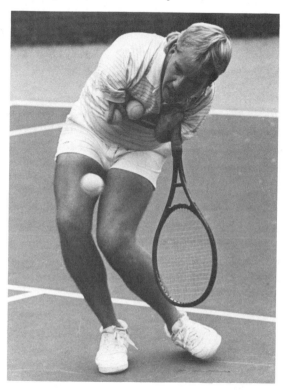

definitely teratogenic in rats, but its effect on developing human embryos is still uncertain. Because it is difficult to determine what substances are teratogenic in humans and to what degree, pregnant women are advised to forgo the use of all drugs, including nicotine, alcohol, and caffeine, especially during the first few months.

The Overmedicating of Americans

Americans consume an enormous quantity of drugs. Persons in our society have a total of about 1.5 billion drug prescriptions filled a year, which amounts to an average of five prescriptions for

TABLE 15.2

Drugs That Have Been Proved to Be Teratogenic

Alcohol	Streptomycin
Anticonvulsant drugs	Tetracyclines
Chemotherapeutic drugs	Thalidomide
Folic acid antagonists	Thiourea drugs
Lithium	Trimethadione
Sex steroids	Warfarin

every man, woman, and child in the country (Wertheimer, 1983). The total annual cost of prescription drugs is about $16 billion, and another $8 billion is spent on over-the-counter (OTC) medications and remedies (Table 15.3). In 1982, the per capita expenditure for drugs in the United States was almost $100, which is two and a half times the amount that was spent 12 years ago.

In 1980 the U.S. Department of Health and Human Services carried out an extensive survey of drug use in office-based medical practices, covering which drugs a doctor recommends for a patient, how often, and for what reason. The survey found that in 1980 Americans made a total of 575,745,000 visits to doctors' offices and that about 60 percent of the time one or more drugs were recommended. It may come as a surprise that in 1981 the top-selling prescription drugs were for stomach ulcers and for high blood pressure—chronic conditions for which nondrug therapies are also quite effective if people are willing to modify their lifestyles.

The use of drugs in our society has become so commonplace and accepted that many people automatically turn to drugs to solve their mental, physical, and emotional problems. So positive and trusting are people's attitudes toward drugs that many fail to appreciate the dangers and health hazards of ingesting drugs. As pointed out by Silverman and Lee (1974): "Much of the blame must be placed on the multibillion-dollar-a-year prescription drug industry and its incredibly effective promotional campaigns. But reprehensible as some of its huckstering has been, the industry cannot be made the only whipping boy. Others—physicians and patients in particular—must share in the responsibility."

It is in the area of drug use that holistic views of health differ most significantly from those of conventional medicine. When people have even minor complaints such as headache, backache, fatigue, upset stomach, colds, and allergies, most believe and expect that taking drugs is the only solution to their problem. This belief is encouraged by drug companies and physicians, but in the final analysis, it is people who demand, purchase, and use the drugs. Thus, you can ignore or resist advertising that is contrary to your health goals. You can reduce or eliminate the amount and kinds of drugs you take, especially for minor complaints. Learning how drugs affect your body and mind and how they can be harmful is the first step to wise drug usage. The next step is to discover possible nondrug solutions to your health problems.

The Effects of Drug Advertising on Health

Drug companies spend approximately $2 billion each year promoting their products both to the general public and to physicians. During the winter months, the TV screen and the pages of pop-

TABLE 15.3

Retail Sales of Prescription and OTC Drugs in 1982

Drugs	Sales (millions of dollars)
Prescription drugs	$16,154
Over the counter pain relievers including aspirin and nonaspirin products	2,451
Digestive aids such as antacids, laxatives, and antidiarrheals	1,996
Cough and cold remedies	1,326
Vitamin supplements	1,031
First aid remedies	839
Diet aids	381
Foot care remedies	278

Data from Statistical Abstracts of the U.S., 1984.

ular magazines are loaded with inducements to buy products for coughs and colds. In the summer it's ads for creams and lotions for sunburn and tanning. Ads for pain relievers and upset stomach remedies are ubiquitous and incessant (Figure 15.3).

Because the lion's share of drug sales comes from prescription medications, it is no wonder that most drug advertising is directed toward physicians, the only persons in the United States who can legally dispense these drugs. Drug companies spend thousands of dollars per year per physician (allopathic and osteopathic) trying to persuade them to prescribe particular drugs. Drug companies send sales representatives to doctors' offices to inform them of the company's products and to leave free samples. Drug companies sponsor seminars and courses to update physicians on the diagnosis and treatment of diseases (for which the company usually manufactures a drug). And drug companies deluge physicians with pharmaceutical junk mail. One doctor found that the drug company junk mail that he had saved weighed nearly 503 pounds at the end of the year.

FIGURE 15.3
OTC pain relievers' share of $1.7 billion market in 1985.

ASPIRIN	
Anacin	8%
Excedrin	7
Bayer	7
Bufferin	6
Other	18

ACETAMINOPHEN	
Tylenol	35%
Anacin	5
Panadol	2
Datril	1
Other	3

IBUPROFEN	
Advil	6%
Nuprin	3

Drug company advertising is a major source of revenue for professional medical journals. In 1984, the *Journal of the American Medical Association* was accused of publishing an article favorable to a particular drug (Procardia) to appease Pfizer Laboratories, one of the journal's major advertisers. Indeed, publication of results that are unflattering to a drug company's product can lead to withdrawal of advertising and loss of revenue for a journal.

Although drug company advertising undoubtedly inflates drug costs, a worse consequence is that it may influence a doctor's clinical judgment. Many doctors haven't the time or the inclination to investigate and evaluate the benefits and safety of a new drug, so they use drug company courses and advertising literature as the sole basis for prescribing the drug.

In 1984 a new pain reliever, *ibuprofen,* was introduced into the OTC drug market. Because aspirin and acetaminophen command over 90 percent of the $1.7 billion market, manufacturers of the new drug have been heavily promoting it in medical journals. The purpose of these ads is to get physicians to recommend or prescribe the new drug. One advertisement shows that after four hours Nuprin relieves headaches about 8 percent more effectively than acetaminophen (Figure 15.4). From a holistic perspective, however, the more significant result is that 40 percent of headache sufferers get the same relief with no drug whatsoever. These people were given a pill that contained no active ingredient. Remember the power of the placebo next time you think you need a pill for minor relief.

The Pharmaceutical Manufacturers Association regularly runs full-page ads in popular magazines to convince the public of the necessity, effectiveness, and safety of drugs. A recent ad opened with this headline: "I'LL HAVE TO TAKE THESE FOR THE REST OF MY LIFE. THANK GOD." Below the headline was a picture of a concerned man holding a bottle of pills. What was this man's problem? High blood pressure, a condition that is often caused by stress. Relaxation techniques have been shown to reduce stress and to relieve high blood pressure. Yet the pharmaceutical industry recommends to the public that people take drugs for this condition for the *rest of their lives.* No mention is

A study of the effectiveness of ibuprofen (Nuprin) versus acetaminophen in relieving headaches. Note that 40 percent of headache sufferers get relief with no drug at all.

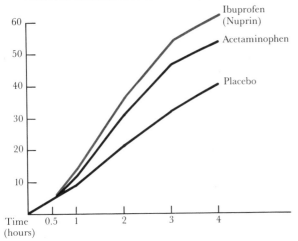

Percent of individuals free of headache pain

Ibuprofen (Nuprin)

Acetaminophen

Placebo

Time (hours)   0.5   1   2   3   4

made of other methods for reducing stress or of the serious side effects of these drugs.

An ad in a medical journal shows a photograph of a sad-looking elderly man sitting alone on a park bench. The ad suggests to the physician that the company's antidepressant drug is an appropriate treatment for elderly patients who are depressed because they are alone much of the time. Of greater benefit might be to get the persons involved in activities and social interactions.

Another medical journal ad shows a man sitting at the console of a complicated electronic device with hundreds of buttons and switches. The man's sleeves are rolled up to indicate he's ready for action, and he's wearing earphones to indicate he is at work. The ad promotes a tranquilizer that promises relief from job anxiety— from the pressure that accompanies this man's responsibility as an electronics expert. If the stress of a job is causing illness, then it is the stress that must be dealt with. Still another drug company ad for a tranquilizer recommends that the physician prescribe this drug for patients who aren't hungry, who feel guilty, who can't calm down, or who can't sleep. None of these

conditions necessarily has anything to do with disease, yet drugs are recommended as the appropriate treatment.

It is easy to be angry over the abuses of drug advertising; it is harder to do something about it. We believe that as people become better informed and aware of the undesirable consequences of taking drugs, and of how frequently drugs do little to promote wellness, they will elect to cope with the symptoms of stress and anxiety in ways that do not involve drugs.

When confronted with a person who is in distress but who is not physically sick, most physicians feel obligated to offer some remedy, even if a medically legitimate one does not exist. People *expect* the doctor to prescribe something. The answer to this dilemma has been neatly provided by pharmaceutical companies that manufacture and advertise mood-altering drugs for just this situation. If a person is anxious, the drug ads tell the physician, prescribe a tranquilizer. If depression is a problem, give an antidepressant. If the person cannot sleep, prescribe a barbiturate or hypnotic.

The giving and receiving of a drug prescription certifies that a therapeutic interchange has taken place. Indeed, the tranquilizer or sleeping pill may help temporarily. Sometimes people become so depressed or upset over a life situation that they cannot muster the clear thinking and action necessary to deal with the problem. In such instances, a drug-induced night's sleep or lift from the fog of depression may help achieve a psychological state from which appropriate action can be taken. Unfortunately, too many people and their doctors assume that taking the drug in itself will solve the problem, whereas it may instead be preventing proper help and treatment.

Drugs and medications are highly useful substances. But as with so many products of modern technology, benefits also bring problems and risks. We have vaccines to help prevent such dread diseases as polio, antibiotics to help cure infections, and a variety of medications that help people deal with serious illnesses. The availability of so many medications has fostered the belief that drugs can help solve just about any health problem. As recipients of medical care, most people expect some form of medication to signify that their illness is being properly treated. And doctors prescribe medications that may be unnecessary in order to signify to their patients and to themselves that they are giving treatment and care.

To their credit, many physicians recognize this problem and do not like it. They would prefer to deal only with physically ill people—the people whose problems they were trained to treat. However, many patients resist the suggestion that they do not have a legitimate medical problem and insist that they receive some form of treatment, usually a tranquilizer or other drug. In our view this is the most serious form of drug abuse, not the illegal use of drugs that receives most of the attention on television and in the press. Being healthy means, among other things, being responsible for the drugs you use. You do not have to resort to "chemical coping" with emotional problems. You can resist being programmed into pill popping by a drug company advertising. You can refuse to accept a drug for a condition that results from anxiety, stress, or emotional problems. Saying no to a drug may be the most healthful action you can take.

When to Take Drugs

Almost everyone takes drugs of one kind or another at one time or another. People take drugs to relieve headaches, heartburn, tension, cramps, fatigue, and anxiety. Drugs are used to get to sleep and to stay awake. They are used for everything from skin problems to emotional problems. Many people who don't consider themselves dependent on drugs still need several cups of coffee a day to wake up or to keep themselves going.

Drugs play a vital role in the treatment and prevention of disease. Used with caution, drugs provide relief from occasional minor complaints. Used in moderation, certain drugs may occasionally enhance enjoyment of social interactions or increase pleasurable sensations.

The fact remains that as a society we are overmedicated and overdependent on drugs. The healthiest approach to living is to be as free

of drugs as possible. Wellness is not achieved by taking drugs. No drug should ever be taken casually, whether prescribed, obtained over the counter, or offered in a social setting. It is everyone's responsibility to treat his or her body with respect. Each person can learn when drugs are necessary to maintain or restore health and when the benefits of drug taking outweigh the risks.

PSYCHOACTIVE DRUGS: USES AND ABUSES

People use drugs not only for legitimate health reasons—relief of pain and disease symptoms—but also for reasons that have nothing to do with illness. Some drugs are taken for "fun" or to increase pleasurable sensations. Drugs that produce pleasurable changes invariably contain psychoactive substances and are often referred to as *recreational drugs*. Most people associate psychoactive recreational drugs with illegal substances such as marijuana, LSD, and cocaine, but recreational drugs also include legal substances such as alcohol, tobacco, and caffeine, as well as many legal prescription drugs, such as amphetamines and tranquilizers.

More than one-fourth of legal drugs sold in the United States and virtually all illegal drugs are *psychoactive;* that is, they alter thoughts, feelings, perceptions, and moods. Millions of Americans use both legal and illegal psychoactive drugs to cope with mental and emotional problems as well as to alter moods and behaviors. Psychoactive drugs include *tranquilizers*, which function to calm people; *stimulants*, which increase energy and physical activity; *narcotics*, which block central nervous system activity, thereby preventing pain and inducing sleep; *sedatives*, which slow down the nervous system and induce sleep; *analgesics*, which block pain; and *hallucinogens*, which alter moods and perceptions. A partial list of the many psychoactive substances people use—legally and illegally—to change thoughts, feelings, and behaviors is given in Table 15.4, along with a summary of the drugs' effects.

TABLE 15.4

Classifications of Drugs That Affect the Central Nervous System (Psychoactive Drugs)

Drug classification	Common and trade names	Medical uses	Effects of average dose	Physical dependence	Tolerance develops
Narcotics	Codeine Demerol Heroin Methadone Morphine Opium Percodan	Analgesic (pain relief)	Blocks or eases pain; may cause drowsiness and euphoria; some users experience nausea or itching sensations	Marked	Yes
Analgesics	Darvon Talwin	Pain relief	May produce anxiety and hallucinations	Marked	Yes
Sedatives	Amytal Nembutal Phenobarbital Seconal Doriden Quaalude	Sedation, tension relief	Relaxation, sleep; decreases alertness and muscle coordination	Marked	Yes
Minor tranquilizers	Dalmane Equanil/ Miltown Librium Valium	Anxiety relief, muscle tension	Mild sedation; increased sense of well being; may cause drowsiness and dizziness	Marked	No
Major tranquilizers (phenothiazines)	Mellaril Thorazine Prolixin	Control psychosis	Heavy sedation, anxiety relief; may cause confusion, muscle rigidity, convulsions	None	No
Alcohol	Beer Wine Liquor	None	Relaxation; loss of inhibition; mood swings; decreased alertness and coordination	Marked	Yes
Inhalants	Amyl nitrate Butyl nitrite Nitrous oxide	Muscle relaxant, anesthetic	Relaxation, euphoria; causes dizziness, headache, drowsiness	None	?

The legality or illegality of a drug has nothing to do with its proven pharmacological action or even with personal and social dangers associated with its use. The use of tobacco, for example, is both legal and encouraged, yet it is a major cause of disease and death. The use of alcohol is also legal and encouraged and a major contributor to disease and death. Tranquilizers such as Valium and Librium, which are among the most widely used prescription drugs, are as physically addicting as narcotics. Some prescription sedatives, and pain relievers also cause physical dependence.

The legal status of drugs changes with social customs and beliefs. For example, alcohol was illegal in the 1920's and 1930's, whereas mari-

TABLE 15.4
Classifications of Drugs That Affect the Central Nervous System (Psychoactive Drugs)— cont'd

Drug classification	Common and trade names	Medical uses	Effects of average dose	Physical dependence	Tolerance develops
Stimulants	Benzedrine Biphetamine Desoxyn Dexedrine Methedrine Preludin Ritalin	Weight control, narcolepsy; fatigue and hyperactivity in children	Increased alertness and mood elevation; less fatigue and increased concentration; may cause insomnia, anxiety, headache, chills, and rise in blood pressure; organic brain damage after prolonged use	Mild to none	Yes
Cocaine	Cocaine hydro- chloride	Local anesthetic, pain relief	Effects similar to stimulants	None	No
Cannabis	Marijuana Hashish	Relief of glaucoma, asthma, nausea accompanying chemotherapy	Relaxation, euphoria, altered perception; may cause confusion, panic, hallucinations	None	No
Hallucinogens	LSD PCP Mescaline Peyote Psilocybin	None	Altered perceptions, visual and sensory distortion; mood swings	None	Yes
Nicotine	(In tobacco)	None	Altered heart rate; tremors; excitation	Yes	Yes

juana was legal; during the early years of this century, opium, morphine, and cocaine were openly advertised and sold in the form of tonics and cough syrups. Coca-Cola, concocted by a Georgia pharmacist in 1886, was sold as both a remedy and an enjoyable drink. "Coke" contained cocaine until 1906, when the cocaine was replaced by caffeine.

Thomas Szasz (1974), a psychiatrist at the State University of New York, argues that our society's views of drug use and abuse are largely based on religious beliefs and on ideas of good and evil rather than on the pharmacological facts. In his view,

. . . the important differences between heroin and alcohol, or marijuana and tobacco—as far as "drug abuse" is concerned—are not chemical but ceremonial. In other words, heroin and marijuana are approached and avoided not because they are more "addictive" or more "dangerous" than alcohol and tobacco but because they are more "holy" or "unholy"—as the case may be.

Szasz contends that our confusion regarding drug abuse is associated with our confusion regarding religion. He defines religion as "any act or idea that gives men and women a sense of what their life is about or for—that, in other words, gives their existence meaning and purpose."

People's motives for taking drugs vary enormously and include curiosity, thrill seeking, relaxation, increased sense of well-being, peer acceptance, and religious experiences. Many people use drugs to escape from the reality of their lives or to achieve happiness and provide meaning to their existence.

In this chapter we discuss the recreational drugs that are widely used (and frequently abused) in American society in the 1980s, without undue emphasis on their legality or illegality. Surveys conducted in 1981 indicate that at least 50 million Americans have some experience with smoking marijuana and 10 million Americans have used cocaine at least once. An estimate of the extent of recreational drug use among high school seniors is shown in Table 15.5. While alcohol and cigarettes lead the way, marijuana and cocaine are not far behind. Obviously, nothing we can say here is going to change the widespread use of recreational drugs in the United States or solve the problems associated with illegal drug use. As with all other aspects of health,

we believe that each individual should have access to as much correct information as possible so that he or she can make an informed decision about whether to use recreational drugs.

Psychoactive Drugs Change Consciousness

Why do people seek out and use substances that are not needed for any health reasons? The answer seems to be that people enjoy changing their state of consciousness and are eager to ingest substances that promote mental and emotional changes, particularly if the changes seem to be pleasurable. Some drugs are able to produce ecstatic feelings in certain individuals, and psychoactive drugs have been used in religious ceremonies for thousands of years.

Consciousness can be broadly defined as the state of being aware of one's internal mental processes—that is, one's thoughts, feelings, moods, and so on. Each of us has a "normal" state of consciousness, although many people would have difficulty describing what they mean by "normal." However, every person knows when his or her state of consciousness deviates from normal—for example, during drunkenness, moods of extreme anger or sorrow, or periods of depression or apathy. High fever during illness can change a person's consciousness even to the point of hallucinating or feeling dissociated from reality.

Many activities that we do not generally regard as consciousness-altering do, in fact, produce changes comparable in many respects to the changes produced by psychoactive drugs. Long-distance runners may experience a change of consciousness that is described as "high"; dancing can produce psychic highs and even ecstatic states of consciousness, which is the goal of whirling dervishes, who practice particular forms of Sufi dancing. Food fasts can produce profound changes in consciousness, which is why prolonged fasts are often part of religious training. Many thrill activities, such as riding a roller coaster or shooting the rapids on a river raft, change consciousness and presumably are enjoyed partly for that reason. Put into this per-

TABLE 15.5
National Drug Use Among High School Seniors, 1982

Drug	Percent ever used
Alcohol	93
Cigarettes	70
Marijuana	59
Stimulants	28
Tranquilizers	14
Cocaine	16
Sedatives	15
Hallucinogens	15
PCP	13
Inhalants	18
Heroin and other opiates	12

spective, ingesting psychoactive drugs is only one of many ways to change consciousness.

Drug Abuse

The human body is capable of tolerating and eliminating small quantities of virtually any substance or drug with no permanent harmful effects. However, if a large dose is ingested or if a drug is used frequently, even though in small quantities, harmful effects on the person's physical or mental health may appear. Generally, any use of a drug to a point where one's health is adversely affected or one's ability to function in society is impaired can be defined as *drug abuse.*

Drug abuse is not so much a problem of the kind or amount of a drug taken but rather of whether the drug is used to cope with problems. If a drug is used to mask anxiety or undesirable behavior, it is being misused or abused. If a drug is used continually to combat the effects of stress, it is being abused. If pleasure is experienced only when the drug is taken, the drug is being abused. Serban (1984) has analyzed the difficulties of eradicating drug abuse:

Due to the complexity of the problems involved in drug abuse, encompassing psychological, sociological, not to mention the biological aspect of it, the prevention is not necessarily successful, as proven by research, by the simple presentation to the public of the unfavorable consequences of drug use. This approach is not a deterrent for the use of drugs in a hedonistically oriented society. It requires, as well, a change in the attitude of people, a reorientation of life toward work, and toward facing and coping with the inherent adversities of life.

Drug Tolerance and Dependence

The dangers of using a particular drug are often associated with the drug's ability to cause addiction, or *physical dependence,* as it is usually called nowadays. Many legal drugs, including barbiturates, tranquilizers, analgesics, opiates, alcohol, and tobacco, cause physical dependence. Among the illegal drugs, only heroin causes se-

vere physical dependence, which means that complex physiological changes result from using the drug, so that *withdrawal symptoms* occur if the addict abstains from using it. The withdrawal from a physically addicting drug invariably causes moderate to severe physical and mental symptoms.

Besides physical dependence, drugs can create psychological dependence, called habituation, and a second kind of physiological condition referred to as tolerance. *Habituation* is the repeated use of a drug because the user finds that each use increases pleasurable feelings or reduces feelings of anxiety, fear, or stress. Habituation becomes injurious when the person becomes so consumed by the need for the drugged state of consciousness that too much energy is directed to drug-seeking. Physically addicting drugs such as heroin and alcohol invariably produce habituation as well, so that the person is trapped into overusing energies and resources for obtaining the drug. As a consequence, relationships, jobs, and families can be destroyed. Many of the widely used recreational drugs, including marijuana, cocaine, LSD, and PCP, do *not* create physical dependence (addiction), but people do become habituated to their use. There are no physical symptoms of withdrawal from stopping use of these drugs, but people may experience uncomfortable psychological symptoms because of the habituation.

Drug tolerance is adaptation of the body to a drug so that ever larger doses are needed to gain the same effect. Because not all regions of the body become tolerant to the same degree, these higher doses may cause harmful side effects to some parts of the body. For example, a heroin or barbiturate user can become tolerant to the psychological effects of the drug, but the brain's respiratory center, which controls breathing, does not. If the dose of heroin, barbiturate, or other depressant becomes high enough, the brain's respiratory center ceases to function and the person stops breathing.

With these general comments on drug use and abuse as background, we devote the rest of the chapter to brief discussions of the most commonly used recreational drugs: cocaine, marijuana, psychedelics, amphetamines, caffeine, inhalants, PCP, and opiates. Alcohol and tobacco are discussed in separate chapters.

Cocaine

Cocaine is a stimulant obtained from the leaves of the coca shrub, *Erythroxylum coca,* a plant indigenous to the Peruvian Andes. For thousands of years, inhabitants of Peru, Bolivia, and Columbia have been chewing coca leaves to obtain the stimulant effects. After the conquest of the Incan Empire in the sixteenth century, coca was introduced to Europe and later to North America. In the late nineteenth century, Angelo Mariani, a Corsican, received a medal from the Pope for manufacturing an extract of coca leaves that "freed the body of fatigue, lifted the spirits, and induced a sense of well-being." In the United States in the 1880s, pharmacist J. C. Pemberton mixed extracts of coca leaves and kola nuts to produce Coca-Cola, claimed at the time to be not only refreshing but also "exhilarating, invigorating, and a cure for all nervous afflictions." Today, of course, Coke no longer contains cocaine, although cocaine-free extracts of coca leaves are still used for flavoring. Sigmund Freud extolled the use of cocaine as a mood elevator, a possible antidote to depression, and a treatment for morphine addiction. However, witnessing a friend's severe and terrifying psychotic reaction to cocaine tempered Freud's enthusiasm for the drug.

In the doses common to recreational use today, cocaine induces euphoria, a sense of power and clarity of thought, and increased physical vigor. These effects usually occur within 15 minutes after the drug is taken, either by sniffing ("snorting") a cocaine-containing powder, by injection, or by smoking. A typical cocaine high lasts 30 minutes to an hour, after which the user usually feels a letdown and a craving for another dose of the drug.

Cocaine increases heart rate and blood pressure. Overdose may induce seizures, heart stoppage, and cessation of breathing. Continued use of the drug can result in loss of appetite, weight loss, malnutrition, sleep disturbance, and altered thought and mood patterns. Frequent cocaine sniffing can inflame the nasal passages and possibly cause permanent damage to the nasal septum (see Table 15.6).

In a strict sense cocaine does not induce tolerance, physical dependence, or withdrawal symptoms. However, the potential for psychological dependence is great, and some people develop such a strong craving for the drug that their lives and fortunes are consumed by their cocaine habit.

In today's society, cocaine use is associated with a lifestyle of high status, wealth, glamour, and excitement. In 1980, cocaine sales in the United States were estimated to have a value of over $30 billion, making the cocaine business one of the biggest industries in the country. From the mid-1970's to the mid-1980's cocaine use increased enormously. In the United States in 1982 about 22 million people admitted to having tried cocaine and about 4 million were current users. In 1985 the cocaine hotline (800-COCAINE) received nearly a thousand calls a day requesting help. The use of cocaine is a national public health emergency.

One of the factors that contributes to the problem is "free base" forms of cocaine known as "crack," which can be smoked or added to tobacco and inhaled along with the smoke. The cocaine that is generally snorted through the nose consists of cocaine hydrochloride and is sold in the form of a powder. Crack is sold in small quantities costing $10 to $20, making it available to a great number of people, especially young

TABLE 15.6
Symptoms of Cocaine Use

- Blurred vision
- Panic attacks
- Crushing headaches
- Debilitating nausea
- Paranoia
- Convulsions
- Depression
- Hallucinations
- Respiratory arrest
- Cardiac arrest
- Death

persons who previously could not afford to buy cocaine. People who use crack either by inhalation or injection become psychologically addicted and dependent on it very quickly. In animal experiments, monkeys that are fed cocaine will choose it over available food and water until they die. Awareness of the dangerous symptoms of cocaine use should deter any sensible person who values his or her health from trying or experimenting with cocaine in any form.

Marijuana

Marijuana and *hashish* are products of the plant *Cannabis sativa* and other *Cannabis* species that grow in temperate climates all over the world. *Cannabis* has been cultivated for thousands of years, principally as a source of hemp fiber used in rope. A number of ancient cultures, including those of China, India, Japan, Greece, and Assyria, used marijuana for its psychoactive properties. In the United States today, marijuana is the most widely used illegal recreational drug, with an estimated one third of all persons between 18 and 25 years of age using it.

The principal psychoactive ingredient in marijuana and hashish is a chemical compound called delta-9-tetrahydrocannabinol, or THC. Ingestion of THC usually occurs either by inhaling the smoke from a cigarette or pipe or by taking a pill or eating a substance (such as cookies or brownies) that contains THC. Once inside the body, THC is absorbed rapidly in the tissues. In most individuals, low doses of THC produce a high characterized by euphoria, a sense of relaxation, and occasionally altered perception of space and time. Speech may be impaired and short-term memory is affected (Nicholi, 1983b). Because perception, motor coordination, and reaction time are also impaired, driving a car or operating other machines while intoxicated with THC is considered unsafe.

Sometimes marijuana use, especially among first-time or naive drug users, evokes such psychological reactions as confusion, anxiety, panic, hallucinations, and paranoia. Marijuana may also worsen a prior mental health problem or negative mood. Long-term use does not cause permanent changes in brain function or impaired cognitive abilities. Some of the possible health dangers of chronic, long-term marijuana use include the risk of developing bronchitis caused by marijuana smoke, increasing heart rate and blood pressure, and possibly a slight depression of immune system functions.

In an exhaustive study, *Marijuana and Health,* conducted by the National Academy of Sciences, a panel of experts concluded that "the verdict of the experts is—that there is no verdict . . . Marijuana cannot be exonerated as harmless, but neither can it be convicted of being as dangerous as some have claimed" (Relman, 1982). The study did state with some conviction that there was no evidence supporting the belief that marijuana use inevitably leads to the use of any other drug.

Marijuana sold illegally used to consist of a mixture of leaves, stems, and seeds. In the past few years, however, sophisticated marijuana growers in California, Hawaii, and elsewhere have begun producing *sinsemilla* (literally, "without seeds") marijuana that consists exclusively of mature dried flowers of female plants (Figure 15.5). Sinsemilla marijuana is usually about ten times more potent than marijuana mixtures containing leaves and seeds. Persons who smoke a joint of this high-potency marijuana may hallucinate or experience a severe anxiety attack. Frequently, just one or two puffs (hits) of a potent marijuana cigarette are sufficient to produce a high; if one is not certain of a drug's potency, it is wise to take one or two hits and wait 15 to 20 minutes to see what the effects are.

In some studies marijuana has been shown to be effective in treating glaucoma (by reducing ocular fluid pressure) and in relieving the symptoms of nausea and vomiting that frequently accompany cancer chemotherapy. The federal government cultivates a limited amount of marijuana to supply physicians who prescribe it for patients and for medical research. However, the widespread illegal cultivation of marijuana is intended solely for sale to those who use it as a recreational drug. A survey by drug enforcement officials in California estimated that the 1981 marijuana crop in that state had a value between $5 billion and $6 billion; nationwide estimates of

FIGURE 15.5

Sinsemilla marijuana cultivation in California. a, A label used by a marijuana grower. b, A field of mature female marijuana plants.

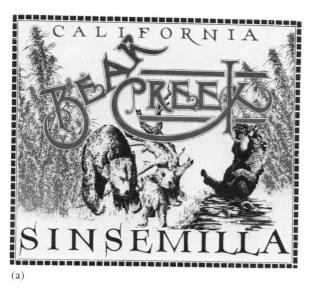

(a)

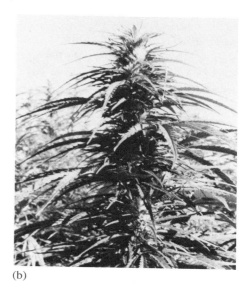

(b)

marijuana sales are in excess of $50 billion, which equals the amount of money Americans spend each year on alcohol and tobacco combined.

By many health criteria, marijuana is a safer substance than either alcohol or tobacco in terms of morbidity and mortality. (Keep in mind that no drug is entirely harmless.) That is why many people believe that the time has come to legalize or decriminalize marijuana use. If 50 million Americans have indeed broken the law, it is argued, it may be time to consider the possibility that something is wrong with the law. Despite the fact that marijuana is a relatively safe substance in a pharmacological sense does not mean that it is without danger to individuals who use it or to society as a whole. People can become dependent on marijuana use just as they become dependent on many other substances. Marijuana affects brain and motor functions and decreases alertness and intellectual abilities. Its use can adversely affect the performance of students and workers and can be a threat to public safety. For example, marijuana use by pilots, bus drivers, ship officers, physicians, and others clearly is a threat to persons who depend on their skills and judgment.

Tests for illegal drugs such as marijuana and cocaine are extremely sensitive and have become relatively inexpensive ($15 to $50). Cocaine can be detected in urine samples up to 48 hours after ingestion; marijuana usually can be detected up to a week after use and in heavy, chronic users traces may persist for a month or more after use has stopped.

Psychedelic Drugs

Drugs whose primary effects are to produce changes in perceptions and thoughts and that may evoke dreamlike and mystical experiences are called *hallucinogens*, or *psychedelic drugs*. The most potent psychoactive drug known is the hallucinogen D-lysergic acid diethylamide, commonly called LSD. As little as a few millionths of a gram of pure LSD can produce hallucinations; 50 to 100 micrograms is an average dose that produces an "acid trip" lasting several hours. The psychedelic effects of LSD were discovered accidently by a Swiss chemist, Albert Hofmann, who subsequently described the experience:

Last Friday, April 16, 1943, I was forced to stop my work in the laboratory in the middle of the afternoon and to go home, as I was seized by a peculiar restlessness associated with a sensation of mild dizziness. Having reached home, I lay down and sank in a kind of drunkenness which was not unpleasant and which was characterized by extreme activity of imagination. As I lay in a dazed condition with my eyes closed (I experienced daylight as disagreeably bright) there surged upon me an uninterrupted stream of fantastic images of extraordinary plasticity and vividness and accompanied by an intense, kaleidoscope-like play of colors. This condition gradually passed off after about two hours.

The hallucinogens comprise a wide variety of chemical substances derived from as many as 100 different kinds of plants as well as from chemical synthesis in the laboratory (Table 15.7). Despite their variety, these substances are able to alter perception, thought, mood, sensation, and experience. The similarity of their effects to psychotic hallucinatory experience is one reason they are called hallucinogens, but in many respects the psychedelic drug experience is not the same as a psychotic hallucination. Psychotic hallucinations are generally auditory and frightening, and the hallucinator believes them to be real. Drug-induced hallucinations tend to be visual, they are usually enjoyable or fascinating, and the individual is aware that the experience is exceptional or unusual and is not part of his or her normal state of consciousness.

Regardless of the specific substance, hallucinogens are most often ingested orally, either by eating the plant itself or by ingesting powder containing the active chemical. Normally, a hallucinogenic drug begins to take effect in 45 to 60 minutes, with the first effects being physical: sweating, nausea, increased body temperature, and pupil dilation. These symptoms eventually subside, and the psychological effects become manifest within an hour or two after ingestion. Depending on the particular substance and the amount ingested, the "trip" will last anywhere from 1 to 24 hours.

A common feature of the hallucinogenic experience is that the drugs suspend the normal psychic mechanisms that integrate the self with the environment. This makes the user extremely open to conditions in the surroundings. For this reason, experience in any particular drug episode is highly influenced, for better or worse, by the setting in which the trip takes place and by the psychic set—the expectations and attitudes—of the user.

Some of the more common effects induced by hallucinogenic drugs:

1. *Changes in mood.* Hallucinogenic drugs can induce mood changes ranging from euphoria and giddiness to terror and deep despair. In the worst case, a person can experience a complete loss of emotional control, becoming frightened, anxious, and paranoid. At the other extreme, some users occasionally experience a state of complete joy, blessedness, and inner peace.

TABLE 15.7
Substances Considered to Be Hallucinogenic or Psychedelic

Substance	Common name
D-lysergic acid diethylamide	LSD
Trimethoxyphenylethylamine	Mescaline (peyote)
2,5-Dimethoxy-4-methyl-amphetamine	STP
Dimethyltryptamine	DMT
Diethyltryptamine	DET
Tetrahydrocannabinol	Marijuana (*Cannabis*), hashish
Phencyclidine	PCP
Psilocybin	Mushrooms
Atropine	
Bufotenin	
Datura	
Harmine	
Ibogain	
Kava	
Khat	
Morning glory seeds	
Nutmeg	

2. *Changes in sensation.* While a person is tripping, colors may seem brighter, sounds richer and louder, and tastes more intense and pleasurable. There may be a sensation of the merging of the senses (synesthesia), such that sounds are experienced as colors or vice versa.

3. *Changes in perception.* The hallucinogenic experience may involve time distortion: seconds may seem like an eternity. Vivid colors and shapes may be seen with the eyes closed. Things that normally go unnoticed, such as pores in concrete, may seem fascinating. Small objects may seem unusually large or plain objects strikingly beautiful. The tripper may visualize intricate geometric forms and patterns.

4. *Changes in relations.* The hallucinogenic drug experience often brings a sense of depersonalization—the user feels simultaneously outside and within. The user's ego boundaries are suspended, so there is a sense of merging with others or with objects in the environment. Occasionally there is a sense of complete merging—oneness with the universe. There may be a sense of profound understanding, and many diverse aspects of life suddenly become clear and meaningful.

Hallucinogenic drugs produce tolerance to the psychedelic effect but do not create physical dependence or produce symptoms of withdrawal, even after long-term use. However, as with most psychoactive drugs, there is danger of psychological dependence. There is no evidence that hallucinogens have permanent harmful effects on health, and they do not cause genetic damage or birth defects in humans, contrary to what is often stated (Grinspoon, 1979).

Many psychedelic drugs have chemical structures quite similar to those of normal brain neurotransmitters. Serotonin, a brain neurotransmitter, is synthesized from tryptophan, an amino acid obtained from proteins in food. LSD and DMT have chemical structures derived from the basic ring structure of tryptophan or serotonin. Because of this chemical similarity, hallucinogens are able to bind to neurotransmitter receptor sites on brain cells or to alter the pattern of binding of neurotransmitters normally synthesized in the body. Even slight changes in brain chemistry can result in profound changes in brain activity and thought patterns.

Hallucinogenic drugs are powerful mediators of brain function and can dramatically alter perceptions and thoughts. They can precipitate psychotic reactions and behavior in persons who are mentally unstable or who fear the effects of the drug. Because they are illegal, hallucinogenic drugs can be obtained only from unreliable sources. Most hallucinogenic drugs sold as LSD or mescaline, for example, contain other psychoactive drugs, and the buyer has no way of knowing what is being ingested.

Amphetamines

Amphetamines are manufactured chemicals that act as stimulants of the central nervous system. The most commonly used amphetamines are dexedrine ("dexies," "footballs," "orange"), benzedrine ("bennies," "peaches"), and methedrine ("meth," "speed"). Another psychoactive amphetamine that is manufactured and sold illegally is called MDA (*m*ethylene*d*ioxy*a*mphetamine), which produces a hallucinogenic state lasting several hours. This drug is not safe and has been shown to cause destruction of brain cells as well as less severe symptoms (Ricaurte, 1985). Amphetamines are usually taken orally but they can also be injected ("mainlined"). The effects of an oral dose usually last several hours.

Although amphetamines are sometimes prescribed to suppress appetite or to counteract fatigue, they are by and large useless as therapeutic agents. Overweight and fatigue are not illnesses that require drug intervention. Both conditions are better managed by improved diet and exercise and in the case of fatigue, by less work, better time management, and more sleep. Another dubious use of amphetamines is to counteract the effects of drugs that depress the central nervous system.

The principal uses of amphetamines are recreational. These drugs produce euphoria, increased energy, greater self-confidence, an increased ability to concentrate, increased motor and speech activity, and improved physical performance. Besides being used by those wishing for the amphetamine high, these drugs are frequently abused by people who fight sleep, such as truck drivers, students who cram for exams all night, and nightclub entertainers. Athletes often use amphetamines to improve physical performance and self-confidence.

Excessive use of amphetamines can produce headaches, irritability, dizziness, insomnia, panic, confusion, and delirium. After extensive amphetamine use, the user often "crashes," or sleeps for long periods, feels very tired, and is depressed.

Prolonged use of amphetamines can lead to tolerance, especially for the euphoric effects and for appetite suppression. Amphetamines do not cause physical dependence, but they can create a psychological dependence and a particular pattern of use called the yo-yo, a cycle of drug abuse in which a person uses amphetamines for the stimulatory effect and then uses a depressant to calm down enough to sleep, only to be followed with more amphetamines in order to get going the next day. Chronic use can cause an amphetamine psychosis, which consists of auditory and visual hallucinations, delusions, and mood swings.

Caffeine

Caffeine is a natural substance found in a variety of plants. Nearly all Americans regularly ingest caffeine in one form or another: coffee, tea, chocolate, and soft drinks (Table 15.8). These beverages and foods are such an integral part of American eating habits that it cannot be argued that they are consumed solely for the pharmacological effects of the caffeine. Nevertheless, these products do have psychoactive properties and in addition to caffeine contain theophylline (principally in tea) and theobromine (principally in cocoa).

The effects of caffeine are familiar to most people. They include a lessening of drowsiness and fatigue (especially when performing tedious or boring tasks), more rapid and clearer flow of thought, and increased capacity for sustained performance (for example, typists work faster with fewer errors). In higher doses, caffeine produces nervousness, restlessness, tremors, and insomnia. In very high doses (10 grams or 60 cups of coffee) it can produce convulsions and be lethal.

Caffeine used to be prescribed for a variety of complaints, but it is rarely used therapeutically nowadays. However, it is still compounded into over a thousand over-the-counter drugs (Table 15.8). For example, many "energizers" and "stay-awake" products are pure caffeine. Analgesics, cough medicines, and cold remedies contain caffeine to counteract the drowsiness produced by the other ingredients in those medications. Caffeine is also put into weight control and menstrual pain products because it is a potent diuretic (it increases urine output and water loss).

A mild psychological dependence can result from the chronic use of caffeine, and tolerance to the stimulant effect can gradually develop. Mild withdrawal symptoms (headache, irritability, restlessness, and lethargy) may occur in habituated persons.

Central Nervous System (CNS) Depressants

Central nervous system depressants comprise a vast number of drugs that reduce a person's level of arousal, awareness of the environment, and level of motor activity, and that increase drowsiness and sedation. The CNS depressants include alcohol, drugs that affect sleep, *sedatives, tranquilizers,* and *hypnotics* (Table 15.9). A number of other drugs, such as opiates, antihistamines, and some medications used in the treatment of high blood pressure or heart disease, may also depress the activity of the central nervous system.

The CNS depressants have effects similar to those of alcohol. In low doses, they may produce a mild state of euphoria, reduce inhibitions, or induce a feeling of relaxation and lessened tension. In high doses they may impair mood, speech, and motor coordination.

CNS depressants are dangerous. All carry the potential for physical and psychological de-

TABLE 15.8
Caffeine Content of Beverages, Foods, and Drugs

Item	Milligrams caffeine (average)	Item	Milligrams caffeine (average)
Coffee (5 oz. cup)		Dark chocolate, semisweet (1 oz.)	20
Brewed, drip method	115	Baker's chocolate (1 oz.)	26
Brewed, percolator	80	Chocolate-flavored syrup (1 oz.)	4
Instant	65	Soft drinks	
Decaffeinated, brewed	3	Mountain Dew	54.0
Tea (5 oz. cup)		Mello Yello	52.8
Brewed, major U.S. brands	40	Tab	46.8
Brewed, imported brands	60	Coca-Cola	45.6
Instant	30	Diet Coke	45.6
Cocoa beverage (5 oz. cup)	4	Shasta Cola	44.4
Chocolate milk beverage (8 oz.)	5	Dr. Pepper	39.6
Milk chocolate (1 oz.)	6	Pepsi-Cola	38.4
Weight-control aids		RC Cola	36.0
Dex-A-Diet II	200	Cold/allergy remedies	
Dexatrim, Dexatrim Extra Strength	200	Coryban-D capsules	30
Dietac capsules	200	Triaminicin tablets	30
Alertness tablets		Dristan decongestant tablets and	16.2
Nodoz	100	Dristan A-F decongestant tablets	
Vivarin	200	Prescription drugs	
Analgesic/pain relief		Cafergot (for migraine headache)	100
Anacin, Maximum Strength	32	Fiorinal (for tension headache)	40
Anacin		Soma Compound (pain relief, muscle	32
Excedrin	65	relaxant)	
Diuretics		Darvon Compound (pain relief)	32.4
Aqua-Ban	100		
Maximum Strength Aqua-Ban Plus	200		

SOURCE: *FDA Consumer*, March 1984.

pendency, tolerance, unpleasant withdrawal symptoms, and toxicity from continual use or overuse. Acute overdose may produce coma, respiratory or cardiovascular collapse, and even death. Aggravating the potential for toxic and possibly lethal overdose is the synergistic actions of CNS drugs. That is, when taken together, two or more CNS depressants can produce a much stronger effect than either drug would produce if taken alone. The most commonly seen synergistic effect occurs when people drink alcohol while taking depressant drugs such as barbiturates.

CNS depressants are the largest class of med-ically prescribed drugs—more prescriptions are written for tranquilizers than for any other class of drugs. Although many depressants are medically useful in the treatment of seizure disorders and insomnia, preparation for anesthesia, and alleviation of acute anxiety that may accompany certain severe mental or emotional problems, the extent of their use far exceeds appropriate therapeutic indications. Millions of prescriptions for depressant drugs are handed out for complaints that are more effectively and safely handled by counseling or changes in lifestyle. CNS depressants are among the most abused of drugs, but because they are not illegal, their abuse receives

TABLE 15.9
Central Nervous System (CNS)
Depressant Drugs

Minor Tranquilizers (benzodiazepines)	*Nonbenzodiazepine—Nonbarbiturates*
Chlordiazepoxide (Libritabs, Librium)	Hydroxizine (Atarax, Orgatrax, Vistaril)
Chlorazepate (Tranxene)	Meprobamate (Equanil, Meprospan, Miltown)
Diazepam (Valcaps, Valium, Valrelease)	*Hypnotics*
Flurazepam (Dalmane)	Chloral hydrate
Halazepam (Paxipam)	Ethchlorvynol (Placidyl)
Prazepam (Centrax)	Ethinamate (Valmid)
Lorazepam (Ativan)	Glutethimide (Doriden)
Oxazepam (Serax)	Methaqualone (Mequin, Parest, Quaalude)
Temazepam (Restoril)	Methyprylon (Noludar)
Barbiturate Sedatives	Paraldehyde (Paral)
Butabarbital (Butisol)	Diphenhydramine (Sominex Formula 2)
Phenobarbital	Doxylamine (Unisom)
Mephobarbital (Mebaral)	Pyrilamine (Nervine, Nytol, Sleep-Eze, Sominex)
Amobarbital (Amytal, "blues")	
Pentobarbital (Nembutal, "yellow jackets")	
Secobarbital (Seconal, "reds")	

little attention from the media or from government regulatory agencies.

Inhalants

Inhalants include a wide variety of chemical substances that vaporize readily and that, when inhaled, produce various kinds of intoxicating effects similar to the effects of alcohol. Like alcohol, inhalants are depressants of the central nervous system. Generally, their intended effect is to produce a sense of euphoria, a loss of inhibition, and a sense of excitement. Some of the unintended effects include dizziness, amnesia,

inability to concentrate, confusion, postural imbalance, impaired judgment, hallucinations, and acute psychosis (Nicholi, 1983a).

Some inhalants that are commonly used for recreational purposes:

1. Commercial chemicals such as model airplane glue, nail polish remover, paint thinner, and gasoline, and substances such as acetone, toluene, naphtha, hexane, and cyclohexane.
2. Aerosol spray products.
3. Anesthetics such as amyl nitrate, nitrous oxide ("laughing gas"), diethyl ether, and chloroform.

Because they are vaporous, these substances get into the body quite rapidly. The fumes are usually inhaled from plastic bags. The intoxicant effects are often felt within minutes, and the high lasts less than an hour. Regular users tend to be preteens and teenagers of low socioeconomic status whose home lives are unstable and often violent. They use inhalants because they do not have the money to buy other drugs. Some adults use amyl nitrate ("poppers") during sexual relations, believing that the drug enhances the sexual experience. Some medical personnel are frequent users of nitrous oxide because it is so easily available to them.

The inhalant chemicals do not produce tolerance or withdrawal, nor do they induce physical dependence. However, they are quite dangerous. In addition to any harm that may ensue because of uncontrolled behavior (such as driving while intoxicated), these chemicals damage the kidneys, liver, and lungs and can upset the normal rhythmic beating of the heart. Some users have suffocated while inhaling the fumes from the plastic bags, and the potential for explosion is everpresent.

Phencyclidine (PCP)

Phencyclidine, also known as PCP, angel dust, hog, crystal, killer weed, and by a variety of other names, was developed originally for medical use as an anesthetic. Because of the drug's many adverse effects, it was taken off the market and became an illegal recreational drug. In the 1960's, phencyclidine was called the *PeaCePill*—a serious misnomer in light of what the drug does to the user.

The effects of PCP are quite variable. Depending on the dose and the route of administration, PCP can be a stimulant, a depressant, or a hallucinogen. Some of the intended effects are heightened sensitivity to external stimuli, mood elevation, relaxation, and a sense of omnipotence. Some of the unintended and frequent effects are paranoia, confusion, restlessness, disorientation, feelings of depersonalization, and violent or bizarre behavior. In high doses the drug can cause coma, interruption of breathing, and psychosis. Many admissions to psychiatric emergency rooms are for PCP intoxication. The drug impairs perception and muscular control, and users are prone to accidents such as falling from heights, drowning, walking in front of moving vehicles, and collisions while driving under the influence of the drug. PCP does not induce tolerance or physical dependence, but because it is eliminated slowly from the body, chronic users may feel the drug's effects for an extended period.

The effects of PCP are unpredictable and frequently unpleasant, if not actually horrible and life-threatening. PCP produces more unwanted and dangerous symptoms of drug intoxication than any other psychoactive substance (Table 15.10). Persons who sell illegal recreational drugs often surreptitiously mix PCP with marijuana or cocaine or sell PCP while claiming it to be LSD, DMT, or some other drug. Because PCP is relatively easy to manufacture, it is one of the more readily available and dangerous of the illegal recreational drugs.

Opiates

The *opiates* are a group of chemically similar drugs that depress the central nervous system (Figure 15.6). These substances do cause physical dependence, habituation, tolerance and produce serious withdrawal symptoms. The opiates are derived from the opium poppy, *Papaver somniferum*, extracts of which have been used for thousands of years in a variety of cultures to produce euphoria, to relieve pain, and to treat various diseases.

TABLE 15.10
Common Signs and Symptoms of Drug Intoxication

Signs and symptoms	PCP	Stimulants	Hallucinogens	Sedative-hypnotics	Narcotics
Aggressive and violent behavior	X	X			
Ataxia	X			X	
Coma	X			X	X
Confusion	X		X		
Convulsions	X	X			
Drowsiness	X			X	X
Hallucinations	X		X		
Hyperreflexia	X	X			
Nystagmus	X			X	
Hypertension	X	X			
Paranoia	X	X	X		
Psychosis	X	X	X		
Respiratory depression				X	X
Slurred speech	X			X	

FIGURE 15.6

Chemical structures of opiate drugs. Morphine and codeine occur naturally in opium extracts of poppies. Heroin is synthesized by chemically modifying morphine. Opiates bind to receptor sites on brain cells (different from hallucinogen receptor sites) and change consciousness.

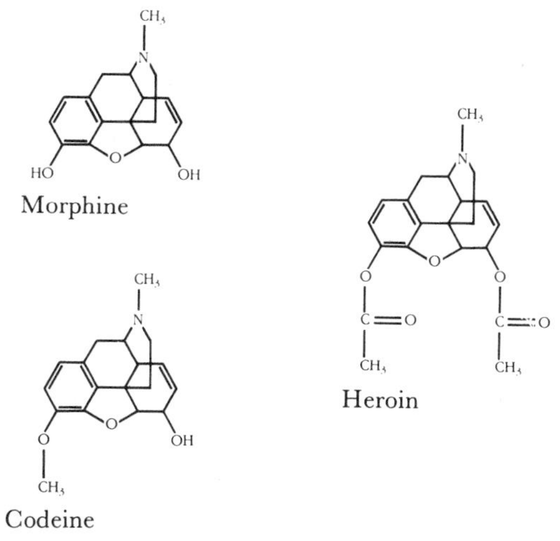

Morphine

Heroin

Codeine

Opium is a complex mixture of plant alkaloids; its principal psychoactive substances are morphine and to a much lesser degree codeine. Heroin is derived from morphine. Morphine and other opiates block nerve transmission in the central nervous system, thereby suppressing mental and physiological functions. Opiates bind to the nervous system cell receptors and mimic the actions of the body's natural pain-relieving substances, endorphins, and enkephalins (Chapter 3). Morphine and codeine are used medically for pain relief, while heroin is used primarily as an illegal recreational drug.

The sensations produced by injecting heroin into the circulatory system are markedly different from those of morphine and codeine, even though the opiate drugs have similar structures. As one heroin user described the sensation: "It's so good, don't even try it once" (Smith, 1972). Regular use of opiates can produce in addition to the psychological high constipation, loss of appetite, depression, loss of interest in sex, constriction of the pupil of the eye, disruption of the menstrual cycle, and drowsiness. Very large doses or prolonged use can be lethal because of respiratory failure.

Street heroin may contain as little as 1 percent to 3 percent heroin; the rest is sugar, cornstarch, cleansing agents, strychnine, or almost any white powder. Heroin is converted to morphine in the body, and the morphine is eventually excreted in the urine, saliva, sweat, and the breast milk of lactating women. Because morphine crosses the placenta, a fetus can become addicted and will experience withdrawal symptoms after it is born.

In 1983 researchers at Stanford University School of Medicine observed that people who used a synthetic heroin acquired a Parkinson-like disease that involved destruction of the brain and nerve cells leading to irreversible neurological damage. The substance in the synthetic heroin that was responsible for these serious symptoms was identified as MPTP (1-methyl-4-phenyl-1,2,3,6-tetrahydropyridine). For scientists the neurotoxic effects of MPTP provided a powerful tool for investigating the chemistry of brain diseases and brain functions. However, for the unfortunate users of MPTP the consequences are irreversible brain damage and destroyed lives.

Recreational Drugs Are Not Always Fun

No one knows why people use drugs. Peer pressure seems to be a strong motivating force. The fact is that drugs have been used by people in all cultures since recorded history and probably much earlier. The following imaginary interview probably contains all the relevant information on why people use drugs:

Question: Why do you use drugs?

Answer: Why not?

Question: What would convince you to stop?

Answer: Show me something better.

All drugs are dangerous, and illegal recreational drugs are especially so, since one cannot be sure of either the drug or the dose. While it may be true that marijuana is less dangerous than either alcohol or cigarette smoking, that does not make it safe. Some persons may benefit psychologically or feel spiritually uplifted by hallucinogenic drugs; others may freak out or suffer a mental breakdown. It is impossible to predict the experience any individual will have with a particular drug.

Recreational drugs are not essential to health and well-being. Yet most people, especially young people, experiment with one or more illegal drugs. For those who are determined to experiment, we offer the following cautions:

1. All illegal drugs are dangerous because of the uncertainty of the drug and the dose. Never use an illegal drug that has not already been taken by someone you know and trust.
2. Never forget that use of illegal drugs can lead to arrest, a criminal record, jail, costly legal defense, and unnecessary stress.
3. Never take an illegal drug to solve personal problems or to try to alleviate anx-iety or depression. All psychoactive drugs enhance negative feelings and can produce severe anxiety attacks or psychotic behavior.

As we get older we are less inclined to experiment with drugs, particularly illegal recreational drugs; we have found other ways to make our lives satisfying and interesting. The earlier in life we discover how to be healthy and happy without drugs, the more satisfied with ourselves we will become. One sign of maturity is being able to say no to the use of drugs.

LESSON PLANS

In light of this discussion, peruse the following lesson plans, keeping in mind that they are the type of lesson plans that you will likely be expected to implement in your classroom. Remember that they by no means encompass a complete unit of instruction. They are simply offered as a guide for the formation of a comprehensive unit.

TOPIC: HOW TO USE MEDICINES SAFELY

Grade Level: Primary

Concept: Medicine can help us get healthy when we use it properly.

Expected Pupil Outcome: The student will be able to summarize the safe ways to use medicines.

Content: Proper ways to use medicines:
1. Take under doctor's care.
2. Identify medicine in lighted room.
3. Have Mom or Dad read directions on label.
4. Follow directions.
5. Take exact amount.
6. Let Mom or Dad give it to you.
7. Keep in safe place.
8. Never share your medicine with others.
9. Don't borrow someone else's medicine.

Learning Experiences
1. *Storytelling:* "How Snoopy Got Better." Teacher reads story to class.
2. Teacher conducts short question/answer.

Key Questions   a) Why didn't Lucy want to give Snoopy an aspirin?

b) Why didn't Lucy want to give Snoopy the medicine that tastes like cherries?

c) Why did the doctor say that the special medicine would make Snoopy's sickness go away?

d) Why did the doctor give Snoopy a shot?

e) Did Snoopy get better?

f) Would you like to be Snoopy?

Short Story: **"How Snoopy Got Better"**

It is Saturday morning and Charlie Brown wants to play baseball. He goes out to wake up Snoopy so that they can practice. Snoopy is the shortstop for the team. He finds Snoopy sick and does not know what to do. Then the other children come.

1. Sally offers aspirin.
2. Lucy says that only grown-up people should give medicine and only if the doctor says to do so.
3. Linus offers cherry-flavored medicine.
4. Lucy says that medicine should not be shared with others. Medicines are not toys even if they sometimes taste good.

Lucy suggests taking Snoopy to the doctor. Perhaps the doctor can help him. Charlie, Charlie's mother, and the other children take Snoopy to the doctor.

1. The doctor helps Snoopy. He gives Snoopy a special medicine and gives special directions to Charlie and Charlie's mother.
2. The doctor says the medicine will make Snoopy's sickness go away because it will kill the bad germs.
3. The doctor says that the medicine will help Snoopy to feel much better.
4. The doctor gives Snoopy a shot so that the sickness will not come back.

Charlie's mother helps him give Snoopy the medicine, following the doctor's directions carefully. Soon Snoopy is all better and is playing baseball with the team once more.

Evaluation Procedures   After the storytelling session and during the question session, the teacher evaluates the appropriateness of the student responses. If the students respond with the appropriate answers to the questions, the objective has been attained.

TOPIC: EFFECT OF DRUGS ON THE BODY

Grade Level: Intermediate

Concept: Drugs can depress or stimulate the body.

Expected Pupil Outcome: The student will be able to describe the different ways drugs affect the body.

Content

1. Ways drugs can slow down or depress the body:
   a) Destroy vitamins A, B_6, C, and E; make you feel depressed and tired
   b) Make nerves sluggish
   c) Make you lose your balance
   d) Difficult to hear and see
   e) Slow down heart rate
   f) Slow down breathing
   g) Lower blood pressure
   h) Make you feel like sleeping
2. Ways drugs can speed up or stimulate the body:
   a) Get nerves excited
   b) Speed up heart beat
   c) Speed up body use of energy
   d) Increase blood pressure
   e) Speed up breathing
   f) Make you tired after a while
   g) Stimulate adrenal glands

Learning Experiences

1. Students *simulate* depressed effects by:
   a) Relaxing their muscles
   b) Closing their eyes and relaxing
   c) Recording their pulse rates (at rest) for one minute

2. Students *simulate* stimulant effects by:
   a) Running in place for two minutes
   b) Recording their pulse rates for one minute immediately after running
   c) Comparing rest and work pulse rates

3. Have students complete crossword puzzle in order to learn the symptoms of drug use.

Crossword Puzzle

A. Depressants—*ACROSS*
1. Mixed up
2. When one slides one's words together, one talks with slurred _____.
3. Sleepiness
4. Walks crookedly
5. Unable to concentrate
6. Too much alcohol will make one _____.
7. Unable to stand without swaying (two words; first word is a contraction)

B. Stimulants—*DOWN*
8. Usually when one gets "butterflies" in one's stomach, it is because one is _____.
9. Craving a drink of water
10. Uneasy
11. Perspire
12. Talky
13. When the dots in the middle of the eyes get big, one has _____. (two words)

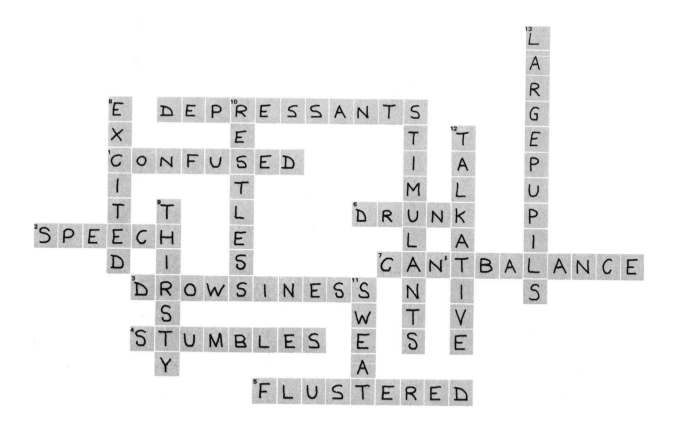

Evaluation Procedures   Successful completion of the crossword puzzle will constitute fulfillment of the objective.

REFERENCES and BIBLIOGRAPHY

Edlin, G., and E. Golanty. *Health and Wellness,* Third Edition (Boston, MA: Jones and Bartlett, 1988).

Grinspoon, L., and J. B. Bakalar. *Psychedelic Drugs Reconsidered* (New York: Basic Books, 1979).

Nicholi, A. M., Jr. "Recent Patterns of Psychoactive Drug Use Among College Students: The Inhalants," *Journal of American College Health* (April 1983):197-200. (a)

Nicholi, A. M., Jr. "The College Student and Marijuana: Research Findings Concerning Adverse Biological and Psychological Effects," *Journal of American College Health* (October 1983):73 (b)

Relman, A. S. "Marijuana and Health," *New England Journal of Medicine* 306 (1982):603-605.

Serban, G. (Ed.). *The Social and Medical Aspects of Drug Abuse* (New York: Spectrum Publications, 1984).

Silverman, M., and P. R. Lee. *Pills, Profiles, and Politics* (Berkeley: University of California Press, 1974).

Smith, D. E., and G. R. Gay. *It's So Good, Don't Even Try Once* (New York: Prentice-Hall, 1972).

Snyder, S. "Matter Over Mind: The Big Issues Raised by Newly Discovered Brain Chemicals," *Psychology Today* (June 1980).

Steel, K., et al. "Iatrogenic Illness on a General Medical Service at a University Hospital," *New England Journal of Medicine* 304 (1981):638-642.

Szasz, T. *Ceremonial Chemistry* (New York: Anchor Books, 1974).

Wertheimer, A. I. "An Empirical Overview of the Prescription Drug Market." In J. P. Morgan and D. V. Kagan (eds.): *Society and Medication: Conflicting Signals for Prescribers and Patients* (Lexington, Mass.: D.C. Heath, 1983).

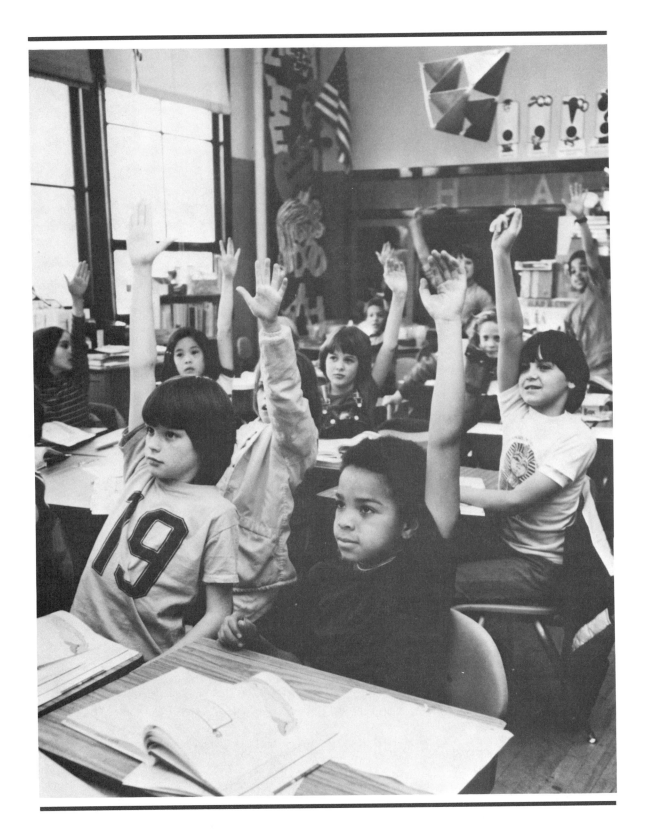

Chapter 16　Teaching About Tobacco

INTRODUCTION

Smoking causes lung cancer. That's right, smoking *causes* lung cancer. In fact, if you're a chronic smoker, your chances of dying before your life expectancy is up are enhanced sevenfold. You have a seven in ten chance of never reaching your life expectancy, because you will most likely die as a result of a cigarette-related chronic disease. This is indeed tragic when you realize that cigarette smoking is one of the most easily preventable causes of illness, disability, and premature death in the United States today.

The question is *why;* why do so many people smoke in light of all the evidence linking smoking with ill health? What entices the smoker to risk longevity and good health for the meager benefits derived from smoking? Certainly some smokers are ignorant of the facts. Some choose to ignore the evidence or rationalize their behavior; others assume a devil-may-care attitude and throw caution to the wind. Whatever the case may be, it is obvious that smoking gives many Americans an indispensable pleasure.

Further analysis discloses that most smokers acquire their habit early in life. Smoking is likely to begin during the late intermediate or early junior high years. In most cases these youngsters have received very little, if any, formalized instruction about the ramifications of smoking. All too often we are content to wait until high school before teaching students about smoking. In most instances we are four or five years too late.

Smoking is most often described as a form of coping behavior that can easily become habitual. Everyone has habitual coping behavior. Some are positive, whereas others may be harmful, like smoking. After a time these habits become a part of our nature and are next to impossible to change. How many times have you heard a person say, "I want to quit (smoking), but somehow I just don't have the perseverance

to do it once and for all"? This type of person is most difficult to help. Unless she or he wants to quit and is willing to pay the emotional price, there is little chance that the habitual smoker will ever completely give up smoking.

Our effort might be better directed at attempting to discourage youngsters from starting to smoke. This is difficult, but it is possible to have a positive influence on children's initial smoking behavior. Unbiased, sound, and scientific information about smoking that is skillfully and creatively imparted can go a long way to motivate children to consider smoking as an "out" thing to do. The earlier such a program starts, the more likely it is to be successful. We must realize that much of the information once considered appropriate for the high school level is now more appropriate at the intermediate level. Smoking and its relationship to health is one of these subjects.

SMOKING

In recent years antismoking efforts in this country have increased markedly, but America still has a long way to go to become a "smokeless society by the year 2000," a goal of the Surgeon General of the United States. Many towns, cities, and states have enacted legislation prohibiting smoking in public places and have mandated no-smoking areas in restaurants and working areas. Some companies have designated no-smoking areas and have used various incentives to encourage their employees to stop smoking. American society as a whole seems to be moving toward less acceptance of tobacco and smoking; however, as of 1986, about 50 million Americans still smoked cigarettes.

The health costs of smoking are staggering. Each year about 350,000 Americans die as a direct result of smoking. Almost one third of all cancer deaths—about 125,000 each year—are caused by smoking. Alan Dershowitz (1986), a professor of law at Harvard University, defends the right of tobacco companies to advertise and

Much of the material in this chapter is from Gordon Edlin and Eric Golanty, *Health & Wellness: A Holistic Approach,* Third Edition (Boston: Jones & Bartlett Publishers, 1988).

sell cigarettes so long as they are legal, but he also says:

Cigarettes kill, maim, and sicken. Anyone who doubts the truth should have his (and increasingly her) head (and probably lungs) examined. There really is no longer any room for rational debate about the dangers of smoking, both to those who inhale and to those upon whom they exhale.

It is estimated that cigarette smoking costs our society about $26 billion per year in lost man-power and $13 billion in direct medical costs (U.S. Surgeon General, 1984). Yet tobacco companies continue to deny that smoking is harmful and continue to advertise vigorously. In 1984 cigarette companies spent $2.1 billion on advertising; cigarette companies rank first in newspaper advertising and second in magazine advertising (Davis, 1987). Few newspapers or magazines can afford to turn down cigarette ads. Kenneth E. Walker (1987) of the University of Michigan School of Public Health points out the irrationality of tobacco advertising:

Ironically, the object of the nation's most expensive marketing campaign is also the only legal product that is hazardous when used as intended. It is the leading cause of premature death, a product so pervasive and lethal that it causes more deaths than the combined total caused by all illicit drugs and alcohol, all accidents, and all homicides and suicides.

More and more people realize that the time has come to ban cigarettes and smoking despite personal motivations or economic hardship (tobacco-growing regions of the country will suffer). The consequences to health justify the statement by Richard Peto (1985), a renowned epidemiologist: "The reason one wants to prevent smoking is not just because it is dangerous—lots of things are dangerous—but because it is *so* dangerous." In this chapter we discuss smoking and its health hazards. We will also attempt to alert you to the dangers of smokeless tobacco and to the blandishments of tobacco advertising.

Tobacco

The use of tobacco in our culture probably originated in sixteenth-century Europe through Spanish sailors returning from voyages to the New World. Apparently the sailors had learned about smoking from American Indians, who used tobacco in much the same way it is used today. In fact, the word "tobacco" is an Indian word signifying the pipe used to smoke the minced or rolled leaf of the tobacco plant.

The smoking habit spread quickly in Europe, fueled by tobacco imports from Spain's New World colonies. By the nineteenth century, changing social customs had largely replaced smoking with tobacco chewing—and by the even more popular habit of sniffing it in the form of snuff. It wasn't until the 1880's, when the cigarette-making machine was invented in the United States, that cigarette smoking became popular. Today about 3 trillion cigarettes are smoked worldwide each year, and in the United States, the number of cigarettes smoked annually is about 600 billion.

Tobacco used for smoking, chewing, or snuff is a processed product of the leaves of the plant *Nicotiana tabacum*. This plant is indigenous to the Western Hemisphere, where it grows best in semitropical climates. Since its discovery by European explorers, it has been cultivated in many regions of the world. In the United States tobacco is grown primarily in 13 states, and the tobacco industry is vital to their economies.

The preparation of tobacco involves harvesting the leaves and drying them by any one of several methods. The cured tobacco leaves are shredded, and various strains of leaves are blended to give a commercially desirable mixture. Often flavorings and colorings are added, as well as chemicals that facilitate even burning. Finally, the mixture is made into cigarettes, pipe tobacco, and chewing tobacco or is wrapped in specially cured tobacco leaves to make cigars.

The most familiar chemical constituent of tobacco is *nicotine*, but when tobacco is burned, approximately 4,000 other chemical substances are released and carried in the smoke—including acetone, acrolein, carbon monoxide, methanol, ammonia, nitrous dioxide, hydrogen sulfide, traces of various mineral elements, traces of radioactive elements, acids, insecticides, and other substances (Table 16.1). Besides these chemical compounds, tobacco smoke contains countless microscopic particles that contribute to the yellowish brown residue of tobacco smoke known as *tar*.

Most of the physiological effects of tobacco smoking are attributable to nicotine. The most prominent effects include increased heart rate, increased release of adrenalin, and a direct stimulatory effect on the brain. These effects combine to produce the "rush" cigarette smokers experience when they light up. Nicotine is also responsible for the nausea and vomiting experienced by most beginning smokers. Habituation to nicotine is probably responsible for the perpetuation of many a smoker's habit, either by causing a psychological dependence—a wish for the immediate psychological effects of the drug—or by causing actual physiological dependence (addiction).

The harmful effects of cigarette smoking probably come from nicotine and carbon monoxide, which are thought to contribute to the development of heart and blood vessel disease (Kaufman, 1983), and from a host of other chemicals that contribute to the development of cancer and diseases of the respiratory tract. Among these chemicals are benzo(a)pyrene, aza-arenes, N-nitrosamines, the radioactive isotope of the element polonium (^{210}Po), and the radioactive isotope radon with its decay products, known as "radon daughters." Polonium-210 is a product of the breakdown of radioactive lead (^{210}Pb), a natural constituent of soil. Radioactive particles in the soil are deposited on sticky tobacco leaf hairs and eventually become part of tobacco smoke. Radon and radon daughters are present in soil and building materials and from these sources condense on airborne particles in tobacco smoke that is inhaled.

Smokeless Tobaccos

An alternative to smoking cigarettes that has gained popularity in recent years is the use of smokeless tobaccos such as snuff and chewing tobacco. This form of tobacco is used by placing a pinch of snuff or plug of chewing tobacco in the mouth. The tobacco mixes with saliva and the nicotine and other chemicals are absorbed into the bloodstream. Dr. Gregory N. Connolly (1986) and other researchers have concluded

---

TABLE 16.1
A Partial List of Chemical Substances in Cigarettes

Aromatic hydrocarbons	Radioisotopes	Phenols	Insecticides
Benzo(a)pyrene	Polonium-210	Phenol	Arsenic
Dibenz(a,b)anthracene	Radium-226	o-Cresol	DDT
Dibenzo(a,l)pyrene	Radon-222	m + p-Cresol	TDE
Dibenzo(a,i)pyrene	Potassium-40	Dimethyl phenols	Endrin
Chrysene	**Aldehydes and ketones**	**Acids**	**Fungicides**
Methylbenzo(a)pyrene	Formaldehyde	Formic acid	Dithiocarbamates
Methylchrysene	Acrolein	Acetic acid	**Vapor phase components**
N-Nitrosamines	Crotonaldehyde	Propionic acid	Hydrogen cyanide
Diethylnitrosamine	**Esters and alcohols**	Lauric acid	
Methyl-n-butylnitrosamine	Solanesol		
Nitrosopiperidine	Phytosterol		
Nitrosopyrrolidine	Phytol		
Other nitrosamines	Oleic alcohol		
	Long-chain unsaturated alcohols		

Adapted from E. Wynder and D. Hoffman, *Tobacco and Tobacco Smoke* (New York: Academic Press, 1967).

that smokeless tobacco causes oral and pharyngeal cancer and is associated with cancers of other organs as well. Despite what tobacco companies say, smokeless tobaccos are not safe.

In 1986 Congress passed a law banning TV advertising of smokeless tobaccos (cigarette advertising was already banned from TV). Congress also required companies to put warning labels on packages. Despite these efforts, the use of smokeless tobaccos has increased markedly in recent years due to advertising and people's belief that chewing tobacco is less dangerous than smoking it.

Sales of snuff rose from 23 million to 37 million pounds between 1978 and 1984. During the same period sales of chewing tobacco increased from 80 million to 87 million pounds. The increase has occurred largely among teenage boys. Surveys show that 8 percent to 36 percent of high school males use smokeless tobacco; one study showed that more than 10 percent of eight- and nine-year-olds were using it.

Besides causing various kinds of cancer, smokeless tobaccos cause less serious diseases of the mouth, such as hard white patches *(leukoplakia)* and inflammatory lesions of the gum *(gingivitis)*. Some users show a marked increase in blood pressure, a major factor in heart disease. There is good evidence that smokeless tobacco products produce dependence on and possibly addiction to nicotine. Smokeless tobacco ads have been all too successful in getting a young, suggestible group to use these dangerous products.

Smoking and Illness

Almost from the beginning of tobacco's use in Europe and colonial America, people have been concerned about the harmful effects of smoking. Several articles in the medical literature of the eighteenth and nineteenth centuries claimed tobacco smoking as a cause of cancer of the lip, tongue, and lung. Twentieth century research into the consequences of cigarette smoking has provided widely accepted evidence that among smokers the incidence of certain diseases is greater—sometimes very much greater—than among people who do not smoke. Smoking is cited as a factor in coronary artery disease; lung cancer; bronchitis; emphysema; cancer of the larynx, lip, and oral cavity; cancer of the bladder and stomach; duodenal ulcer; and allergies (Surgeon General, 1979).

An enormous amount of data demonstrates that the death rate from causes such as cancer, heart disease, and respiratory diseases is higher among cigarette smokers than among nonsmokers (Figure 16.1). The data also show that the death rate for smokers is greater than for nonsmokers whatever the listed cause of death. The death rate from lung cancer for adult male smokers is 8 to 10 times that for nonsmokers. For heart disease, the death rate for smokers is almost twice that for those who do not smoke. Although the data vary somewhat for adult women, a similar pattern is observable.

Other studies indicate that babies born to mothers who smoke have lower birth weights than babies born to nonsmoking mothers and that smokers' babies show a higher risk of dying early in infancy. There is also evidence that pregnant women who smoke are more likely to have spontaneous abortions than those who do not.

One feature that emerges from these studies is that the risk of developing smoking-related diseases and other complications depends in part on the type as well as the extent of exposure to tobacco smoke. For example, pipe and cigar smokers show an incidence of death and disease for the smoking-related illnesses somewhere between that for cigarette smokers and nonsmokers—presumably because pipe and cigar smokers inhale less smoke than cigarette smokers. Light smokers (4 to 10 cigarettes per day) are at less risk than heavy smokers (more than 25 cigarettes per day). The mortality rates for heart disease and cancer for those who stop smoking for 15 years are about the same for nonsmokers. Cessation of smoking also improves breathing and reduces the chance of premature death from noncancerous respiratory disease.

Smokers' apparent concern for their health has produced a tremendous demand for low-tar/low-nicotine cigarettes. Approximately 60 percent of the cigarettes now sold in North America are of the low-yield variety. Whereas the use of low-tar/low-nicotine cigarettes may reduce

FIGURE 16.1
Death rates per 100,000 population of smokers versus nonsmokers. (Data from National Cancer Institute Monograph No. 19.)

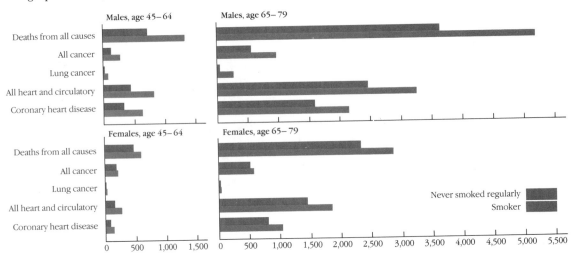

somewhat the risk of developing lung cancer, smoking these kinds of cigarettes apparently does not lessen the risk of developing heart disease (Rickert, 1983). One principal reason is that smokers of low-yield cigarettes change their smoking behavior: They increase the depth of inhalation, increase the frequency of puffing, increase the time that smoke is held in the lungs, and increase the number of cigarettes consumed. Consequently, smokers of low-nicotine cigarettes do not consume less nicotine than smokers of brands with a higher nicotine yield (Benowitz, 1983), and they increase their consumption of other constituents of tobacco smoke, including carcinogens and tar.

Lung Cancer

Lung cancer has long been the most common form of cancer among men, and in recent years, among women also. In 1986 approximately 125,000 persons died of lung cancer in the United States. The number of men dying of lung cancer has increased steadily since 1940 (Figure 16.2). While the rate of increase among men is beginning to decline (fewer men are smoking cigarettes), the increase in lung cancer among women is still rising (more women are smoking cigarettes). In 1984, for the first time

in U.S. history, lung cancer surpassed breast cancer as the leading cancer-related cause of death in women.

As shown in Figure 16.3, the increase in lung cancer deaths is the principal reason that the overall death rate from cancer continues to increase. If lung cancer rates are excluded from the statistics, the actual death rate from cancer has been falling steadily for many years, principally because of preventive efforts and improved diagnosis and treatment of cancers not associated with cigarette smoking. This situation is ironic as well as tragic, for lung cancer is one of the most easily preventable of all diseases. Most people simply need to stop smoking cigarettes.

Not all lung cancer deaths are attributable to cigarette smoking. The data suggest that about 80 percent of lung cancer deaths are related to smoking; the other 20 percent may be due to any number of environmental factors, including air pollution (some studies indicate that twice as many city dwellers die of lung cancer as do people who live in rural areas) and airborne substances encountered at work such as particles of chromate, iron, and asbestos.

A full biological explanation of how smoking causes lung cancer (and contributes to cancer in other body sites) is not yet available. A number

FIGURE 16.2

Lung cancer rates per 100,000 population in the United States. (Data from U.S. National Center for Health Statistics and U.S. Bureau of the Census.)

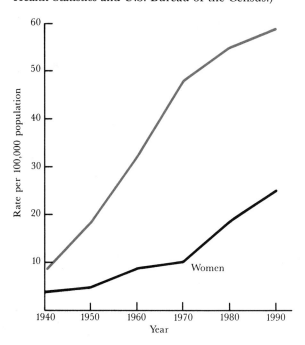

FIGURE 16.3

Death rates per 100,000 population from all cancers, lung cancer, and all cancers other than lung cancer, 1950–1978. (From "Health Consequences of Smoking: Cancer." U.S. Department of Health and Human Services, 1982.)

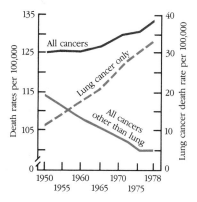

of known *carcinogens*—cancer-causing chemicals—are found in tobacco smoke, and it is thought that they are at least partly responsible for the onset of the cellular changes leading to the disease. For example, some evidence suggests that lung cancer may be caused by deposition of radioactive particles such as ^{210}Po, radon, or radon daughters in lung tissues (Martell, 1983). These radioactive elements, which are known to be present in tobacco smoke, become trapped in the lungs and accumulate over the years. The long-term exposure to the radioactivity at specific sites in the lungs may eventually trigger the conversion of normal cells into cancer cells. Transfer of the radioactive particles or of cancer cells to other parts of the body could also account for the increased risk smokers have of developing cancers in other organs as well.

Bronchitis and Emphysema

Bronchitis and emphysema are respiratory diseases that are sometimes classified along with asthma as *chronic obstructive pulmonary disease*

(COPD). Each of these maladies is associated with difficulty in breathing caused by obstruction of some part of the respiratory system. Many persons suffer from more than one of these conditions at the same time.

Bronchitis is an inflammation of the upper part of the respiratory tract, principally the trachea or the larger bronchial airways. It is characterized by an excessive production of mucus by cells that line the airways, which is the cause of the major symptoms of bronchitis—a continual cough (smoker's cough) and the production of large amounts of sputum. Some affected people also experience shortness of breath, particularly during exertion.

Unquestionably, smoking is a factor in the development of chronic bronchitis, although air pollution and the breathing of hazardous chemicals and particles encountered in certain occupations are also suspected of contributing to it. Apparently the excessive production of mucus by the glands of the bronchi is a reaction to the irritation caused by cigarette smoke and other air pollutants.

The pathology that produces the symptoms of bronchitis can be almost completely reversed by giving up smoking, reducing one's exposure to polluted air, or both. It is not uncommon, however, for people to "live with" their persistent cough for many years and not be concerned with the message their body is giving them. If the disease is left to run its course, the person increases the vulnerability to other respiratory illnesses, and the airways may become irreversibly blocked.

Emphysema is the result of the destruction of the tiny air sacs deep in the lungs called *alveoli* (Figure 16.4). Each lung contains millions of alveoli. It is across their thin membranes that the function of breathing is accomplished—the exchange of the respiratory gases, oxygen and carbon dioxide.

Upon inhaling, about 500 ml of air (which is 20 percent oxygen) flows through the nose and mouth into the trachea and bronchial tubes to the lungs, where it fills the approximately 300 million alveoli. Oxygen diffuses through the membranes of the alveoli into tiny blood vessels in the lung tissue. Having entered the bloodstream, it is carried by red blood cells throughout the body, where it is used to provide energy for cellular activities. One of the by-products of cellular energy production is carbon dioxide, which is carried by the blood to the lungs, where it diffuses into the alveoli and is eliminated from the body upon exhalation.

FIGURE 16.4

The respiratory system, which provides the body with oxygen and removes carbon dioxide. Oxygen enters and carbon dioxide leaves the body via tiny air sacs in the lungs called alveoli. The rest of the respiratory system facilitates gas exchange in the alveoli. The rate and depth of breathing is controlled by the brain, which receives impulses from sensors in the heart, blood vessels, and lungs telling it how much oxygen the body needs or how much carbon dioxide is present. The brain regulates breathing by sending messages to the diaphragm; when the diaphragm contracts, the lungs expand, drawing in oxygen-laden air. When the diaphragm relaxes, the lungs deflate, and air containing carbon dioxide is expelled.

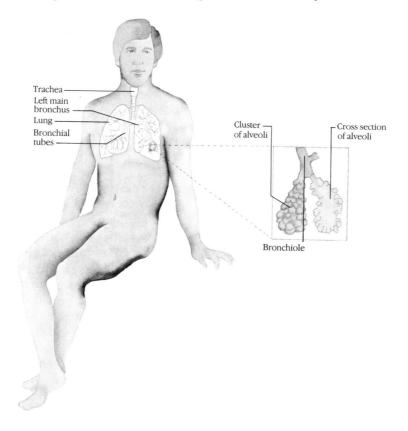

In emphysema, the alveoli lose their shape and become distended with trapped air, which ultimately results in the impairment of gas exchange. Emphysema involves a slow, irreversible process of alveoli destruction; thus, as the disease progresses, affected people have greater and greater trouble breathing.

As with lung cancer, the mechanism by which tobacco smoking or air pollution contributes to emphysema is still under investigation. One hypothesis suggests that body cells in the lung normally engaged in the destruction of material foreign to the body release large amounts of destructive enzymes in response to respiratory pollutants, and these enzymes inadvertently destroy lung tissue, causing emphysema. Normally, a protein in the blood called alpha-one-antitrypsin, or AAT, inhibits the destructive enzymes. Some studies have shown that people with emphysema have low levels of AAT, either because of genetic factors that increase their susceptibility to emphysema or because of some as yet unknown correlation between respiratory pollution and the impaired production of AAT.

Tobacco Smoke's Effects on Nonsmokers

Many people are surprised to learn that nonsmokers who are exposed to tobacco smoke run some health risk as well. People who work or live in environments that are heavily laden with tobacco smoke inhale the same smoke-borne substances as do smokers. In fact, about two thirds of the smoke from a burning cigarette enters the environment, and anyone who has been in a roomful of smokers can attest that such an environment is considerably more polluted than the worst smoggy day in a big city. A nonsmoker in a smoke-filled room can inhale in one hour the equivalent of a cigarette's worth of nicotine, carbon monoxide, and other substances. Many people are allergic to tobacco smoke, and such an environment can bring about eye irritation, headache, cough, nasal congestion, and asthma. Nonsmokers forced to inhale tobacco smoke for long periods, such as those who work in enclosed environments routinely filled with tobacco smoke, can suffer impairment of the lungs equivalent to that of smokers who inhale 10 cigarettes

a day (White, 1980). A study of the risks of passive smoking among Japanese adults found that the wives of men who smoked had a one-third higher cancer mortality rate than wives of nonsmoking men (Hirayama, 1981).

Passive cigarette smoking also affects children. Studies have shown that the children of parents who smoke are more prone to bronchitis, episodes of pneumonia, chronic cough, more missed school days, and more hospital admissions (Weis, 1983). Substances in tobacco smoke have been found in the urine of infants whose parents smoke (Greenberg, 1984). Maternal cigarette smoking has been shown to hinder the development of the lungs of children and to impair respiratory function, which may predispose these children to respiratory illnesses later in life (Tager, 1983).

Following an exhaustive review of the evidence for and against the effects of passive smoke on health, the 1986 Surgeon General's report concluded that involuntary smoking *is* a cause of disease and that "it is certain" that some nonsmokers' lung cancers are caused by exposure to tobacco smoke. Despite numerous studies demonstrating the harmful effects of passive smoke, the Tobacco Institute steadfastly maintains that "proof of harm to nonsmokers from passive smoking remains as wispy as cigarette smoke itself" (Stapf, 1987). We believe that a smoke-free environment will benefit both nonsmokers and the millions who desire to quit smoking.

Why People Smoke

Most people begin to smoke in their teens, emulating parents or celebrities who smoke. Teenagers also smoke to attain acceptance in their peer group. About half of the people who experiment with smoking continue the habit into adulthood. There must be some very compelling reasons that people continue to smoke despite the unpleasant taste, the initial adverse physiological reactions, and the knowledge—now widespread—that tobacco smoke can cause serious, even life-threatening, illness.

The reasons people give for smoking are

many and varied. According to the American Cancer Society, the motivations of smokers can be grouped into six general categories:

1. *Stimulation*—some people get a psychological lift from smoking. They say that smoking helps them to wake up in the morning and organize their energies. They often report that smoking increases their intellectual capacities.
2. *Handling*—some people enjoy the mere handling of cigarettes and smoking paraphernalia, such as lighters.
3. *Pleasurable relaxation*—some smokers say they smoke simply because they like it. Smoking brings them true pleasure and is often practiced to enhance other pleasurable sensations, such as the taste of a good meal.
4. *Reducing negative feelings* (crutch)—approximately one third of smokers say they smoke because it helps them deal with stress, anger, fear, anxiety, or pressure.
5. *Craving*—some people crave cigarettes and have no other explanation than frequent needs to smoke, irrespective of the pleasurable or tension-relieving effects that smoking might bring.
6. *Habit*—some smokers light up only because of habit. They no longer receive much physical or psychological gratification from smoking; they often smoke without being aware of whether or not they really want the cigarette.

The American Cancer Society has developed a self-administered test to help smokers determine their strongest motives for smoking.

The question that still eludes a definitive answer: What distinguishes people who smoke from those who do not? The list of suggested answers includes a biological susceptibility to dependence on nicotine, a variety of personality and sociological traits, and a need for an effective way to deal with stress. There may be as many reasons as there are smokers. Whatever the case, people smoke because they want to. Many biological, psychological, and sociological explanations of smoking have been offered by various researchers, but in the final analysis, smoking—

like any other habitual, non-life-supporting behavior—is a matter of choice.

Quitting

There's an old joke among smokers: "It's easy to quit. I've done it over fifty times!"

Each year millions of smokers try to kick their habit. The major problem they face, as the little joke recognizes, is that stopping for awhile is not nearly as difficult as permanently eliminating the habit. Each year, however, thousands of people successfully quit smoking. They do so for a variety of reasons: to reduce the risk of early death from heart or lung disease, to enjoy once again the unpolluted taste of food, to please nonsmoking loved ones, to eliminate the ever-present ashes and smell of cigarette smoke from the house, and to fulfill a simple commitment to get healthy. Frequently a positive change in other aspects of one's lifestyle leads to an unplanned cessation of smoking. For example, many people who take up meditation, t'ai chi ch'uan, jogging, or other physical activity automatically stop smoking. They simply lose the desire to smoke cigarettes.

In recent years many psychologists and human behavior specialists have been involved in a search for a "quitter's magic bullet"—a single therapeutic approach that will help people stop smoking, not only during the several weeks of the treatment, or the six months to a year after the treatment has stopped, but for the rest of their lives.

There are now a dozen or more different therapeutic strategies to help people stop smoking. Often these strategies are applied in special smoking clinics, where smokers are exposed to health information, encouragement, moral support, social pressure, and suggestions about how to resist the temptation to light up.

A chemically based therapy makes use of the idea that people smoke because they are addicted to the effects of nicotine. Thus, the therapy provides smokers with nicotine or a nicotine-like drug that satisfies their dependence on nicotine while eliminating the tar and other harmful chemicals in tobacco smoke from their system.

Still other therapies are based on the idea

WHY DO YOU SMOKE?

Here are some statements made by people to describe what they get out of smoking cigarettes. How often do you feel this way when smoking? Circle the number for each statement.

Important: Answer every question.

	Always	Frequently	Occasionally	Seldom	Never
A. I smoke cigarettes in order to keep myself from slowing down.	5	4	3	2	1
B. Handling a cigarette is part of the enjoyment of smoking it.	5	4	3	2	1
C. Smoking cigarettes is pleasant and relaxing.	5	4	3	2	1
D. I light up a cigarette when I feel angry about something.	5	4	3	2	1
E. When I have run out of cigarettes I find it almost unbearable until I can get them.	5	4	3	2	1
F. I smoke cigarettes automatically without even being aware of it.	5	4	3	2	1
G. I smoke cigarettes to stimulate me, to perk myself up.	5	4	3	2	1
H. Part of the enjoyment of smoking a cigarette comes from the steps I take to light up.	5	4	3	2	1
I. I find cigarettes pleasurable.	5	4	3	2	1
J. When I feel uncomfortable or upset about something, I light up a cigarette.	5	4	3	2	1
K. I am very much aware of the fact when I am not smoking a cigarette.	5	4	3	2	1
L. I light up a cigarette without realizing I still have one burning in the ashtray.	5	4	3	2	1
M. I smoke cigarettes to give me a "lift."	5	4	3	2	1
N. When I smoke a cigarette, part of the enjoyment is watching the smoke as I exhale it.	5	4	3	2	1
O. I want a cigarette most when I am comfortable and relaxed.	5	4	3	2	1
P. When I feel "blue" or want to take my mind off cares and worries, I smoke cigarettes.	5	4	3	2	1
Q. I get a real gnawing hunger for a cigarette when I haven't smoked for a while.	5	4	3	2	1
R. I've found a cigarette in my mouth and didn't remember putting it there.	5	4	3	2	1

(Continued on next page.)

How to Score

1. Enter the numbers you have circled in the spaces below, putting the number you have circled to Question A over line A, to Question B over line B, etc.
2. Add the three scores on each line to get your totals. For example, the sum of your scores over lines A, G, and M gives you your score on *Stimulation*, lines B, H, and N give the score on *Handling,* and so on.

Totals

___ + ___ + ___ = ___				
A	G	M	Stimulation	
___ + ___ + ___ = ___				
B	H	N	Handling	
___ + ___ + ___ = ___				
C	I	O	Pleasurable relaxation	
___ + ___ + ___ = ___				
D	J	P	Crutch: tension reduction	
___ + ___ + ___ = ___				
E	K	Q	Craving: psychological addiction	
___ + ___ + ___ = ___				
F	L	R	Habit	

Scores of 11 or above indicate that this factor is an important source of satisfaction for the smoker. Scores of 7 or less are low and probably indicate that this factor does not apply to you. Scores in between are marginal.

Smoker's Self-testing Kit developed by Daniel Horn, Ph.D. Originally published by National Clearinghouse for Smoking and Health, Department of Health, Education, and Welfare.

that smoking is a response to personal stress—and so stress-reduction techniques such as meditation and biofeedback are employed to give the smoker another, healthier way to deal with stress.

Some basic tips for smokers who want to quit are presented in the box on p. 315. Whatever the specific technique, most people involved in helping smokers quit agree that the major factor in stopping smoking is the personal resolve of the smoker to do so (Schwartz, 1978). There is no magic bullet. No single therapeutic technique stops the smoking habit. This does not mean that smokers have to exercise will power or employ unusual behavior like putting money in a piggy bank each time they resist the urge to smoke. Such artificial practices rarely stop smoking permanently. Successful elimination of the smoking habit can be accomplished by becoming aware of one's personal motives for smoking. It is possible to reprogram the mind to eliminate the thoughts and behavior that lead to smoking. A person can then integrate positive and rewarding activities, thoughts, and feelings in place of those that lead to smoking. In so doing, people stop smoking because they feel good without having to smoke, and in fact, feel better by not smoking at all.

The War of Words Between the Pros and the Antis

There exists a long-standing war of words between antismoking groups (most notably the American Cancer Society and The American Heart Association) and the tobacco industry (tobacco growers and other businesses involved in the production and sale of smoking products). At stake are the loyalties of millions of smokers and prospective smokers. The health groups try

---

TIPS FOR SMOKERS WHO WANT TO QUIT

When Thinking About Quitting . . .
1. List all the reasons you want to stop smoking.
2. Keep a diary of the times of the day and the circumstances of your smoking behavior. Be particularly mindful of feelings that lead you to light up.
3. Tell your family and friends you are going to quit and ask for their support.
4. Switch to a brand of cigarettes you dislike. Try not to smoke two packs of the same brand in a row.

Cut Down the Number of Cigarettes You Smoke
1. Smoke only half of each cigarette.
2. Don't smoke when you first experience a craving. Wait several minutes. During this time change your activity or talk to someone.
3. Do not buy cigarettes by the carton. Wait until one pack is empty before buying another.
4. Make cigarettes difficult to get. Don't carry them with you.
5. Don't smoke automatically. Smoke only when you really *want* to.
6. Reward yourself in some way other than smoking.
7. Reach for a glass of juice instead of a cigarette for a pick-me-up.

Immediately After Quitting
1. Whenever you feel uncomfortable sensations from having stopped smoking, remind yourself that they are signs of your body's return to health and that they will soon pass.

2. If you miss the sensation of having a cigarette in your hand, play with something else—a pencil, a paper clip, a marble.
3. Instead of smoking after meals, get up from the table and brush your teeth or go for a walk.
4. Temporarily avoid situations you strongly associate with the pleasurable acts of smoking.
5. Develop a clean, fresh nonsmoking environment around yourself—at work and at home.
6. Until you are confident of your ability to stay off cigarettes, limit your socializing to healthful outdoor activities or to situations in which smoking is prohibited.
7. Look at cigarette ads more critically. Remind yourself that cigarette companies are making money at the expense of your health and well-being.

Find New Habits
1. Change your habits to make smoking difficult and unnecessary.
2. Keep a clean-tasting mouth.
3. Substitute relaxation and deep breathing for stressful situations.
4. Absorb yourself in activities that are meaningful to you.
5. Never allow yourself to think that "one won't hurt"—it will!

Based on *Calling It Quits*, U.S. Department of Health, Education, and Welfare Publication No. (NIH) 79-1824.

---

to persuade these people not to smoke; the tobacco industry encourages them to smoke more and more. Legal experts such as Alan Dershowitz (1986) reluctantly concluded that "in the end, the cigarette industry's right to free speech may well cost lives. The First Amendment requires us all to tolerate views we find offensive as the price of being able to present views we deem essential."

The medical war of words takes place in relative obscurity compared with that of advertising. Each year the tobacco industry spends hundreds of millions of dollars to promote its products and to recruit smokers. Perusal of many major magazines and newspapers reveals that

cigarette advertising relies heavily on imagery that portrays smoking as healthful and enjoyable and smokers as attractive, sexy, slim, and of high social status (see box on p. 316). Most magazines depend heavily on the financial rewards of cigarette advertising. When cigarette advertising was banned from radio and television in 1970, tobacco companies actually increased their advertising budgets and began spending hundreds of millions of dollars on newspaper and magazine ads. They also developed costly promotional campaigns (such as the Virginia Slims Tennis Tournament) that attempt to associate smoking cigarettes with health, fun, and fitness. Tobacco companies began to support health research, ex-

WOMEN AND CIGARETTE ADVERTISING

For over 50 years tobacco companies have tried to entice women to smoke cigarettes by emphasizing sexiness, slimness, elegance, and fun in advertisements. (The Lucky Strike ad is from 1931; the other ad is from the 1980's.) The success of such ads over the years in getting women to smoke is borne out by the number of lung cancer deaths among women who smoke. About 23 million American women smoke cigarettes. Between 1935 and 1983 the percentage of women who smoked increased from 18 percent to 30 percent. (During the same interval the percentage of men who smoked decreased from 52 to 35 percent.)

The female group that increased its smoking most dramatically in 1986 was white women in their twenties. In 1983 tobacco companies spent $329 million on advertising cigarette brands designed exclusively for women. As one observer put it: "The cigarette industry has mastered the art of sending the subliminal message to the susceptible consumer."

In 1985 about 40,000 women died of cigarette-caused lung cancer. Lung cancer has surpassed breast cancer as the leading cause of cancer deaths among women. Smoking also increases women's chances for heart disease and cervical cancer. If that's not enough, the beauty editor of *Harper's* magazine points out that "smokers' skin wrinkles up to 10 years sooner than that of nonsmokers." Not believing cigarette ads and not smoking are the individual's responsibility. As long as tobacco is legal, companies have a right to advertise. You also have the right not to smoke, which is one of the single most important health decisions you can make.

otic travel excursions, rock concerts, and major athletic events to promote smoking. To combat this promotional blitz by the tobacco industry, antismoking groups put forth hundreds of messages each year about the health consequences of smoking, using not only the printed media but also radio and television.

In other parts of the world, particularly the developing countries of Africa and Asia, cigarette advertising is having an enormous impact. In Africa, for example, per capita cigarette consumption in the 1970's increased 33 percent. Many Third World governments do not warn their citizens of the health risks of smoking, and some are in economic partnership with tobacco companies. If this trend continues, the World Health Organization fears that "smoking disease will appear in developing countries before communicable disease and malnutrition have been controlled, and the gap between the rich and poor countries will thus be further widened."

People would benefit if the land and resources used for the cultivation of tobacco were used to grow food crops, and if the desire to eradicate worldwide hunger were as important to governments and corporations as the promotion of tobacco use.

The federal government plays a paradoxical role in the war of words. It supports both sides. Through the Department of Agriculture, the government provides price supports and other financial aids to tobacco growers and other members of the tobacco industry. Through the Public Health Service the government supports antismoking programs and finances research into the health effects of smoking. Given the pluralistic nature of our governmental system, one could hardly expect anything else, which points up once again that it would be foolish to depend entirely on the federal government—or on any other organization—to be the guardian of your personal health.

LESSON PLANS

In light of our preceding discussion in this chapter, peruse the following lesson plan examples, keeping in mind that they are indicative of the type of lesson plans that you will likely be expected to implement in your classroom. Remember that they are only exemplary in nature and by no means encompass a complete unit of instruction. They are simply offered as a guide or basis for the formation of a comprehensive unit dealing with the topic in question.

TOPIC: EFFECTS OF CIGARETTE SMOKING ON THE BODY

Grade Level: Intermediate, junior high

Concept: Cigarette smoke affects all systems of the body.

Expected Pupil Outcome: The student will be able to describe how cigarette smoke affects all bodily systems.

Content: Effects on each body system are:

1. Respiratory system:
   a) Anesthetizes cilia and eventually destroys them.
   b) Stimulates overproduction of mucus.
   c) Uses up vitamin A and causes irritation of trachea, causing coughing.
   d) Increases susceptibility of bronchial tube to infection.
   e) Puts carbon monoxide into blood, decreasing oxygen in blood, thereby making it difficult to breathe.
   f) Reduces circulation in lung.
   g) Enhances destruction of alveoli.
   h) Greatly increases the chances of contracting lung cancer, emphysema, and chronic bronchitis (see Figure 18.2).

2. Cardiovascular system:
   a) Nicotine increases heart rate.
   b) Constricts superficial blood vessels.
   c) Raises blood pressure.
   d) Accelerates atherosclerosis.
   e) Decreases clotting time.

3. Nervous system:
   a) After a short period of stimulation, nicotine depresses the sympathetic and parasympathetic nerves.
   b) Nicotine depresses the functions of taste and smell.

4. Other systems:
   a) Smoking reduces appetite and stimulates peristalsis.
   b) Nicotine is actively and rapidly metabolized. The resulting metabolites are excreted in the urine and may cause irritation and bladder cancer.
   c) Ulcers are greatly irritated by smoking.
   d) Your risk of death from cirrhosis is doubled.

Learning Experiences

1. Demonstration of the effect of cigarette smoke on the cilia of a fresh chicken's trachea or on a salamander. (Directions for conducting this demonstration are included in accompanying section on experiments and demonstrations.)

2. Demonstration of the effect of nicotine on the heart of a live frog. (For directions on how to conduct this experiment, see the accompanying section on experiments and demonstrations.)

3. Demonstration of the effect of nicotine on a live fish in a bowl. (See accompanying section for details.)

4. Tic-tac-toe game to reinforce facts.

e) Nicotine causes stress to the liver and destroys vitamins B_6, C, and E. One cigarette destroys about 25 mg of vitamin C, or about one-half the recommended minimum daily allowance. Smoking jeopardizes the liver's ability to function.

f) Smoking one pack of cigarettes depletes 500 mg of vitamin C.

g) Smoking causes facial wrinkling at early age; it speeds up the aging process.

Evaluation Procedures The day following instruction the students will be given a twelve question short answer quiz. Three questions will be devoted to each of the four body systems. If the students are 80 percent correct on the average in their responses, successful completion of the objective will be assumed.

Alternative Experiments and Demonstrations

The following experiments may help teachers to demonstrate the effects of cigarette smoke on living things and particularly on the human body. These may be used as alternatives to those suggested in the lesson plans. Teachers should select experiments that are feasible for their teaching situations. Experiments and demonstrations should be tried out by the teacher first before they are conducted with children. Such an approach helps the teacher to anticipate "hang-ups" as well as to avoid them.

Effects of cigarette smoke on living things

1. Wipe a cotton pellet that has been saturated with tobacco tars on the tongue of a live frog and observe temporary collapse.

2. Using a cotton pellet that has been saturated with tars from the smoking machine, wipe the stems of several growing plants. Keep some plants as controls to observe the differences.

3. Place a drop of solution containing paramecia on a microscope slide. With the low power of a microscope, observe the movement of these one-celled organisms. Blow smoke from collection flask on the preparation and note the effects on the paramecia.

4. Make a nicotine insecticide by soaking cotton pellets from the smoking machine or cigarette tobacco in water. Test and use as a spray on insects.

5. *Purpose:* To demonstrate the effect of the toxic compounds in cigarette smoke on fish.

   Procedure: Set up a smoking machine (Figure 16.5). As the vacuum is applied, the smoke from the cigarette will bubble through the water. By the time three to ten cigarettes have been consumed, the toxic agents in the smoke, primarily nicotine, should begin to affect the fish, causing them to lose their equilibrium. As soon as the fish lose their equilibrium and begin to roll to one side, they should be removed from the water and

FIGURE 16.5

How to set up equipment to show effects of cigarette smoke on fish.

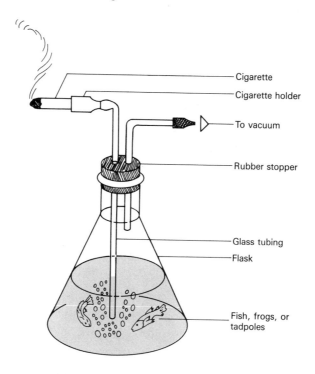

placed immediately in fresh water. If fish are not transplanted into fresh water immediately, they will die.

6. *Purpose:* To observe the biological effects of cigarette tars on white mice.

   Procedure: Hook a vacuum line (from an aspirator or water pump) to a burning cigarette in such a manner that the cigarette is consumed in about four to six minutes. In the line attach a trap containing glass wool moistened with acetone (Figure 16.6). This will collect most of the tobacco tars. The distillation of the tar can be facilitated by placing the bottle in an ice water bath during the course of the experiment.

After the cigarettes (about 40 per day) have been smoked, the tar can be removed with additional acetone—using as little as possible to dissolve the tar. This solution should be allowed to stand for several hours in a fume hood to concentrate the tar. A vacuum distillation method in a warm water bath without flame is effective.

The backs of six to ten mice should be trimmed with electric clippers to remove heavy hair growth. The tars from about three cigarettes can be applied by eye dropper twice daily to the clipped area, five days a week.

FIGURE 16.6
How to set up equipment to collect coal tar.

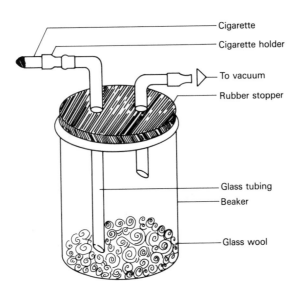

Tumors can be expected to appear in about 40 percent of the mice in six to nine months. The tumors will be both benign and malignant.

To demonstrate effects of cigarette smoke on the respiratory system

1. *Purpose:* To demonstrate the tars that are inhaled into the mouth and lungs of a cigarette smoker. Of particular interest will be the difference in the amounts of tar in the inhaled smoke and in that which is exhaled.

   Equipment: 1 white handkerchief, 1 smoker

   Procedure: Have the smoker inhale from a lighted cigarette, making every attempt to hold the smoke in his or her mouth without allowing it to go into the lungs. As rapidly as possible, after inhaling from the cigarette, stretch a handkerchief over the mouth as firmly as possible and blow the smoke back through the handkerchief. This will cause quite a dark stain.

   Now have the smoker inhale once more from the cigarette, this time allowing the smoke to go well into the lungs. Now place a different area of the handkerchief firmly over the mouth and exhale back through the handkerchief. The second stain will be much lighter than the first stain. Theoretically, the difference between the two stains represents the amount of tar that remains in the lungs with each puff of the cigarette.

2. *Purpose:* To demonstrate the effect of cigarette smoke on ciliary action.

a) This may be demonstrated on the trachea of a chicken or salamander lung. Slit two fresh chicken tracheas upward from below and pin them on two separate stiff cardboards or plywood, so that the inside of the trachea, with cilia, may be viewed.

Put a small drop of India ink or dye in the middle of the trachea. Lay the tracheas flat. Place one near a source of fresh air. Place the second trachea far away from the first and blow smoke on it. In both samples of trachea observe to see how far the ink has moved. The ink on the trachea that received cigarette smoke has not moved (see Figure 16.7). This may be explained by noting that nicotine in the smoke paralyzed the cilia. An analogy can be made with the effect cigarette smoke has on the cilia in the human respiratory tract. When the cilia are inactivated, the mucus collects and becomes a fertile place for numerous pathogens. Hence a smoker becomes much more susceptible to respiratory infections than does a nonsmoker.

b) Put a salamander to sleep by soaking it in (1) a solution of saturated chloretone diluted by adding nine parts of water, or (2) a one-percent aqueous solution of tricaine methanesulphonate. As soon as the salamander is asleep, cut off the head, open the chest and abdominal cavity, slit the lung longitudinally, and snip it off. Keep the specimen wet with Ringer's solution. Examine the lung surface under the microscope to study the cilia beating. Blow a little smoke from the collection flask over the tissue and observe the effect it has on the cilia.

To demonstrate the effect of cigarette smoke on the cardiovascular system

1. *Purpose:* To demonstrate the effect of smoking on the heart and the circulatory system.

   Procedure: It is recommended that students do this experiment on their parents at home and record their findings. The arterial

FIGURE 16.7

The effects of cigarette smoke (nicotine) on fresh chicken trachea that have been slit and pinned to a board. Ink was placed in the lower end of the trachea (nearest the lung). Smoke was blown over the entire area surrounding the ink.

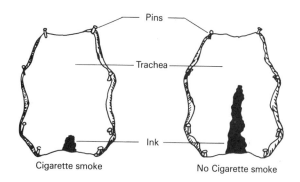

pulse, taken at the wrist, is an accurate indication of the heart rate. One can take the pulse of a subject by placing two middle fingers of the right hand on the thumb side of the wrist of the patient (see Figure 16.8).

The subject's pulse should be taken two or three times to establish a baseline accuracy. In each instance record your pulse rate as the number of pulsations felt per minute.

Have your subject light a cigarette, then take the pulse after he or she has concluded the third or fourth puff. When the cigarette is finished, take the pulse every 15 minutes until the pulse rate returns to normal. Chart your findings on a graph and determine how many extra beats one pack of cigarettes causes the subject. Since with each beat, the heart pumps approximately 70 cc of blood, calculate the extra volume of blood that is pumped by the heart induced by smoking one package of cigarettes.

2. The slowing down of blood circulation can be tested with a clinical thermometer. Have the nonsmoker, or someone who has not smoked for several hours, hold the thermometer. Then have a smoker hold the thermometer. Smokers show a drop of about six degrees or more, even when using filter cigarettes.

3. *Purpose:* To test the effects of carbon monoxide in tobacco smoke on animal blood. (The blood can be obtained from a butcher shop. Keep the blood from coagulating by adding one part of sodium oxalate solution to nine parts of blood. Place in bottle.)

FIGURE 16.8
How to take pulse.

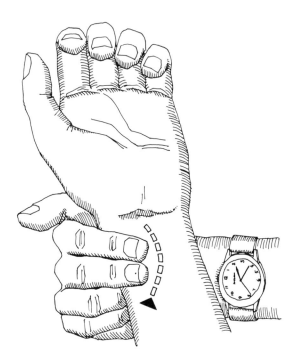

Procedure: Smoke a cigarette or tobacco in the manner described for smoking machines (see Figure 16.9). Smoke coming through the tube from bottle A to bottle B will cause the blood to turn a deeper red as the hemoglobin takes on carbon monoxide. As a result carboxy-hemoglobin is formed. This is what happens in carbon monoxide poisoning. The hemoglobin loses its ability to release oxygen.

Add a fresh yeast culture to the blood. Also add a yeast culture to a control batch of blood. In the control, yeast enzymes cause the hemoglobin to release oxygen, which comes off as bubbles in a foam at the surface. In the experimental bottle, this oxygen release is impaired. (Bottle C is simply a trap, to keep blood from frothing into the pump or aspirator.)

4. *Purpose:* To demonstrate the effect of smoke on the circulatory system.

Procedure: Pith a frog and place it on its back on a frog board. Spread and pin the web of a foot over an opening in the board and examine the blood vessels under low power on a microscope. Keep the specimen moist with Ringer's solution. Place a tube from the smoke bottle in the frog's mouth and blow smoke in while someone is watching the rate of blood flow. If it is possible to count the blood cells going past a given point, you may notice several rate changes; faster, then back to normal, perhaps faster again, and back to normal a second time.

FIGURE 16.9

How to set up an experiment to study the effects of cigarette smoke on animal blood. (From *Smoking and Health,* Washington, D.C.: U.S. Department of Health, Education and Welfare, 1964.)

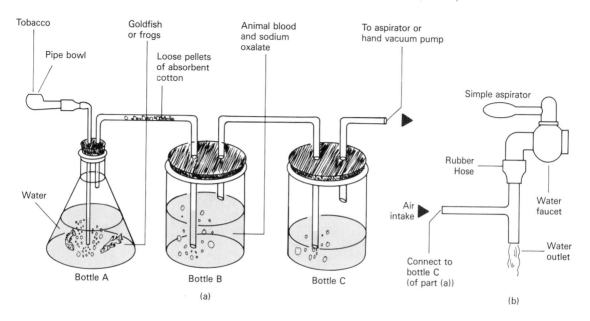

5. *Purpose:* To demonstrate the effect of cigarette smoke on the heart.

   Procedure: Pith a frog and place the frog on its back on a frog board. Spread and stretch the legs and pin them rigidly to the frog board. With a scalpel, open up the chest cavity, and carefully expose the heart. Carefully remove the pericardium, or protective sac, around the heart. Observe the heart rate, time it, and record. Place a drop of pure nicotine solution on the heart. Observe, time the heart rate, and record. Compare the pre- and postrates.

   The frog's heart may be attached to a kymograph and the heart rates recorded as a kymograph.

Smoking machines

Numerous smoking machines are sold commercially. The two most popular ones are "Nicotina" and "Smoking Sam." The kind of smoking machine to be used should be relevant to the purpose of the demonstration or experiment. "Nicotina" is excellent for demonstrating that tar is part of cigarette smoke and that it is inhaled. "Smoking Sam" does much the same thing, except that the two glass jars, filled with white angel hair, simulate human lungs. When these commercial machines are not available, the amount of tar in one or more cigarettes may be demonstrated by collecting tar on cotton pellets, angel hair, or filter paper placed in the tubing of a teacher-made machine. Tar can also be observed as a residue on the

FIGURE 16.10
How to design a classroom smoking machine.

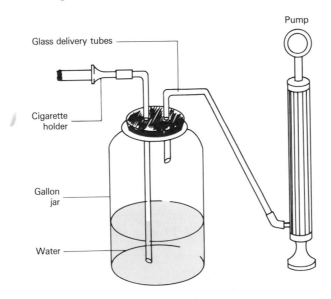

Glass delivery tubes

Cigarette holder

Gallon jar

Water

Pump

tubing and containers and as a discoloration of water through which cigarette smoke has been filtered. Smoking machines may be adapted to a variety of demonstrations. The following machine may be constructed for classroom demonstrations and experiments.

Equipment: A large gallon jar with a two-hole stopper, cigarettes, delivery tubes (glass), cigarette holder, vacuum pump.

Procedure: Assemble cigarette tar separating apparatus, as shown in Figure 16.10. Fill the gallon jar half full of water. Place cigarette in intake and light. Pump vacuum pump so as to draw smoke from cigarette into gallon jar and water. Pump until cigarette is burned completely. Replace with additional cigarettes until tars can be seen in water. Examine color of water; smell and taste the liquid.

TOPIC: WHY DO TEENAGERS SMOKE?

Grade Level: Intermediate

Concept: Students start smoking for many wrong reasons.

Expected Pupil Outcome: The student will be able to state why students often take up smoking.

Content: Reasons why students often start smoking.
Peer pressure
Feel grown up
Identify with idol
Rebellion
Experiment—find out for self what something is like

Learning Experiences

1. Students are given scripts and asked to role play the following situations:
   a) *Situation 1.* Three students are off in a corner playing. A fourth student is playing alone, but decides to play with the others. The child walks over to the group, sees that they are smoking, and decides to join them.
   b) Interactive Discussion:
      Key Questions
      1. Why do you think that the fourth student decided to smoke?
      2. Does one have to smoke if his or her friends smoke?
   c) *Situation 2.* Bob's mother is furious with Bob because he never obeys her. He is fed up with hearing her nag and scream at him all the time. He goes off to a place where she won't see him. He starts to smoke.
   d) Interactive Discussion:
      Key Questions
      1. Why do you think Bob was smoking?
      2. What else could Bob have done to release his anger?
   e) *Situation 3.* Dad comes home after a long day of work and sits down in his favorite chair. He takes off his shoes and reads the newspaper. His daughter sits near his chair and watches television. After reading for a while, Dad lights up a cigarette and smokes for a while. He then gets up to get something from the other room. The daughter goes to the chair, picks up a cigarette, and takes a few drags from it.
   f) Interactive Discussion:

Key Questions

1. Why did the daughter decide to smoke?
2. Does smoking mean that one is grown up?

Evaluation Procedures   Teacher subjectively evaluates the quality of the student responses to the key question interactive discussion sessions following each role play situation. If the student comments are generally on target the objective will be considered accomplished.

REFERENCES AND BIBLIOGRAPHY

Benowitz, N. L. "Smokers of Low-Yield Cigarettes Do Not Consume Less Nicotine." *New England Journal of Medicine,* 309 (1983), 139-142.

Connolly, G. N., et al. "The Reemergence of Smokeless Tobacco." *New England Journal of Medicine,* 314 (1986), 1020-1027.

Davis, R. M. "Current Trends in Cigarette Advertising and Marketing." *New England Journal of Medicine,* 316 (1987), 725-732.

Dershowitz, A. "Bad Ideas Have Rights Too." *San Francisco Chronicle,* September 7, 1986, This World Section, p. 19.

Greenberg, R. A., et al. "Measuring the Exposure of Infants to Tobacco Smoke." *New England Journal of Medicine,* 310 (1984), 1075-1078.

Hirayama, T. "Nonsmoking Wives of Heavy Smokers Have a Higher Risk of Lung Cancer: A Study from Japan." *British Journal of Medicine,* 282 (1981), 183-185.

Martell, E. A. "Alpha-Radiation Dose at Bronchial Bifurcations of Smokers from Indoor Exposure to Radon Progeny." *Proceedings of the National Academy of Science,* 80 (1983), 1285-1289.

Kaufman, D. W. "Constituents of Cigarette Smoke and Cardiovascular Disease." *New York State Journal of Medicine,* December 1983, 1267-1268.

Rickert, W. S. "Less Hazardous Cigarettes: Fact or Fiction?" *New York State Journal of Medicine,* December 1983, 1269-1272.

Schwartz, J. L. "Successes and Failures in Smoking Cessation: Insights from Personal Interviews." *World Smoking and Health,* 3 (1978), 11-18.

Surgeon General of the United States. *Report on Smoking and Health.* Washington, D.C.: U.S. Government Printing Office, 1979. (b)

Surgeon General of the United States. *The Health Consequences of Smoking: Cancer.* Washington, D.C.: U.S. Government Printing Office, 1982.

Stapf, S. E. "A Propaganda War Against Cigarettes." *New York Times,* January 4, 1987, Section 3, p. 2.

Tager, I. B., et al. "Longitudinal Study of the Effects of Maternal Smoking on Pulmonary Function in Children." *New England Journal of Medicine,* 309 (1983), 699-703.

Weis, W. L. "Clearing the Air on Office Smoke." *Business Week,* February 7, 1983, 4.

White, J. R., and Froeb, H. F. "Small Airways Dysfunction in Nonsmokers Chronically Exposed to Tobacco Smoke." *New England Journal of Medicine,* 302 (1980), 720-723.

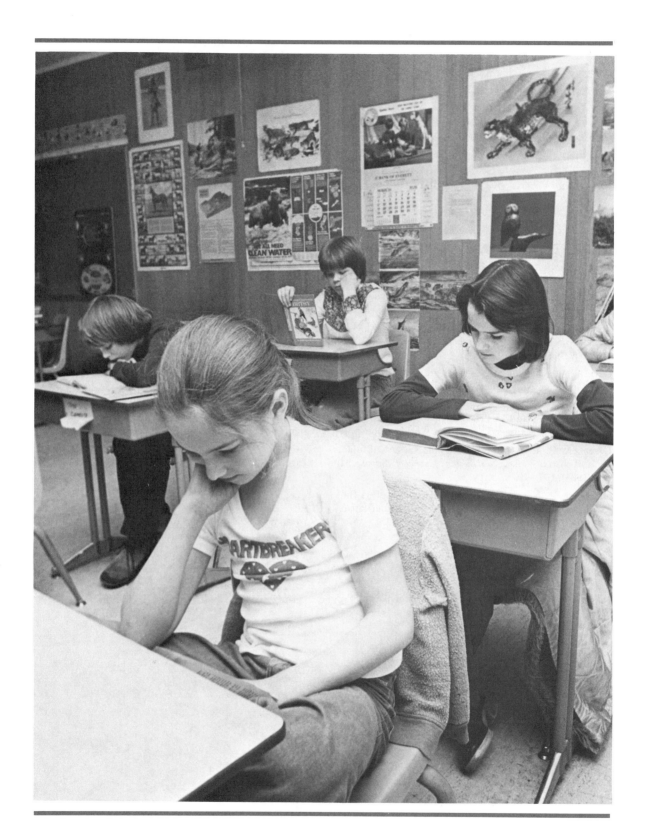

Chapter 17   **Teaching About Alcohol**

INTRODUCTION

The consumption of alcoholic beverages is an age-old custom. Except for some uncertain times during Prohibition, alcoholic beverages have enjoyed immense popularity with the American public. This is evidenced by the fact that approximately 71 percent of the total adult population in the United States consumes alcohol with regularity. The yearly per capita consumption of alcoholic beverages by adults 21 and older averages approximately 26 gallons.

In addition to being popular, drinking supports a most lucrative industry. Production of alcoholic beverages is a $13 billion industry in the United States, and approximately half of the total revenues go to state, federal, and local taxes.

Without reservation, alcohol is the most widely used and accepted *drug* in our society today. Alcoholic beverages are addicting drugs. Over time, the drinker will develop a tolerance to alcohol, can become psychologically dependent on alcohol, and may even become physiologically addicted to the point of suffering withdrawal symptoms during attempts to give up drinking. However, only a tenth of those who choose to drink are, or will be, adversely affected by their drinking habits. The overwhelming majority of those who indulge do so in moderation. It is the small minority of problem drinkers who have created an American nightmare.

For example, there are some 9 million to 10 million chronic alcoholics in this country. They cause untold harm to their loved ones and to society in general. They are responsible for countless lost hours in business and industry, not to mention their burden on the taxpayer in the form of court costs, hospitalization, and rehabilitation. Alcoholism is a very serious affliction, as anyone who has been touched by it knows. In addition to the alcoholic, the problem drinker and the overzealous occasional drinker present a serious problem to society. Nearly 60,000 people are killed every year on the highway, and in

approximately half the accidents, one or both of the drivers were under the influence of alcohol.

Alcohol consumption at high levels affects the body in numerous destructive ways. The depressant effects on the brain and central nervous system are well documented elsewhere, but the disruption of metabolic processes in the liver and the killing of brain cells are not too well reported. These are of greater importance to survival than the affects of alcohol on other parts of the body. Small blood vessels all over the body become clogged when the blood alcohol level becomes too high (Williams, 1973). This results in partial deprivation of oxygen and food in the nerve cells of the brain. Brain cells apparently also lose their ability to use glucose as a fuel, become impaired, and die off with greater rapidity than normal (Williams, 1973). Alcohol inhibits metabolic conversions in the liver, causing a deficiency of vitamins B_1 (thiamine), B_2 (riboflavin), B_3 (nicotinic acid), B_6 (pyridoxine), B_C (folic acid), B_{12} (cobalamin), biotin, vitamins C and E, and the minerals magnesium, potassium, and zinc (Di Cyan, 1974; Williams, 1973). The vitamins B_1, B_6, and biotin support the oxidation-inducing enzymes; nicotinic acid and B_2 are needed to overcome the inhibition of metabolic conversion caused by alcohol; vitamin E is needed to prevent the increased peroxidation of fats in the liver; more folic acid and vitamins B_6 and B_{12} are needed to repair the damage alcohol causes; and vitamin C is needed to keep connective tissue in healthy condition (Di Cyan, 1974). Thus consumption of alcohol at high levels undoubtedly damages brain cells and inhibits liver function (Figure 17.1).

ALCOHOL USE AND ABUSE

Alcohol abuse is one of the most significant health-related drug problems in the United States and in many other countries. Although the use of heroin, marijuana, cocaine, and other illegal drugs receives much more attention from governments and the news media, these drugs affect far fewer people and cause far fewer health problems than alcohol. In 1986, over

Much of this material in this chapter is from Gordon Edlin and Eric Golanty, *Health & Wellness: A Holistic Approach*, Third Edition (Boston: Jones & Bartlett Publishers, 1988).

FIGURE 17.1

Effects of alcohol on the central nervous system of a person weighing 150-160 pounds.

Alcohol concentration in blood stream	No. drinks* per hour	Part of brain affected	Area of brain affected
0.03%	1 bottle beer (12 oz.) 1 cocktail (whiskey) (90% proof)	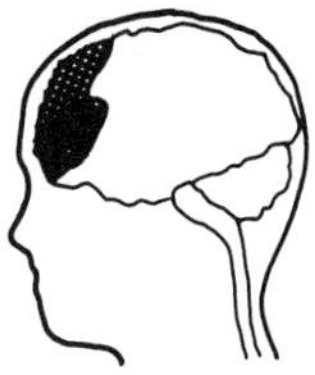	1 reason/judgment (minor)
0.05%	2 bottles beer 2 cocktails	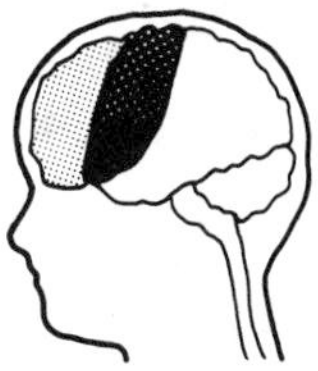	2 coordination 3 self-control
0.10%	4 bottles beer 4 cocktails	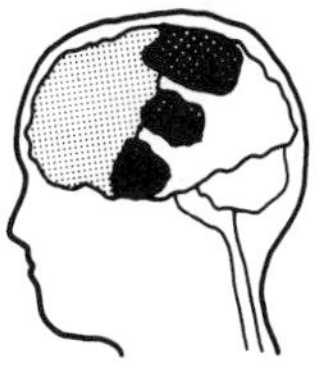	4 vision 5 speech 6 hearing 7 reaction time
0.15%	6 bottles beer 6 cocktails	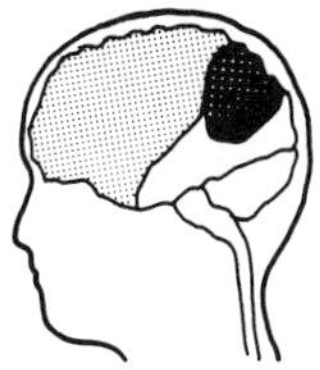	8 balance 9 coordination 10 judgment
0.30%	12 bottles beer 22 cocktails	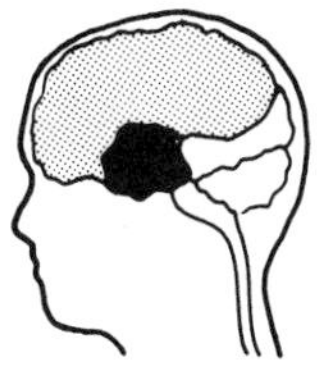	11 memory 12 unconsciousness
0.60%	24 + bottles beer 24 + cocktails	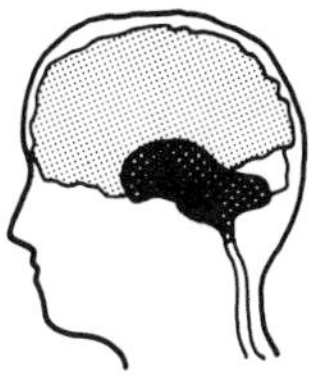	13 respiratory center inhibited 14 DEATH possible

*4% alcohol in beer; 90% proof distilled beverage

100,000 U.S. deaths were alcohol related, and alcohol abuse was responsible for approximately $120 billion in health and social costs. Excessive alcohol use is associated with thousands of divorces, perhaps as many as 50 percent of the incidents of family violence, and millions of hours of school and job absenteeism. Alcohol abuse is also linked to a long list of diseases and disorders (Figure 17.2).

Alcohol use has long been a part of social events such as parties, dinners, weddings, ball games, and picnics. The liquor industry encourages alcohol use by spending over $1 billion per year advertising its products in newspapers and magazines and on radio and television. No direct link between advertising of alcohol-containing products and alcohol abuse has been established. However, public health authorities and organizations believe advertising that associates drinking with athletic prowess, wealth, prestige, relaxation, and sex encourages irresponsible drinking. Breweries and distributors are especially active on college campuses, spending approximately $2 million per year on advertising in campus newspapers and promoting their products by sponsoring "pub nights" and drinking contests, giving away items with product logos, and underwriting some of the costs of college athletic events.

Alcohol's positive public image makes many people skeptical that they can benefit from learning about alcohol use and abuse. Most people who drink believe they can "hold their liquor" and that alcoholic beverages, especially beer, are no more harmful to health than soft drinks. It is not our intention to argue that all consumption of alcohol is unhealthful. As with so many other aspects of health, for most people responsibility and moderation are more desirable than fanatical adherence to a single course of action. Everyone can benefit from knowing more about the effects of alcohol on the brain and body.

History of Alcohol Use

It is likely that humans have been drinking alcohol since someone accidently noticed the psychological effects of drinking fermented liquids.

Anthropological evidence indicates that Stone Age people drank the fermented juice of berries. Perhaps this first fruit wine was produced when some berry juice was left too long in a covered earthen jar and yeasts in the mixture converted the sugar in the juice to alcohol by *fermentation*. The first recorded use of alcohol dates from the Mesopotamian agrarian cultures of around 5000 B.C.

Through the ages, the drinking of fermented grains (beer); fermented berries, grapes, and fruits (wine); and the distilled products of natural fermentations (brandies and hard liquors) has become commonplace in almost every human society. Alcohol is used in some religious ceremonies, is given as medicine, is used to ratify contracts, agreements, and treaties, and is offered to display hospitality. Alcohol consumption has been an integral part of American life since the landing of the Mayflower at Plymouth Rock. Yet over the years many people have regarded drinking as a social evil and drunkenness as a sin. The United States government tried to prohibit alcohol use in 1919 by the Volstead Act, a Constitutional amendment that prohibited the sale and consumption of alcoholic beverages. This attempt to control alcohol consumption failed, however, and in 1933 prohibition was ended by another amendment to the Constitution.

Today, alcoholic beverages come in many varieties. Not only are there the old standbys beer, wine, and the traditional hard liquors, but beverage manufacturers also market a variety of premixed cocktails, often sweetened and containing various flavors to make the drink more palatable.

Alcohol and the Body

The alcohol in beverages is *ethyl alcohol*. There are many other kinds, such as methyl (wood) alcohol and isopropyl (rubbing) alcohol. Most alcohols are poisonous in small amounts. In large amounts even ethyl alcohol is toxic, but the body has ways to detoxify and eliminate some of it.

The amount of ethyl alcohol in any commercial product is listed on the label. The

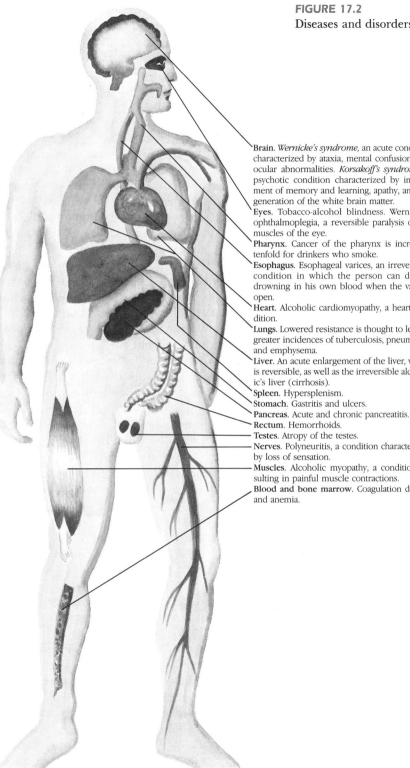

FIGURE 17.2
Diseases and disorders associated with alcohol abuse.

Brain. *Wernicke's syndrome,* an acute condition characterized by ataxia, mental confusion, and ocular abnormalities. *Korsakoff's syndrome,* a psychotic condition characterized by impairment of memory and learning, apathy, and degeneration of the white brain matter.

Eyes. Tobacco-alcohol blindness. Wernicke's ophthalmoplegia, a reversible paralysis of the muscles of the eye.

Pharynx. Cancer of the pharynx is increased tenfold for drinkers who smoke.

Esophagus. Esophageal varices, an irreversible condition in which the person can die by drowning in his own blood when the varices open.

Heart. Alcoholic cardiomyopathy, a heart condition.

Lungs. Lowered resistance is thought to lead to greater incidences of tuberculosis, pneumonia, and emphysema.

Liver. An acute enlargement of the liver, which is reversible, as well as the irreversible alcoholic's liver (cirrhosis).

Spleen. Hypersplenism.

Stomach. Gastritis and ulcers.

Pancreas. Acute and chronic pancreatitis.

Rectum. Hemorrhoids.

Testes. Atropy of the testes.

Nerves. Polyneuritis, a condition characterized by loss of sensation.

Muscles. Alcoholic myopathy, a condition resulting in painful muscle contractions.

Blood and bone marrow. Coagulation defects and anemia.

amount of alcohol in beer and wine is given as the percentage of the total volume. Beer is generally about 4 percent alcohol, although some beers may contain more and some less (so-called light beers have nearly the same alcohol content as regular beers); wine is about 12 percent alcohol. The amount of alcohol in distilled liquors (scotch, vodka, bourbon, tequila, rum, and so on) is given in *proof,* a number that represents twice the percentage of alcohol in the product. Thus, 80 proof whiskey is 40 percent alcohol; 100 proof vodka is 50 percent alcohol.

Most standard portions of alcoholic drinks contain about half an ounce of ethyl alcohol. For example, a 12-ounce can of beer that is 4 percent alcohol contains 0.48 ounces of alcohol. The same amount of alcohol is contained in a 4-ounce glass of wine. The alcohol content of a cocktail mixed with 1 ounce of 100 proof bourbon is 0.5 ounce. A can of beer, a glass of wine, and a highball contain approximately the same amount of alcohol.

Alcohol is readily absorbed into the body through the gastrointestinal tract. About 20 percent of ingested alcohol is absorbed by the stomach and the rest by the small intestine, then carried by the blood to all the body's tissues and organs. Although not strictly a food (it contains no protein, vitamins, or minerals), alcohol does contain calories—in fact, almost twice as many calories per gram as sugar.

Several factors affect the rate at which alcohol is absorbed into the tissues. For example, food in the stomach—especially fatty foods or proteins—slows the absorption of alcohol. Nonalcoholic substances in beer, wine and cocktails slow absorption of alcohol. Carbon dioxide in beverages such as champagne, sparkling wines, beer, and carbonated mixed drinks increases the rate of alcohol absorption. That is why people feel intoxicated more quickly when drinking champagne or beer, especially on an empty stomach. The higher the alcohol content in a drink, the faster it is absorbed.

The concentration of alcohol in the blood is called the *blood alcohol content* (BAC). A simple way to estimate BAC is to assume that ingesting one standard drink per hour (one beer, one glass of wine, one mixed drink), which contains ap-

proximately half an ounce of ethyl alcohol, gives a BAC of 0.02 in a 150-pound man. Thus, the BAC of an average-sized man who drinks five beers during the first hour at a party will be 0.10; this is the level of alcohol in the blood that violates the drinking-and-driving laws of most states. This shorthand method of approximating BAC changes with body size, body composition, and gender. All other things being equal, the BAC of a large person is less than that of a smaller person who has drunk the same amount because the alcohol is diluted more in the large person's tissues. According to Jones and Jones (1976), women tend to have a higher BAC from the same number of drinks as men because they generally weigh less than men, have proportionately more body fat (which does not absorb alcohol as readily as muscle and other tissues), and have sex hormones that tend to increase alcohol absorption and decrease its elimination.

Alcohol is eliminated from the body in two ways. About 10 percent is excreted unchanged through sweat, urine, or breath (hence the use of breath analyzers to test for drinking). Alcohol that is not excreted is broken down, primarily by the liver, winding up as carbon dioxide and water. The liver detoxifies alcohol at a rate of about half an ounce per hour, and there is no way to speed up the process. Sobering-up remedies, such as drinking a lot of coffee, taking a cold shower, or engaging in vigorous exercise, do not accelerate the rate at which the liver removes alcohol from the body.

Alcohol and Behavior

Alcohol is a central nervous system depressant, which means that it slows certain functions in some parts of the brain. In moderate amounts, alcohol may affect the parts of the brain that control judgment and inhibitions, which is why many people have a drink or two at a party—drinking may help them loosen up, become less shy and interact more freely with others. They may talk or laugh more than usual. Unfortunately, the effects of alcohol are unpredictable, and some people become boisterous, argumentative, irritable, or depressed after drinking.

The effects of alcohol on sexual desires and performance vary from person to person and with the BAC. Pinhas (1980) points out that in some individuals small amounts of alcohol may dispel uncomfortable feelings about sex and therefore may facilitate sexual arousal. Higher amounts of alcohol, however (0.10 BAC), may produce problems getting and maintaining an erection or ejaculating in males and a reduction in vaginal lubrication and difficulty reaching orgasm in females. Even at moderate BAC, some individuals are too intoxicated to give and receive sexual pleasure.

The behavioral effects of alcohol depend on the BAC (Table 17.1). At a BAC of 0.05, the loosening-up effects of alcohol become manifest. At a BAC of 0.10, the depressant effects of the drug become pronounced, the person may become sleepy, and motor coordination is affected. Speech may become slurred and postural instability may become noticeable. Alcohol's effects on motor skills, judgment, and reaction times make driving after drinking extremely dangerous (see box). Approximately *half* of highway fatalities each year involve people who are intoxicated with alcohol. Highway accidents are among the 10 leading causes of death in the United States.

Physical and psychological tolerance to the effects of alcohol can be acquired through regular use. The nervous system can adapt over time so that higher amounts are required to produce the same physiological and psychological effects. Some people learn to modify their behavior so that they appear sober even though their BAC is quite high. This phenomenon is called *learned behavioral tolerance*. In general, the more experience a person has with certain acts, the less likely alcohol will be to impair them, although not all behavior is affected by alcohol to the same degree.

Studies indicate that some people may feel

TABLE 17.1
Behavioral Effects of Alcohol

Number of drinks	Ounces of alcohol	BAC (g/100 ml)	Approximate time for removal	Effects
1 beer, glass of wine, or mixed drink	½	0.02	1 hour	Feeling relaxed or loosened up
2½ beers, glasses of wine, or mixed drinks	1¼	0.05	2½ hours	Feeling high; decrease in inhibitions; increase in confidence; judgment impaired
5 beers, glasses of wine, or mixed drinks	2½	0.10	5 hours	Memory impaired; muscular coordination reduced; slurred speech; euphoric or sad feelings
10 beers, glasses of wine, or mixed drinks	5	0.20	10 hours	Slowed reflexes; erratic changes in feelings
15 beers, glasses of wine, or mixed drinks	7½	0.30	15–16 hours	Stuporous, complete loss of coordination; little sensation
20 beers, glasses of wine, or mixed drinks	10	0.40	20 hours	May become comatose; breathing may cease
25–30 beers, glasses of wine, or mixed drinks	15–20	0.50	26 hours	Fatal amount for most people

intoxicated without ingesting alcohol. This placebo effect can occur in individuals who are familiar with the state of being high or drunk from previous experiences. On the other hand, some people who drink can decide they do not want to feel drunk even after several drinks and, in fact, feel and act sober. Most people who drink alcohol know that the psychological and behavioral effects of alcohol are strongly influenced by their mental and emotional states.

Other Effects of Alcohol

Alcohol can impair the functioning of body organs other than the brain. Alcohol can irritate the organs of the gastrointestinal (GI) tract—the esophagus, stomach, intestine, pancreas, and liver—causing upset or irritability, nausea, vomiting, or diarrhea. Alcohol can dilate arteries and cause bloodshot eyes. Dilation of arteries in the arms, legs, and skin can cause a drop in blood pressure and loss of body heat. This is why people occasionally feel flushed and their faces redden when they drink. Giving people alcohol to warm them up can produce the opposite effect.

Alcohol should not be ingested with other CNS depressant drugs such as tranquilizers and sedatives. In many instances, alcohol and the other drug interact so that the combined effect of the two drugs is greater than the simple additive effects. What may seem like reasonable amounts of alcohol, when taken with another drug, can dangerously suppress brain function and respiration (Table 17.2).

The Hangover

One consequence of drinking alcohol is a *hangover*, which may involve stomach upset, headache, fatigue, weakness, shakiness, irritability, and sometimes vomiting after a drinking episode. The frequency and severity of hangovers vary. The particular factors in alcohol that cause a hangover are unknown, but several causes have been suggested:

1. When alcohol is present in the body, normal liver function may slow in order to

TABLE 17.2
Alcohol and Drugs That Don't Mix
Alcohol should not be consumed when taking drugs such as those listed below.

Drug	Dangerous interaction
Acetaminophen (Tylenol, Anacin-3)	Heavy use plus alcohol can cause liver damage.
Aspirin (Anacin, Excedrin)	Heavy use plus alcohol can cause bleeding of stomach wall.
Antihistamines (Chlor-Trimeton, Benadryl)	Drowsiness and loss of coordination increased by alcohol.
Tranquilizers, sedatives (Valium, Dalmane, Miltown)	Alcohol increases their effects.
Painkillers (codeine, Percodan, morphine)	Alcohol increases sedation and reduces ability to concentrate.
Barbiturates (Amytal, Seconal, phenobarbital)	Potentially FATAL. Don't ever use with alcohol.

break down the alcohol. This may reduce the amount of sugar the liver releases into the blood, resulting in temporary hypoglycemia and its resultant fatigue, irritability, and headache.

2. Alcohol may inhibit REM sleep, resulting in fatigue, irritability, and trouble concentrating.

3. *Congeners*, other chemical substances in an alcoholic beverage, or the breakdown products produced in the liver may cause a hangover.

4. Acetaldehyde, a toxic intermediate produced when the liver breaks down alcohol, may be responsible for hangover symptoms.

The best way to deal with a hangover is to sleep, to drink juice to replace the lost body fluid and blood sugar (alcohol increases urine output), and perhaps to take an analgesic for headache. Ingesting more alcohol will only prolong the hangover.

Fetal Alcohol Syndrome

Alcohol can harm the health of anyone, man or woman, young or old. Even the unborn fetus can be damaged by alcohol. Over the last 10 years accumulated evidence has shown that numerous kinds of birth defects and mental retardation may result from ingestion of alcohol by pregnant women—a condition known as *fetal alcohol syndrome*. Fetal alcohol syndrome is estimated to be the third leading cause of birth defects and mental retardation among newborns. Since the harmful effects are believed to occur during the first few weeks or months of prenatal development, a time during which much of the nervous system is being formed, it is important that women refrain from drinking if they are trying to become pregnant or if they suspect that they are pregnant. Studies have also shown that the level of alcohol in the fetus's blood may be 10 times greater than the BAC of the mother. This explains why even a couple of drinks during pregnancy can endanger normal fetal development.

Alcohol Abuse and Alcoholism

Alcohol abuse is the principal drug problem in the United States. Approximately 12 million Americans of different ages, religions, races, educational backgrounds, and socioeconomic status have problems with alcohol. Over 3 million American teenagers (ages 14–17) have a drinking problem. More than a third of all suicides involve alcohol. Approximately 6 million adults have personal and health problems with alcohol that are severe enough to warrant the label "alcoholic" and to suffer alcoholism (see Figure 17.3). These people are unable to control their drinking. Some are physically dependent on alcohol and may experience withdrawal symptoms, including *delirium tremens* (DT's), when deprived of alcohol. Delirium tremens is characterized by hallucinations and uncontrollable shaking.

FIGURE 17.3

Percentage and types of drinkers among adults age 18 and older, 1981. (Data from National Institute of Alcohol Abuse and Alcoholism.)

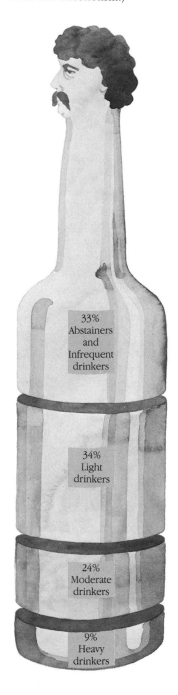

33% Abstainers and Infrequent drinkers

34% Light drinkers

24% Moderate drinkers

9% Heavy drinkers

Problem drinking can cause many problems in a person's life. Job and school performance can be impaired, family relationships and friendships can be destroyed, and drunk driving may cause legal problems. Because alcohol supplies calories, constant drinkers are rarely hungry, and they may suffer from vitamin deficiency, which results in loss of muscular coordination and mental confusion. After years of heavy drinking, a person may suffer serious liver, stomach, heart, and neurological damage.

The causes of problem drinking and alcoholism are unknown, although hypotheses abound. Before the advent of modern psychology and medicine, alcohol abuse was thought to be a manifestation of immorality and irreligiousness. Some people still hold that view, but most professionals (and problem drinkers) interpret alcohol abuse as a behavioral disorder or a medical disease. For example, some people with low self-esteem or seemingly unmanageable conflicts may drink in order to feel better about themselves or to try to cope with life. Instead they may add a drinking problem to their other problems.

There is some evidence that at least for some people, alcoholism may have a biological basis, either because people metabolize alcohol differently or because their brains respond differently to alcohol. Some experts resist considering alcohol abuse a disease because doing so may remove the sense of personal responsibility for problem drinking. Others argue that calling alcohol abuse a disease fosters successful treatment because it removes the stigma and lessens guilt associated with such behavior and offers a supervised and presumably scientifically based plan for treatment.

The Development of Alcoholism

Alcoholism usually develops from a prealcoholic stage of needing to drink to relieve tensions and anxieties. The prealcoholic phase may last for years, during which tolerance to alcohol gradually develops. Progression to a state of alcoholism is characterized by three phases (Jellinek, 1960):

1. *The warning phase.* In this first stage, problem drinkers have an increased tolerance to alcohol and a preoccupation with drinking. For example, when they are invited to a party they may ask what alcoholic beverages will be served rather than who is going to be there. In this stage problem drinkers may sneak drinks often and may deny that they are drinking too much. Blackouts may also occur. Blackouts are not periods of unconsciousness. Others observe the drinker as behaving normally, but he or she has no recall of events that happened while drinking. Some of the signs of the warning phase of alcoholism are presented in Table 17.3.

2. *The crucial phase.* This phase of alcoholism is characterized by the problem drinker's loss of control over how much he or she drinks. The person may not drink every day, but he or she cannot control the amount of alcohol consumed once drinking has begun. In this stage, the problem drinker may rationalize his or her drinking and actually believe that there are

---

TABLE 17.3
Warning Signs of Problem Drinking or Alcoholism

---

1. Gulping drinks.
2. Drinking to modify uncomfortable feelings.
3. Personality or behavioral changes after drinking.
4. Getting drunk frequently.
5. Experiencing "blackouts"—not being able to remember what happened while drinking.
6. Frequent accidents or illness as a result of drinking.
7. Priming—preparing yourself with alcohol before a social gathering at which alcohol is going to be served.
8. Not wanting to talk about the negative consequences of drinking (avoidance).
9. Preoccupation with alcohol.
10. Focusing social situations around alcohol.
11. Sneaking drinks or clandestine drinking.

good reasons for heavy drinking. An alcoholic may still carry out his or her responsibilities (housework, job, doing well in school) for some time and may employ a series of strategies to keep the family from rejecting him or her. These may include promising to stop drinking. Often the alcoholic's extravagant measures to prove he or she doesn't have a drinking problem appear successful, and eventually the person begins drinking heavily again. Perhaps at this point the problem with alcohol is blamed on the kind of drinks that the person prefers or on the usual place of drinking; so the problem drinker changes to a different form of alcoholic beverage or to a different place in which to drink.

3. *The chronic phase.* In this phase, the alcoholic is usually totally dependent on the drug, and drinking behavior has consumed all aspects of life. Friends and family have resigned themselves to the problem and may be angry and ignore the alcoholic. The person may be unable to work or attend school. The health consequences of alcohol abuse may intensify and the person may need medical attention and even hospitalization. If physical addiction to alcohol has occurred, continual drinking is needed to prevent withdrawal symptoms. Drinking may go on for days at a time, which is called a *bender*. The great majority of alcoholics do not wind up on skid row but instead struggle with their problem within their families and communities.

Alcoholism and the Family

Alcoholism can severely disrupt marriage and family relationships. One family member's drinking problem can cause all the other family members mental and emotional suffering and sometimes financial hardship. Alcoholism is costly to many persons, not just the alcoholic.

Close relatives of a problem drinker can experience a variety of emotions, ranging from joy and relief when the problem drinker stops drinking for a time to feelings of failure and depression when the problem drinker begins actively drinking again. In between the highs and lows, family members can feel rage, shame, guilt, pity, and constant anxiety. They may try to cope with the situation in different ways. Some may try to assume responsibility for the problem; others may be blamed for it (scapegoats). Some may withdraw in silence, while others try to maintain their sense of humor. These are all defense mechanisms against the family's psychological pain.

Like the problem drinker, family members may deny the problem, try to rationalize it, isolate themselves from friends and relatives, and in some cases feel responsible for the other's drinking problem. This enabling or protection process keeps the alcoholic from feeling responsible for drinking—which is part of the paradox experienced by families of alcoholics. In their attempts to protect, family members may unwittingly be contributing to the problem and may even protect the alcoholic from some of the serious social consequences of drinking too much (such as making excuses for absenteeism from work or school).

Family members of alcoholics may attend Alanon, an organization that helps spouses, families, and friends of alcoholics. Alateen is a similar organization that helps children of alcoholics. Alanon and Alateen help family members understand how alcoholism has affected their lives and explore the family relationships that contribute to the problem. Family therapy (with or without the problem drinker's participation) may help find ways to cope with the problem and regain a harmonious family life.

Seeking Help

The situation of problem drinkers and alcoholics is serious but not necessarily hopeless. Recovery is possible if the person is strongly motivated to stop drinking. Moreover, as in other aspects of health, an ounce of prevention is worth a pound of cure.

Sometimes the motivation to stop drinking

comes in the form of a threat—a drinking-related legal problem, severe disruption of the family life, loss of job, or a serious drinking-related illness. The motivation can also come from the person's own resolve to stop his or her self-destructive behavior and to stop feeling helpless, hopeless, and confused.

Alcoholics Anonymous (AA), the worldwide nonprofit self-help organization, has assisted many people to get on the road to wellness and enjoyment of life again. AA bases its program on total sobriety, anonymity, and a step-by-step program of recovery. The environment at AA meetings is relaxing, caring, and open. Members share their experiences, strengths, and hopes with each other, with the goal of helping new and old members identify and learn more about their own problems with alcohol. Practical tips on how to remain sober are shared, and telephone numbers are exchanged so that a member can contact another member if stressful situations arise that previously led to drinking.

Alcoholics Anonymous emphasizes that sobriety is a state of mind, which means that recovering from a drinking problem involves changing values, attitudes, and lifestyles. The AA program helps problem drinkers examine their feelings, recognize their limitations, and accept responsibility for past wrongs. For problem drinkers, remaining sober is an ongoing process that involves finding new ways to satisfy emotional, spiritual, and environmental needs. Of course, AA may not be the answer for everyone who has a drinking problem. Individual and group psychotherapy with a therapist skilled in helping problem drinkers can also be successful.

Responsible Drinking

Each person has the option of drinking or abstaining from alcohol. Each of you has responsibility for determining the occasions for drinking and the amounts of alcohol that you consume. If you are one of the millions of people who already enjoy drinking, here are some guidelines to remember:

1. Make sure that alcohol use improves your social interactions and does not harm or destroy them.
2. Drink slowly and avoid mixing alcohol with other drugs.
3. Be sure that using alcohol enhances your general sense of well-being and does not make either you or other persons feel disgusted with your actions.
4. If you plan to drink, decide beforehand that you will not drive and designate someone who will not drink to be the driver.

In addition to being responsible for your own drinking habits, you can also help other people to drink responsibly. Respect the wishes of the person who chooses to abstain from drinking and don't push drinks on people at parties. If you are giving a party, be sure to provide alternatives to alcohol. You may also offer places to sleep for those who have been drinking and should not drive home. Remember to eat when you drink and to provide food at parties.

There is no evidence to indicate that abstaining from alcohol is necessary to health. On the other hand, there is a great deal of evidence showing that excessive alcohol use can destroy personal health and family relationships, can cause traffic deaths and suicides, and can produce birth defects in newborns. We believe that you can significantly improve your health and happiness by developing responsible drinking habits while you are young and maintaining moderate drinking habits throughout life.

LESSON PLANS

In light of this discussion, peruse the following lesson plans, keeping in mind that they are indicative of the type of lesson plans that you will likely be expected to implement. Remember that they by no means encompass a complete unit of instruction. They are a guide for the formation of a comprehensive unit.

TOPIC: EFFECTS OF ALCOHOL ON THE BODY

Grade Level: Intermediate

Concept: Alcohol depresses bodily systems.

Expected Pupil Outcome: The student will be able to summarize how alcohol depresses bodily functions.

Content: Alcohol depresses various systems of the body:

1. Central nervous system

a) *Brain*	*Quantity*
Reasoning, memory	1–2 drinks
Judgment, self-control	3–4 drinks
Speech	5–6 drinks
Hearing	5–6 drinks
Sight	5–6 drinks
Touch	5–6 drinks
Coordination	5–6 drinks
Balance	7–8 drinks
Breathing	10+ drinks

2. Cardiovascular system
   a) Heartbeat affected
   b) White blood cells destroyed? function?
   c) Vitamins C and E destroyed; vitamin C is essential for building and maintaining collagen, which holds cells together; vitamin E deficiency results in abnormal collagen, which constricts blood vessels and chokes off adequate blood supply to the tissues, eventuating in cell death.
3. Respiratory system
   a) Rate reduced
4. Digestive system
   a) Interferes with absorption of food
   b) Stimulates gastric secretions?
   c) Stimulates flow of saliva
5. Liver
   a) Vitamins B_6, C, and E destroyed, impairing liver function
   b) May become inflamed
6. Skin
   a) Rosy glow
   b) Increased perspiration

Learning Experiences

1. *Rat Demonstration (Experiment)*
   Material
   1. One or two rats weighing about 200 grams and not fed for about six hours
   2. A mixture of 0.5 ml (cc) 190-proof pure grain alcohol and 0.5 ml distilled water
   3. Hypodermic syringe marked off in cc
   4. Hypodermic needle (Yale B-D 26 gauge, 3/8 in.)
   5. Several cotton balls
   6. A small bottle of rubbing alcohol
   7. Boiling water
   8. A small saucepan
   Procedures
   1. For each 18 grams of body weight, inject 0.1 cc of the distilled water-alcohol solution into the peritoneal (abdominal) cavity of the rat. The rat will probably die from an injection that is too large.
      a) Secure the rat by either tying its hind legs to a table or a board or having someone hold its legs.
      b) Support the rat in one hand and place your thumb and forefinger about its neck and against its lower jaw.
      c) The needle should not be injected any deeper than 1/4 of an inch; the needle should not enter straight into the rat's body, but rather at an angle such as one would use when removing a splinter from the hand. The object of the injection is to get just beneath the outer layer of the skin.
      d) Care should be taken not to puncture the viscera by going too deep or the diaphragm by going too near to the rib cage.

7. Other:
   a) Increased cholesterol in the body
   b) Increased triglycerides, which are associated with heart disease.

   e) Two to three minutes after the injection, the rat behavior tests may be tried. If the rat has been fed sooner than the six hours recommended, it will take longer for behavior to be affected.

Observation
1. Normal rat behavior
   a) If held by the tail and brought near an object, the rat will reach for the object.
   b) If placed on its back, the rat will right itself immediately.
   c) Place your finger near the rat's eye, and it will blink.
   d) If held several inches above a table and spun around, the rat will, when released, land on its feet, like a cat.
   e) After a few trials, the rat will be able to find its own way out of a maze without difficulty.
   f) If placed on a balancing pole (any round pole) above the table, a rat will balance itself.
2. Alcoholic. rat behavior: An alcohol-injected rat will be unable to perform the actions in the tests. The rat may be able to duplicate the actions after a considerable lapse in time and much effort.

Conclusion
This experiment will show the students of various grade levels the effect alcohol has on the human body. The rat is like a miniature human. Both eat and drink similar things, and one day in the growth pattern of the rat is equivalent to about one month of human growth (12 days is equal to one year). It is important to establish this analogy successfully so that the student will be readily able to relate the effect he or she observes the alcohol to produce in the rat to the effect of alcohol on the human being.

Evaluation Procedures   The day following instruction the students will be asked to respond to a short essay question, which will solicit their understanding of how alcohol serves to depress bodily functions. An 80 percent correct response by a majority of the class will indicate that the objective was accomplished.

TOPIC: WHY PEOPLE DRINK

Grade Level: Intermediate

Concept: People often drink alcohol for the wrong reasons.

Expected Pupil Outcome: The student will be able to discuss the reasons why people drink alcohol.

Content: Poor reasons people drink:
1. To get a high
2. To deal with unhappiness
3. To imitate others
4. To develop a feeling of importance
5. To escape from worry or self-pity
6. To be more sociable
7. To satisfy curiosity
8. To escape frustration
9. To feel grown-up
10. To seek social status and approval for indulging in a customary activity

Learning Experiences
1. *Role playing:* Pupils act out three or four situations, with follow-up after each one:
   a) *Situation 1:* Dad and his friends gather around the TV to watch a football game and drink beer.
   b) *Situation 2:* Each member of a group at a party begins to drink for different reasons: John to feel grown up, Mary to escape feeling inadequate, and Rusty to conform, etc.
   c) *Situation 3:* Sam, a married man with three children, is in debt. On the way home, he stops at the local bar and gets drunk with a friend.
2. Have class suggest other reasons; teacher uses these suggestions to initiate class discussion (list on blackboard).

Evaluation Procedures During the discussion periods following each role playing, the teacher will subjectively evaluate the quality of the student responses. If the students tend to respond with the correct comments, the objective will be considered achieved.

REFERENCES AND BIBLIOGRAPHY

Edlin, G., and E. Golanty. *Health and Wellness*, Third Edition (Boston: Jones and Bartlett, 1988).

Jellinek, E.M. *The Disease Concept of Alcoholism* (New Haven: College and University Press, 1960).

Jones, B.M., and M.K. Jones. "Women and Alcohol: Intoxication, Metabolism, and the Menstrual Cycle." In M. Greenblatt and M.A. Schuckit (Eds.): *Alcoholism Problems in Women and Children* (New York: Grune & Stratton, 1976).

Pinhas, V. "Sex Guilt and Sexual Control in Alcoholic Women in Early Sobriety," *Sexual and Disability Journal*, 3 (Winter 1980).

Williams, R.J. *Nutrition Against Disease* (New York: Bantam, 1973): 169-189.

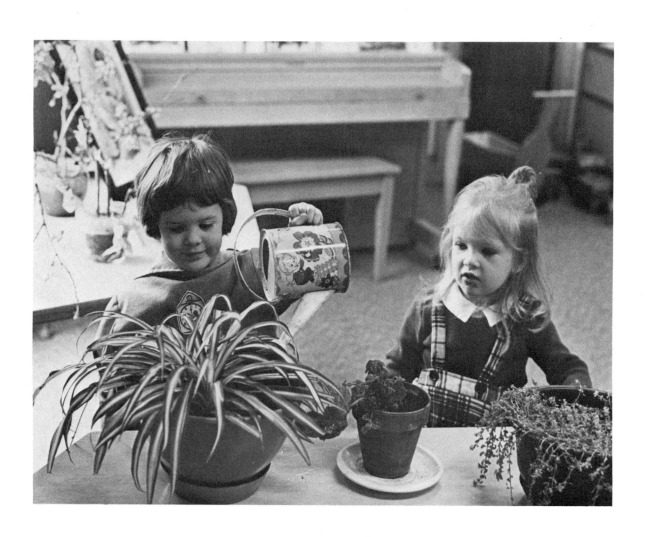

Chapter 18 **Teaching About Environmental Conservation**

INTRODUCTION

The concern for our environment is mounting. Best that it should, because there is precious little time left to atone for past ecological sins. Nature is very forgiving, as history has proved, but our senseless disregard for the environment has reached such proportions that the damage done is just now beginning to have catastrophic consequences. The inevitable is obvious. People simply cannot continue to rape their environment. If they do, human existence will be threatened in the near future.

Progress and pollution are the horns of a dilemma. On the one hand, humans have been tremendously successful in overcoming the restraints that their environment and competing organisms have imposed on them throughout history. Modern technological advances have turned science fiction into reality. On the other hand, the by-products of technology have the unique capacity for creating ecological mires which may be instrumental in human destruction.

It is difficult to comprehend why people continue to abuse the ecosystem. Perhaps the answer lies in the fact that humans have never really been anything but polluters. At no time have men and women ever learned to deal with their overzealous needs and waste materials.

This makes sense when you consider that early humans were somewhat kept in check by nature's own selection process. The environment was able to assimilate humans and to accept their thoughtless acts because they were few in number. As time passed and humans became more effective in overcoming the many restraints imposed by the environment, the population increased rapidly. It follows that as the population increased, so did demands on the environment. These unchecked demands have taken their toll and are now at an intolerable level. Even to the most naive, it should be obvious that the environment can no longer continue to meet human needs if present practices are continued.

There are too many people. The relationship between population growth and the environmental nightmare is direct. All ecological problems are closely related to population levels. If we continue to populate the earth at our present rate, there will be 1,000 people per square foot of the earth's surface some 900 years from now. In just 1,000 years, the world's population will equal the weight of the earth. More people require more goods and services. Increased demand for goods and services prompts even more waste material. The by-products of this vicious cycle are air, water, noise, pesticide, and radiation pollution.

Pollution can best be described as any human-caused change in the ecosystem that renders the environment less desirable for sustaining life. Beyond a shadow of a doubt, countless ecological atrocities are the cause of the major pollutants as we know them today. These pollutants inhibit the natural functions of the highly interdependent ecosystem. Once one aspect is set askew, one or more other phases are also affected. In essence, nature's system of checks and balances has been usurped.

The answer is simple; people must quickly learn to live within the natural limitations of the environment. To accomplish this goal requires that each person realize and accept the fact that the environment does *not* belong to humans, but rather that they belong to the environment. The human organism is simply not *independent* of the environment, but in the truest sense of the word is *interdependent* with all other forms of life on our planet. Like all organisms, a person is the product of both heredity and environment and needs to be aware that all organisms and environments are continually changing. Indeed, the social and physical environments in the last hundred years have changed dramatically. In trying to cope with many rapid changes, people have been progressively degrading their environment. Unfortunately, the world has not fully committed itself to fostering a sensible program of global environmental conservation. The consequences will be catastrophic unless there is productive action in the near future. Education at

---

Much of the material in this chapter is from Gordon Edlin and Eric Golanty, *Health & Wellness: A Holistic Approach,* Third Edition (Boston: Jones & Bartlett Publishers, 1988).

an early age is one approach that answers this urgent call for conservation.

The basic goal of environmental education should be to make everyone aware that everyone is absolutely dependent on the environment, and everyone affects it. At the primary school level, the emphasis should be on the environment in the school and neighborhood. In the intermediate grades, the teacher should progress to the community and region. The teacher should guide the children to discover problems by forcing them to examine their interaction with the environment. How do we use the environment to satisfy our needs? These and other questions should be answered during the discovery process. In lieu of these learning experiences, there should be a twofold program in the elementary schools. The indirect approach is for the teacher to plan and facilitate a physical environment in the classroom, and in the school generally, that is conducive to positive learning and sound personality development. It would reinforce the second, or direct, approach.

ENVIRONMENTAL HAZARDS TO HEALTH

The environment includes everything to which we are exposed, both internally and externally. The term *environment* in this chapter refers to all external factors, natural and man-made, that affect health and well-being. In order to survive, all animals, including humans, have certain basic biological needs that must be met, including adequate air, water, food, and shelter. To the extent that individuals are deprived of any of these factors, or that the factors are impure or toxic, health is adversely affected. Anyone who has had difficulty breathing or persistent eye irritation from smoggy, dusty, or pollen-laden air realizes that health is diminished by poor air quality. Anyone who has become sick from inhaling chemical fumes, drinking contaminated water, or eating spoiled food knows how important to health is the quality of air, water, and food.

Optimizing health means keeping the quality of the environment high. Magazine and news-paper headlines tell us almost daily that the environment is becoming increasingly polluted and unhealthy and that people's lives are becoming increasingly affected by this pollution. The effects are widespread and some damage may be long-lasting or even irreversible. It may be many more years before our society realizes the extent of air, water, and land pollution and before we are prepared to pay the price, both in money and lifestyle changes, that will be required to clean up and maintain a healthy environment. For example, the pesticides DDT and 2,4,5-T were introduced into wide use in the mid-1940s, but it wasn't until the 1970s that the health hazards became so apparent that further use of these chemicals was banned in the United States.

Environmental health hazards stem from many causes—which is the reason why solutions to environmental problems are not easily found. Many factors have to be considered in assessing pollution and deciding what to do about the problems.

The United States is making progress in reducing environmental pollution, preserving natural resources, and protecting plant and animal wildlife, but much remains to be done to restore the environment to a healthier condition. Despite enactment of environmental protection bills, six of which were modified and renewed in 1984, much of this country's air, water, and land is becoming increasingly polluted. At least 700 toxic industrial chemicals have been identified in underground and surface water supplies, and it is estimated that 30 percent of all groundwater systems used to supply drinking water are contaminated. In checking almost 1,000 hazardous waste sites, the Environmental Protection Agency (EPA) found that 90 percent of the sites had caused some contamination and that about 25 percent of them were health hazards.

We cannot expect the government—or any organization, for that matter—to solve this country's pollution and health problems. As the character Pogo the possum declared a number of years ago in the comic strip of the same name created by Walt Kelly: "We have met the enemy and he is us!" Each of us must assume responsibility for living in a manner that brings the greatest personal health and satisfaction while at the same time causing the least damage to the environment that we share with all living organisms. Environmental hazards and accidents frequently result in death (Table 18.1).

Our dependence on the automobile and the

TABLE 18.1
Causes of Death in the United States by Rank Order (1984)
Note that 9 of the 16 most frequent causes of death are accident or self-inflicted injury.

Number of deaths	Cause
738,000	Heart disease
328,000	Cancer
209,100	Stroke
55,350	Motor vehicle accidents
38,950	Diabetes
24,600	**Suicide**
21,730	Emphysema
18,860	Homicide
7,380	Drowning
7,380	Fire
3,690	Tuberculosis
2,563	Poison
2,255	Firearm accident
1,886	Asthma
1,517	Motor vehicle collisions with trains
1,025	Electrocution
902	Appendicitis
677	Infectious hepatitis
451	Pregnancy, birth, and abortion
410	Syphilis
334	Excess cold
205	Flood
129	Nonvenomous animal
107	Lightning
90	Tornado
48	Venomous bite or sting
17	Polio
15	Whooping cough
8	Smallpox vaccination
6	Fireworks
5	Measles
2	Botulism
1	Poisoning by vitamins
0	Smallpox

vast amount of gasoline and oil we use provide a graphic example of how people's lifestyles contribute to pollution and endanger the health of everyone (Figure 18.1). The emissions from millions of gasoline engines pollute the air with lead and other harmful chemicals. Every year the giant petrochemical industries that manufacture gasoline, oil, plastics, and chemicals dump uncounted tons of toxic wastes into the environment. Highways, parking lots, and new housing destroy millions of acres of fertile land each year. About 50,000 people die and another 2 million are seriously injured in automobile accidents every year in the United States. Still, our lifestyles and physical comforts depend on automobiles, on trucks, and on petroleum products. Therein lies the dilemma: How can each one of us achieve a healthy lifestyle and at the same time live in ways that pollute the environment and that create health hazards for everyone? Solutions to environmental problems will require major changes in the values of our society.

Air Pollution

Every person breathes about 35 pounds of air a day—more than 6 tons over the course of a year. Pure, unpolluted air is essential for all body functions and for health. Fresh, clean air consists of about 21 percent oxygen, 78 percent nitrogen, and trace amounts of seven other gases. It is the oxygen in air that is essential to human life. If the oxygen content of air drops below 16 percent, body and brain functions are affected. If breathing stops for more than a very brief period, the person becomes unconscious and will die within a few minutes unless breathing is restored.

Air pollution reduces the quality of the air we breathe by limiting the availability of oxygen and by forcing us to breathe substances that are harmful to the lungs, blood, and tissues. The American Lung Association estimates that one out of five people suffers from chronic obstructive pulmonary disease (COPD), which includes asthma, emphysema, bronchitis, and chronic cough.

In addition to causing breathing problems

FIGURE 18.1

Automobiles produce air, water, and land pollution. (Courtesy Environmental Protection Agency.)

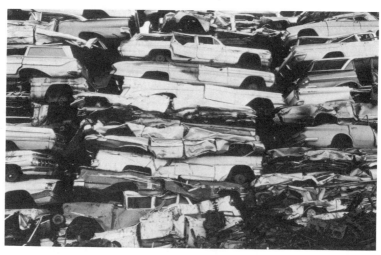

and serious illness, air pollution can damage vegetation, can diminish the growth of vegetables, grains, and flowers, and can even reduce milk and egg production. It can also corrode metal and erode stone and cause paper, leather, and rubber products to disintegrate.

Everybody has heard of *smog* (Figure 18.2). The term was first used in England to describe a hazardous combination of smoke and fog (hence "smog") that is largely responsible for the chronic cough and bronchitis that affected many British citizens. In many U.S. cities smog is not associated with fog but results from the action of sunlight on various airborne chemicals and from particles and gases in the air emitted by automobiles, electricity generating plants, blast furnaces, oil refineries, and many other sources. The major kinds of "aerial garbage" are described in Figure 18.3. The EPA has developed a numerical scale for measuring air pollution called the Pollutant Standards Index (PSI). The hourly concentration of six constituents of polluted air are measured and the total amounts are expressed as a number from zero to 500. Values below 100 are regarded as safe, whereas values above 100 are increasingly unhealthful. Values above 300 mean that the air is hazardous to the health of people breathing it.

Smoggy, polluted air not only is irritating to the eyes and lungs but also contributes to more serious health problems such as allergies, lung infections, and heart disease. Carbon monoxide, one of the components of smog, interferes with the binding of oxygen to the hemoglobin in red blood cells. If the air contains 80 ppm (parts per million) of carbon monoxide, the body's supply of oxygen is reduced about 15 percent. In heavily congested traffic the levels of carbon monoxide may reach 400 ppm, and people are frequently stuck in traffic jams for hours at a time. It is no surprise that many commuters in large cities arrive home with headaches. Car mechanics and parking lot attendants are often exposed to high levels of carbon monoxide for extended periods and may develop health problems as a consequence.

Sulfur oxides are produced when coal or oil containing sulfur is burned. If the air is damp, sulfuric acid, a very corrosive substance, is formed. Damp air laden with sulfur oxides can pit metals and erode stone buildings as well as damage lung tissue. Acid rain is produced in air containing sulfur oxides and can damage crops and forests far from the site of the initial air pollution.

Most scientists and environmentalists who are familiar with the facts concerning the dispute over acid rain agree that forests, lakes, and rivers

FIGURE 18.2
New York City smog. (Courtesy Environmental Protection Agency.)

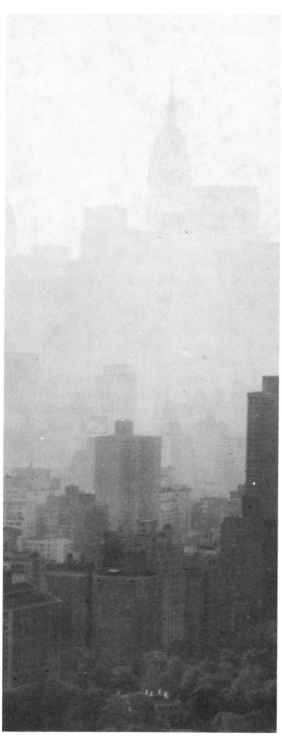

are damaged by acid rain. Many kinds of fish are finding it more and more difficult to survive and reproduce in water that is increasingly acidic. Fish eggs are damaged and fish hatchlings develop abnormally in water whose pH is below 5.0. Water that is neutral—that is, neither basic nor acidic—has a pH of 7.0. Since pH values are based on a logarithmic scale, a pH change from 7.0 to 5.0 means that the acidity has increased 100 times.

Canada began to monitor the acidity of rain in 1976, and the United States, two years later. In 1982 the United States spent almost $20 million on research into the acid rain problem (Figure 18.4). However, despite the expenditure of vast amounts of time and money, no acceptable federal policy or solution to the acid rain problem is in sight. Ore smelters and related industries in the U.S. spew millions of tons of sulfur dioxide, the principal cause of acid rain, into the atmosphere each year. Acid rain consists of about 70 percent sulfur dioxide; the remaining 30 percent is derived from nitrogen oxides. The sulfur and nitrogen oxides released into the atmosphere react with water to produce sulfuric and nitric acids that fall into lakes and rivers, raising their acidity. Worldwide about 130 million tons of sulfur dioxide is put into the atmosphere annually, which makes acid rain a global problem.

Solutions to the acid rain problem involve difficult economic and political decisions and require the cooperation of many countries. Acid rain can fall thousands of miles from the source of the sulfur dioxide emissions, which explains why it is difficult to assign the blame. Meanwhile, forests continue to be damaged and many forms of animal life will suffer and die because of acid rain.

Nitrogen oxides, which are produced mostly by automobile exhausts, interfere with the oxygen-carrying capacity of the lungs and blood cells. Photochemical smog, containing nitrogen oxide, is formed over large cities such as Los Angeles by the action of sunlight on the various nitrogen compounds in the polluted air. This gives the air a hazy, brownish appearance, limits visibility, and irritates eyes and lungs.

In addition to widespread outdoor pollution,

FIGURE 18.3

Components of smog. Almost 200,000 tons of aerial garbage are released into the air annually in the United States. (Data from Environmental Protection Agency.)

Carbon Monoxide
A poisonous gas from car exhaust that drives out oxygen in the bloodstream. Large amounts can kill; small amounts can cause dizziness, headaches, and fatigue. Often exists in tunnels, garages, and heavy traffic. Especially dangerous for people with heart disease, asthma, anemia, and so on.

Hydrocarbons
Unburned chemicals in combustion, such as car exhaust, which react in air to produce smog. Hydrocarbons have produced cancer in animals.

Sulfur Oxides
Poisonous gases that come from factories and power plants burning coal or oil-containing sulfur. Forms sulfur dioxide, a poison that irritates the eyes, nose, and throat, damages the lungs, kills plants, rusts metals, and reduces visibility.

Particulates
Solid and liquid matter in air such as smoke, fly ash, dust, and fumes. They may settle to the ground or stay suspended. They soil clothes, dirty window sills, scatter light, and carry poisonous gases to lungs. They come from autos, fuels, smelters, building materials, fertilizers, and so on.

Nitrogen Oxides
A result of burning fuels that convert the nitrogen and oxygen in the air to nitrogen dioxide. Can cause a stinking brown haze that irritates the eyes and nose, shuts out sunlight, and destroys the view.

Photochemical Smog
A mixture of gases and particles oxidized by the sun from products of gasoline and other burning fuels. They irritate the eyes, nose, and throat, make breathing difficult, and damage crops.

FIGURE 18.4

Acidity of rain in North America. On the average, rain in the eastern part of the country (pH 4.1 to 4.6) is five to ten times more acid than the rain falling in other parts of the country (pH 5.0 to 5.6). Winds tend to blow from west to east and carry industrial emissions eastward. These data were compiled by various U.S. and Canadian agencies in 1982.

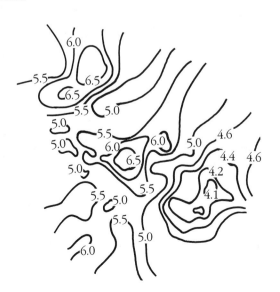

the lungs are assaulted by indoor pollutants. Not only is cigarette smoking harmful to the person who smokes, but second-hand smoke often creates indoor air pollution that is more harmful than all but the worst forms of outdoor smog. Carbon monoxide indoors may be increased by cigarette smoking to levels that are regarded as hazardous to workers in industry and that are prohibited by law. For example, factories are not allowed to exceed carbon monoxide levels of 50 ppm, and the Federal Air Quality Standard Act sets the allowable level in outdoor air at 9 ppm. Yet the air in bars, conference rooms, and other places where many people are smoking may contain levels of carbon monoxide as high as 50 ppm.

Experimental animals that were exposed for several months to 50 ppm to 100 ppm of carbon monoxide showed heart and brain damage, and it is necessary to assume that people also suffer some adverse effects from these levels (Table 18.2). Particulate matter such as dust, soot, lead, and asbestos in polluted air also creates serious public health problems but is of particular concern to workers who are exposed to these substances in large amounts.

TABLE 18.2
Symptoms of Carbon Monoxide Poisoning

Percentage of CO in hemoglobin	Symptoms
0–2	No symptoms.
2–5	No symptoms in most people, but sensitive tests reveal slight impairment of arithmetic and other cognitive abilities. Levels of 2 percent to 5 percent are found in light or moderate smokers.
5–10	Slight breathlessness on severe exertion. Levels of 5 percent to 10 percent are found in smokers who inhale one or more packs of cigarettes per day.
10–20	Mild headache, breathlessness on moderate exertion. These levels are sometimes seen in smokers who are exposed to additional CO from other sources.
20–30	Throbbing headache, irritability, impaired judgment, defective memory, rapid fatigue.
30–40	Severe headache, weakness, nausea, dimness of vision, confusion.
40–50	Confusion, hallucinations, ataxia, hyperventilation, and collapse.
50–60	Deep coma with possible convulsions.
Above 60	Usually results in death.

The human lungs have a remarkable capacity for extracting vital oxygen from the air and for expelling unwanted gases and contaminants. Tens of millions of *cilia,* tiny hairlike projections in the breathing passageways, sweep out airborne microorganisms and particulate matter before the air reaches the lungs. Within the lungs, special macrophage cells scavenge the foreign substances that reach the alveoli, the tiny air sacs that exchange incoming oxygen for carbon dioxide produced by the body. Years of breathing polluted air and smoking tobacco can weaken and destroy cilia, alveoli, and other lung cells.

Air pollution is not confined to the immediate vicinities of factories, oil refineries, or cities. The air supply is global, and eventually air pollutants are carried all over the planet. This fact is dramatically demonstrated by the increase in lead content in the Greenland snowpack. The amount of lead in the snowpack has increased sharply since 1900 because of the lead that is carried in the air and falls from it onto this isolated area of the world. Most airborne lead is presumed to have originated from automotive exhausts. (This is one reason why auto manufacturers are now required to design cars that run on lead-free gas.)

Since pre-Roman times the amount of lead in the atmosphere has increased two thousand-fold. It has been suggested that the decline and fall of the Roman empire could have been caused, at least in part, by lead poisoning of its leaders and citizens (Nriagu, 1983). It is thought that the physical and mental deterioration exhibited by Roman emperors including Claudius, Caligula, and Nero could have been the result of alcoholism and chronic lead poisoning. In Roman times, lead was widely used to store food and wines and in plates and wine goblets. In short, Romans ate a daily dose of lead.

Today, the primary source of lead pollution is lead-contaminated air. There is evidence that the introduction of lead-free gasoline several years ago has reduced blood levels of lead in the U.S. population to a significant degree (Figure 18.5). In 1984, after ten years of studies, hearings, and legal maneuvering by lead and gasoline companies, the EPA proposed reducing the amount of lead in gasoline by a factor of 10. The long-term goal would be to eliminate lead in gasoline. The decision was based mainly on a cost

FIGURE 18.5

Total lead used in gasoline versus the average level of lead in people's blood. The chart shows that blood lead levels have declined at about the same rate as the use of lead in gasoline. The EPA decided in 1985 to phase out lead in all gasoline.

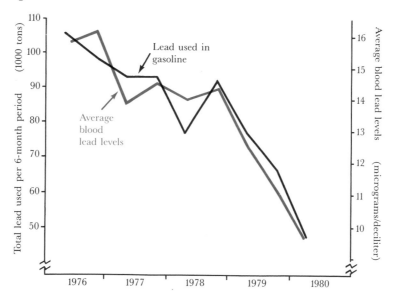

analysis showing that by 1988 the country would save almost $800 million, partly from longer engine life and reduced wear and tear on exhaust systems, but more than half from children who would not require treatment for lead poisoning or remedial education because of their diminished capacity to learn.

Water Pollution

After air, water is the body's most immediate requirement. We can survive without air for only a few minutes and without water perhaps several days. The human body is about 60 percent water, which is essential to every function carried out by the body, including digestion, blood circulation, and excretion.

Agriculture and industry in this country are enormous consumers of water. Several hundred gallons of water are necessary to produce a pound of flour; brewing a barrel of beer consumes a thousand gallons; a ton of newspaper takes about a quarter of a million gallons; a ton of steel requires more than half a million gallons; and irrigating an acre of orange trees requires a

million gallons of water a year. Plentiful water is vital to the maintenance of our lifestyle, as it is to the body's health.

Water is continuously recycled in the environment by evaporation and rain. However, as more and more water becomes polluted from pesticides, chemicals, oil spills, and sewage, less and less water is suitable for human consumption and agricultural use. Of special concern is the chemical contamination of rivers, lakes, and underground water supplies, which provide most of our water needs.

Waterborne diseases such as cholera, typhoid fever, and dysentery have been virtually eliminated in North America through sanitation and water treatment. In many communities the water supplied to homes is purified by sedimentation filtration and/or chlorination, although adding chlorine to water to kill dangerous bacteria may create other health hazards. Interaction of chlorine with other chemicals in the water produces toxic substances such as chloroform and chloramines, which are carcinogens. The widespread use of detergents, herbicides, pesticides, fertilizers, and other chemicals has also contributed to increased water pollution.

WIDESPREAD CONTAMINATION OF DRINKING WATER EXISTS IN THE UNITED STATES

Over one hundred chemicals potentially hazardous to health have been introduced into drinking water supplies across the country as a result of environmental pollution from various sources. The Environmental Protection Agency (EPA), which is responsible for monitoring our drinking water and for setting standards, has established safe levels for about 20 of the more common pollutants in drinking water (table).

In many areas other compounds have seeped into underground water supplies from nearby industrial complexes or toxic waste dumps. Other hazardous substances found in drinking water are benzene, carbon tetrachloride, dioxin, ethylene dibromide (EDB), polychlorinated biphenyls (PCBs), and vinyl chloride. All of these chemicals are carcinogens. Children are usually more vulnerable to ingestion of toxic substances than adults because of their smaller size and because they are still growing.

Many kinds of home water purifiers are now on the market, but many of them are not very efficient at filtering out hazardous substances despite manufacturers' claims. Safe drinking water is going to be increasingly hard to find in the future.

Pollutant	Maximum level (mg/l)	Pollutant	Maximum level (mg/l)
INORGANIC CHEMICALS			
Arsenic	0.05	Lead	0.025
Barium	1.0	Manganese	0.05
Cadmium	0.01	Mercury	0.002
Chromium	0.05	Nitrites and nitrates	10.0
Copper	10.0	Selenium	0.045
Detergents	0.5	Silver	0.05
Fluoride	1.4	Sulfate	250.0
Iron	0.3	Total dissolved solids	500.0

ORGANIC CHEMICALS		RADIOACTIVE SUBSTANCES	
Endrin	0.0002	Radium 226 and 228	5 pCi/l
Lindane	0.004	Gross alpha particle activity	15 pCi/l
Methoxychlor	0.1		
Toxaphene	0.005		
Total trihalomethanes (THM)	0.1*		

*EPA has slated a future goal of 0.01–0.025 mg/l for THM.

The federal government recently declared Love Canal, formerly a charming waterway in New York near Niagara Falls, a disaster area. Between 1947 and 1952, the Hooker Chemical Company disposed of its chemical wastes in the area around Love Canal. Years later, as the chemicals oozed to the surface of the land and into the canal, the incidence of cancer and birth defects among people living in the area was found to be unusually high. No one knows for certain how much it will cost to clean up Love Canal, and some areas near the canal may remain a health hazard. Recent studies have found that small field mice called voles living around the canal have a reduced life expectancy compared to voles living some distance from the canal. The closer to the canal the voles live, the younger they die (Christian, 1983). Many of the voles that have been trapped, especially those living close to the canal, show evidence of liver damage and have high tissue levels of the pesticides that were dumped into the canal years ago.

Analysis of drinking water from communities across the United States has shown that much of the water is unsafe and unhealthful (Box). In the early 1970's, the Environmental Protection Agency found the water supplies of many towns and cities were dangerously contaminated with pathogenic organisms and toxic chemicals. (It found 66 organic chemicals in the drinking water of New Orleans, for example.) As a result of these findings, Congress passed the Safe Drinking Water Act of 1974, which covers 40,000 community water supply systems and another 200,000 private systems. The law requires that these systems meet new federal drinking water safety standards, but it is one thing to pass such a law and another thing to enforce it, and many community water supplies are still contaminated. Many people today are forced to drink bottled, distilled, or spring water to protect their health.

Land Pollution

Until recently, little public attention has been given to the disposal of solid wastes. Each year in the United States we junk about 7 million autos; 75 billion cans, bottles, and jars; and 200 million tons of trash and garbage. The U.S. Public Health Service has labeled over 90 percent of the thousands of authorized hazardous waste disposal sites as posing "unacceptable" health risks. Hazardous wastes consist of materials that are flammable, corrosive, toxic, or chemically reactive, and about 35 million tons of such wastes are produced each year in the United States. In 1979, the EPA documented 400 cases of health and environmental damage due to improper hazardous waste disposal, and this number is thought to represent only a tiny fraction of the actual health problems caused by disposal of toxic substances. The magnitude of the environmental pollution and of health problems posed by disposal of hazardous chemicals is indicated by the data in Table 18.3. Because most of these toxic substances are not readily broken down or inactivated in the environment, the health problems resulting from such wastes may increase in the years ahead.

TABLE 18.3
Annual Disposal of Some Hazardous Chemicals in the United States, 1977

Substance	Amount (millions of pounds)	Source	Health effects
Mercury	2.6	Sludge from chloralkali plants; electrical equipment, fluorescent lights	Tremors, mental retardation, loss of teeth, kidney damage, neurological damage
Arsenic	110.0	Arsenic trioxide from coal combustion and from metal smelters	Diarrhea, vomiting, paralysis, skin cancers
Cadmium	1.8	Waste from electroplating industry; paint containers, nickel-cadmium batteries	Lung diseases
Cyanide	21.0	Electroplating industry waste	Poisoning, interference with cellular energy metabolism
Pesticides	230.0	Solid wastes and wastes in solutions	Rashes, respiratory and gastrointestinal symptoms, neurological disorders, hemorrhages

Data from Janice Crossland, "The Wastes Endure," *Archives of Environmental Health*, 19 (1977), 9.

Pesticides and Related Chemicals

Soil and water in America have become increasingly polluted by chemicals used to control weeds, insects, and plant diseases. Any substance capable of killing or limiting the growth of living organisms is called a *pesticide*. Chemicals that are specific for certain classes of organisms are called insecticides, rodenticides, fungicides, herbicides, and so on. Pesticides are important to the agricultural industry of this country, which claims it could not produce such an abundant food supply without them, although some experts disagree (Van den Bosch, 1978). Billions of pounds of DDT and other polychlorinated hydrocarbons have been used in the last 20 years to kill insects and other pests that destroy valuable crops. Pesticide use has been beneficial to agriculture, but it has also created serious environmental and health problems, which are not easily resolved. DDT, probably the most widely disseminated pesticide in the world, was banned from use in the United States.

The principal danger from continued widespread use of pesticides is that most are carcinogens and teratogens (cause damage to developing embryos). Pesticides are found in farmland and forest soils, and because they are washed out of the soil by rain and irrigation, are found in rivers, lakes, and oceans. Their harmful effects are enhanced because they accumulate in animal and human tissues. The chemicals become more and more concentrated in organisms as they move up the food chain. The fish, fowl, and beef that people eat nowadays may contain high levels of pesticides, which become part of human body tissues. Several agencies of the federal government monitor pesticide contamination in various foods, and the government must determine what levels should be regarded as dangerous to health. It is easy to understand how government decisions can provoke heated controversy between consumers concerned with health and producers of food who are concerned with productivity (Box).

Recent studies by the National Cancer Institute (NCI) show that farm workers exposed to the weed killer 2,4-D have 5 to 10 times higher risk of cancer than farm workers not exposed to it. After several farm workers died following exposure to Dinoseb, a widely used, highly toxic herbicide, the EPA issued an emergency ban on its use. About 10 million pounds of Captan, a potent fungicide, are used in the United States each year, primarily on fruits such as grapes and apples. Captan is a carcinogen, a mutagen, and a teratogen, but because it is not acutely toxic like Dinoseb, it has been regarded as safe. However, increased public pressure may force EPA to ban the use of Captan also.

The lesson from these and numerous other studies is that no pesticide is safe and most can cause short- or long-term health problems (Figure 18.6). Evidence is also beginning to show that common pesticides used around the home and garden can cause headaches, allergies, and flu-like symptoms. Everyone needs to be aware that pesticides are dangerous, and if they must be used, all precautions against exposure should be observed.

Dioxin, a contaminant in some herbicides, is an extremely potent carcinogen. It has been detected in human breast milk, which creates a problem for mothers who have to decide whether to nurse their babies or not. The U.S. Forest Service still sprays forests with herbicides to control brush, although there is some evidence suggesting that the health of people living near forests that are sprayed is adversely affected. Some veterans of the Vietnam War believe that their health was impaired by the herbicides (such as Agent Orange) they were exposed to in Vietnam, and some have sued the government for damages. In 1984 the U.S. military agreed to establish a fund of $180 million to be distributed over the next 25 years to Vietnam veterans and their families who were affected by exposure to Agent Orange (Raloff, 1984). Despite this enormous settlement, the official policy of the federal government and chemical companies is that no adverse health effects have been proven except for the occurrence of skin rashes (chloracne) among people who are exposed (Tschirley, 1986).

Because of extensive chemical contamination of their town, about 800 residents of Times Beach, Missouri, will never return to their homes

SOME COMMON PESTICIDES AND PRECAUTIONS FOR THEIR USE

Organophosphates
diazinon
malathion

Organophosphates have a relatively short persistence in the environment. They can cause acute nervous system poisoning in people. Malathion is less acutely toxic than many other pesticides.

Carbamates
carbaryl (Sevin)
aldicarb (Temik)

These chemicals are similar to the organophosphates in their persistence and toxic effects on the nervous system. The chemical involved in the mass poisonings in Bhopal, India, has been used in manufacturing these pesticides.

Organochlorines
DDT
chlordane
lindane

Compared to the previous groups, organochlorines have relatively long persistence in the environment and low acute toxicity. Each of these three chemicals has been shown to cause cancer in experimental animals. Chlordane is widely used to control termite infestations. Lindane has been used in home pesticide vaporizers and as a drug in treating scabies (mite infestations). DDT is no longer used in the United States but is used in other countries to control insects that spread disease such as malaria.

Phyenoxyacetic acids and related compounds
2,4,5-T
2,4-D
pentachlorophenol

This group of compounds is generally used to kill weeds. Several have been found to be contaminated with dioxins, chemicals that are deadly both on an acute and a long-term basis.

Pesticides derived from plants
pyrethrum
nicotine
rotenone

Exposure to some of the botanical pesticides can cause allergic reactions and other adverse reactions. Pets and people may be affected. These chemicals have fairly long persistence in the environment.

1. *Before you buy* a pesticide, read the instructions for use and any health and safety warnings. Do not purchase the product if you can't use the pesticide properly; you may not have the right equipment. If you don't understand or feel completely comfortable with the health and safety information provided, get more information before you buy the product. Also, consider whether you have adequate storage for the pesticide. A bigger bottle may be cheaper, but can you store it safely?

2. Use the least toxic pesticide available for your problem. Try to strike a balance between effective pest control and the safety of people, pets, and other nontarget organisms.

3. Minimize skin and respiratory contact with pesticides. Wear protective gloves. When you select gloves, consider both the solvent used in the pesticide and the possibility that the pesticide itself can penetrate skin. A local safety equipment store (check the telephone directory) can be helpful. You may want to use a respirator to guard against inhaling pesticide spray or dust.

4. Use pesticides only as intended. For instance, some wood preservatives are meant for outside use only, so don't use them inside the house!

5. Don't leave seemingly empty pesticide containers where children can get them. Children have been poisoned by drinking from "empty" containers that actually contained leftover pesticide.

FIGURE 18.6

Cholinesterase levels in five office workers exposed to pesticides. After their office was sprayed by an exterminator, all five workers became ill within an hour. They were told that they had the flu. Cholinesterase is an enzyme essential for functioning of the brain and nervous system. Their enzyme levels remained abnormal for over a month after pesticide exposure. (Data from Hodgson and Parkinson, 1985.)

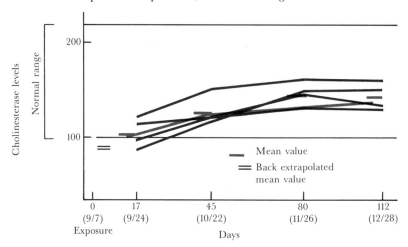

(Sun, 1983a,b; Garmon, 1983). These people had to abandon their town because dirt roads and other dusty areas had been sprayed over years with oil that was heavily contaminated with dioxin (2-3-8 tetrachlorodibenzopara dioxin, TCDD). Horses, dogs, cats, birds, and insects died after coming into contact with sprayed areas. Children broke out in rashes and came down with other medical problems. The residents of Times Beach were eventually compensated for the loss of their homes, and continuing efforts are being made to decontaminate the area.

Ethylene dibromide (EDB) is widely used to fumigate fruit and to control insect infestation in stored grain. For the past 20 years it has been assumed that EDB is safe despite many studies showing it to be a highly toxic chemical and a potent carcinogen in mice and rats. After almost seven years of deliberation, in 1984 the EPA finally decided to ban further use of EDB (Sun, 1984a).

Polybrominated biphenyls (PBBs) were widely used in the 1970's as fire retardants. In 1973 several thousand pounds of PBBs were accidentally added to livestock feed and distributed to about 800 dairy farmers in Michigan. Some months later, when cattle became sick and calves began to die, the accident was discovered. In the meanwhile, people had eaten PBB-contaminated milk and meat and had assimilated the substance into their tissues. Public health scientists are continuing to monitor these people to see whether their health is adversely affected over the long term.

Polychlorinated biphenyls (PCBs) are compounds used in electrical transformers, hydraulic fluids, paints, and many other products. Although the EPA banned the manufacture of PCBs a number of years ago, the chemicals continue to find their way into the environment. It is estimated that there are still 340 million pounds of PCBs in air, water, and soil and another 750 million pounds of various pieces of equipment still in use (Garmon, 1982).

What is certain in the controversy over the use of pesticides is that billions of pounds of chemicals have been diffused into the environment and that these chemicals will continue to pollute the land and water for generations to come. Increased rates of cancer, stillbirth, and birth defects tomorrow may be the terrible harvest of the widespread use of pesticides, herbicides, and toxic chemicals now and in the past.

Heavy Metal Pollution

Many heavy metals are toxic to living organisms when they are in the body in more than minute amounts. These metals include beryllium, cadmium, nickel, arsenic, manganese, and especially lead and mercury. Because these heavy metals are vital to many manufacturing processes and industries, the amounts entering the environment have increased sharply in recent years. Heavy metals affect health in a variety of ways—all of them detrimental. They inhibit many essential enzyme reactions in body cells. They damage blood cells, producing symptoms of anemia. And they damage cells of the nervous system, causing headaches, loss of coordination, drowsiness, mental retardation, and even death.

Lead

Lead is a cumulative cellular poison and presents the most serious health hazard because of the enormous amounts that are used and because it contaminates air, food, and water. Early symptoms of *plumbism* (lead poisoning) are loss of appetite, weakness, and anemia. Because such general symptoms can result from many causes, a diagnosis of plumbism often is not made until more serious symptoms develop (Table 18.4).

One of the tragedies of lead poisoning is that children are the chief victims. In 1970 the Surgeon General estimated that 400,000 children in the United States had dangerous levels of lead in their blood, and that number may be higher today. More than one-fourth of those children will suffer some brain damage. The number of children suffering lead poisoning is particularly high in city slums (Berwick, 1982).

In addition to airborne lead pollution poisoning, small children become poisoned because of a condition known as *pica*, an appetite for unusual substances or abnormal kinds of food. Many older paints contain lead and are sweet to the taste. As paint flakes off walls in old buildings, children crawling around are apt to eat the

TABLE 18.4
The Effect of Lead Accumulation in People

Amount of lead in blood (micrograms/100 ml)	Observable effects
10	Enzyme inhibition, learning disabilities
15–40	Red blood cells affected
40–50	Anemia
50–60	Central nervous system affected, cognitive disabilities
60–100	Permanent brain damage

Data from "Air Quality Criteria for Lead," Environmental Protection Agency 600/8-77-017, pp. 13–25.

paint flakes. Mothers do not usually notice any unusual symptoms until the lead poisoning has advanced to a stage where brain damage has already occurred. Studies of children with learning disabilities suspected to have been caused by lead poisoning have shown them to have more than five times the normal amount of lead in their bodies (Pihl and Parkes, 1977).

In 1975, about 900,000 tons of lead were used in the manufacture of batteries and other metal products. An additional 200,000 tons of lead were used in the production of gasoline as an antiknock additive. The lead added to gasoline is the more serious source of pollution because almost all of it ends up in the air. It is estimated that without man-made lead pollution, the natural body burden of an adult would be about 0.25 mcg of lead per 100 ml of blood. Today the average adult living in a large city has a blood level *100 times* that amount, or 25 mcg of lead per 100 ml of blood. Because pregnant women share materials in their blood with the developing embryo, babies are sometimes born already suffering from lead poisoning.

Although polluted air is the main source for lead entering the lungs and blood, food may also contribute significant amounts of lead, since plants and animals also assimilate lead from the air and soil. Food may add 50 mcg to 200 mcg of lead a day to the body.

Lead in the environment is one of the most serious pollution problems facing our society. Elevated blood levels of lead in children may be partly responsible for learning disabilities, hyperactivity, and even mental retardation. Needleman of Harvard Medical School and Piomelli of New York University Medical Center (1978) have written a report describing and documenting the many health hazards of lead exposure, especially from low levels. They conclude: "Lead in the air is a product of man's activity and can be controlled by man. Rarely do important biomedical problems offer themselves to such available remedy."

Mercury

In 1953, an epidemic of methylmercury poisoning occurred in several villages around Minamata Bay in Japan. Since the first epidemic, mercury poisoning has become known as "Minamata disease." Another outbreak occurred in Japan in 1965. In 1970, high levels of methylmercury were found in Lake St. Clair in Canada, where a chemical plant had been discharging its wastes. In 1970, the U.S. Food and Drug Administration began to determine which bodies of water in the United States were contaminated by mercury, and as a result of their investigation, fishing limitations were imposed in 18 states because of unsafe mercury levels in fish.

Mercury poisoning is characterized by muscle weakness, lack of coordination, paralysis, progressive blindness and deafness, and mental retardation. Like many other toxic substances, methylmercury is concentrated as it moves up the food chain. Children and developing embryos are the ones most strongly affected by mercury and lead poisoning because their body and brain cells are still growing rapidly.

Radiation

The cells of the body are continuously exposed to various forms of electromagnetic radiation, such as gamma rays, x-rays, ultraviolet light, and subatomic particles from nuclear disintegrations—all of which go undetected by any of the senses. These are all forms of ionizing radiation and can cause permanent changes in cells that may result in cancer or an increased risk of birth defects, may destroy molecules, and may affect chemical reactions in living cells. Much of the potentially harmful radiation from the sun and stars is filtered by the earth's atmosphere. However, as anyone who has had a sunburn should know, too much radiation is dangerous.

Electromagnetic radiation and radioactivity result from natural processes, but technologies developed in recent years have produced a marked increase in overall exposure to radiation, especially for certain occupational groups such as x-ray technicians and nuclear industry workers.

Radiation hazards tend to remain more localized than those stemming from chemical pollution of air and water. A medical x-ray exposes the patient and persons in the immediate vicinity, such as the doctor or technician. Exposure to radioactivity is usually limited to persons who live or work near radioactive materials, such as those produced in nuclear power plants and those found in uranium mines or in places where radioisotopes are used. However, radioactive materials can be spread over large areas as fallout from atomic explosions and from uranium mining. There has been concern that the higher incidence of leukemia reported among children in southern Utah might have been due to atomic test explosions carried out in neighboring Nevada in the 1950's. In 1984 a federal judge ruled in a suit filed by leukemia victims that the federal government was liable for damages where the evidence appeared convincing that the leukemia was caused by radioactive fallout. Also, at least seven states in the southwest have large areas polluted with millions of tons of radioactive debris resulting from uranium mining. The radioactive materials are spread further by wind and rain, which wash the radioactivity into the rivers.

Any exposure to x-rays or radioactivity carries with it some degree of risk. There is no such thing as a safe dose of radiation. One can argue that the risks are greatly outweighed by the benefits for particular circumstances—taking an x-ray to facilitate setting a fractured bone or using radiation to treat an inoperable tumor. Nonetheless, we should not forget that even the brief

ESTIMATING YOUR ANNUAL EXPOSURE TO RADIATION

The recommended maximum dose of radiation from all sources is 500 millirems per year. Use this chart to estimate your annual exposure to radiation.

Source of radiation	Approximate annual dose in millirems
Cosmic rays from space: 40 mrem average at sea level; add 1 mrem for each 100 feet above sea level	_____
Radioactive minerals in rocks and soil: ranges from 20 to 400 mrem; *U.S. average* = 55	_____
Radioactivity from air, water, and food: ranges from about 20 to 400 mrem; *U.S. average* = 25	_____
Medical and dental x-rays and tests: 22 mrem for chest x-ray, 500 for x-ray of lower gastrointestinal tract, 910 for whole-mouth dental x-ray film, 1500 for breast mammogram, 5 million for radiation treatment of a cancer; *U.S. average* = 80	_____
Living or working in a stone or brick structure: 40 mrem for living and an additional 40 for working in such a structure	_____
Smoking one pack of cigarettes a day for one year: 40 mrem	_____
Nuclear weapons fallout; *U.S. average* = 4	_____
Air travel: 2 mrem per year for each 1500 miles flown	_____
TV or computer screens: 4 mrem per year for each 2 hours of viewing a day	_____
Occupational exposure: 100,000 mrem per year for uranium ore miner, 600–800 for nuclear power plant worker, 300–350 for medical x-ray technician, 50–125 for dental x-ray technician, 140 for jet plane crews; *U.S. average* = 0.8	_____
Normal operation of nuclear power plants, nuclear fuel processing, and nuclear research facilities; *U.S. average* = 0.1	_____
Miscellaneous: luminous watch dials, smoke detectors, industrial wastes, etc.; *U.S. average* = 2	_____
Your annual total	_____
Average annual exposure per person in the United States	230

Chart adapted from *Living in the Environment* by G. Tyler Miller, Jr. (Wadsworth, 1984).

exposure from a diagnostic x-ray poses some health risk (Bross, 1979). Some studies have indicated that certain people may be particularly sensitive to low levels of radiation and that children who develop leukemia are often in this "susceptible" group (Bross, 1972). As more data became available in recent years, the allowable radiation standards established by federal regulatory agencies have been steadily lowered (see box, above).

Each person has the responsibility for minimizing his or her exposure to radiation and radioactivity. You are entitled to a complete explanation from your doctor or dentist as to the necessity for any x-ray or radiation. You should ask yourself whether you really need a routine annual chest or dental x-ray if there are no symptoms present. Many dentists routinely take an x-ray with every checkup because it was an accepted practice when they were trained. Many cavities can be detected by a careful visual exam, and if a person has had no cavities for several years, an x-ray is probably unwarranted. Discuss with your dentist the pros and cons of routine x-ray examination. If you are unsatisfied, you may prefer to find a dentist who is more conservative in the use of x-rays.

Many companies and government agencies require annual chest x-rays. Most companies require new employees to have a chest x-ray as part of their physical exam. If a person changes jobs frequently, he or she may be exposed to several unnecessary x-rays each year. Often companies, doctors, and hospitals will not accept x-rays taken elsewhere, which adds to a person's radiation exposure.

Some medical x-ray machines, because they are defective or adjusted improperly, expose patients to unnecessarily high doses of radiation. During x-ray examination or treatment, the reproductive organs should be protected by a lead apron or screen. During pregnancy, no x-rays should be taken unless absolutely necessary for the diagnosis of some serious abnormality of the mother or fetus. Caution regarding your exposure to ionizing radiation over a lifetime will help preserve your health and minimize damage to your body.

Other forms of nonionizing electromagnetic (EM) radiation, such as radio, television, radar, and microwaves, are widespread in the environment. Indeed virtually all forms of electronic communication and other aspects of our technological society depend on using low-level EM radiation. Over the years various concerns have been raised regarding possible deleterious biological effects of long-term exposure to this kind of radiation. Despite considerable research into the biological consequences of such exposure, no harmful effects have been consistently observed or documented (Foster, 1986). However, despite the low risk it probably is advisable to avoid ongoing exposure to powerful transmitters of nonionizing EM radiation.

ever found yourself thinking, "If that noise doesn't stop, I'm going to scream"?

Most of us are disturbed daily by some kind of noise. We usually dismiss our annoyance by accepting noise as part of the environment. Yet noise interferes with sleep and causes fatigue, irritability, anger, tension, and anxiety. High levels of noise, such as exposure to high-intensity rock music, jet planes, and jackhammers, can cause permanent hearing loss as well as physiological changes that are detrimental to health.

Sound activates the nervous system and in so doing affects functions of the endocrine, cardiovascular, and reproductive systems (Raloff, 1982). Noise is a stressor and can increase blood pressure, alter hormone levels, constrict blood vessels—in short, can contribute to the development of disease, just as do other kinds of stress. Many people live and work amidst the din of urban life and tend to forget how necessary to health and how comforting silence can be to one's state of mind. When you have the good fortune to spend time in the woods or mountains, you become aware of the quiet. The human need for stillness was expressed most eloquently in 1854 by Chief Seattle, after whom the modern city is named:

There is no quiet place in the white man's cities. No place to hear the unfurling of leaves in spring or the rustle of insect's wings. But perhaps it is because I am a savage and do not understand. The clatter only seems to insult the ears. And what is there to life if a man cannot hear the lonely cry of the whippoorwill or the arguments of the frogs around a pond at night? I am a red man and do not understand. The Indian prefers the soft sound of the wind darting over the face of a pond, and the smell of the wind itself, cleansed by a midday rain or scented with the pinion pine.

Noise Pollution

Have you ever been kept awake during the night by a dripping faucet? Do fire and ambulance sirens put you on edge? Does the persistent pounding of rock music affect you? Have you

Nuclear Winter

In 1945 atomic bombs were dropped on the cities of Hiroshima and Nagasaki in Japan. An estimated 140,000 people died in Hiroshima and another 70,000 in Nagasaki from the blasts and fires that resulted. Since then the world's nations and citizens have been concerned with the possibility of nuclear war and the consequences to the environment and life. The term "nuclear winter" was introduced to describe the global destruction that some scientists believe would result from a large-scale nuclear war (Turco, 1983).

A nuclear war would cause the social and economic fabric of societies to collapse. Food and water would be contaminated or destroyed. Starvation would be widespread. Some experts believe that the earth's temperature would change and that the environment could be changed so drastically that human life might eventually die out. Even if this view is extreme, physicians have predicted dire consequences for human health following a nuclear war (Leaf, 1986). However, even these predictions have been contested by critics who argue that estimates of destruction and problems are overblown. They also argue that discussions of nuclear winter are inappropriate for both scientific and political reasons (Nuclear War Letters, 1987).

Nuclear war and nuclear winter are events that everyone hopes can be avoided. Yet the disturbing reality is that nations (and individuals) have not learned how to resolve differences without violence or the threat of violence. Until people learn how to live and interact without violence, nuclear war and nuclear winter remain as the ultimate threat to the environment. Perhaps the slogan of the peace activists says it more clearly than all the arguments: "No one is right if no one is left."

Accidents

Most people don't think of accidents as health problems, but accidents affect the well-being of millions of people every year (Figure 18.7). When people think of accidents, they usually think of something over which they have no control. Accidents are commonly described as occurring by chance, for no specific reason, or because God made it happen. It is true that the victims of some accidents have no control over the occurrence: passengers on a train or airplane

FIGURE 18.7
Percentages of years of potential life lost before age 65. Injury causes more loss than cancer and heart disease combined. Some facts to remember: injury is the fourth leading cause of death; injury caused 143,000 deaths in 1983; injury causes about half of all deaths in children 1 to 14. Be careful!

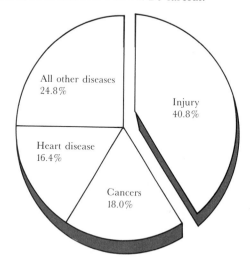

that crashes, those who take food or water that contains poisons, those who are hurt in a tornado or flood. But the overwhelming majority of accidents are caused by poor judgment, inattention, or confusion.

People cause accidents and are the victims. For example, alcohol abuse is known to be a primary cause of all kinds of accidents. That drinking is responsible for most automobile fatalities has been shown in many studies. A recent study in Texas showed that 72 percent of the drivers killed in auto crashes in Houston had blood alcohol levels over the legal index of intoxication. Psychological tests given to persons who survived an auto accident showed that 76 percent had an alcohol or personality problem, while in a nonaccident control group, 88 percent of the people were classified as normal by the same psychological criteria. Among young people between the ages of 15 and 24, accidents claim more lives than all other causes of death combined, and automobile fatalities are a major contributor to teenage deaths (Figure 18.8).

Some authorities single out September 13, 1899, as a memorable day in the history of the

FIGURE 18.8

Teenage male drivers have the highest percentage of deaths from motor vehicle accidents. Male and female drivers below age 25 have the most accidents and the greatest number of deaths. (Data from the Insurance Institute for Highway Safety.)

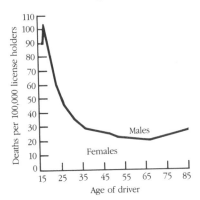

automobile. On that day it was reported that Mr. H. H. Bliss was struck and killed by an electric taxi at 74th Street and Central Park West in New York City. Bliss may have been this nation's first automobile fatality, culminating in what has today become carnage on the highways. Traffic fatalities in the United States have accounted for more deaths than have been recorded in all of the wars that the United States has fought since the country was founded. One drink too many, a moment's inattention, a reckless decision, or simply a brief joyride can result in a lifetime of regret and pain.

Safety in the broadest sense means being in harmony with oneself and with the environment. Usually when the bread knife slips and cuts a finger or when you stumble and fall, it is because you are upset or angry or distracted in some way that allows the mishap to occur. If a person has been trying to cope with life's problems by using alcohol or drugs, the capacity for judgment, as well as muscle coordination, is impaired and the chances for an accident are significantly increased. People not only endanger their own physical safety and health when they become intoxicated with alcohol or take drugs, they endanger the lives of other people as well. A philosophy of safety that fits in with the ideas of holistic health was expressed 40 years ago in a classic article by Herman H. Horne (1940). His broad view of accidents is that:

the universe of which we are a part, that is, the cosmos, is characterized, so the astronomers tell us, by law, harmony, symmetry, and rhythm and order. Nothing happens in the world at large by chance, everything occurs according to law. Safety for man means only that he is catching step with the universe of which he is a part and which explains his being here at all.

Accidents do not just happen. They are caused. Fatalism is an incorrect philosophy of life. Self-determinism is better. Man himself in his choices is a cause, and in a measure man can control external causes and situations.

Ultimately, health and well-being depend on how people interact with the environment. If you strive to establish harmonious interaction with all of nature, it becomes clear that you cannot tolerate pollution, contamination, noise, or accidents, for they all result from people's negative actions and destructive states of mind. If people are feeling positive and loving, they will not think of throwing a bottle at the earth, much less at another person or animal. So we must find ways to live more gently on the earth. Our health and safety depend on it.

LESSON PLANS

In light of this discussion, peruse the following lesson plans, keeping in mind that they are indicative of the lesson plans that you will likely be expected to implement in your classroom. Remember that they by no means encompass a complete unit of instruction. They are simply a basis for the formation of a comprehensive unit.

TOPIC: ECOLOGY

Grade Level: Intermediate, junior high

Concept: We should live within the limitations of our environment.

Outcome: The student will be able to describe how ecology is a way of keeping the human web of life in balance with nature.

Content: Ways people keep a balance with nature, not polluting the environment:

1. *Food chains*
   a) Animals
   b) Insects
   c) Birds
   d) Fishes
   e) Plants

   Consumers—original sources need to be in balance for food chain to continue.

   f) Human—a polluter, a destroyer, and consumer

Learning Experiences

1. *Stimulate* with pictures and interactive discussion using the flannel board and the ecosystem of a pond (Figure 18.9).
2. *Suggested alternative experiences*
   a) *Which America do you choose?* Pupils identify what people have done right and wrong in their environment (Figure 18.10).
   b) *Film: Ecology,* 22 min, 16 mm, B & W. Relationships of people, plants, and animals to their environments. Order from Academy Films, 748 North Seward St., Hollywood, Calif.
   c) *Sound filmstrip set: Ecology; Interaction Environments:* set of seven to study the interaction of living things with one another and with their environments. Order from Scott Educational Division, Holyoke, Mass. 01040.
   d) *Filmstrips & record/cassette:* Series of film strips identifying and describing current ecological-pollution problems from a biological viewpoint. Order from Holt, Rinehart and Winston Inc., 383 Madison Ave., New York, N.Y. 10017
   e) *Filmstrips: Man is the Biosphere. Introduction to Human Ecology,* plus Teacher's Guide (70w4100). Order from Ward's Natural Science Establishment, P.O. Box 1749, Monterey, Calif., 93940.
   f) *AEP Ecology Program:* Weekly reader practice books to make students aware of delicate balances between all forms of life and their supportive habitats. Four ecological concepts stressed: diversity, adaptations, interrelationships, and change. Order from *My Weekly Reader,* Education Center, Columbus, Ohio 43216.

FIGURE 18.9
Suggestions for a pond ecosystem, demonstration, or field trip. Can you show food chains in this pond?

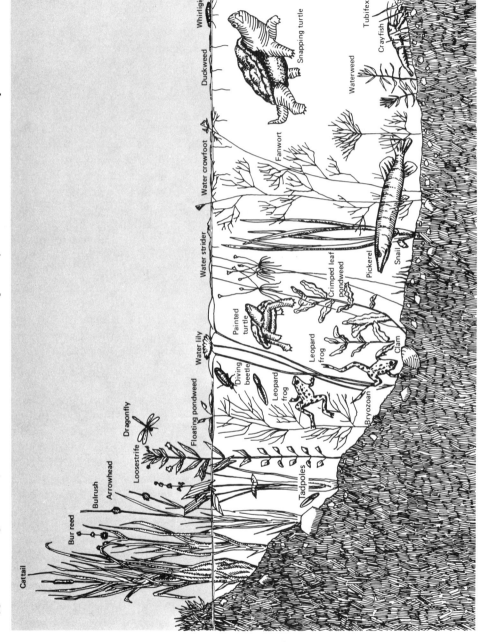

A POOR PLACE TO LIVE

Abuse of land, air, and water create problems that turn appealing areas into ghettos of ugliness and decay. The accompanying illustration tells the story of a watershed area where users of resources have sacrificed their environment for the quick profit—the short-term gain. Follow the keys below to condition depicted by related keys in the illustration.

1. Lack of Water Control

A rampant stream destroys valuable land, fails to recharge ground water supplies, and jeopardizes lives. Usually it goes through periodic low-water cycles that make it an unreliable source of supply for cities. Not all streams should be dammed, of course, but some must be.

2. Ruinous Forestry Practices

Here, cut-and-get-out logging operations, inadequate fire protection, and other short-sighted actions have led to watershed soil erosion, downstream flooding, and loss of habitat for wildlife. Recreation opportunities are destroyed.

3. Poor Farming Methods

Overuse of land and repeated planting of the same crops have exhausted the soil's fertility. The absence of contour farming leads to rapid runoff and results in erosion by wind and water.

4. Uncontrolled Growth of Suburbs

Lack of effective zoning and building regulations speeds decay. Open green space is chopped up into inadequate patches. "Bedroom" suburbs like this produce monotony, blight, and high crime rates.

5. Upstream Industrial Pollution

Industries that disregard downstream and downwind pollution degrade the entire watershed. Rural areas often encourage industrial parks without requiring adequate pollution controls.

6. Pollution from Mines

Mining companies abandon underground working without a thought that eventually they will cave in and create surface pockets or feed deadly acid water into streams. Others strip off valuable topsoil and leave ugly scars which add to stream pollution and deterioration of the area.

7. & 9. Faulty Industrial Zoning

Unregulated placing of industry pollutes city's air and water and downgrades value of adjacent property.

8. Improper Waste Disposal

Sewage treatment and waste disposal facilities lag behind population growth, hastening the poisonous suicide of the city.

10. The Polluted River

Pollution the full length of the river has made it an open sewer. Fish cannot live in it, people dislike drinking it even after costly purification. Swimming is impossible and boating unpleasant.

11. Poorly Managed Traffic

A source of air pollution, frustration, and sudden death, poorly planned traffic facilities—added to substandard mass transportation—strangle the central city.

12. Trapped by Towers

As the population grows and open space is lost to monstrous high-rise apartments, city dwellers become imprisoned by their own "progress." They live elbow-to-elbow. The more fortunate breathe filtered air at home and at work. Others sneeze and sniffle through smog-filled days and nights.

A GOOD PLACE TO LIVE

The balance of Nature and the quality of man's environment can be maintained in an increasingly popular watershed if sound conservation practices are followed. Some of the benefits are listed below and are keyed to the right half of the illustration.

1. Proper Forestry and Mining

Good forest management means selective cutting, fire protection, and planting new trees. Such practices promote continuing yields of forest products. Stripmined areas have been re-covered with topsoil. Planting holds the soil in place and keeps streams silt-free.

2. Space to Roam

Wilderness areas are protected, providing assured wildlife habitat, a healthy forest base for the watershed, and outdoor recreation for all.

3. Multipurpose Reservoir

Flood control, power generation, municipal and industrial water supply source, and outdoor recreation facilities are some of the benefits of this reservoir.

4. Farm Land Management

Rotation of crops and grasslands, contour strip planting, wildlife hedgerows, all make this farm flourish while protecting the health and quality of the land.

5. Irrigation

Water provided by a diversion dam and a high-line canal turns normally non-productive land into fertile farms.

6. Industrial Parks

Planning and zoning provide attractive and efficient clustering of industry, to the benefit of both industry and city. Sources of industrial water and air pollution are controlled within the regulated industrial park complex.

7. Fish Hatchery

Hatcheries provide fish to supplement stocks in reservoirs, streams, and lakes.

8. Satellite Communities

Self-contained communities like this offer the services and advantages of close-in suburban living. The beauty of the natural terrain and setting is carefully preserved.

9. Waste Disposal

Efficient sewage plants treat effluents from city systems, keeping the river clean. Refuse is burned to generate power in plants equipped with air pollution abatement devices.

10. The Beautiful City

Careful planning and development provide a beautiful, livable Central City environment. Area-wide master plans control the city's growth, provide a smooth traffic flow, and promote work and living patterns oriented not to technology but to people.

11. & 13. Highways and Rapid Transit

Recessed and underground superhighways, combined with a rapid transit system that extends to the suburban satellite communities, provide efficient movement of people and goods to and from the Central City. With home-to-work rapid transit, private car use is reduced. Combining highway and rapid transit operations uses less open space and requires fewer river crossings.

12. City Park and Recreation Areas

Planned parks like this provide the Central City with large wedges of open space and afford many forms of recreation and cultural facilities for the city dweller.

14. Footpaths and Bicycle Trails

Trails follow the natural terrain of the river banks from city to headwaters.

15. Green Spaces

Through proper planning and zoning, abundant open space in and around the city is preserved. This green space provides a natural source of beauty and recreation opportunities.

16. The Clean River

Pollution control and good watershed management keep the river clean, making it a recreational delight.

17. Scenic Easements

Scenic easements along river banks protect the natural beauty of the river. Pollution control is made easier and bank erosion prevented. Outdoor recreation opportunities abound in the natural areas preserved.

FIGURE 18.10

Which America do you choose? (a) A poor place to live—why? (b) A good place to live—why? (From *Conservation Chart: Which America Do You Choose?* Washington, D.C.: U.S. Department of the Interior.)

g) *Filmstrips:* Order from Life Filmstrips
   (1) *Water Pollution, Part 1: The Great Lakes—History and Ecology.* Pollution problems of the Great Lakes.
   (2) *Water Pollution, Part II: The Causes of Pollution.* Shipping pollution, municipal sewage landfill, agricultural pesticides, detergents, industrial wastes, and new pollutants.
   (3) *Water Pollution, Part III: The Results of Pollution.* Closed beaches, ruination of fishing, decline in tourism, stinking marshes, threatened dunes, endangered health and what can be done about it.

Evaluative Procedures   After the formal instruction, the students will be asked to write a short essay addressing the following questions:

1. Define ecology

2. How do food chains help maintain a balance of all living things?

3. Describe the basic kinds of environments.

4. How does the food chain become disrupted?

If the average grade of the class is 80 percent or better, the objective will be considered accomplished.

TOPIC: ECOSYSTEMS

Grade Level: Intermediate

Concept: Pollution results when ecosystems are disturbed or disrupted.

Outcome: The student will be able to describe how pollution results when ecosystems are disturbed.

Content: Ecosystems are dependent on food chains

1. First-order consumers—plankton, tadpoles —feed on plants.
2. Second-order consumers—bass—feed on tadpoles.
3. Third-order consumers—those living things that feed on bass, plankton, and tadpoles; humans.
4. Examples of food chains
   a) grass→zebra→lion
   b) grass→cattle→person
   c) meadow→grass→cricket→frog→hawk
   d) pond algae→protozoa→insects→larger insects→black bass→pickerel→person

Learning Experiences

1. *Game:* Bass Ecosystem (Figure 18.11)

Bass Ecosystem Game

Objective: To have each pupil evolve a balanced pond ecosystem and avoid a polluted pond.

Description: This game allows each pupil to play. Teacher has pupils duplicate the original board and makes enough organism-exchange pieces and pollution-result cards for all in class to participate. Pupils can also make their own die. For best results, have four or five players per card and a banker or a card for each pupil and a banker. (An adaptation of an Urban Systems ecological game.)

Rules of the Game

1. High throw of die determines starting player.
2. All players place token in the START space on the board.
3. Each player throws die to determine number of spaces to move on board.
4. Each player interprets the consequence of his or her move:
   a) A player who lands on an ORGANISM space (sunfish, rotifers, algae, bass, weeds, bacteria, minnows, worms, and copepods) takes an organism of the species and places it in his or her lake.
   b) A player who lands on an ORGANISM EXCHANGE space may exchange extra pieces for others that are equal to or higher than his or her original organism. The player may exchange one piece for an organism (from the banker).

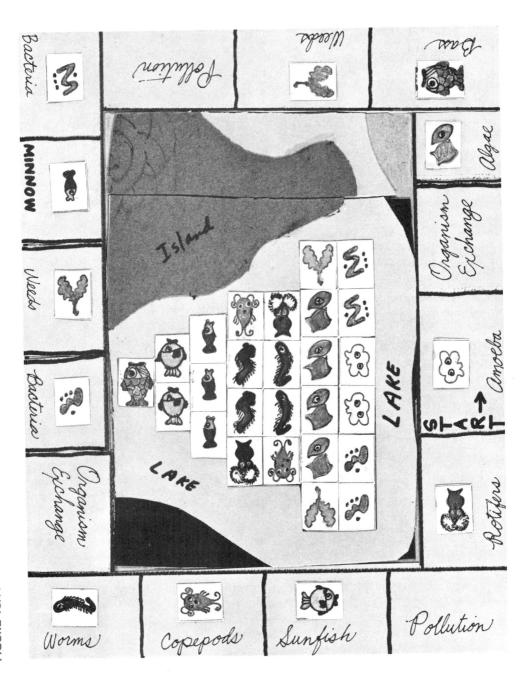

FIGURE 18.11

c) A player who lands on a POLLUTION space throws the die to determine the source of pollution and suffers the consequences outlined on the POLLUTION RESULT card (teacher can draft cards).

5. Overpopulation occurs when the player gains more than the number provided for in the lake. For example, there are three minnows in the lake, so although the player may keep more than three minnows, he or she may not make an exchange for any more than three. If the lake becomes overpopulated, the player returns all the extras of that species and pays the penalty (series of consequences of overpopulation, which the teacher can draft).

6. A player wins by covering each organism in his or her lake with an organism exchange card. The player has constructed an ecosystem.

2. *Demonstration:* Evolve an ecosystem in two identical *aquariums* over a period of several months. Keep one healthy and balanced. Disrupt the ecological balance of the other and compare the consequences.

AN ECOSYSTEM AQUARIUM

Purpose: To learn about the balance of life in an aquatic ecosystem.

Procedure: The teacher and pupils may plan their own aquarium. Help may be obtained by referring to "Life in the Water" kit and conducting suggested experiments on food sources of brine shrimp and plankton (algae). Kit No. 71354 may be ordered from Edmund Scientific Co., 100 Edscorp Building, Barrington, New Jersey 08007.

A filmstrip, *Keeping An Aquarium,* may be obtained from Scott Education Division, Holyoke, Mass. 01040.

3. Study the history of Lake Erie and identify how the ecosystems were disrupted by human activity.
4. Field trip to a nearby lake or pond.
5. *Alternative learning experiences*
   a) *Pupil Project:* Making a jam jar aquarium.
   b) Making an aquarium for larger water animals.

AN AQUARIUM FOR LARGER WATER ANIMALS

In a glass aquarium 50 cm by 25 cm is a useful size (Figure 18.12). Old accumulator cells are suitable, but the glass is not very clear.

To prepare an aquarium, get some fine silt from an aquarium shop or the bottom of a clear stream or pond. Wash it carefully in running water. Cover the floor of the aquarium with it to a depth of about 2 cm. Plant a few reeds in this, weighting the roots with a stone or lead ring. Then put in a layer of coarse sand or gravel and

FIGURE 18.12
Water aquarium.

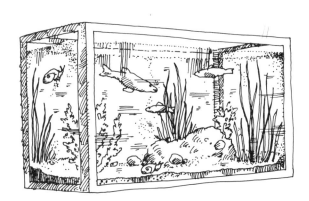

some large stones to serve as hiding places for the water insects. Fill with a slow stream of water and allow to stand for a day or two until clear. Plants from clean water should be introduced. There is no need for elaborate aeration if plenty of water weeds are present. If tap water is used, some live food such as daphnia should be added and the water must stand for at least two days to lose the chemical "purifiers."

The animals can now be introduced. Add a few snails to keep the glass clean. Very little feeding will be necessary. Fish will eat the snails' eggs, and enough small water organisms can be found in the average pond to supply other needs. If worms are used as food, they should be given only once a week, freshly cut into pieces small enough to be eaten. Unless unconsumed food is removed immediately, fungi will grow and infect the fish.

The aquarium must be covered with a glass plate or perforated zinc lid to keep out dust. If frogs or newts are kept, a floating piece of cork must be provided for them to sit on; the glass or zinc cover will prevent their escape.

    c) *Film: Lakes—Aging and Pollution;* 15 min., color, 1971; Underwater photography to show aging of lakes, life cycles, and changes of water quality with emphasis on human input. Order from Centron Educational Films, 1621 West Ninth St., Lawrence, Kansas 66044.

    d) *Film: Energy and Living Things;* 11 min., color, 1972. The relationship of energy and matter is brought out by tracing solar energy through plants, herbivores, and carnivores to fossil fuels. Order from Centron Educational Films.

Evaluation Procedures

After the formal instruction, ask the students to write a short essay addressing the following questions:

1. Define an ecosystem.

2. How can an ecosystem be thrown out of balance?

3. How can a human ecosystem be kept in balance?

If the average grade of the class is 80 percent or better, the objective will be considered accomplished.

TOPIC: PROPER TRASH DISPOSAL

Grade Level: Primary

Concept: Proper disposal of trash makes a healthier world for us to live in.

Expected Pupil Outcome: The student will demonstrate the proper way to dispose of trash.

Content: Proper ways of disposing of garbage:
1. Wrap garbage in a paper or plastic bag.
2. Wash garbage can periodically.
3. Elevate can six inches above the ground.
4. Use a tight-fitting lid.
5. Have regular pick-up.
6. No dirt or rocks in garbage can.

Learning Experiences
1. *Demonstration:* Teacher invites custodian to bring a can and some actual trash, which they spread around classroom. Children take turns disposing of various items of trash, with class expressing approval or disapproval.
2. *Alternative learning experience:*
   Role-play situations depicting right and wrong ways of garbage disposal.

Evaluation Procedures Teacher observes students during the demonstration. If they properly dispose of trash, the objective will be considered accomplished.

TOPIC: SOURCES OF NOISE POLLUTION

Grade Level: Intermediate

Concept: There are many human-made sources of excessive noise.

**Expected Pupil
Outcome:**   The student will be able to identify sources of noise pollution.

Content: Sources of noise pollution:
1. Automobiles
2. Airplanes
3. Industrial machines
4. Crowds
5. Home appliances: radios, TVs, vacuum cleaners, can openers

Learning Experiences
1. *Demonstration survey:* Have several pupils assist in recording different sound sources in the community on a tape recorder and simultaneously monitoring noise levels with a noise meter. Replay the tape in the classroom.
2. Develop a histogram depicting the extent of noise pollution from each recorded source.

Evaluation Procedures   If the students are successful in both recording and accurately measuring the source noise levels, then constructing a histogram of the results, the objective will be considered accomplished.

REFERENCES AND BIBLIOGRAPHY

Berwick, D. M., and A. L. Komaroff. "Cost Effectiveness of Lead Screening," *New England Journal of Medicine* 306 (1982): 1392-1398.

Bross, I. D. J., and J. Natarajan. "Leukemia from Low-level Radiation," *New England Journal of Medicine* 287 (1972): 107.

Bross, I. D. J., M. Ball, and S. Falen. "A Dose Response Curve for the One Rad Range: Adult Risks from Diagnostic Radiation," *American Journal of Public Health* 69 (1979): 130-136.

Christian, J. J. "Love Canal's Unhealthy Voles," *Natural History* (October 1983): 8-16.

Edlin, G., and E. Golanty. *Health and Wellness,* Third Edition (Boston, Mass.: Jones and Bartlett, 1988).

Foster, K. R., and A. W. Guy, "The Microwave Problem," *Scientific American,* September 1986.

Garmon, L. "Puzzled Over PCBs," *Science News* (May 29, 1982): 361-363.

Garmon, L. "Dioxin in Missouri: Troubled Times," *Science News* (January 22, 1983): 59-62.

Horne, H. H. *A Philosophy of Safety and Safety Education* (New York: Safety Education Digest, 1940).

Needleman, H. L., and S. Piomelli. *The Effects of Low Level Lead Exposure* (New York: National Resources Defense Council, 1978).

Nriagu, J. O. "Did Lead Poisoning Contribute to the Fall of the Empire?" *New England Journal of Medicine* 308 (1983): 660-663.

Nuclear War Letters. *New England Journal of Medicine* 316 (1987), 688-690.

Pihl, R. O., and M. Parkes. "Hair Element Content on Learning Disabled Children," *Science* 198 (1977): 204-206.

Raloff, J. "Agent Orange: What Isn't Settled," *Science News* (May 19, 1984): 314-317.

Sun, M. "Missouri's Costly Dioxin Lesson," *Science* 219 (1983), 367-369. (a)

Sun, M. "Dioxin's Uncertain Legacy," *Science* 219 (1983), 468-469. (b)

Sun, M. "EDB Contamination Kindles Federal Action," *Science* 223 (1984), 464-466. (a)

Tschirley, F. H. "Dioxin," *Scientific American,* February 1986.

Turco, R. P., et al. "Nuclear Winter: Global Consequences of Multiple Nuclear Explosions," *Science* 222 (1983), 1283-1292.

Van den Bosch, R. *The Pesticide Conspiracy.* New York: Doubleday, 1978.

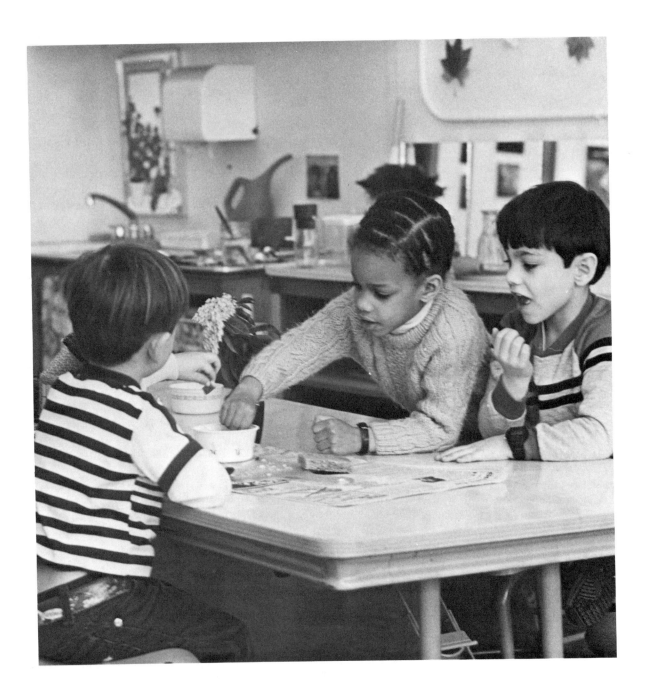

Chapter 19   Teaching About Nutrition

INTRODUCTION

Eating is both a vital function and a cherished experience. However, the quantity and quality of foods that Americans consume vary to a great extent. Even though the United States is the leading food producer in the world, many Americans, rich and poor, still die of a lack of food, malnutrition, or chronic diseases caused by poor nutrition. In too many cases, ignorance of the principles of nutrition prevents many people from eating well. This is unfortunate, for the principles of nutrition are few and easily understood.

Food intake is essential to the building and repairing of body tissue. It also fuels energy production for warmth and strength. The challenge is to match our needs with the essential ingredients found in foods. This brings us to the key aspect of nutrition: balance. The well-fed person is not necessarily well-nourished. Without the proper balance of vitamins, proteins, minerals, carbohydrates, essential fatty acids, fiber, and water, one is not well nourished.

While it is easy to theorize about good nutrition, it is most difficult to attain it. Many people practice sound nutritional habits and maintain a good diet without ever thinking about it, following the principles of nutrition that were presented in school. These include eating a balanced and varied diet on a regular schedule. On the other hand, many others fulfill their need for food but consume nutrient-deficient diets.

LIFESTYLE AND NUTRITION

What sounds simple presents a major problem for many people. The lifestyle most Americans lead is not conducive to sound nutritional habits and optimal well-being. Most people attempt to eat a variety of foods and hope their meals are balanced. They assume that they are getting the proper amounts of vitamins, minerals, and other essential nutrients. This is not always true.

Americans consume many convenience and snack foods (french fries, potato chips, sweets, soft drinks). These kinds of foods are termed "empty calorie" foods—rich in sugar and/or salt and deficient in other nutrients. Eating such foods regularly not only develops poor eating habits and problems related to overweight, but can also lead to chronic deficiency diseases.

Other aspects of lifestyle may contribute to vitamin and mineral deficiencies. Supermarkets abound in convenience foods. Thus poor food choice is compounded by availability of numerous snack and convenience foods. In order to retard spoilage and to lengthen shelf life, some foods are processed in a variety of ways that lead to loss of much of their nutrient value. For example, high-speed milling of wheat into white flour removes vitamin E, bran, wheat germ, and most trace minerals. Although breads and cereals are often enriched, or fortified, by the addition of vitamins B_1, B_2, and niacin, 12 other essential B vitamins and most trace minerals are not returned (Passwater, 1976).

Another habit that may contribute to nutritional deficiencies is eating in restaurants and cafeterias, where food is often kept warm in steam tables for many hours. Although such prolonged heating prevents the growth of germs, it also destroys a large portion of the vitamins B and C of most meats and vegetables. Yet we eat in such establishments on the assumption that cooked and preheated food does retain its original vitamins.

Additionally, nutrients in the body are depleted when the liver makes enzymes to detoxify the more than 2,000 chemicals that may find their way into our bodies (Nutrition Research, 1975). These chemicals include food preservatives, coloring agents, and sweeteners as well as insecticides, antibiotics, and so forth. Ingesting these chemicals adds to the detoxification load of the liver. The liver, in order to rid the body of these chemicals, uses extra amounts of vitamins B_6, C, and E and minerals such as selenium to make detoxicant enzymes. If these micronutrients are not present in sufficient quantities, fatigue sets in and the body functions poorly. Such reactions often reflect nutrient deficiency.

Another burden to the liver arises from pollution. The body is continually exposed to pollutants in food, in air, and in water. Human metabolic processes eliminate these chemicals. Removal of ozone and nitrous oxide by the liver creates additional nutrient demands. Likewise, nutrient demands are also raised in those who smoke; drink colas, coffee, and alcoholic beverages; and work under emotional stress.

In summary, significant losses of nutrients occur during cooking, storage, transportation, and processing of foods. The lifestyles of many people further deplete vitamins and minerals in their bodies. Nutrient losses in foods and depletion in the body weaken the natural resistance to stress, diseases, and other disorders. Many children, teenagers, and adults have nutrient deficiencies and do not know it. Consequently, their potential for optimal health is suppressed, and they function with a lowered level of well-being.

There is mounting evidence, both in this and in foreign countries, that many health problems and diseases stem from vitamin and mineral deficiencies and from eating too many of the wrong foods. The prevention and treatment of heart disease, cancer, obesity, diabetes, arthritis, emotional disturbances, allergies, and other diseases may very well be found in nutrition; food provides for everything that the body synthesizes and uses. Without food, life cannot go on. Shortage of vitamins and minerals leads to a subsistence life. We should think of nutrition as helping us to attain optimal health. In general, we focus on counting calories and eating a diet balanced in terms of proteins, carbohydrates, and fats. Thus a person who eats the required number of calories each day is thought of as well fed. However, such a person may not be well nourished. Many persons eat a lot of calories but not enough vitamins and minerals.

The major consequence of poor eating is lowered immunity. Research throughout the world (Cheraskin, 1976; Clark, 1973; Chandra, 1979; Chandra, 1986) points out that resistance is lowered when one does not eat properly. Malnourished persons have more frequent colds, respiratory infections, and diseases (Chandra, 1986). Malnourished children are sick longer, more frequently, and more severely than well-fed children. Good nutrition during childhood is especially important, as good diet fortifies young bodies against many respiratory illnesses and helps to build natural immunity to such illnesses. A well-balanced diet is the child's best way to resist diseases and stay healthy.

In the sections that follow, we discuss proper eating habits, nutrients, nutritional needs, and some common food problems.

EATING HABITS

Good eating habits are best begun at an early age. The best way to maintain ideal weight and eat well throughout life is to learn how to eat and exercise early in life (Mayer, 1977). Teachers should help parents teach children proper exercising and eating. Of all the habits of living, the most important to good health is eating properly.

Eating a Balanced Diet

One way to eat a balanced diet is to *select a variety of foods each day.* Foods have been traditionally classified into four groups. The four groups are milk and milk products, meats and equivalents, fruits and vegetables, breads and cereals. However, recent literature often contains a discussion of more than the traditional four food groups. Some authors mention five, while others will discuss as many as seven (i.e., dairy products, meats, vegetables, fruits, grains, seeds, oils, and fats).

Milk and Milk Products

It is recommended that each day children under 9 consume *two or more cups* of fluid whole milk or its equivalent. Children 9 to 12 need three cups per day, and teenagers require four or more cups. The choice should be made from fluid or dry milk, whole, low fat, skim or fat free; evaporated or condensed milk; milk products such as yogurt, cheese and cottage cheese; and alternates such as soy milk and soy cheese.

Milk is one of few foods that comes close to being perfect. Although almost every nutrient is found in milk, its major nutrients are calcium, protein, and vitamin B complex. Milk's nutrients are essential to growth. However, in recent years, changing tastes and concerns over dietary fat have led to the development of imitation cream, cheese, and canned milk. These products do not contain any milk solids—only nondairy ingredients—and do not contribute milk's nutrients to the diet. Adding to the confusion about milk products is concern about the amount of fat and cholesterol in milk and its products. To lower fat intake, eliminate or reduce processed foods such as potato chips and french fries, red meats (steak, pork) and preserved cold meats (weiners, sausages, bologna) before reducing milk intake. One way to lower fat intake is to substitute low-fat milk for whole milk, but milk should not be eliminated from the diets of children for it contributes too many nutrients essential for growing.

Meats and Equivalents

Two or more servings a day from this group are recommended. Although the choices are many, making choices to lower fat consumption in the American diet to less than 30 percent is difficult. Meats and equivalents include high-fat items such as beef, veal, lamb, and pork; fish, shellfish, chicken, and turkey; navy beans, lima beans, lentils, split peas, pinto beans, and chickpeas; high-fat nuts and nut butters; textured vegetable proteins; and moderate-fat meat equivalents such as eggs and cheese. Two meat servings per day provide approximately 50 percent of the protein; 25 percent to 50 percent of the iron; 25 percent to 30 percent of vitamins B_1 and B_2; and 35 percent of the niacin needed daily. Meat is not a good source of vitamins C or A, calcium, or fiber.

Various meats and meat equivalents provide varying amounts of protein, ranging from about 12 percent in pork to 30 percent in some fish. The alternatives such as eggs, cheese, beans, and peas contain less protein than meat but are inexpensive sources, especially when eaten with other protein foods.

Fruits and Vegetables

The food guides recommend *four or more servings of fruits and vegetables each day*. Fruits and vegetables are major sources of iron and vitamins A and C. They contain many necessary trace elements. Most fruits and fresh, green, leafy vegetables are rich in vitamins and minerals, low in calories, low in fat and high in roughage or fiber. One should eat two servings of fresh, green, leafy vegetables and two kinds of fruit each day.

A variety of fruits and vegetables should be chosen from these sources: for vitamin A, dark green leafy vegetables (broccoli, spinach), orange vegetables (carrots, pumpkin), and orange-fleshed fruits (apricots, mangoes); for vitamin C, citrus fruits (grapefruit, lemons, oranges), watermelon, strawberries, raw sweet peppers, broccoli, cauliflower, cabbage, and tomatoes.

Cereals and Cereal Products

Four or more servings of grain products are recommended for each day. Whole grain foods provide iron; vitamins B_1, B_2, and niacin; trace minerals; and fiber. Choose from whole-wheat breads, rolls, and muffins; whole-grain cereals, ready to eat or cooked; and whole-wheat pasta and rice. Whole-wheat products are preferred to refined products (those made with white flour).

The protein in grains is incomplete and should be completed by eating protein-rich foods (macaroni and cheese, milk on cereal) at the same meal. Cereals provide trace minerals—selenium, iron, copper, cobalt, and molybdenum—that are hard to find in sufficient amounts. Proteins also provide an essential kind of fiber.

Digestion of Nutrients

Food provides us with important chemicals needed by the body and also supplies us with energy. Food is composed of six basic types of chemical substances: carbohydrates, proteins, water, minerals, vitamins, lipids (fats). Proteins, most carbohydrates, and most lipids cannot be used by the body until they are broken down into smaller chemical units. Vitamins, minerals, and water need not be broken down; they are absorbed into the body as is. This breakdown of food substances and the absorption of nutrients is termed "digestion."

Carbohydrates

Carbohydrates are the principal source of the body's energy. There are two principal types of carbohydrates: *simple sugars* which are found predominantly in fruit, and the *complex carbohydrates,* found in grains, fruit, and the stems, leaves and roots of vegetables.

Our diets contain several kinds of simple sugars. The most common is glucose. Others include fructose, sucrose, and lactose.

There are two major classes of complex carbohydrates: *starch* and *fiber.* Much of the starch in our diet comes from foods made from wheat flour, such as bread, pastries, and noodles.

The other major form of complex carbohydrate in our diet is cellulose, which is obtained from the nondigestible vegetable matter called fiber, or roughage.

Fiber has been greatly overlooked in the typical American diet of "meat, bread, and potatoes." Most American diets are deficient in fiber, and most Americans do not understand the role of fiber in the human body.

Fiber, or roughage, is mostly plant cell wall that cannot be digested in the human gut. There are two kinds of fiber. The water soluble kind, found *inside plant cells,* includes pectin in apples and beans and gum in oat bran and vegetables. Water insoluble fiber, found in plant *cell walls,* comprises cellulose in vegetables; hemicelluloses in wheat bran, corn bran, skins of potato, beans, and peanuts; and lignin in peas and whole grains. Overall, vegetables make up 45 percent, cereal fibers 35 percent and fruit fibers 29 percent of the typical American diet. Most Americans need to double their intake of all kinds of fiber. All three fiber sources—vegetable, cereal, and fruit—need to be ingested regularly each day. An average adult should eat five to six grams of crude fiber per day (or 100 mg of fiber per kilogram of body weight).

Over the past 15 years, persuasive evidence has linked increased fiber intake to the prevention and treatment of certain common Western diseases. Fiber may help in the fight against diabetes, obesity, hyperlipidemia, hypertension, and cancer. Lack of fiber has also been implicated in diverticulitis and constipation. Fiber increases fecal bulk and stool frequency, shortens transit time and alters microflora. Fiber affects large bowel functions.

Proteins

Protein is essential to human life. The human body is approximately one-fifth protein, and the protein content constantly changes. In a child the absence of protein will terminate growth; major functions of protein are growth, repair, and maintenance of the body. Protein helps to control body fluid balance and has a special role in detoxifying the body. If protein intake is inadequate, the body's ability to detoxify foreign substances is impaired.

Fat

Only a small amount of fat is needed in the daily diet. Fats transport the fat-soluble vitamins A, D, E, and K. Fats are concentrated sources of energy, stored in the body against illness and starvation. Fat insulates the body, protecting it from cold and the vital organs from injury. Additionally, fats satisfy the appetite and make foods more tasty and attractive.

Water

Water accounts for 45 percent to 60 percent of the content of all living organisms. A person can live much longer without food than without water. The body uses water for digestion, absorption, circulation, transporting nutrients, excretion, building tissue, and maintaining body temperature. Since children tend to be more active than adults, they generally need more water. Six to 12 glasses daily are recommended, although much of this may be obtained from solid food.

Minerals

Minerals serve two important functions in the body: they are structural components such as the calcium in teeth and bones, and they regulate important body processes such as digestion, metabolism, and muscle contraction. Since these body functions vary, minerals are needed in varying amounts. *Megaminerals*—calcium, phosphorus, magnesium, and potassium—are needed in amounts of one gram or more per day. *Trace minerals,* such as zinc and selenium, are needed in smaller amounts (milligrams). Mineral deficiencies cause malnutrition and lower the immunity level. For example, severe iron deficiency causes deficiency of red blood cells. The richest sources of minerals are fish and fresh green vegetables although the minerals available in the daily diet seldom supply FDA's recommended daily amounts.

Vitamins

Vitamins are organic compounds other than fats, carbohydrates, and proteins that are *essential to human life.* They help enzymes digest, absorb, and metabolize fats, carbohydrates and proteins. They encourage chemical reactions but are not changed or incorporated into the products of the reaction.

Water-soluble vitamins include B-complex and C vitamins. *Fat-soluble* vitamins A, D, E and K are found in butter, cream, vegetable oils, seeds, and the fats of meats and fish. Water-soluble vitamins are not stored in the body and must be ingested daily. Fat-soluble vitamins are stored in body tissues, primarily the liver.

All vitamins can be destroyed by exposure to heat, light, oxygen, or radiation. Fat-soluble vitamins are more stable than water-soluble vitamins and are less likely to be destroyed in processing and cooking of foods.

Vitamins in ordinary foods are readily absorbed into the body and are seldom at toxic levels. Excessive water-soluble vitamins are usually excreted by the kidneys. Excess fat-soluble vitamins are stored in the liver. Toxicity from overdose of vitamins seldom occurs, although vitamin A toxicity is possible if 30,000 or more international units (IU) per day are ingested over two or more months. Children are especially susceptible to vitamin toxicity.

Eating a variety of foods and a balanced diet

is the best way to provide the body with vitamins it needs. The best source of vitamins are fresh leafy green vegetables. Legumes, nuts, and whole grains are also good sources of vitamins. Root vegetables and fruits have lesser amounts of vitamins. Lean meats are good sources of B-complex vitamins. A few vitamins (D, K and several B-complex) are synthesized by bacteria in the large intestine.

In addition to choosing the right amounts from the basic food groups, these habits are important for optimal well-being. Eating regularly contributes to good health. Research indicates the body can adjust to any pattern of eating: three meals, or five or six. Research also indicates that eating a nutritious breakfast increases a person's efficiency throughout the day. Since the stomach empties every three to five hours, it is wise to get on a pattern of regular eating and getting a good start with breakfast.

Lipids (Fats)

Lipids are a group of diverse chemical substances that have the common property of being relatively insoluble in water. Perhaps the most familiar lipid is *triglyceride,* otherwise known as body fat. Excess calories, whether obtained from too much sugar or too much fat, are converted by the liver into triglycerides, which are stored in all too obvious places in the body.

Other lipids, such as cholesterol and lecithin, are essential constituents of cell membranes. The steroid hormones produced by the reproductive organs and adrenal glands are lipids; vitamins A, D, E, and K are lipids; and substances in liver bile that help digest fats, the bile acids, are lipids.

Dietary lipid comes in three principal forms: cholesterol, saturated fat, and unsaturated fat. Saturated fat differs from unsaturated fat by having more hydrogen atoms in each fat molecule. Saturated fats tend to be solid at room temperature, whereas unsaturated fats tend to be liquid.

The amounts of cholesterol, saturated fat, and unsaturated fat taken into the body depend on what kinds of foods are eaten. Some foods, such as egg yolk, contain large amounts of cholesterol, whereas others, such as vegetable oils, are high in unsaturated fat and contain no cholesterol. There is considerable controversy about the health effects of eating high amounts of certain kinds of fats, although the present consensus among nutritionists and medical researchers seems to be that diets containing more than 600 milligrams per day of cholesterol and 50 grams per day of saturated fat may contribute to heart and blood vessel disease.

The body requires one type of unsaturated fat, *linoleic acid;* not getting enough of it may lead to a deficiency disease characterized primarily by skin lesions. For this reason, you should not attempt to eliminate all lipids from your diet. Furthermore, fats provide energy. If you were to eliminate nearly all fat from your diet and not compensate with increased amounts of carbohydrate or protein, your body would break down its protein to supply energy.

Exercise

More and more researchers realize that exercise is very important to nutrition and proper body weight. *Physical activity stabilizes and regulates the appestat* in the hypothalamus of the brain. The appestat determines appetite, psychological satisfaction from eating, and body weight. In addition to keeping the body healthy, exercise also aids the body in using nutrients. It may also help prevent some diseases and illnesses. A minimum of 15 to 30 minutes of exercise three times a week is recommended for good health.

Dietary Goals and the RDA

Are Americans nutrient-deficient? Should elementary school teachers be concerned about this? The answer to both is yes. Several intensive dietary surveys in the late 1960's studied the nutritional status of the American people. The U.S. Department of Agriculture in 1965 discovered that only 50 percent of American households had diets that were rated "good" by their standards (Passwater, 1976). A 1970 follow-up study by the U.S. Public Health Service revealed gross vitamin and iron deficiencies (Labuza, 1975).

Numerous vitamin C deficiencies were also found among the 18-to-25 age group and the elderly.

These and other studies point out that since 1946 our food and eating habits have been deteriorating. *Dietary Goals for the United States* (1977), a study prepared by the United States Senate's Select Committee on Nutrition and Human Needs, lends support to the concerns:

The simple fact is that our diets have changed radically within the last 50 years, with great and often very harmful effects on our health. These dietary changes represent as great a threat to public health as smoking. Too much fat, too much sugar or salt, can be linked directly to heart disease, cancer, obesity, and stroke. In all, six of the ten leading causes of death in the United States have been linked to our diet.

In the early 1900s, almost 40 percent of our caloric intake came from fruit, vegetable, and grain products. Today, only a little more than 20 percent of calories comes from these sources.

The six recommended dietary goals and changes in food selection and preparation are summarized in Figure 19.1. The goals are as follows:

1. *Increase carbohydrate consumption* to account for 55 percent to 60 percent of the energy (calorie) intake.
2. *Reduce overall fat consumption* from approximately 40 percent to 30 percent of energy intake.
3. *Reduce saturated fat consumption* to account for about 10 percent of total energy intake, and balance that with polyunsaturated and monosaturated fats, each of which should account for about 10 percent of energy intake.
4. *Reduce cholesterol consumption* to about 300 mg a day.
5. *Reduce sugar consumption* by about 40 percent to account for about 15 percent of total energy intake.
6. *Reduce salt consumption* by about 50 percent to 85 percent, to approximately three grams a day.

FIGURE 19.1

Composition of average American diet in the 1980's as contrasted to the recommended dietary goals. (Select Committee on Nutrition and Human Needs of United States Senate, *Dietary Goals for the United States.*

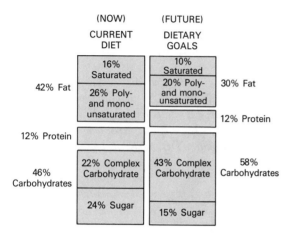

These goals suggest the following changes in food selection and preparation:

1. *Increase consumption of fruits, vegetables, and whole grains.*
2. *Decrease consumption of meat* and increase consumption of poultry and fish.
3. *Decrease consumption of foods high in fat* and partially substitute polyunsaturated fat for saturated fat.
4. *Substitute nonfat milk for whole milk.*
5. *Decrease consumption of butterfat, eggs, and other high-cholesterol sources.*
6. *Decrease consumption of sugar and foods high in sugar.*
7. *Decrease consumption of salt and foods high in salt.*

The national dietary recommendations raise the question of how much of a vitamin or mineral one needs for one day. The stock approach is to refer to the 1980 *Recommended Daily Allowances (USRDA)* of vitamins and minerals. Although intended to guard against disease deficiencies and to maintain the undefined health of

most people, the RDAs fail to consider the variances in lifestyle and eating habits or the destruction of nutrients in foods through storage, preservation, freezing, and cooking. Rather, RDA levels are minimal intakes of nutrients that meet the needs of healthy adults living under nonstressful conditions; they do not take into account special needs arising from infections, metabolic disorders, chronic diseases, or other abnormalities (National Academy of Sciences, 1984). This report states that continued use of antibiotics, antidepressants, insomnia and headache medications, and oral contraceptives will greatly deplete essential nutrients. The report suggests making nutrient allowances whenever such conditions exist or whenever food intake is curtailed or the diet is marginal in specific nutrients (e.g., overloaded with bread, cereal, and pastries made with refined white flour). There are many times, often continuous, when some nutrients are depleted in a person. At other times, skipping meals, eating junk foods, or eating without any idea of balance results in insufficient intake of nutrients. RDA levels are only guidelines at best and have definite limitations. As stated in the National Academy of Sciences report (National Academy of Sciences, 1984):

RDAs have been established for only about one third of the essential nutrients, that foods are ordinarily analyzed for only a small number of nutrients, and that interactions of various types between nutrients and food constituents may reduce the availability of some nutrients and, hence, the accuracy of information about food composition . . . RDA are recommendations for the amounts of nutrients that should be consumed daily, not for the nutrient content of foods.

Moreover, Pauling (1976) and Roger Williams (1973) have postulated that in many individuals the constitutional need may be 10 or more times the recommended daily allowances. Biochemical individuality takes into account the genetic, metabolic, and biochemical variability among individuals, that each person has a unique physiological and nutritional norm, and that nutritional needs must be geared for the individual and not the general public.

FOOD PROBLEMS

Undernutrition

This is the lack of essential nutrients in the human body caused by insufficient food intake. The causes of undernourishment are many: lack of food, insanitary living conditions, poor housing, unsafe and inadequate drinking water, unemployment, lack of parental education, and other social, geographic, and cultural factors. The majority of documented cases of undernourishment in the United States involve newborn infants, children, adolescents, college students, and the elderly. The symptoms of undernourishment include dry and lusterless hair, pale skin, edema, depressed cardiovascular function, lowered immunity, and in some cases, anemia. A balanced diet, high in complex carbohydrates and low in sugars, salt, and fat, can help correct undernutrition.

Obesity

Obesity frequently is a problem among children and adolescents. Studies have shown that over 80 percent of youth who are obese by age 10 to 13 will be so 20 years later. If not corrected early, obesity causes health problems such as low self-esteem; predisposition to high blood pressure, heart disease, and diabetes; and discrimination in school, employment, and society in general. Perhaps the major contributing cause of obesity in a child is the lifestyle of parents. Children copy the behavior and values of their parents. Inactive parents often have inactive children who overeat. Some parents who are insecure or need to relieve guilt overfeed their children to alleviate their own anxieties. Many parents also use food as an award or pacifier; their children tend to overeat and become obese. Overweight and obesity generally result when energy intake exceeds

the energy used for body maintenance, growth, and activities.

Snacking

Snacking among children has been one of the most controversial topics in nutrition. It is well confirmed that excess snacking, especially close to mealtime, decreases appetite for meals. However, since children have small stomachs, they cannot eat much during regular meals even if they have not been snacking. Children may not be able to eat enough at meals, especially during rapid growth. In this case, snacks solve part of the problem. The teacher should help children become aware that some snacks are nutritious and others are not. Persistent nutrition education of children and their parents can mold the child's snacking patterns in healthful ways.

Snacks loaded with sugar, salt, and fat but low in protein, fiber, vitamins, and minerals are bad. If children snack on nutritious foods, especially any that are lacking in their regular meals, then snacking is a great idea. A slice of cheese, a wheat cracker, or a banana at midmorning or midafternoon can help keep children from tiring.

Myths About Nutrition

Many nutritional problems and diseases arise from misinformation or lack of information about food. Here are some misconceptions about nutrition:

1. *Everyone should take vitamin and mineral supplements.* There is considerable controversy about this practice. Much of the rationale to support it has been substantiated. One way to bolster a poor diet is to take nutrient supplements. However, one should never pop vitamin pills as a substitute for a balanced diet. The best way to get your vitamins and minerals is in the food itself, not in supplements.

2. *Sugar is a good source of energy and is good for us.* Although refined white sugar is a source of energy, it lacks the B vitamins and minerals necessary to assimilate it. This means that the liver must leach out from the other cells the vitamins and minerals needed to use the sugar. Sugar is the leading flavoring in the United States today. It is used in almost all fruit drinks, salad dressings, many baby foods, sauces, canned and dehydrated soups, frozen foods, bacon and other cured meats, canned and frozen vegetables, fruit yogurt, and breakfast cereals. Tomato ketchup contains as much as 29 percent sugar, and coffee creamer as much as 65 percent sugar (Consumer Reports, 1978). Sugar is used as a preservative and to improve appearance and taste of food. Taken alone or in other foods, it displaces natural complex starches essential to the body. A six-ounce bottle of cola contains about four and a half teaspoons of sugar (Airola, 1977). Sugar masks the bitter taste of cola.

There is a real danger of children ingesting too much sugar in chocolate bars, soft drinks and sweets, unknowingly becoming sugar addicts. In this country sugar usage is 125 pounds per person per year (Select Committee on Nutrition and Human Needs of the United States, 1977; Consumer Reports, 1978). Eating refined sugar is one of our worst food habits.

3. *Vitamins regulate specific parts of the body;* for example, vitamin A regulates the eyes; vitamin E, reproduction. This misconception stems from the outdated idea of "a specific cause for a specific disease." Although still not clearly understood, there is ample evidence that vitamins, minerals, and amino acids work collectively to affect the body as a whole. Vitamins and minerals need each other to be absorbed and used in the body. For example, for a cell to build a particular protein molecule, all eight essential amino acids that make up that protein have to be available at the same time.

Otherwise the protein cannot be built. The same is true for the B vitamins, all of which must be taken together. Vitamins A, B_6, C, and E and selenium have been identified as essential for the liver to detoxify polluted air and cigarette smoke. Vitamins A, B, C, D, and E have all been found essential for good eye health. Although vitamin C has been characterized as affecting almost all body functions, it is probably aided in its functions by the presence of other vitamins and minerals. Although these few examples do not paint a complete picture, they should reinforce the concept that nutrients work together. Perhaps these examples will also help you to understand that only a balanced diet can provide all the essential nutrients.

4. *We can substitute soft drinks and beer or wine for water.* We need to replace water lost in normal body functions and physical activities. Soft drinks contain one or more of the addictive chemicals caffeine, salt, and sugar. Besides robbing the body of essential vitamins and minerals, all three distort the ability to taste. Water does not taste good to those who use lots of sugar and caffeine. Soft drinks and alcoholic beverages are no substitutes for water.

5. *We should not eat cholesterol foods because they cause heart disease.* Cholesterol foods do not cause heart disease (Williams, 1973). The early statistical and medical evidence linking heart disease to cholesterol was misleading, but nonetheless the wisdom of eating cholesterol continues to be controversial.

6. *One can avoid overweight and obesity by not eating fats and carbohydrates.* The secret of avoiding obesity and maintaining desirable weight lies not in avoiding any food group but in eating the nutrients necessary for optimal well-being, ingesting an appropriate number of calories, exercising regularly, and fulfilling one's emotional needs. Nutrients and exercise are both essential for proper functioning of the appestat, which controls hunger,

thirst, appetite, body weight, and emotions. Regular exercise keeps the appestat tuned up and maintains its regulatory function. Along with resetting the appestat, one should correct faulty eating habits. Counting calories may not be as important as exercising regularly and ensuring a balanced intake of vitamins and minerals.

7. *Poor nutrition causes overweight and obesity.* Poor nutrition fosters worse nutrition. People who eat poorly tend to consume too much starchy and sugar-rich food. Lack of B-complex vitamins disrupts and upsets the appestat and predisposes one to obesity. Poor nutrition usually reflects poor eating habits.

SUMMARY

A revolution in nutrition is on in this country. Indeed, there are numerous controversies among physicians, nutritionists, biochemists, and the lay public about the many aspects of nutrition, weight control, and eating practices. Often the patient knows more than the physician about nutrition. With new information on nutrition published daily, we can expect the revolution to gain momentum and to continue for some time. As Sheldon Margen, professor of human nutrition at the University of California at Berkeley and a major consultant to the 1977 Senate Select Committee on Nutrition and Human Needs, put it (Rice, 1978): "Can a change in the nation's diet reduce the rate of the killer diseases such as cancer, arteriosclerosis, and diabetes? We don't know for sure, but we can't afford to spend another 20 to 30 years finding out."

We believe in bringing the nutrition controversy out in the open. The nutrition revolution is just beginning. Nutrition therapy may even replace drug therapy and surgery as the medical mode of treating and preventing many of today's diseases and disorders. We can expect the field of nutrition to gain greater public recognition and our eating habits to change when medical schools begin to include nutrition courses in the preparation of physicians, when the medical community begins to recognize the importance of nutrition to health and in the treatment and prevention of diseases, and when the food industry stops destroying nutrients in foods. Meanwhile, teachers should continue to offer up-to-date information on nutrition and not wait for miracle changes in medicine and the food industry.

LESSON PLANS

In light of this discussion, peruse the following lesson plans, keeping in mind that they are the type you will likely be expected to implement in your classroom. Remember that they by no means encompass a complete unit of instruction. They are simply a basis for the formation of a comprehensive unit.

TOPIC: A GOOD BREAKFAST

Grade Level: Primary

Concept: Breakfast is the most important meal of the day.

Expected Pupil Outcome: The student will recognize the importance of a good nutritious breakfast.

Content: A good, nutritious breakfast is important for the following reasons:
1. A long time has passed since the last meal.
2. It gives us energy to go to school.
3. It gives us energy to learn.
4. It gives us energy to work.
5. It gives us energy to play.

Learning Experiences
1. *Survey:* How many ate breakfast? What did you have for breakfast?
2. *Picture simulation:* Pictures of different people and discussion of how they feel and possible relationship to a good breakfast.
3. Storytelling using the picture simulation. Students are asked to react to the different pictures and story line, which reinforces why a good breakfast is important.

Evaluation Procedures   The teacher subjectively evaluates the quality of the student responses during the storytelling/picture simulation session. If the students are correct in their comparison of the different pictures to the notion of a good or poor breakfast, the objective will be considered accomplished.

TOPIC: EATING A BALANCED DIET

Grade Level: Intermediate

Concept: A balanced diet includes foods from the four food groups, plus water.

Expected Pupil Outcome: The student will select a balanced diet.

Content: Food groups contributing to a balanced diet:
1. Dairy products (2 plus glasses for young children)
   a) Milk
   b) Butter
   c) Eggs
   d) Ice cream
2. Fruits and vegetables (4 plus servings)
   a) Orange-tomato juice
   b) Lettuce
   c) Cabbage
   d) Carrots
   e) Peas
   f) Potatoes
   g) Celery
3. Breads and cereals (4 plus servings)
   a) Bread
   b) Cereals
4. Meats (2 plus servings)
   a) Beef
   b) Pork, ham
   c) Chicken
   d) Fish
5. Water

Learning Experiences
1. *Self-survey:* Pupils start out by listing foods they ate the previous day and then reporting results.
2. *Results:* Isolate a pupil with a well-balanced diet and another with a poorly balanced diet. Match their diet to picture cut-outs of foods they ate on large pie plates representing breakfast, lunch, and dinner. Let class decide which is balanced. Do not criticize student. Offer constructive comments on how diet might be improved.
3. *Handout:* Worksheet for planning a balanced school lunch and ask students to independently complete for a turn in assignment.

Evaluation Procedures   The teacher goes over the following turned in assignment to determine if the students were capable of planning a balanced lunch. If the majority of the students were successful, the objective will be considered accomplished.

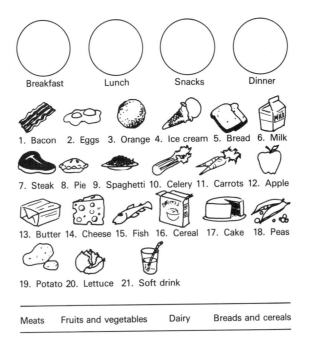

| Breakfast | Lunch | Snacks | Dinner |

1. Bacon 2. Eggs 3. Orange 4. Ice cream 5. Bread 6. Milk

7. Steak 8. Pie 9. Spaghetti 10. Celery 11. Carrots 12. Apple

13. Butter 14. Cheese 15. Fish 16. Cereal 17. Cake 18. Peas

19. Potato 20. Lettuce 21. Soft drink

| Meats | Fruits and vegetables | Dairy | Breads and cereals |

Are My Meals Balanced?

Directions: Using the list of foods, write in the circles the foods you ate yesterday. Do these foods form a balanced diet? To help you answer this question, regroup your foods in the bottom four food groups.

ALTERNATIVE CLASSROOM LEARNING EXPERIENCE FOR NUTRITION EDUCATION

Rat Nutrition Experiment*

Planning the Demonstration

1. Objectives of the experiment
   a) Demonstrate the importance of good nutrition in the growth and development of rats
   b) Relate the growth of the rats to growth in other living things
   c) Include as many students and groups as possible in the experiment
   d) Create awareness of eating habits
   e) Create interest in nutrition
   f) Help students learn to organize and evaluate a project from beginning to end with as little help as possible
2. Plan the committees that will be needed
   a) Consider the Committee for Care of Rats
      (1) Fasten the cages securely
      (2) Cover the floor of cages with newspaper strips, sawdust, shavings
      (3) Water and food cups—cold cream jars
      (4) Temperature—no drafts; even temperature—70° to 80°

---

*Adapted from *Animal Feeding Demonstrations for the Classroom* (pamphlet), National Dairy Council, Chicago, 1963.

(5) Cover the cages with blankets or newspapers at night and on weekend

(6) Daily care: change floor material; remove left-over meals; clean food and water cups

(7) Weekly routine: wash cages with soap, water, and brush

(8) At all times: handle the rats quietly and gently; do not excite them with shrill, loud voices or loud noises

b) Committees needed

   (1) Equipment Committee: Obtain the following equipment
      (a) Rat cage—may be obtained through health department
      (b) Feeding cups—heavy enough not to tip over
      (c) Wood shavings for covering bottom of cage (newspapers)
      (d) An old pair of gloves for handling the rats
      (e) Cloth for covering the cage at night
      (f) Container for holding the rat while he is being weighed (oatmeal box)
      (g) Gram scales for weighing rats
      (h) Utensils for cutting up food

   (2) Food Committee
      (a) Prepare food for feeding the rats
      (b) Feed the rats; food kept in cages at all times. Follow this routine
         i) Daily—fill cups with food; fill cups with liquid
         ii) Weekends—provide extra cups of food and water
         iii) Cage food (dry bread crumbs with salt) at all times
         iv) Display the contrasting diet in food models near the cages

   (3) Committee for Weighing Rats
      (a) Weigh weekly
      (b) Use same box for each weighing

   (4) Committee for Cleaning Cages
      (a) Daily clean-up
      (b) Weekly washing of cages

   (5) Committee to Observe Changes in Rats
      (a) Well nourished rat
         i) Clean, smooth, glossy fur
         ii) Smooth tail, free from roughness
         iii) Firm nails
         iv) Quick, alert movements; good muscle control
         v) Clean and tidy habits
         vi) Easily handled, good natured
         vii) Bright pink eyes, pink nose, ears, feet, and tail
      (b) Poorly nourished rat
         i) Shaggy, dull, and possibly thin fur
         ii) Rough, dry, scaly ears, feet, and tail
         iii) Possibly soft nails
         iv) Restless, irritable, and cross
         v) Whiskers not long and sharp, possibly dirty
         vi) Breathing difficult, susceptible to sniffles

vii) Eyes not clear, pinched look in face

   (6) Publicity Committee

      (a) Posters

      (b) Talks

      (c) Radio and newspaper articles

      (d) Photographing the demonstration

      (e) School paper and assemblies

   (7) Chart and Graph Committees

      (a) Plot the growth of rats

      (b) Each pupil may keep individual weight graphs on rats, which the committee may check for accuracy

3. Establish guidelines for each committee to follow
4. Plan the extra activities
   a) Puppet show—open house or assembly program
   b) Flannel-board story for second graders
   c) Diaries
   d) Rat race
   e) Poster
   f) Business places
5. Plan other subjects to emphasize in demonstration
   a) Arithmetic—graphs, bar graphs, line graphs

Compare ages of human with ages of rats:

Human in years—	2½	3	3½	4	4½	5	5½
Rats in weeks—	4	5	6	7	8	9	10

---

   b) Language—newspaper articles, plays, diaries, scrapbook

   c) Art—scrapbook, posters, bulletin boards

   d) Spelling

   e) Science

   f) Family life

6. Problems
   a) Acquiring the white rats
   b) Cages
   c) Scales
   d) Local situation—water
   e) What to do with rats on weekends
   f) Pets
   g) How to dispose of animals when demonstration is completed
7. Plan your evaluation

REFERENCES AND BIBLIOGRAPHY

Airola, Paavo. *Hypoglycemia* (Phoenix: Health Plus Publishers, 1977).

Chandra, R.K. "Nutrition and immunity—Basic considerations: Parts 1 & 2," *Contemporary Nutrition* 11, Number 12 (1986).

Chandra, R.K. "Nutritional deficiency and susceptibility to infection," *Bulletin of the World Health Organization* 57 (2) (1979):167-177.

Cheraskin, Emanuel, and William Ringsdorf. *Psychodietetics* (New York: Bantam, 1976).

Clark, Linda. *Know Your Nutrition* (New Canaan, CT: Keats, 1973).

Labuza, Theodore P. *The Nutrition Crisis: A Reader* (St. Paul, MN: West, 1975):104, 105.

Mayer, Jean. *A Diet for Living* (New York: Pocket Books, 1977):298, 444.

National Academy of Sciences. *Recommended Daily Allowances* (Washington, DC: National Academy of Sciences, 1984).

Nutrition Research Inc. *Nutrition Almanac* (New York: McGraw-Hill, 1975).

Passwater, Richard A. *Supernutrition* (New York: Pocket Books, 1976).

Pauling, Linus. *Vitamin C, The Common Cold and the Flu* (San Francisco: Freeman, 1976).

Rice, Marjorie. "Physician Feels Diet Could KO Killer Diseases," *San Diego Union*, March 21, 1978.

Select Committee on Nutrition and Human Needs of the United States. *Dietary Goals for the United States,* 2nd ed. (Washington: U.S. Printing Office, December, 1977).

"Too much sugar?" *Consumer Reports*, March, 1978, 136-142.

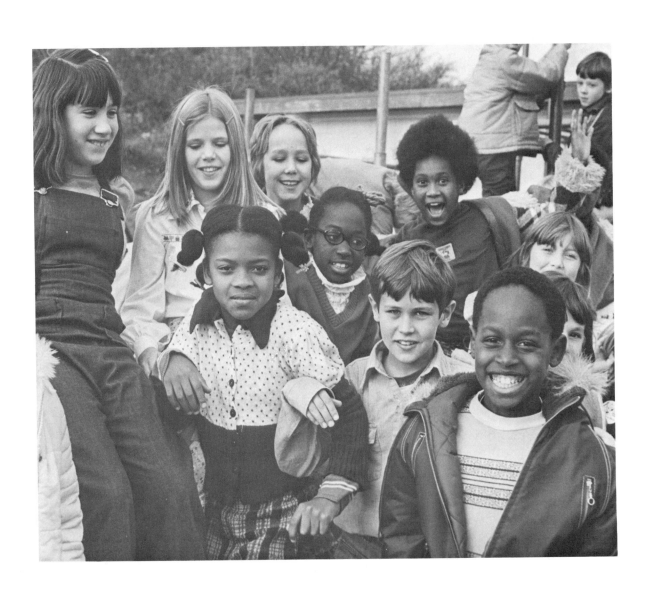

Chapter 20

Teaching About Dental Health

INTRODUCTION

One of the pressing health problems facing us today is dental disease. Although it does not receive the headlines that drug abuse, sex education, and some other health issues do, it deserves a great deal of attention. Ninety-five percent of the American population lives with dental problems. Many of your students will never have visited a dentist. The average youngster in your class will have one to three decaying teeth, and this number will increase as the child grows older. In many instances ignorance accompanies tooth decay.

The most common dental problem in adults is periodontal disease. "Periodontal" comes from two Greek words meaning "around the tooth." Hence diseases of the gums and other supporting structures of the teeth are known as periodontal disease. Such diseases should be given instant preventive attention. Unfortunately, most people are unable to care properly for their teeth, do not know how, don't care, or ignore good dental hygiene. In addition, most of us have been trained in ineffective brushing techniques that were in vogue 20 to 30 years ago. We tend to teach these practices to children.

Two major factors affecting dental caries and periodontal disease are (1) nutrition of the mother during pregnancy, and (2) nutrition of the infant and oral hygiene in control of dental plaque once teeth appear. A third factor is heredity, which determines the color, hardness, shape, and size of teeth, thickness of enamel, and resistance to dental caries.

A child's and an adult's teeth are only as healthy as the nutrients available during the mother's pregnancy. Prevention of dental caries begins during pregnancy if the expectant mother eats the proper amounts of essential nutrients. The formation of teeth begins very early; the permanent teeth begin to grow five months before a child is born (Williams, 1973). The cells responsible for tooth production during these early stages need complete nutrition, not only at that time but for many years to follow. When prospective mothers follow inferior diets, their infants grow up to have teeth that are subject to decay. Adequate nutrition (vitamins, minerals, and other micronutrients) remains critical throughout childhood, when teeth develop and mature. Infants and children who are well nourished grow teeth resistant to dental caries. Genetic susceptibility to tooth decay can be overcome by providing teeth with adequate nutrition, including vitamins and minerals (Table 20.1). Refined sugar and foods rich in sugar, such as soft drinks, candy, and pastries, should be eliminated from the diet. There follows an eating guide (Table 20.2) to help children balance the four major food groups for dental health.

Most persons need to cut down on hidden sugar in foods. It is much easier to reduce table sugar (adding sugar to iced tea) than hidden sugar (see Table 20.3).

Most children and adults fail to take proper care of the areas where the gums meet the teeth. In addition to brushing as the teeth grow, dental hygienists suggest that the soft bristles be hand-vibrated in these areas. Such bristle action, if properly used in the way described by your dentist, at least once a day, not only disrupts bacterial plaques, but also massages the gums. If not removed regularly, the bacteria in plaque produce acids that may dissolve tooth enamel and cause cavities. Bacterial plaque can cause periodontal disease by producing chemicals that irritate the gums. In addition, when plaque accumulates over a long period, it may harden to become calculus or tartar. Calculus dams up the toxins produced by plaque, heightening gum irritation, causing swelling of gums and periodontal disease. (Topical application of fluoride or drinking fluoridated water helps prevent dental caries in children.)

These are new ways of conserving teeth and a healthy mouth. New research suggests that brushing teeth once a day with proper and regular use of dental floss may be more effective than brushing teeth after every meal. Mouthwashes have no effect on the bacteria in the mouth and do not prevent tooth decay. Dental hygienists are most optimistic about a new kind of chewing gum and serum that may help develop immunity to dental caries when used as an adjutant to more effective dental care.

(Text continues on page 402.)

TABLE 20.1
Vitamins and Minerals Essential for Healthy Teeth

Vitamins	Function	Best Sources

A
  RDA = 3,500 IU children 7-10
        4,000 IU females
        5,000 IU males
	Protects mucous membranes in mouth	Green vegetables, broccoli, sweet potato, liver, cantaloupe

B-complex	Maintains health of mouth and gums	Whole-wheat bread and cereals, green vegetables, lean meats, milk, yeast

C
  RDA = 45 mg children 7-10
       60 adults
	Helps heal gums, prevents bleeding
	Helps maintain hard teeth and bones
		Citrus fruits, fruit juices, cauliflower, cantaloupe

D
  RDA = 400 IU children 7-10
       400 IU adults
	Helps build strong teeth and bones	Sunshine for 30 min/day
		Milk, cod liver oil

K*	Helps stop fermentation of food in mouth	Cauliflower, root vegetables, kelp, green leafy vegetables, fruits

Minerals	Function	Best Sources

Calcium
  RDA = 800 mg children 7-10
       1200 mg females
       800 mg males
	Helps build strong teeth and bones
	Maintains bone strength
		Dairy products (milk), dolomite, bone meal, sardines with bones

Fluorine RDA = 0.4-0.5 mg adults	Maintains strong teeth and bones	Seafoods, fluoridated water, gelatin
Iodine RDA = 0.9 mg adults	Helps maintain healthy teeth	Seafoods, kelp, iodized salt

Magnesium
  RDA = 200 mg children 7-10
       300 mg adults
	Forms hard tooth enamel (fights tooth decay)	Wheat germ, whole-wheat bread, seeds, nuts, soybeans, leafy green vegetables

Phosphorus
  RDA = 800 mg children 7-10
       800 mg adults
	Helps growth of teeth and bones
	Strengthens teeth
		Meats, fish, poultry, eggs, seeds, whole grains, nuts

Vanadium*	May prevent tooth decay	Seafoods, kelp, gelatin
Molybdenum*	Helps build strong teeth	Green beans, oatmeal, wheat bread, meats

*No RDA established.

EATING BETWEEN MEALS

Snacking between meals greatly increases your risk of dental caries.

Eating sugary foods and drinking soft drinks between meals are major contributors to dental caries. Sugary foods such as chocolate bars, sugary cereals, cookies, candies, and soft drinks feed the bacteria in your mouth. Bacteria eat the sugar and excrete acids which combine with saliva to form a very strong acid that dissolves the enamel of teeth.

Eating habits are important to slow down tooth decay. First, don't snack on sweets. The less sugar you eat, the less food there is for bacteria. You are most likely to get cavities when you regularly eat sugar between meals.

Next, do not leave sugar acids on your teeth for long periods. Continually eating sweets increases exposure to sugar acids.

Do not eat sweets alone. If you are going to eat sugary foods, have them with meals rather than alone. The presence of other foods will get saliva flowing to help buffer and dilute any sugar acid.

Regardless of when you eat sweets, it is most important that you brush your teeth and mouth immediately afterward. Bacteria begin eating sugar immediately, and harmful acid levels build up within 15 minutes. By brushing immediately after eating, you reduce the amount of sugar available for bacteria.

After brushing for three minutes or longer, rinse your mouth with water to wash out loose food particles, sugar acid, and bacteria. If you cannot brush your teeth and mouth, refrain from eating sweets. Swishing with water lowers the risk of sugar acid forming in your mouth and hence, lowers the risk of cavities.

You are at very high risk for dental caries if you are under 25 and snack on sweets between meals.

When and how often you eat sweets affect your risk of dental caries. Eliminate sweet snacks immediately. If you must snack, then eat unsweetened foods such as celery, cucumbers, cauliflower, and fresh fruits.

TABLE 20.2
Four Major Food Groups and Serving Amounts

Group	Food Sources	Nutrients	Servings per Day
MILK AND MILK PRODUCTS	Milk (2% fat), cheese	Calcium, B-complex, D, phosphorus, proteins	2
MEATS AND EQUIVALENTS	Fish, poultry, beef, eggs, cheese, yeast, soy-beans, nuts	Proteins, iron, niacin, trace minerals, iodine, phosphorus, choline, biotin, B_5, B_6	2
FRUITS	Orange, banana, pear, watermelon, canta-loupe, peach, grapes, apple	C, trace minerals, fiber, potassium	2
AND			
VEGETABLES	Fresh green leafy, seed vegetables (peas)	Fiber, trace minerals, iron, potassium, phosphorus, magnesium, biotin, A, B_6, C	2
BREADS/CEREALS	Wheat bread, cereals, bran muffins	Fiber, B-complex, trace minerals, iron, incomplete proteins	2

EATING SWEETS

Eating sweets is a major risk factor for dental caries for all of us.

Tooth decay is caused by sugar. Bacteria in the mouth feed on sugary foods and produce acids that dissolve the enamel of teeth. To reduce your chances of developing cavities, or dental caries, reduce the frequency of eating sweets and eating sweets alone. You are most likely to get cavities when you regularly eat sugar between meals and expose your teeth to sugar for long periods. Children, adolescents, and adults under the age of 25 have the highest risk of cavities, while those over 25 have a high risk to periodontal disease, such as gingivitis, in which plaque forms on the surface of teeth next to the gums, causing irritation of the gums, or gingivae.

Some people think their teeth are safe from decay if they brush their teeth each time they eat sweets. This may not be entirely correct, as it is difficult to brush the teeth well enough to overcome all the effects of sugar. You would have to brush your teeth for three minutes within five minutes after eating sugary food. Since most persons find it inconvenient to brush teeth properly when they eat sugary foods, it is wise to limit sweets as much as possible. When you do eat sugary foods, have them with meals rather than alone. Other foods get saliva flowing to help buffer and dilute acids. It is always wise to brush as soon as you can after eating.

Sugar-rich foods are low in vitamins and minerals and are often high in fats. Such foods are called empty calorie foods because they are high in calories but low in essential nutrients. This is another reason to not eat too many sweets.

How much sugar is acceptable in your diet? The U.S. Dietary Goals suggest that refined sugars should make up no more than 10 percent of the total calories you eat each day. Your body does *not* need sugar! It needs complex carbohydrates for energy. Complex carbohydrates (from potatoes, rice, whole-grain spaghetti, and vegetables) provide more vitamins and minerals and longer-lasting energy than do sugary foods. Therefore, the official guide for sugar is too high. Think of displacing sugar foods with fresh fruits and vegetables.

How can you tell if a food has sugar in it? Most processed and refined foods have sugar, since sugar is both a sweetener and a preservative. The best thing to do when you are shopping is to read the label. If sugar, sucrose, dextrose, corn syrup, fructose, maltose, honey, molasses, turbinado, confectioner's sugar, monosaccharides, or disaccharides is one of the first few ingredients in the list on the package, assume sugar is a major part of the food. If it is listed toward the end, it may be present in smaller amounts. ALWAYS READ THE LABEL!

Refer to the list below to identify the sugar content of a few foods. To lower your risk for dental caries, consider substituting unsweetened, unprocessed foods for the sugar-rich foods. A few unsweetened foods are suggested on the right side of the list.

TABLE 20.3
Hidden Sugar Content of Some Common (Processed) Foods

Food	Serving Size	% Sugar Calories	Sugar Substitute Foods
BEVERAGES (ounces)			
Cola	12 oz	99	Water
			Orange juice
Grape juice (Welch's)	6 oz	55	
Hi-C orange	6 oz	81	
Kool Aid (sugar flavored)	6 oz	98	
Sprite, Coca-Cola	12 oz	100	
CEREALS (cups)			
All bran (Kellogg)	0.33	26	Natural rolled oats
Apple jacks (Kellogg)	1	56	
Cherios (General Mills)	1.25	3.5	
Cocoa puffs (General Mills)	1	39	
Corn flakes (Kellogg)	1	7	Shredded wheat
Fruit loops (Kellogg)	1	99	Cracked wheat
Life (Quaker)	.67	18	
Lucky charms (General Mills)	1	39	
Natural rolled oats	1	00	
Oatmeal with cinnamon and spice	.63	35	
Post alphabits	1	39	
Post raisin bran	.5	39	
Rice crispies (Kellogg)	1	17	
Sugar pops (Kellogg)	1	46	
Sugar frosted flakes	.67	39	
Sugar smacks (Kellogg)	.75	56	
Total (General Mills)	1	11	
Wheaties (General Mills)	1	11	
CONDIMENTS (tablespoons)			
Bleu cheese dressing	1	5	Oil + vinegar (with spices)
French salad dressing	1	18	
Italian dressing	1	4.5	
Catsup	1	61	Tomato
Sugar (white & brown)	1	50	Raisins, dates, bananas
FOOD (ounces)			
Chocolate bar (Hershey)	1.2	37	Fresh raw fruits
Chocolate pudding	4	37	
Graham cracker	2	25	
Ice cream (vanilla)	4	36	
Jello (cherry)	4	87	
Milkshake (vanilla)	12	37	Low-fat milk; juices
Peas (sweet canned)	4	20	Fresh/frozen peas
Pears (canned with syrup)	4	50	Fresh pears
Hot dogs	1.6	4	Chicken, fish
Yogurt (lowfat)	8	33	Fresh fruit
Yogurt (fruit)	8	50	Fresh fruit

WAYS TO MAINTAIN ORAL HYGIENE

1. Brush your teeth properly for three or more minutes after each meal (or at least once a day).
2. Use a soft-bristle toothbrush.
3. Floss each day the surfaces of teeth that brushing cannot clean.
4. Drink plenty of water and rinse your mouth out each time. Doing so reduces bacterial content in the mouth.
5. Do not crack nuts or hard objects with your teeth.
6. Massage the gums each day with a toothbrush while brushing and with your fingers.
7. Have a dental checkup every six months.
8. Avoid drinking extremely hot or cold liquids.
9. Eat a balanced diet each day.
10. Avoid tobacco.
11. Drink fluoridated water.
12. Do not eat refined sugar (sucrose) products.
13. Assess your mouth for plaque once a month.
14. When playing contact sports that may injure your teeth, wear protective equipment.
15. See a dentist immediately if you injure your teeth or mouth.

WHAT TO DO ABOUT BAD BREATH

Almost everyone has bad breath (halitosis) at one time or another. However, a clean, healthy mouth (California Medical Association, 1978) gives a fresh, clean breath. For years advertisers have taken advantage of this with a barrage of advertising for mouthwashes, breath sweeteners, and toothpastes.
Bad breath may be caused by:

Food (garlic or onions)

Tobacco

Alcoholic beverages

A dry mouth and throat, as when you wake up in the morning

Poor flow of saliva

Indigestion

Poor nutrition

Poor mouth hygiene

Tooth or gum infection

Infected tonsils

Lung infection

Diabetes

Liver disease

Brushing with a toothpaste and using a mouthwash are temporary and ineffective ways of dealing with halitosis. Drinking plenty of water will help control bad breath. If bad breath persists, see your doctor or dentist or both so that you can identify the cause.

Many dentists believe that one can strengthen the tooth against bacterial plaque. Dr. Aslander perceives dental caries as a deficiency disease and not a bacterial infection (Adams, 1977). He perceives the nourished tooth as being immune to dental caries. Only nutrient-starved teeth are attacked by disease. Just as mineral deficiency contributes to tooth decay, so a deficiency of fluorine and molybdenum in the regular diet makes teeth especially sensitive to dental caries (Adams, 1977). Adequate dental nutrition can be aided by a dental checkup every six months and by drinking fluoridated water. Adding one part fluoride to 1 million parts of drinking water cuts dental decay in children and teenagers in half.

How should the teacher approach dental health in the classroom? The answer is twofold. First, since most children suffer from dental caries and since children tend to receive most of their permanent teeth between 6 and 12 years of age, reinforce proper brushing technique early in the primary grades. The brushing technique and the correct technique for using dental floss should be introduced at the preschool age. Emphasis at all levels should be on regular dental habits and sound nutrition, not on education. Teachers will do far more good by providing time each day for dental care, as after the noon meal, than offering a once-a-year instruction. Good habits should be cultivated each day and ingrained before the child has reached age 12.

LESSON PLANS

In light of this discussion, peruse the following lesson plans, keeping in mind that they are the type you will likely be expected to implement in your classroom. Remember that they by no means encompass a complete unit of instruction. They are simply a basis for the formation of a comprehensive unit.

TOPIC: BRUSHING THE TEETH CORRECTLY

Grade Level: Primary

Concept: Correctly brushing your teeth requires skill.

**Expected Pupil
Outcome:** The student will be able to brush his or her teeth correctly.

Content

Proper brushing requires:

1. Top inside surfaces—left, front, right
2. Bottom inside surfaces—left, front right
3. Top outside surfaces—left, front, right
4. Bottom outside surfaces—left, front, right
5. Chewing and biting surfaces—top, left, right
6. Tongue

Learning Experiences

1. *Demonstration:* Teacher demonstrates steps in brushing teeth correctly on a large model of teeth, using a large toothbrush. Stress brushing action and organized approach so all surfaces will be brushed (Figure 20.1).

2. *Practice—simulation session:* Two students work together as buddies. One uses popsicle stick or tongue depressor and pretends to brush his or her teeth, and the other corrects. Reverse. Teacher walks around and also corrects.

3. The techniques of brushing teeth should be repeated until children have acquired correct brushing skills and the practices become habitual. To add variety to the repetition, the following alternatives are suggested:

   a) Teacher and children recite the brushing-teeth rhyme while brushing teeth. (Note: This rhyme stresses areas of teeth to brush; it does not stress correct technique for plaque removal.)

   The Brushing Teeth Rhyme (sing to melody of "Around the Mulberry Bush")
   This is the way we brush our teeth
   Brush our teeth
   Brush our teeth
   This is the way we brush our teeth
   So early in the morning
   Upper teeth, upper teeth
   Brush them downward
   Lower teeth, lower teeth
   Brush them upward
   Brush upper teeth, Brush lower teeth
   Brush also the grinders
   This is the way we brush our teeth
   Brush our teeth
   Brush our teeth
   This is the way we brush our teeth after every meal

FIGURE 20.1
Correct method of brushing teeth. (From "Effective Oral Hygiene," pp. 2-6, developed by the USAF School of Aerospace Medicine, Brooks Air Force Base, Texas.

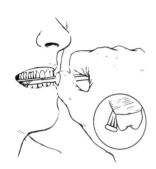

Place brush where teeth and gums meet.

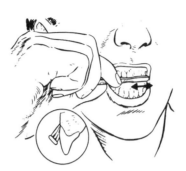

Look at the arrows on the brush. (VIBRATE, using short back-and-forth strokes, without disengaging the bristles from the edge of the gum.)

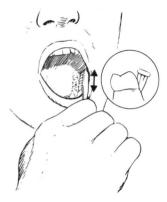

Keep brush where teeth and gums meet. VIBRATE.

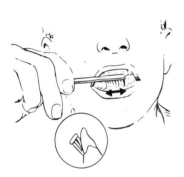

Use short *vibrating* strokes.

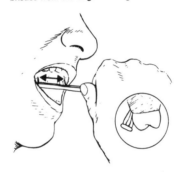

Use same method on inside surfaces.

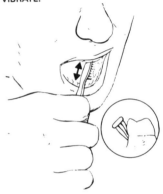

VIBRATE brush *back* and *forth*.

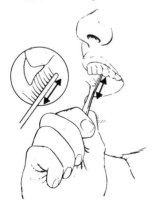

Brush, (vibrate) *up* and *down*.

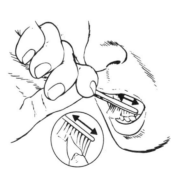

Keep strokes short and vibrate brush.

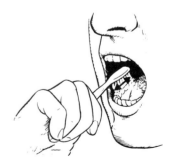

Brush back and forth on biting surfaces.

FIGURE 20.2
A healthy-tooth cleaning idea.

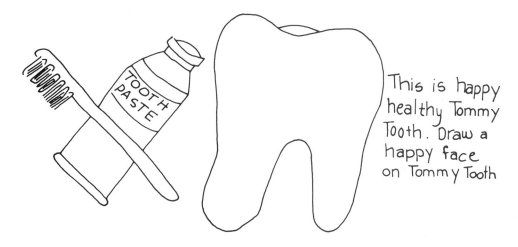

This is happy healthy Tommy Tooth. Draw a happy face on Tommy Tooth

b) Children draw a happy face in Tommy Tooth (Figure 20.2).

c) Children brush to the accompaniment of "My Toothbrush Song" by Ann Lloyd and the Sandpipers, Golden Record R43R.

Evaluation Procedures   During the practice/simulation session the teacher will observe the students and correct any mistakes. Once all students have performed all steps correctly, the objective is accomplished.

TOPIC: USING DENTAL FLOSS PROPERLY

Grade Level: Primary, Intermediate

Concept: Using dental floss once a day helps to prevent dental caries.

Expected Pupil Outcome: The student will be able to demonstrate proper use of dental floss.

Content: Techniques of using dental floss:

1. Pull about 24 inches of floss from dispenser or use toothbrush that has dental flosser.
2. Wrap most of the floss around one finger.
3. Wrap the remaining floss around the same finger of the other hand. This finger can take up the floss as you use it.
4. Use thumbs as guides for flossing upper teeth.
5. Use index fingers for lower ones.

Learning Experiences
Demonstration:

1. Teacher demonstration (Figure 20.3).
2. Practice session: Pupils practice flossing just as they do brushing. Teacher observes and corrects where necessary.

FIGURE 20.3

Correct method of using dental floss. (From "Effective Oral Hygiene," pp. 8-10, developed by the USAF School of Aerospace Medicine, Brooks Air Force Base, Texas.

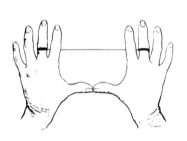
Wrap floss on middle fingers.

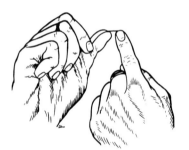
Thumb to the outside for upper teeth.

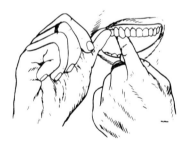
Flossing between upper back teeth.

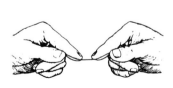
Holding floss for lower teeth.

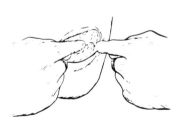
Flossing between lower back teeth.

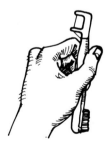
Toothbrush-Flosser

6. Hold floss tightly and work it gently between the teeth (back and forth).
7. Curve floss around tooth and work it under the gum line and scrape.
8. Repeat on adjacent teeth.
9. Follow same pattern each time.
10. Rinse vigorously with water after flossing to remove food particles and plaque that has been cut loose.

Evaluation Procedures During the practice session the teacher observes the students for correct technique. When all students have performed the procedure correctly, the objective will be attained.

TOPIC: VISITING THE DENTIST

Grade Level: Primary

Concept: The dentist helps protect our teeth.

Expected Pupil Outcome: The student will indicate a willingness to accept the dentist as a friend.

Content: The dentist is our friend in the following ways:

1. Shows us how to clean our teeth
2. Cleans our teeth (with special machine)
3. Protects our teeth with fluoride
4. Checks the growth of our teeth
5. X-rays our teeth
6. Finds and fills cavities
7. Corrects crooked teeth and may pull out sick teeth if necessary
8. Shows us how to care for our teeth, gums, and mouth

Learning Experience

1. Skit

A Visit To The Dentist

Characters

Jerry Mahoney, a boy of 5 to 7 who has never been to the dentist. Instead of a pupil playing the part, a dummy, Jerry Mahoney and a dental unit, may be obtained from the local Dental Association (Figure 20.4).

FIGURE 20.4
Kindergarten children simulating a visit to the dentist, using Jerry Mahoney and the dental unit. (Photograph courtesy of the Women's Auxiliary to the San Diego County Dental Society.)

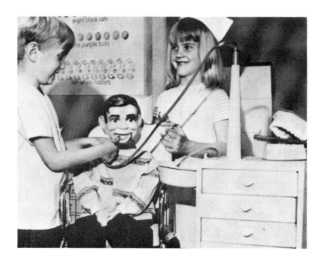

Jerry's mother

Ms. Goodday, receptionist, dressed in yellow, has a sparkling, bubbling disposition, wears hat with "HI" on it.

Ms. Sparkles, dental assistant, dressed in light blue, is neat and a good conversationalist.

Dr. Gums, dentist, wears a light green top jacket, has a great sense of humor, easy-going manner.

Props: The dress as described for the dental team.

Act II: Dental chair and simulated drill, X-ray, spittoon, dental instruments, mirror; explorer; packer; paper cups; paper towels; bib; reception desk.

Suggested Approach: This script may be acted out or the lines ad-libbed by pupils in grades 4 to 6, who could put on the play for the kindergarten or grade 1 pupils. The teacher could help the class ad lib and simulate the scripts.

Act I

Setting: The dentist's office, 10:30 a.m. Mother and Jerry enter the office. The receptionist, with a sparkling, happy disposition, greets them. There is soft music and singing about teeth and dental hygiene. (Set props for Act I.)

Receptionist: Good morning, Mrs. Mahoney, and a special good morning to you, Jerry. Won't you please sit down, and I'll tell Dr. Gums that you are here. [She goes out and comes back immediately.] You are lucky, Jerry, Dr. Gums and his assistant will be able to see you in a few minutes. How are you feeling today?

Jerry: Okay, I guess. Will this visit take long? My friends and I are going to the beach this afternoon.

Receptionist: No, just a few minutes. My, but you have a beautiful smile—and such white teeth. My goodness, you must take good care of your teeth—how do you do it?

Jerry: Naw, I brush them because Mom wants me to. (A bell rings from the inner office.)

Receptionist: Okay, Jerry, they are ready for you now.

Act II

Setting: (Props as described in introduction.) Receptionist takes Jerry by the hand, and they enter Dr. Gum's office, where the dental assistant greets them. Dentist's room has dentist's chair, with simulated drill and spittoon, a small shelf, and an X-ray machine. On the table are small plastic animals, a small rag doll, several comic books, a large set of teeth, a large toothbrush.

Receptionist: Jerry, this is Dr. Gum's assistant. She will help you and Dr. Gums.

Assistant: Hi, Jerry. I am glad you could make it today. I hear you and your friends are going to the beach today—where?

Jerry: Where they swim and the waves are this high.

Assistant: You must be a good swimmer. Jerry, would you like to sit in this big chair?

Jerry: (apprehensive) Okay.

Assistant: Now, make yourself comfortable, and I'll put a bib on you. Do you build sand castles at the beach, Jerry?

Jerry: Gee, what are those?

Assistant: You have heard of castles where kings and queens lived, with large towers and high walls—[she gets a colored picture of a castle]. Here is a picture of an ancient castle where the Sleeping Beauty lived.

Jerry, you hold this picture and look at it if you want to. Meanwhile, I would like to look at your teeth. Would you open your mouth wide—yes, like that, thank you, Jerry. (She examines his teeth with the small mirror.) You have some new teeth, Jerry. And they look real healthy; they could stand a cleaning though. You know, Jerry, Dr. Gums takes his son and daughter, about your age, to the beach on weekends. And they build sand castles. Why don't you ask him how to build sand castles?

Jerry: Gee, I didn't know dentists like to build sand castles. (Dr. Gums enters.)

Assistant: Dr. Gums, this is Jerry Mahoney.

Dr. Gums: (Smiling and thumbs Jerry's hand as a greeting.) Good morning, Jerry. I see from the way you shook hands with me that you and I have a lot in common. What's that picture you have?

Jerry: It's a picture of a Sleeping Beauty's castle.

Assistant: Jerry is going to the beach this afternoon and was thinking of building a sand castle.

Dr. Gums: Why, I build them every time I go to the beach. Building castles is one of my hobbies. Now, Jerry, show me how big and white your teeth are; open wide. Good, let me look at your back teeth. [Dr. Gums readjusts headrest and puts napkin under chin. As Dr. Gums examines Jerry's teeth, they continue to talk.] Castles are a lot of fun to make, and I'll be happy to make one with you this Sunday. Would you like that?

Jerry (nods and smiles).

Dr. Gums: Your teeth tell me you are about 6 years old (continues to examine the teeth). Open your mouth wider.—Oops, not too wide [smiling]; I don't want to fall in. Gee, Jerry, looks like you have a tooth missing on this side. How did you lose it? (Dr. Gums stops and lets Jerry explain.)

Jerry: It came loose last week and just fell out. I have it here in my pocket (pulls it out).

Dr. Gums: That is a very healthy tooth. Don't lose it. [He picks up the set of big teeth and brings it in front of Jerry.] See this big set of teeth—this is what your teeth will look like when you get all new teeth in a few years. This is the tooth that is missing now. (Gives the teeth to his assistant.) May I have an explorer, Ms. Sparkles? Jerry, with this instrument I can find all the secret hiding places of your food and also check to see that your teeth are healthy. Let's see, hum. Ms. Sparkles, would you like to bring that large model of teeth in front of Jerry again? Great. Thank you. [Ms. Sparkles, smiling, holds it.] [Dr. Gums points explorer between teeth.] Do you see the place where these two teeth meet? Food gets in between here. Yes, that's it—Ms. Sparkles [she uses the toothbrush to waft the food out between the crevice]. See how Ms. Sparkles brushed to pull the food particles out? You do that when you brush your teeth. Let's take another look at your teeth.—Hm. I bet you had peanut butter and jam on your toast this morning. I just found a part of a peanut in between your teeth. And I bet you like to eat candy. Do you, Jerry?

Jerry: I like O'Henry bars—they are delicious.

Dr. Gums: What do you do right after you eat a candy bar, Jerry?

Jerry: Play, what else?

Ms. Sparkles: Do you rinse your mouth with water or brush your teeth right after eating the bar?

Jerry: Naw, I don't have time.

Ms. Sparkles: If I can't brush my teeth, then I always rinse my teeth after I eat a bar. Look how clean my teeth are. [She smiles and shows her teeth.]

Dr. Gums: Aren't her teeth clean and white? And she has such a pretty smile. Ms. Sparkles, it's good to work with you. Now, Jerry, let me clean your teeth for you. You have no cavities as yet. You know, some of your teeth are a little dirty—let's clean and freshen them up a bit. Ms. Sparkles, some cleaning compound. Jerry, this is a cleaning machine; it helps to clean your teeth. It won't hurt. [He proceeds to clean the teeth.] There, now sip some water from this paper cup and spit it out. Good. One more sip; swish the water all around—good, now spit. How does that feel, Jerry?

Jerry: That stuff smells better than it feels. It tastes like candy.

Dr. Gums: Yes, it does, it removes the tartar, or slime, that coats the teeth. Jerry, remember the candy bar you like so much?

Jerry: Oh yes, I do.

Dr. Gums: Well, what is on the outside of the bar?

Jerry: Chocolate, and it tastes good.

Dr. Gums: Yes, and if we imagine that the center of the candy bar is your tooth, we can say that the chocolate on the outside is like the slime that coats the outside of your teeth. By cleaning your teeth just now, I removed this slime. Now your teeth can feel healthy again. But, Jerry, let's cut out all these sweets, for they are not good for your teeth. Ms. Sparkles, why don't you take some pictures of Jerry's teeth? He may have some decay that I am not able to see. (He turns to Jerry.) Ms. Sparkles will take an X-ray of your teeth, and that will be all for today. I would like to check your teeth again in about six months. Jerry, would you like to come and see me again?

Jerry: Oh, yes, and where on the beach will we meet to build the sand castles?

Dr. Gums: I will be at Life Guard Station 3 with my son, Mark, and daughter, Wendy. I want you to meet them. Why don't you bring your mom and dad, and we can all have fun building sand castles?

Jerry: Are you coming also, Ms. Sparkles?

Ms. Sparkles: I'm not sure yet, but I'll try.

Dr. Gums: See you Sunday, Jerry.

Ms. Sparkles: Let's have you sit up, Jerry! (She places a negative in

Jerry's mouth and takes X-rays of his mouth. As she does this, she talks to Jerry.) Jerry, you're going to have fun with Dr. Gums on Sunday. Here, now bite this—good. There, that's it! (She removes the bib.) Jerry, would you like this comic book? It has pictures of many kinds of castles. Maybe you'll get an idea for your castle on Sunday.

Jerry: Gee, may I? [Both return to the reception room.]

Jerry: [Runs to his mother exuberantly.] Hey, Mom, Dr. Gums and I are going to build sand castles on the beach Sunday. Would you and Dad like to come?

Mother: Why that's wonderful. We'll plan on it. (Turns to Ms. Sparkles and Ms. Goodday.) Thank you so much for helping Jerry with his teeth. Bye for now.

Ms. Sparkles: See you here in six months' time, Jerry, unless the X-rays show us something that needs to be fixed right away.

Jerry: Okay, Ms. Sparkles. Bye.

Evaluation Procedures

At a later date students will be asked about their most recent visit to the dentist. If the majority of students indicate that it was important to visit the dentist so that they can maintain healthy teeth, the objective will be considered attained.

TOPIC: CAUSE OF TOOTH DECAY

Grade Level: Primary

Concept: Bacteria such as lacti can cause tooth decay.

Expected Pupil Outcome: The student will be able to state what causes tooth decay.

Content: The steps in the decay process:
1. Sugars in the mouth
2. Lacti (germs) in the mouth
3. Lacti eats sugar
4. Lacti produces acid
5. Acid and saliva make more acid
6. Acid attacks tooth
7. Tooth decay is the result

Learning Experience
1. *Matching bee:* Process is identified in formula fashion and conceptualized by illustrations (Figure 20.5).
2. *Alternative experiences*
   a) Perform cola and tooth experiment: drop an extracted tooth in a cola bottle overnight. Observe tooth next day and compare action of lactic acid to cola.
   b) Children color pictures that depict the tooth decay process. A comic-coloring book, *Casper's Dental Health Activity Book,* is available from the American Dental Association.

FIGURE 20.5
Pictures conceptualizing the tooth decay process.

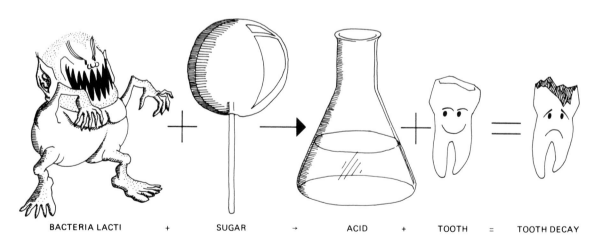

BACTERIA LACTI   +   SUGAR   →   ACID   +   TOOTH   =   TOOTH DECAY

Evaluation Procedures Once the matching bee is complete, the teacher asks the class to respond, in unison, the steps in the tooth decay process. If the class is successful, the objective will be deemed accomplished.

REFERENCES and BIBLIOGRAPHY

Adams, Ruth, and Frank Murray. *Minerals: Kill or Cure?* (New York: Larchmont Books, 1977): 14-17, 49.

Weinstein, Philip, et al. "What to do about bad breath," *Health Tips* (San Francisco: California Medical Association, February 1978).

Williams, Roger J. *Nutrition and Disease* (New York: Bantam, 1973):119.

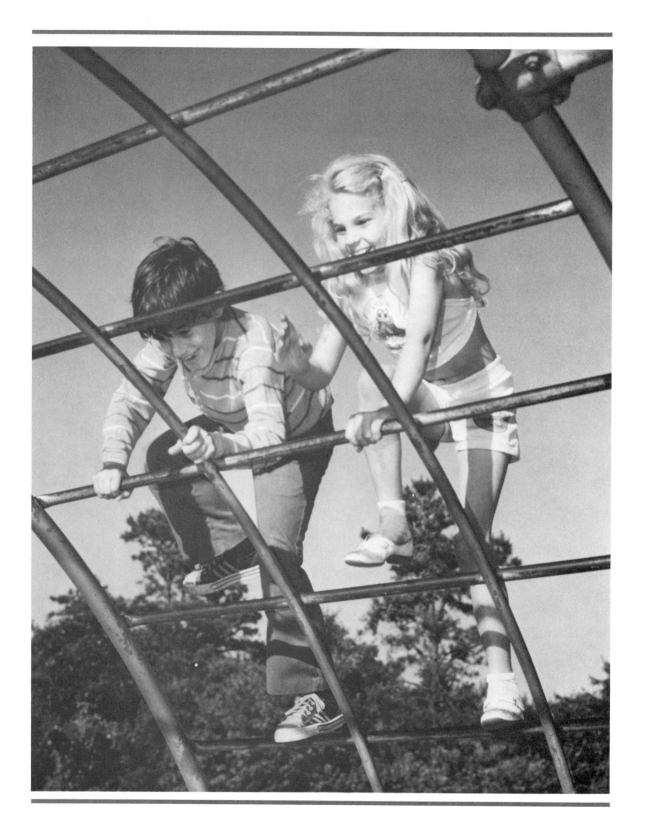

Chapter 21

Teaching About Safety

INTRODUCTION

The need for safety and efforts to provide it have been part of human existence since the beginning of time, when survival and safety were much the same thing. Although the hazards of survival have changed, the fundamental problem is the same. Since primitive people sought shelter and developed weapons to protect themselves from danger, the anticipation of danger and the ability to overcome it have been major keys to safety and survival.

Accidents don't just happen. They result from violations of rules, regulations, procedures, and courtesies that have evolved over the years. Accidents are always a symptom of disorder or failure to adapt. The disorder may be in the habits of an individual, in the customs of the community, or in the breakdown of a machine. An accident or a near-accident, no matter what the degree of severity, is a signal that something or someone is not functioning as it should.

Approximately 15 percent of accidents are caused by hazardous conditions in our environment. The remaining 85 percent have human causes. Among elementary school children the human element responsible for contributing to accidents is fourfold: (1) lack of knowledge of and experience with cause and effect; (2) lack of skill in such activities as swimming, using playground equipment, and crossing busy highways; (3) improper attitudes and personal traits—foolhardiness and taking unnecessary chances; and (4) poor emotional health that results in an accident-prone frame of mind.

This last factor should be of special interest to elementary school teachers. Children lacking physical skills may evolve emotional problems that create an accident habit or behavioral pattern as an adjustment compensation. Such careless children have more emotional outbursts, lack self-control, and are likely to be more impulsive and act more hastily than others. Thus accident prevention in the school involves fostering a safe physical and social environment, promoting emotional and mental well-being, and providing opportunities for children to practice safety precautions.

Participation in a variety of activities, familiar or unfamiliar, always presents possibilities of accidents. Many accidents are not caused by carelessness or poor mental attitudes. Curiosity leads children to explore, and since their curiosity is not checked by fear, they do not perceive the dangers of new objects and situations. With experience and increased insight, they gradually learn to be more cautious. Accidents are the leading cause of death among school children. Approximately two thirds of childhood accidents occur before the child is 9 years old, with 2 and 3 being the most vulnerable and 5 and 6 next. At these ages children are exploring the environment for themselves.

Certain environments are hazardous. Of every five school accidents, two occur in unorganized activities and three in organized activities. The classroom, the gymnasium, and the street are the most common sites for accidents. Elementary school teachers must assume responsibility for providing a safe environment and direct safety instruction.

Safety is a cultural concept. It can also be thought of as a series of habits that should be inculcated during the child's formative years. When integrated with the other essential skills of living, the skills of safety become the basis for a sensible and rational lifestyle. Although the foundation for safety is laid in the home by the parents, it must be reinforced in the school and the community. Today's children must be able to solve problems so as to have safe but nonetheless exciting and challenging adventures.

The elementary school teacher's responsibility is to instill in pupils attitudes that encourage them to act in the interest of their own safety, that of their families, and that of society. It is not only training in conservation of life and in the prevention of accidents, but also instruction in how to be a good citizen. Other responsibilities of the teacher are to guide the students in molding sound values, to direct their thinking and decision making, and to help them regulate their behavior. Education for the elementary school child is an ongoing process of living, and safety education is a continuous process of conserving children's lives and well-being.

Concern for safety in the classroom and in life should not stifle initiative, adventure, and discovery. Indeed, such concern should evolve opportunities for a more abundant and richer style of living. Freedom from accidents and injuries is part of optimal well-being. Children should develop as many dimensions of themselves as possible. In doing so, they acquire the capacity to function more fully. Safety education provides insurance for children to develop in this direction and should be generated by teachers through the school environment and classroom instruction.

SAFETY AT HOME

Young people are frequently the victims of fire in the home. Because of the high incidence of home fires, it is important that children understand how fires start and how to prevent them.

It takes three things to start a fire: oxygen, heat and combustible material. Since oxygen is part of the environment, the only things that can be controlled are the sources of heat and the combustible materials.

Sources of Heat

Several kinds may be found in the home. *Matches* are present in most homes. One of the most common admonitions children hear is "Don't play with matches." Safety matches cannot be ignited without the striker strip provided. Other matches will strike on any surface.

Lighters can be unpredictable. Even when used properly, they may flare up when ignited. Using a lighter should be left to adults, and the lighter should always be pointed away from faces and clothing when put into use.

The *pilot light* on a stove or heater may not seem dangerous, but it can ignite flammable vapors in the air.

Space heaters, fireplaces, and kitchen stoves produce heat or fire that can spread if combustible material is allowed to come too close to them.

Combustible Materials

The third component of fire is combustible material. Flammable liquids such as gasoline, kerosene, lighter fluid, alcohol-based nail polish remover, and rubber cement; natural and synthetic materials, especially lightweight varieties used in clothing; and upholstered furniture, mattresses, and bedding are frequent fuel for home fires.

Preventing Fires

Here are some basic safety habits that children should learn and share with their families and friends:

1. Don't play with matches.
2. Keep matches away from younger brothers and sisters.
3. If lighter fluid or any flammable liquid spills on you or your clothes, wash it off immediately.
4. Don't get too close to a space heater, fireplace, kitchen stove, or oven.
5. Caution any smokers in your family not to smoke while sitting in upholstered furniture or in bed, especially when sleepy, on medication or on alcohol.
6. Keep clothing, especially sleeves and shirt hems, away from stoves, open flames, heaters, and any other source of heat.
7. Never light a fire in the fireplace or wood-burning stove. Always allow parents to do this.
8. Never lean over a fireplace or put hands inside for warmth.
9. Remind parents to inspect working fireplaces and chimneys frequently and keep them in good condition.

Additional Safety Precautions

Smoke detectors are a good idea for homes; installed and maintained correctly, they can save lives. Students should encourage parents to test smoke detectors once a month to be sure they are in working condition.

Home fire drills are also a good idea. The family should plan escape routes and practice what to do in case the smoke detector goes off. There should be alternate exits planned, as the first choice may be blocked by smoke and/or fire. A meeting place outside the house should be selected where everyone can meet to be sure all family members were able to leave the house. In the event of a fire, it may be necessary to pass through smoke-filled halls. Since smoke rises, safe passage requires keeping close to the floor, perhaps even crawling. If it is necessary to open a door during escape, the door should be felt to see if it is hot to the touch. If it is, fire may be just outside and escape should be made by an alternate route.

Reporting Fires

Students should learn how to report a fire. They should know how to dial the emergency number (often 911) and give the correct address and location of the fire.

First Aid in Fires

There are some important things children should know about helping to reduce the seriousness of burns until professional help can be obtained:

1. If clothing catches fire, do not run. Stop! Drop to the ground and roll back and forth to smother the flames.
2. If the skin is burned, hold the burn under cool running water.
3. Never put grease or butter on a burn or try to clean it.
4. Never pull clothing over a burn or try to remove pieces of clothing sticking to it.
5. Never break burn blisters.
6. A burn should be covered with a clean, dry sheet to protect it.
7. Get the patient to a doctor.

SAFETY ON THE PLAYGROUND

The playground is vital to a child's development. Play is natural to children and it is there that they learn many lessons. Some of these are how to interact with others, to take turns, to share, and to cooperate. Children can make a playground anywhere: at school, at home, or at a friend's house. It is important that they learn what is safe and unsafe behavior at a playground.

The Consumer Product Safety Commission (1984) estimated that about 93,000 people were treated in emergency rooms for injuries associated with playground equipment. Four out of five of these injuries were suffered by children 10 years of age and younger. The causes of the accidents were varied, but seven of 10 injuries were caused by falls, the most common playground accident.

It is natural for children to roughhouse, and this often leads to accidents. It is important to teach safety without dampening imaginative play. Children need to be encouraged with positively presented safety concepts.

The Most Frequent Types of Playground Accidents

Falls accounted for 72 percent of the injuries sustained on *climbing apparatus* such as monkey bars and chinning bars. Most often the victims fell when they slipped, lost their grip, or lost their balance.

Sixty-nine percent of the injuries related to *swings* occurred when children fell or jumped from the swings. In 26 percent, a child was struck by a moving swing.

Falls from *slides* (over the side, from the platform, and from the ladder) accounted for 78 percent of slide-related injuries. These falls were caused by roughhousing, walking up and down the slide, losing the grip, slipping, and losing balance. Other injuries resulted from striking protruding bolts, the side rim and edge, or slipping on the ladder and striking the steps.

Injuries associated with *merry-go-rounds* resulted from falls when the children either lost their grip and were thrown from the apparatus, fell down while pushing it, or fell while riding it.

Seesaw injuries for the most part resulted from falls. Other injuries resulted from being struck by a moving seesaw and long splinters from worn and poorly maintained equipment.

Preventing Playground Accidents

Safety on Swings: Sit in the center of the swing. Never stand or kneel. Hold on with both hands. Stop the swing before getting off. Don't walk too close to a moving swing. Have only one person in one swing at a time. Never swing empty swings or twist swing chains. Never put head and feet through exercise rings on swing sets.

Safety on Slides: Hold on with both hands while going up the steps. Take one step at a time. Never go up the sliding surface or the frame. Slide down feet first, sitting up, one at a time. Be sure no one is in front of the slide before sliding down. Be patient and wait for a turn. Leave the front of the slide after taking a turn. Don't use a metal slide that has been in the sun.

Safety on Climbing Apparatus: Use the correct grip. Use fingers and thumbs for climbing and holding. Use both hands. Watch carefully when climbing down and avoid those climbing up. Avoid having too many people on the equipment at once. Everyone should start at the same end of the equipment and move in the same direction. Stay well behind the person in front and avoid swinging feet. Never use equipment when it is wet. Avoid speed contests and trying to cover too large a distance in one move. Drop from the bars with knees slightly bent and land on both feet.

Safety on Seesaws: Sit facing one another, not leaning back. Keep a firm hold with both hands. Never stand or run on the board. Keep feet from under the board as it goes down. Tell partner before getting off. Never jolt the other person by hitting the ground hard with either end of the board.

SAFETY WITH ROLLER SKATES, BICYCLES, AND SKATEBOARDS
Bicycle Safety

In 1981 more than 549,000 people suffered bicycle injuries serious enough to require treatment in the emergency room. Over 70 percent of these injuries involved children under 15. Bicycles are a major form of transportation for children. It's important for children to understand how bicycle accidents happen and how they can be prevented.

There are *five major ways to get hurt on a bicycle.* The first is collision, either with a car or another bicycle. Collisions happen in one of several ways:

1. *Driveway rideout* occurs when a child rides out of a driveway and is hit by a car. This type accounts for about 8 percent of all collisions between a car and a bike.
2. *Running a stop sign* occurs when a bicyclist runs a stop sign. Most of those who get hit riding through stop signs knew they were supposed to stop. They just didn't understand why, didn't feel like stopping, or got distracted. About 10 percent of car-with-bike crashes occur this way.
3. *Turning without warning* occurs when a rider makes a left turn without looking behind for traffic or signaling their intention. This type accounts for another 10 percent of all crashes between bikes and cars.
4. *Nighttime riding* is a risk factor. Certain types of accidents occur most often after dark. A car may come up behind a rider to overtake and instead hit the bicycle and rider. These can be very serious crashes. They account for about 25 percent of fatal car-with-bike collisions. Although most of these accidents involve older riders, children riding bicycles at night should learn to be cautious.
5. *Following the leader* is a dangerous game. Many collisions between cars and bikes occur when children are following each other. The leader may run a stop sign and

get through but the second one gets hit. This is very difficult to counter; children should be urged to watch out for their own safety and everyone's when riding in groups.

Loss of control is the second major cause of bicycling injuries. Faulty brakes; riding too large a bicycle; riding double (for example, on a banana seat, rear fender, handlebars or the horizontal top bar on a boy's bike); stunting; hitting a hole, bump, or other obstacle have all been implicated.

Getting the feet, hands, or clothing caught in the bicycle is the third major cause of these injuries.

The fourth major cause of injuries during bike riding stems from *mechanical and structural problems*. These include brake failure, wobbling or disengagement of the wheel or steering mechanism, difficulty in shifting gears, chain slippage, pedals falling off, and frame breakage.

The final major cause of bicycling injuries is when the *rider's foot slips from one or both pedals, resulting in loss of control*.

To prevent bicycle-related injuries, children need to learn and obey traffic laws. They also need to be taught how to select, maintain, and store a bike.

Here are some tips for bicycle safety:

Know and obey traffic laws and signals. The laws that govern automobiles also apply to bicyclists. Bike riders must show the same courtesy they hope drivers will show them. Always yield the right of way to cars and pedestrians. Be alert for people stepping out from between parked cars. Be prepared to use the bell or horn as a warning, but always be ready to yield. Always stop at stop signs and traffic lights. Know and use hand signals. Always check behind when making a left turn. Walk the bicycle when crossing busy streets. Look carefully in all directions when riding out of driveways.

Don't ride a bike if it is not in *good working condition*.

Ride near the curb in the same direction as traffic. Always ride single file. Don't travel on routes with high-speed or *heavy traffic*. Look for safer, less traveled routes.

Don't stunt or clown on a bicycle. This can result in serious injury. Bikes are fun, but safety is serious business.

Avoid playing *follow the leader* on your bike.
Never *carry a passenger*.
Use a basket or carrier for packages.

Be alert to the *condition of riding surfaces* and what's happening around you. Watch for sewer grates, potholes, rocks, and other bad surface conditions, which can easily throw the best riders. Ride slowly enough to avoid unexpected obstacles such as car doors opening suddenly, or cars backing out of driveways or parking lots.

Avoid *riding in wet weather*. It's hard for cars to see bicyclists in the rain. Wet tires can skid and wet handbrakes may not stop the bike.

Be cautious when *riding at night*. If it's necessary to ride at dusk or in darkness, make sure the lights and reflectors are in good working order. Wear white or light-colored clothing and ride slowly. Reflector tape on clothing also improves visibility.

Avoid skidding. Slow down on rough or slippery roads and when riding downhill. Watch for loose sand and gravel.

Helmets save lives. About 75 percent of bicycle fatalities are from head injuries. Many other people are handicapped as a result of hitting their heads. The cost of a helmet ($25 to $35) is small when compared with that of a head injury. Hard-shell helmets are recommended.

Bicycle fits rider. The rider should be able to straddle the seat with both feet flat on the ground, and with no less than a one-inch clearance between the frame's top tube (on a boy's bike) and the rider's crotch. The rule to buy a bicycle that fits today. Some bikes were manufactured and sold before current guidelines went into effect. Students should watch for these older bikes and the following hazards: sharp edges; a bent or broken frame; protrusions above the top frame or between the seat and the handlebars; faulty brakes; a non-derailleur bike without a chain guard; a bike without reflectors or lights; and tires with thin tread and cracked surfaces or sidewalls.

Maintaining the bike is essential to safety. While most children don't have the skills to repair their own bicycles, they should be aware when something needs repair and alert their parents. It's recommended that bicycles have a tune-up and safety check at least once a year.

Bicycles should be stored indoors to prevent rust and to keep all parts in order. Keeping a bicycle inside also helps prevent theft of the bike.

Roller Skate Safety

Roller skating is very popular with children, but they can fall hard while learning to skate. In 1981 approximately 189,000 persons required emergency room treatment for roller skating injuries. Following are some of the major causes of roller skating accidents:

1. Poor or uneven surface. Cracked or uneven cement sidewalk or street, rocks, tree branches, and other debris can cause tripping or skidding.
2. Structural problems in the skates, for example, a loose axle or wheel.
3. The human factor can play a major role. This includes skating too close to other skaters, inexperience with the skates or doing trick skating, horseplay and pushing, lack of attention, misusing the skates (for example, going up and down stairs with skates on).
4. Roller skating in traffic.

To prevent skating accidents, it is important to learn to select skates properly and to use them properly. Always buy or rent skates that fit well. Buy them for the size the child is now, not to grow into. Check for sharp points and edges that can cut in the event of a fall.

In using roller skates, these points should be kept in mind:

1. Learn to perform basic skating maneuvers well before attempting more complicated ones.
2. Check the skating surface carefully before and while skating. Avoid uneven or broken pavement and branches or rocks in the skating path.

3. Don't roller skate in the streets unless they are closed to traffic to allow skating.
4. Don't hitch a ride while roller skating.
5. Wear safety equipment, such as protective knee and elbow pads, when roller skating. This can help prevent serious injuries. Other equipment includes wrist braces, helmet, and mouth guard, which may prevent knocked-out or broken teeth.
6. Learn how to fall in case of an accident. Try to roll onto fleshy parts of the body such as the buttocks, upper legs, and shoulders. Try to relax rather than going stiff.

Keep roller skates in good condition. Make sure the wheels and straps are in good condition. Keep skates dry and clean. Lubricate them when needed. Keep skates in a dry place away from moisture, which can rust the skates.

Skateboard Safety

Skateboards can be a lot of fun, but skateboarding is dangerous unless precautions are taken. Selecting a proper skateboard is important. Skateboards come in many shapes, sizes, and colors. There is no rule about what is best. Before buying one, gather as much information as possible. Visit stores where skateboards are sold and look at several kinds. Go to a library and read magazines or books on skateboarding.

There are several points to keep in mind when riding the skateboard:

1. Use protective equipment. Closed-toe non-slip shoes as well as helmets, gloves, and padding can reduce the number and severity of injuries.
2. Check the riding surface for holes, bumps, rocks, and other obstacles.
3. Avoid riding in the street.
4. Never hitch a ride from a car or bicycle.
5. Only allow one person on a skateboard at a time.
6. Learn how to fall. This reduces the chances of being severely injured. (See

Roller Skating Safety, above, for details on falling.)

As with all recreational equipment, proper maintenance is important to help make skate-boarding safe. Make sure all parts of the skate-board are in good condition and that nothing is broken, bent, or cracked. Keep skateboard in a dry place to prevent rust and warping of the board.

THREE-WHEEL ATVs

Many families allow their children to ride three-wheelers just as though they were bicycles. Three wheel motor bicycles are called all-terrain vehicles [ATVs] because they can climb up and down all kinds of land terrains. Research shows that these vehicles are extremely hazardous for all ages. They can flip over and cause death, spinal injuries, and permanent disabilities. One driver is injured for every 100 drivers. Since 1980 a total of 640 drivers have been killed—20 per month. There were also 7,000 injuries per month in 1986.

The best safety precaution for ATVs is not to drive or ride one. Elementary school teachers have an obligation to educate both children and their parents about the dangers of ATVs which have proven to be unsafe for persons of all ages.

POISON PREVENTION

The Food and Drug Administration's National Clearinghouse for Poison Control Centers estimates that accidents involving hazardous substances occur to 500,000 children annually. Most poisonings involve preschool children, but there are many hazards to older children as well. It is important for children to understand the sources of poisonous substances in their environments and to know how to avoid accidental poisoning.

There are *three types of poisoning:* drug poisoning, usually from an accidental overdose; household chemical poisoning; and vapor poisoning.

Preventing Drug Poisoning

Overdoses, especially of aspirin, tranquilizers, and iron tablets, kill more children than any other drugs. It is important to teach children the proper attitudes about drugs. They should be taught that medicine is not food or drink. They should understand that pills are not candy, and cough syrups are not syrup for pancakes or waffles even though they look and flow like these substances. No one should use or give another person someone else's medicine. Medicine should always be taken and administered in a lighted room and all instructions should be carefully followed.

Preventing Household Chemical Poisoning

In the home, poisonous substances are stored mainly in the bathroom, kitchen, garage, basement, and storage areas. Children should understand that the substances kept in these storage areas are for special purposes and not for human consumption. A good rule is "always ask first" before eating or drinking anything.

Preventing Vapor Poisoning

Children and adults are often victims of poisoning from vapors in the air. When sprays are being used around the house, keep other people out of the area. These sprays should never be allowed into the eyes or the lungs.

What To Do If Someone Is Poisoned

Students should learn basic emergency and first aid procedures as part of their health studies. For third and fourth graders, getting an adult is the emergency procedure. Some fifth and sixth graders can learn the emergency number for the paramedics. It is important to try to stay calm and act quickly if poisoning is suspected.

SUMMARY: IMPLICATIONS FOR TEACHERS

Although teachers cannot teach all aspects of safety to a child, they should cover major safety topics in the classroom. Although developing skateboard skills is out of the realm of most teachers, all elementary school teachers should teach their students how to fall correctly in physical education (tumbling) classes. This will prepare children to fall safely. Routine school fire drills should produce skills that the child takes home for instituting home fire drills. A simple first aid and safety course provided by the teacher in the school is the best safety and health insurance that a child and parents can receive. The *classroom teacher has three major responsibilities:* to impart information about safety, to develop physical and cognitive safety skills, and to maintain a safe physical environment in the school.

LESSON PLANS

In light of this discussion peruse the following lesson plans, keeping in mind that they are the type you will likely be expected to implement in your classroom. Remember that they by no means encompass a complete unit of instruction. They are simply a basis for the formation of a comprehensive unit.

TOPIC: CROSSING THE STREET SAFELY

Grade Level: Primary

Concept: It is important to stop, look, and listen before crossing the street.

Expected Pupil Outcome: The student will be able to cross the street safely.

Content

1. Stop
   a) At crosswalk
   b) On curb
   c) For green light
2. Look—all four ways
3. Listen—for cars
4. Walk
   a) Use crosswalk
   b) Keep to right
   c) When crosswalk is clear

Learning Experiences

1. *Demonstration—simulation:* An intersection is laid out in the classroom using masking tape. Pupils simulate crossing under different traffic conditions: no cars present, cars present, traffic lights, and patrol person (Figure 21.1).

   Teacher explains briefly how to cross a street safely, while a student demonstrates.

   Students take turns crossing street alone, then in twos.

   A signal light should be introduced. Children cross when the light is green.

   Have three to five students put on a large paper picture of a car and simulate car traffic. Children practice crossing street with simulated traffic.

2. *Practice crossing the street.* After practicing inside, students should try to cross a real street with adult supervision.

Evaluation Procedures   Teacher observes students during demonstration/simulation session and corrects any mistakes. After the practice session, the students proceed to real street corner and cross the street safely with adult supervision. If students do well, the objective will be accomplished.

FIGURE 21.1
Steps for practice session for safety in crossing streets.

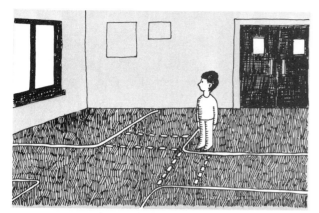

(a) Crossing street by yourself

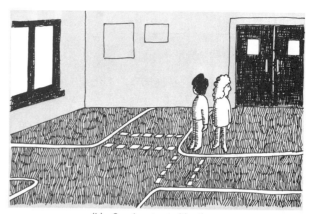

(b) Crossing street with others

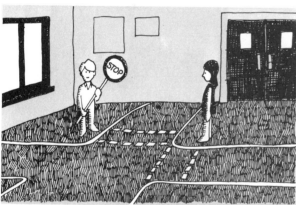

(c) Crossing street with patrol boy

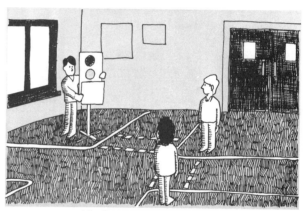

(d) Crossing street with signal lights

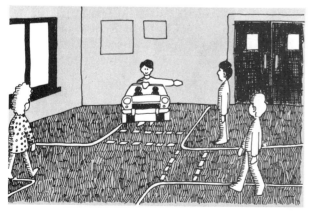

(e) Crossing street with traffic

TOPIC: MAINTAINING A SAFE BICYCLE

Grade Level: Intermediate

Concept: A bicycle in good working order is an important safety measure (Figure 21.2).

Expected Pupil Outcome: The student will be able to describe how to keep a bicycle in good working condition.

Content: Ways of keeping bicycle in good working order:
1. Handlebars
   a) Keep tightened
   b) Adjust to appropriate level

Learning Experiences

1. *Demonstration Skill Discussion:* Have several pupils bring their bicycles into class and have them identify the parts, by name, and describe how to care for each part.

FIGURE 21.2
Parts and their location on a bicycle and suggestions for maintaining a bicycle in good working order.

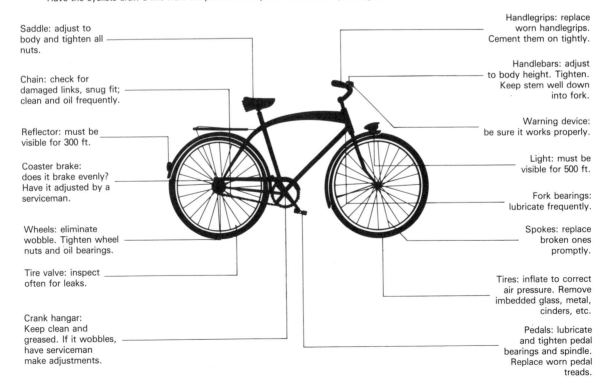

WHAT'S YOUR BIKE MAINTENANCE RATING?

Have the cyclists draw a line from the printed description to the arrow pointing to the corresponding part on the bike drawing

Saddle: adjust to body and tighten all nuts.

Chain: check for damaged links, snug fit; clean and oil frequently.

Reflector: must be visible for 300 ft.

Coaster brake: does it brake evenly? Have it adjusted by a serviceman.

Wheels: eliminate wobble. Tighten wheel nuts and oil bearings.

Tire valve: inspect often for leaks.

Crank hangar: Keep clean and greased. If it wobbles, have serviceman make adjustments.

Handlegrips: replace worn handlegrips. Cement them on tightly.

Handlebars: adjust to body height. Tighten. Keep stem well down into fork.

Warning device: be sure it works properly.

Light: must be visible for 500 ft.

Fork bearings: lubricate frequently.

Spokes: replace broken ones promptly.

Tires: inflate to correct air pressure. Remove imbedded glass, metal, cinders, etc.

Pedals: lubricate and tighten pedal bearings and spindle. Replace worn pedal treads.

2. Saddle
   a) Tilt upward in front
   b) Adjust to body height
   c) Tighten all nuts
3. Wheels
   a) Run freely
   b) Spokes straight
   c) No wobble
   d) Oil bearings
4. Reflector—visible for 300 ft.
5. Brake
   a) Quick
   b) Even
6. Chain
   a) Fits snuggly
   b) Links in good condition
   c) Cleaned and oiled frequently
7. Pedal
   a) Tread in good condition
   b) Lubricate and tighten pedal bearings and spindle
8. Tires
   a) Inflate to correct air pressure
   b) Remove foreign objects
9. Spokes—replace broken ones
10. Light—visible for 500 ft.
11. Warning device—horn or bell in working order
12. Frame—clean

2. Have students take the bike quiz (see Figure 21.3).

FIGURE 21.3
Identifying parts of a bicycle. (Adapted from "Bike Quiz Guide," Bicycle Institute of America.)

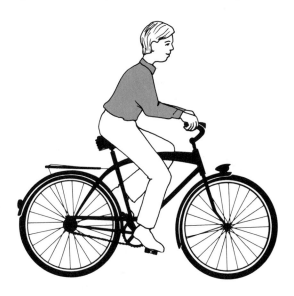

Evaluation Procedures If the students, on the average, can answer 80 percent of the questions correctly, the objective will be accomplished.

TOPIC: RULES FOR SAFE BICYCLE RIDING

Grade Level: Intermediate

Concept: Abiding by safe bicycling rules makes good sense.

**Expected Pupil
Outcome:** The student will be able to state the rules for safe bicycle riding.

Content: Basic bicycle rules of the road:
1. Always ride with the traffic.
2. Ride on the right side of the road.
3. Never hitch a ride.
4. Walk your bike across busy intersections.
5. Ride single file.
6. Don't carry riders.
7. Yield right of way to pedestrians.
8. Do not carry anything in your hands.
9. Keep both hands on the handlebars.
10. Give proper arm signals.
11. Look before changing direction or lane.
12. Obey all traffic signals.
13. Have bicycle inspected for safety twice a year (bike in good condition).
14. Adjust speed to road conditions, weather, traffic, and experience as a rider.
15. Select the safest route to your destination— avoid busy streets and intersections.

Learning Experiences
1. *Picture simulation* of traffic situations. Students pick out what the bicycle rider is doing right or wrong. *Film strip: Perception of Driving Hazards, Urban and Suburban,* by Shell Oil Company.
2. Quiz: Administer bicycle riding in traffic quiz—or—bike riding quiz.

Evaluation Procedures If the class averages 80 percent correct responses on the quiz, the objective will be considered attained.

Quiz on Bicycle Riding in Traffic *Directions:* Circle the letter of the answer that you think *best* answers the statement.
1. When riding a bike at night
   a) Lights in front and back are necessary
   b) A front light and a back reflector are necessary
   c) Only a front light is necessary
   d) Only a back reflector is necessary
2. When making a right turn on your bike, you should
   a) Make the turn from the left lane
   b) Make the turn from the right lane
   c) Ignore the lanes because you are on a bike
3. While riding your bike, you may
   a) Carry a rider if he or she is not too heavy
   b) Carry a rider only when you have a luggage rack
   c) Never carry a rider
   d) Carry a rider on the handlebars

4. If you come to an intersection marked "no left turn," the sign
   a) Applies to cars only and not to bikes
   b) Applies to bikes as well as cars
   c) Can be ignored if there are no cars coming
5. A bike rider in heavy traffic should
   a) Make a hand signal, then turn left
   b) Make a hand signal and make the turn at same time
   c) Force the traffic to stop so that you can make the left turn
6. Signaling to stop is
   a) Helpful but is not always necessary for bike riders
   b) Necessary to let other drivers know what you are going to do
   c) Not necessary because cars pay little attention to bikers
7. When passing a slow-moving car, you should
   a) Go on the sidewalk to pass car
   b) Pass car on the left side
   c) Pass car on the right side
   d) Never pass a car
8. A bike rider should
   a) Always keep both hands on the handlebars
   b) Keep both hands on the handlebars except when carrying things
   c) Keep both hands on the handlebars except when signaling
9. You should
   a) Hitch a ride on a car or truck only if it is going slow
   b) Never hitch a ride on a car or truck
   c) Hitch a ride if you have a strong rope or chain
10. When riding in the street, a group of riders should
    a) Ride double file
    b) Ride single file
    c) Weave across the lanes

Bike Riding Quiz   The correct answers to these 50 true or false questions are circled.

1. A bicycle is considered a vehicle and should be ridden on the right-hand side of the street.   (T) F

2. Bicycle riders should observe and obey all traffic signs, stop signs, and signals and other traffic control devices.   T (F)

3. Bike riders should try to crowd ahead between cars at a stop light so they can be in front when the light changes.   T (F)

4. Pedestrians do not have the right of way on sidewalks or crosswalks.   T (F)

5. The signal for a right turn is extending the right arm straight out.   T (F)

6. Night riding without a white headlight and red taillight or reflector is unsafe.   (T) F

7. Bicycle riders hitching a ride on another vehicle can easily have an accident.   (T) F

8. It is safe and proper for a bike rider to carry a passenger.   T Ⓕ

9. A bike in poor mechanical condition is safe if the rider is skilled.   T Ⓕ

10. It is safe to ride bikes three abreast when riding in a group.   T Ⓕ

11. The roadway is a safe place to park your bike.   T Ⓕ

12. Bikes should be inspected twice a year by a reliable service person.   Ⓣ F

13. The headlight of a bicycle should be seen from at least 500 ft.   Ⓣ F

14. Riding single file is the sensible thing to do.   Ⓣ F

15. The proper way to make a left turn is to cut the corner.   T Ⓕ

16. It is safe to enter the street from the sidewalk without first seeing whether a car is coming.   T Ⓕ

17. When passing a slow-moving car going in the same direction, you should pass to the left.   Ⓣ F

18. Bicyclists should keep to the right while riding in the street.   Ⓣ F

19. Bike riders should give hand signals when stopping or turning.   Ⓣ F

20. Hitching a ride on another vehicle is safe if the rider is careful.   T Ⓕ

21. An icy or slippery street is a dangerous place to ride a bike.   Ⓣ F

22. A bike rider should look only straight ahead when crossing an intersection.   T Ⓕ

23. It is safe for two people to be on a bike if one is on the handlebars.   T Ⓕ

24. Cyclists should ride at least three feet away from parked cars.   Ⓣ F

25. On country roads cyclists should keep to the left, same as pedestrians.   T Ⓕ

26. Broken or loose spokes should be replaced immediately.   Ⓣ F

27. Pedals should not be worn or broken.   Ⓣ F

28. A broken coaster brake can be easily fixed at home.   T Ⓕ

29. Handlebars should be loose so you can change riding positions.   T Ⓕ

30. Your chain should be loose enough to slip off easily.   T (F)

31. The whole bicycle should be cleaned and oiled occasionally.   (T) F

32. Saddle and handlebars should be adjusted to your height.   (T) F

33. Riding bikes off curbs doesn't damage the bikes.   T (F)

34. It is permissible to ride small children in baskets.   T (F)

35. Persons riding bikes are subject to the same traffic laws that govern automobile drivers.   (T) F

36. Blue is a good color to wear when biking after dark.   T (F)

37. It is not necessary to stop at intersections if there is no traffic.   T (F)

38. You can drive a bike, but not a car, in either direction on a one-way street.   T (F)

39. There is danger of skidding on curves even if the road is not wet.   (T) F

40. If you live in the country, you can ride on either side of the road.   T (F)

41. Even a skilled bike rider should walk his or her bike through heavy traffic.   (T) F

42. If you don't ride on busy streets, you don't need a horn or bell.   T (F)

43. Cyclists have the right of way over pedestrians.   T (F)

44. The faster you ride, the safer it is.   T (F)

45. A warped wheel rim can cause an accident.   (T) F

46. When riding at night, ride to the left so you can see approaching headlights.   T (F)

47. A good bicycle really never needs greasing and oiling.   T (F)

48. A loose saddle is a potential danger to the cyclist.   (T) F

49. It is a bad idea to wax the metal finish of your bike.   T (F)

50. When cycling, you should pay strict attention to what you're doing.   (T) F

REFERENCES AND BIBLIOGRAPHY

Accident Facts, 1986 edition. (Chicago: National Safety Council, 1986).

Bike Safety Pamphlet. (San Diego, CA: San Diego Fire Department).

California Driver's Handbook. (Sacramento, 1986).

Consumer Product Safety Commission, *It's No Accident.* (Washington, D.C.: CPSC, 1984).

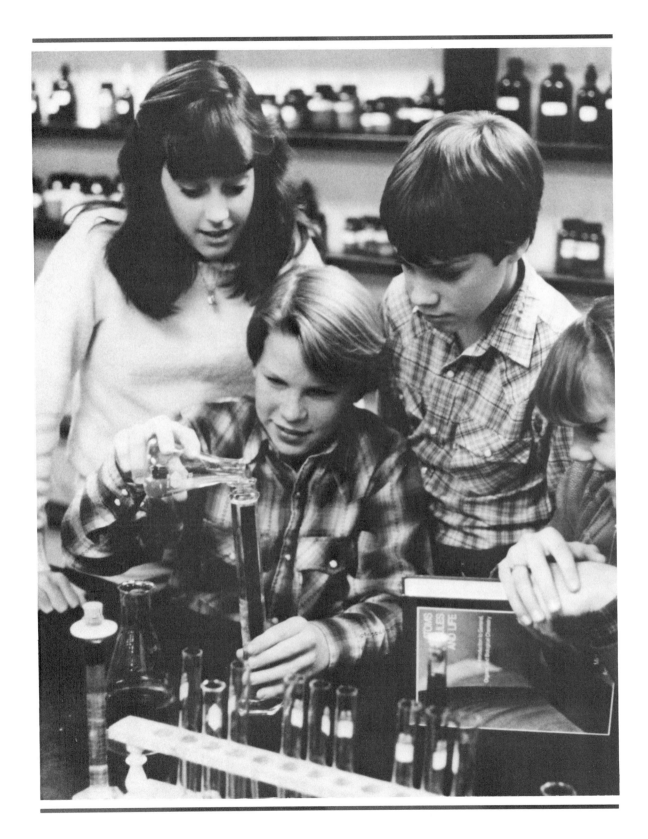

Chapter 22

Teaching About Illness and Disease

INTRODUCTION

Today complete freedom from disease and illness is a dream. However great the benefits of progress, improved sanitation, regular medical care, and a high standard of living, they do not ensure freedom from disease. Children are especially susceptible to infections and ailments.

Almost 50 percent of childhood diseases are respiratory. The common cold, influenza, measles, mumps, diphtheria, and strep throat are just a few of the common infections from which children suffer. Children react emotionally to such infections. They become disabled physiologically and their social life is disrupted. They respond with fear and anxiety, which disrupt learning as well as overall development. Children need help in allaying such emotional stresses. Hence teachers need to be aware that children need not only immunization against diseases, but also general information about illnesses and diseases, how to care for oneself during illness, and how to keep from getting sick.

Illness and disease, like well-being, are cultural concepts, and are interpreted through society's value system. For example, whether one takes a cold to bed or disregards the cold in his or her daily routine is directed by one's cultural perception of illness. Cultural evaluation varies, and we find a great deal of confusion over what disease, infection, and disorder are. The distinctions are discussed below.

For most people, life consists of extended periods of wellness punctuated by occasional illness. It would be foolish to pretend that you will never become sick or that diseases do not exist. Health is achieved not only by preventing illnesses but by having a good attitude during sickness and injury.

Attitudes toward illness are very important. Anger and frustration are common responses to sickness or injury. Some people get angry at their bodies for failing to function or they become frustrated that they are unable to do all the things they want to do. But there are other, more positive ways to deal with illness. One way is to regard times of sickness as unavoidable parts of living. Another way is to recognize that sickness or injury can be your body's way of telling you that you need rest—that perhaps you have been pushing yourself too hard. Yet another is to use periods of illness to reexamine the stresses and habits that may contribute to susceptibility to sickness. Viewed positively, many illnesses may become more tolerable. And by reducing anger, frustration, and worry, you can speed the healing process.

DISTINGUISHING BETWEEN ILLNESS AND DISEASE

There are a number of important distinctions between illness and disease. Illness is felt, whereas disease is diagnosed by the physician. A person may "feel ill" without a disease in evidence; a person may have a disease without any illness or suffering. Millions of Americans have the disease high blood pressure, which may be symptomless until a heart attack occurs. A common example of illness without disease is low back pain. About 5 percent of working Americans suffer from low back pain and about two of every hundred of those are disabled by persistent pain (Williams, 1983). Doctors are rarely able to diagnose any disease or identify a medical cause of pain. The treatment most commonly recommended is aspirin and bed rest to allow the lesion to heal. Hadler (1986) shows that "more than 80 percent of patients will be well or much better within two weeks."

Reading (1977) describes the distinction between illness and disease:

Illness tends to be used to refer to what is wrong with the patient, disease to what is wrong with his body. Illness is what the patient suffers from, what troubles him, what he complains of, and what prompts him to seek medical attention. Illness refers to the patient's experience of ill-health. It comprises

Much of the material in this chapter is from Gordon Edlin and Eric Golanty, *Health & Wellness, A Holistic Approach*, Third Edition. (Boston: Jones & Bartlett Publishers, 1988).

his impaired sense of well-being, his perception that something is wrong with his body, and his various symptoms of pain, distress, and disablement. Disease, on the other hand, refers to various structural disorders of the individual's tissues and organs that give rise to the signs of ill health.

The onset and severity of any illness can be affected by the ways in which a person deals with it. If you become angry or depressed at being sick or excessively concerned about the outcome of the illness, you can interfere with the body's ability to heal. Disturbed emotions may lower resistance to disease by reducing the immunological responsiveness of the body (Chapter 3). Stress and worry can also produce physiological changes that interfere with the natural healing mechanisms of the body and contribute to illness and disease. As Thomas (1979) suggests, worrying about health is not healthy:

Far from being ineptly put together, [people] are amazingly tough, durable organisms, full of health, ready for most contingencies. The new danger to our well-being . . . is in becoming a nation of healthy hypochondriacs, living gingerly, worrying ourselves half to death.

Optimism can reduce the severity of illness and disease as well as one's susceptibility to becoming sick.

CAUSES OF DISEASE

Traditionally, medical practitioners refer to diseases as resulting from specific causes. The cause of a disease is its *etiology*. For example, specific bacteria are said to cause pneumonia or gonorrhea; certain viruses are said to cause measles, mumps, and hepatitis; a broken leg may have been caused by a fall.

Few diseases have a single cause. Whether or not a person gets sick depends on a wide range of modifying factors (Figure 22.1). Dubos (1968) points out that:

all manifestations of human disease are the consequence of the interplay between body, mind and environment. This situation creates a difficult dilemma for physicians and medical scientists. They recognize that the analytic breakdown of the problems of disease into their component parts never results in a true picture; yet they know from practical experience that the artificial reduction of these problems into their constituent parts, or their conversion into simpler models, is an absolute necessity for scientific progress.

The common cold, one of the most widespread human diseases, involves infection of the upper respiratory tract (nose and throat) by any one of hundreds of different cold viruses (see

FIGURE 22.1

Various internal and external factors determine whether or not disease results from infections by viruses, bacteria, fungi, worms, protozoa, and other kinds of infectious agents.

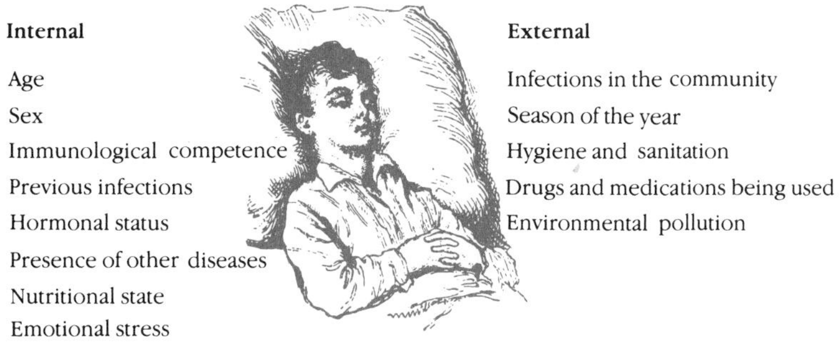

Internal	External
Age	Infections in the community
Sex	Season of the year
Immunological competence	Hygiene and sanitation
Previous infections	Drugs and medications being used
Hormonal status	Environmental pollution
Presence of other diseases	
Nutritional state	
Emotional stress	

THE COMMON COLD

Virtually everybody catches a cold sometime or other. Schoolchildren may contract as many as a dozen colds a year. It is estimated that 100 million serious colds occur each year in the U.S., causing 30 million days lost at school and work. Sales of over-the-counter cold remedies (which do not cure colds but may relieve symptoms) amount to about $1 billion annually. The common cold is clearly something that everyone prefers not to catch or to suffer from.

In 1914 a German scientist, W. Von Kause, first proposed that colds are caused by viruses. However, an actual cold virus (adenovirus R-167) wasn't isolated until 1953. Finally, in 1985, a detailed three-dimensional picture of a cold virus was obtained by using high-energy x-rays. Despite these major advances in cold virus research, a cure for the common cold is still not in sight. Even the development of a vaccine that would prevent colds is doubtful because of the large number of different viruses that can cause colds and the ease with which cold viruses change their antigenic properties.

Six major classes of cold viruses—rhinoviruses, coronaviruses, adenoviruses, myxoviruses, paramyxoviruses, and coxsackieviruses—have been identified. Within the rhinovirus class alone more than 120 different types have been observed. To prevent infection by all 120, many vaccines would have to be developed and administered. Scientists hope to find some common feature shared by most of the cold viruses so that a single vaccine could prevent most colds. However, this prospect is quite remote and may not be possible.

New evidence shows that most colds are not transmitted through the air by sneezing or coughing but by hand-to-hand contact. Infected persons have viruses on their hands and transfer viruses to others by hand-to-hand contact. The second person becomes infected by touching his or her nose with a hand or contaminated object. Frequent washing of hands when around people with colds may reduce chances of catching a cold.

The idea that cold, damp weather or drafts predispose people to catching cold has been disproved in numerous experiments. Volunteers who are deliberately infected with cold viruses and then placed in a cold damp room for two to three hours did not catch cold more easily than a control group. Recent experiments show that a nasal spray containing alpha-interferon can reduce the chances of catching a cold if the nasal spray is used just prior to exposure. The problem with interferon is that it is a potent drug and its safety has not been demonstrated, especially in children, and for the drug to be effective, you would have to spray interferon into your nose daily, since you never know when or where you may become exposed to cold viruses.

The unfortunate conclusion is that a cure for the common cold is uncertain, certainly years in the future.

box, above) yet the presence of a virus does not always cause a cold. In experiments with volunteer subjects in which suspensions of cold virus were sprayed into the nose and throat, not everyone in the study developed symptoms. For a variety of reasons some persons were more resistant to the virus than others.

Similarly, the cause of tuberculosis is not simply the presence of the infecting organism, *Mycobacterium tuberculosis*. Tuberculosis was one of the leading causes of death in the United States at the turn of the century, but today few deaths are attributed to tuberculosis even though the bacterium has not disappeared from the environment. Robert Koch, a famous microbiologist of the nineteenth century, called TB "the disease of poverty" because it tended to be associated with squalor, overcrowding, poor nutrition, and poor sanitation. Many persons today have small tubercular lesions in their lungs, yet they never have any symptoms of illness because poverty, poor nutrition, and an unwholesome environment are as much the "causes" of TB as are bacteria.

Discussing a disease in terms of a single cause is mostly a matter of convenience; many factors contribute to the initiation and course of a disease. It is possible, however, to classify diseases according to the *principal* factor causing them. The principal factors accounting for nearly all disease are (1) heredity, (2) infectious organisms, (3) lifestyle and personal habits, (4) accidents, and (5) poisons and toxic chemicals.

Keep in mind that with rare exceptions, anyone can influence the development of a disease for better or worse. Disease disrupts a person's balance of body, mind, and spirit and interactions with other people. Whatever can be done to restore harmony can help cure most diseases and reestablish health.

INHERITED (GENETIC) DISEASES

About 5 percent of human beings are born with hereditary defects that result in anatomical or physiological abnormalities; these inherited abnormalities are called *genetic diseases.* They result from anomalies in the physical structure of a person's chromosomes, the microscopic structures that contain all the hereditary material (DNA). Changes in the genetic material result from *mutations;* many environmental substances, such as chemicals, x-rays, and atomic radiation can increase the probability of mutations.

Altogether, about 3,000 human genetic diseases resulting from single gene defects have been identified; most, fortunately, are quite rare. Some of the better-known ones are listed in Table 22.1. Serious genetic defects often do not permit the fetus to survive to birth and are the cause of as many as half of all spontaneous abortions (miscarriages).

In order to assign a disease or defect to genetic causes, at least one of three criteria must be met: (1) The disease must show a pattern of inheritance from generation to generation according to the laws of Mendel. (2) The chromosomes of cells in affected individuals must show some observable abnormality. (3) A basic biochemical defect, such as the loss of an essential enzyme, must be demonstrated in cells of the affected individual.

Sometimes a particular disease is said to run in the family. This means that there is a higher frequency of that disease among closely related persons than in the general population. This is called a *familial pattern.* Such diseases are not necessarily due to genetic anomalies; they may be due to some factor in the family's environment. This is an exceedingly important point. People

TABLE 22.1
Some Relatively Frequent Human Genetic Diseases

Genetic Disease	Major Consequences	Genetic Disease	Major Consequences
Albinism	Disturbed vision	Hemophilia	Bleeding—blood does not clot
Phenylketonuria	Mental retardation		
Alkaptonuria	Arthritis	Lesch-Nyhan syndrome	Mental retardation, self-mutilation
Galactosemia	Cataracts, mental retardation	Cystic fibrosis	Respiratory disorders
Porphyria	Abdominal pain, psychosis	Pituitary dwarfism	Short stature
		Hurler's syndrome	Coarse facial features, mental retardation
Homocystinuria	Mental retardation		
Down's syndrome (mongolism)	Mental retardation	Xeroderma pigmentosum	Skin cancers
Tay-Sachs disease	Neurological deterioration	Agammaglobulinemia	Defective immune response
Retinoblastoma	Blindness	Myotonic dystrophy	Progressive muscular weakening
Sickle-cell anemia	Blood disorder		
		Turner's syndrome	Sterility
		Klinefelter's syndrome	Sterility

who are told that a disease is familial and believe that it is inherited often feel they are doomed to get it even though they have no symptoms; believing a disease is genetic can lead to unnecessary feelings of hopelessness and worry that can undermine one's health.

Many common diseases in our society are regarded as hereditary or as having a strong genetic basis even though the disease does not follow any of the rules for inheritance. Examples of diseases with familial patterns are allergies, alcoholism, schizophrenia, diabetes, rheumatoid arthritis, hypertension, and even some rare forms of cancer, but it is incorrect to regard these as genetic diseases in the same sense as those listed in Table 22.1. These diseases are caused by complex interactions of the genes with the environment, and they can be started and affected by nutrition, stress, emotions, hormones, drugs, and other environmental factors. From the standpoint of personal health, it is advisable not to accept a genetic explanation for a disease unless the scientific evidence is unambiguous.

Doctors and other medical scientists sometimes refer to a person's *genetic susceptibility,* meaning that one's overall genetic makeup may make one prone to a particular disease. The term can lead to confusion if a person believes a genetic disease is involved. Many people think of diseases in absolute terms—either one's genes or the environment is at fault. However, the expression of genes is always influenced to some degree by both internal and external environments.

For example, not everyone who smokes two to three packs of cigarettes a day for many years will die of lung cancer. From this fact, some people (especially those who are employed by tobacco companies) would like to argue that cigarette smoking is a relatively harmless habit and that those persons who do contract lung cancer were genetically susceptible in the first place. A similar deceptive argument has been used to support the notion that exposure to radiation and radioactivity is safer for some people than for others because people vary genetically in their ability to repair radiation-damaged cells. To push this kind of argument into absurdity, one could argue that people over seven feet tall

are genetically defective and prone to head injury since they are more likely to hit their heads on doorways and low-hanging objects.

The point is that the environmental factor in question is hazardous, whether it is cigarette smoke, radiation, or low doorways. The fact that people respond differently to these items does not mean that they are genetically handicapped in any way. Each of us can choose and change our environment; we cannot choose or change our genes.

Prenatal Detection of Hereditary Defects

Prevention of hereditary diseases and prenatal detection of genetic defects are important goals of modern medicine. Genetic counseling of parents who are at risk for bearing a child with a hereditary disease can help them reduce their chances of having a genetically handicapped child. Already several hundred hereditary human diseases can be detected by *amniocentesis* and more are being added yearly (Figure 22.2). This prenatal diagnostic procedure is used to test for genetic and developmental defects in the fetus. Around the fifteenth week of pregnancy, a sample of amniotic fluid is removed; fetal cells cultured from this fluid are subjected to various tests, including visual examination (karyotyping) of the chromosomes. Amniocentesis also determines the sex of the fetus, although in the United States it is never performed solely for this purpose.

Inserting a needle into the amniotic sac to remove fluid entails a small but finite risk to the fetus; therefore, amniocentesis is generally recommended only in the following situations: (1) The pregnant woman is 35 or older or the father is over 50. (2) The couple have had a previous child with a chromosomal abnormality or neural tube defect. (3) The pregnant woman may be a carrier of a deleterious X-linked trait. (4) Both parents are known to be carriers of recessive genes that cause a hereditary disease or one parent is a carrier of an abnormal dominant gene.

FIGURE 22.2

In the diagnostic procedure called amniocentesis, a sample of the fluid that surrounds the developing fetus is collected. Both the fluid sample and the fetal cells it contains are then analyzed for biochemical or chromosomal defects. Amniocentesis is performed early in pregnancy, whenever possible, so that the parents can decide whether to continue the pregnancy or abort the fetus. The decision is generally made after discussion and counseling with their physician.

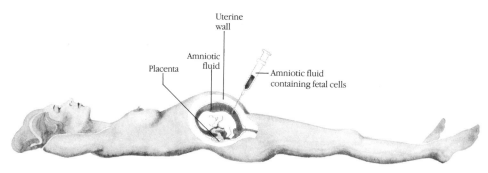

The most frequent chromosomal abnormality detected by amniocentesis is *Down's syndrome,* a hereditary disorder that affects about 5,000 children born in the United States annually (Figure 22.3). Down's syndrome results from an extra chromosome (number 21) present in all cells. Persons with severe Down's syndrome are mentally retarded and require special care and attention through their lives, although mildly affected persons may lead productive lives. Most individuals with Down's syndrome now live 40 to 50 years or longer. Many families are drained both emotionally and financially in caring for Down's syndrome patients, and most affected individuals are eventually placed in institutions.

Amniocentesis is used to detect serious genetic defects in the fetus early enough so that the pregnancy can be terminated if that is the parents' decision after the results of the test are known. Because the fetus must have been developed for four to five months before the test can be given, a test that would permit an earlier diagnosis is desirable. One new test, called *chorionic villi sampling,* can be performed as early as six to eight weeks after conception; however, the safety and reliability of this procedure remain to be proven. Early results with a small sample indicate that the fetal loss rate is unacceptably high and that chorionic villi sampling is therefore not as safe as amniocentesis (Hecht, 1984).

One medical advance that has contributed to the safety of amniocentesis is *ultrasound scanning,* or sonography. This is the use of high-frequency sound waves to outline the fetus's body (Figure 22.4). The sound waves penetrate the womb and are reflected differently from embryonic tissues that differ in composition and density. The reflected sound waves are displayed on a screen, and the pattern is interpreted by the doctor.

Ultrasound can be used to detect multiple fetuses and to reveal the orientation of the fetus in the womb as well as ectopic (tubal or cervical) pregnancy. It can ascertain the location of the placenta, which is particularly important if amniocentesis is to be performed, and gauge the fetus's head size, providing an independent means of determining the age of the fetus and normal or abnormal brain development. Despite the apparent safety of ultrasound scans, pregnant women are advised to expose their fetus only if it is clear that the health of the mother or the fetus is in jeopardy (Williams, 1983).

CONGENITAL DEFECTS

A *congenital defect* is any abnormality present at birth. Some are hereditary. Others result from

FIGURE 22.3

Frequency of children born with Down's syndrome (mongolism) in relation to the age of the mother at the time of birth. Around age 35 the risk begins to rise sharply. (Data from E. B. Hook, 1977.)

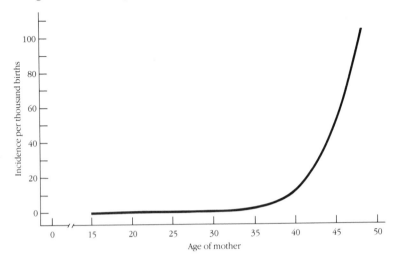

events during pregnancy and are not hereditary. Injury, harmful chemicals, nutritional deficiencies, hormone imbalances, virus infections, and even severe stress can cause developmental defects.

In recent decades a number of tragic occurrences of congenital defects have been caused by drugs prescribed for women during early pregnancy. Thalidomide, a sedative taken as a sleeping pill, interferes with the development of the bones of the arms and legs of the fetus. In Europe and Asia between 1960 and 1962, before the effects of the drug were discovered, several thousand babies were born with deformed arms and legs. Fortunately for Americans, the drug was not distributed in this country.

In the 1950's and 1960's, the synthetic hormone DES (diethylstilbestrol) was prescribed as a fertility drug in women and as a morning-after birth control pill. Many daughters of women who took DES before or during pregnancy are now discovering that they have abnormalities in their reproductive organs. The daughters of women who took this drug also have a higher risk of developing vaginal cancer. It is not yet clear what effects, if any, the drug has had on male offspring.

The congenital defects caused by these drugs are *not* hereditary. Offspring of people with con-

genital defects will not necessarily have the same defects. The lesson is that during pregnancy—especially during the first few months—extra care should be taken and *no* drugs should be ingested, not even caffeine, aspirin, or alcohol, if they can be avoided.

FIGURE 22.4

Image of a fetus obtained by ultrasound scanning. Ultrasound reveals the position of the fetus and may indicate certain physical abnormalities.

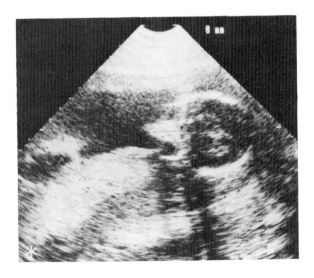

INFECTIOUS DISEASES

A remarkable variety of organisms, ranging from viruses to worms, can infect the human body and under certain conditions cause *infectious diseases.* An organism that can produce a disease in an animal is a *pathogen;* the major kinds of pathogens are illustrated in Figure 22.5. Most can be transmitted from person to person and so cause communicable diseases. Colds, measles, mumps, and gonorrhea are communicable diseases. Pathogenic organisms may be transferred to people from animals, or *vector*—the carrier of the disease. For example, malaria is caused by parasitic protozoa. These microscopic organisms are transmitted to people by infected mosquitoes; the mosquito is the vector. Rabies is caused by a virus that can be transmitted through the bite of an infected dog, bat, or other animal. The animal is the vector for rabies in people. Some types of viruses remain in the body for life (see Table 22.2).

Infectious Diseases in Human History

Throughout history infectious diseases have killed hundreds of millions of people. To ap-

preciate how your health has benefited from the eradication of many infectious diseases, it is worth briefly reviewing some of that history. Keep in mind that while each disease is initiated by a particular organism, epidemics, deaths, and human suffering were also the result of ignorance, poor sanitation, dirt, and malnutrition, among other factors.

During the Middle Ages, *bubonic plague* repeatedly decimated Europe's population. This disease is estimated to have killed more than 150 million persons. Caused by the bacterium *Pasteurella pestis,* plague is primarily a disease of rats and is transmitted to humans by fleas. If populations of rats or other rodents are kept from flourishing, there is no reservoir of the bacterium and people do not become infected—the reason that rodent control is vital to health. Plague is not eradicated; there are still occasional small outbreaks in the United States and other countries. But diligent control measures have kept these outbreaks under control; cases rarely exceed a handful, and fatalities are even rarer.

In 1703, in Philadelphia, 5,000 people died of *yellow fever.* At that time no one suspected the disease was caused by a virus transmitted to people by mosquitoes; viruses were unknown. Now, with control of the mosquito population, yellow

FIGURE 22.5
Different kinds of disease-causing organisms.

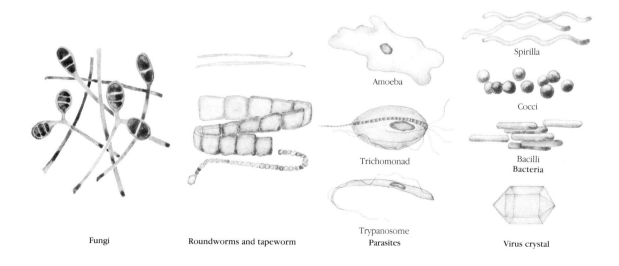

Fungi

Roundworms and tapeworm

Amoeba

Trichomonad

Trypanosome
Parasites

Spirilla

Cocci

Bacilli
Bacteria

Virus crystal

fever has virtually disappeared from most of the United States.

In the sixteenth century the Spanish brought *smallpox* to the American continent. It is estimated that half of the North and South American Indian population was killed by this viral disease; the epidemic greatly facilitated the Spanish conquests. Smallpox is believed to be the first human infectious disease to be eradicated. As a result of a worldwide vaccination program carried out by the World Health Organization (WHO), it now seems that there is not a single person left who is infected with smallpox virus (see box on page 445).

Following the Russian Revolution in 1917, 3 million Russians died of *typhus,* a disease caused by the microorganism *Rickettsia prowazekii.* Typhus is transmitted by body lice; in this instance poor sanitation and personal hygiene were responsible for the typhus epidemic. In 1918, influenza swept the globe, killing more than 20 million people. Every few years a new strain of "flu bug" (influenza virus) appears. Carried from country to country by travelers, it causes outbreaks of influenza that often reach epidemic proportions. Until early in this century, the principal causes of human sickness and suffering were infectious diseases. Since then, the death rates for many infectious diseases—especially those likely to strike in infancy and childhood, such as tuberculosis and typhoid fever—have fallen sharply.

Most infectious diseases are no longer a serious health problem in the United States. This is not the case in other areas of the world, where hundreds of millions of people still suffer from and die of infectious diseases. Roundworm, pinworm, hookworm, and tapeworm infect about 1 billion persons; another 200 million are debilitated by the water-borne parasite that causes *schistosomiasis* (Anderson, 1982). Malaria still attacks 300 million people each year and accounts for at least a million deaths annually in Africa. Even more serious is acute diarrhea in children under 5. Most surveys show that about a billion children suffer from diarrhea in Asia, Africa, and Latin America, and approximately 5 million of them die each year (Holmgren, 1981).

Infectious diseases are a major source of suffering and death in many parts of the world. Hygienic measures such as clean water and safe disposal of sewage would dramatically reduce the death from infectious and diarrheal disease. However, many countries do not have the ca-

TABLE 22.2
Some Types of *Herpes* Viruses Remain in the Body for Life Once Individuals Are Infected

Type	*Symptoms*	*Spread by*	*Remains in*
Herpes simplex I	Cold sores on lips or in mouth	Direct contact; most infectious when lesions are present	Nerve cells
Herpes simplex II	Painful blisters on genital organs	Direct contact; oral-genital sex can transmit type I or II to mouth or genital area	Nerve cells
Cytomegalovirus (CMV)	No symptoms in most children and adults; CMV can cause stillbirth and mental retardation in fetuses	Body fluids: blood, urine, saliva	White blood cells
Varicella-Zoster virus	Chicken pox in children; shingles in adults	Close contact	Nerve cells
Epstein-Barr virus (EBV)	Mononucleosis	Saliva (kissing)	Lymph glands

THE CONQUEST OF SMALLPOX

Smallpox is an ancient disease. The earliest direct evidence of it is found on the mummy of Pharoah Ramses V, who died around 1160 B.C. Written records from China and India indicate that smallpox was known earlier. Apparently a form of vaccination was practiced by the Chinese and Indians thousands of years ago: the inhalation of dried material from pox sores. The drying probably killed the virus without destroying its capacity to stimulate the body's production of antibodies, which provided immunity.

However, in Europe it was not until the eighteenth century that vaccination against smallpox became widespread. You may have heard the expression "a complexion as clear as a milkmaid's." Edward Jenner, an English physician, noticed that milkmaids almost never contracted smallpox. He reasoned that they escaped smallpox because most of them had been infected with the similar, but much milder, disease cowpox, which somehow made them resistant to the more serious smallpox. In 1796, Jenner exposed an 8-year-old boy, James Phipps, to cowpox and subsequently to smallpox. The boy survived. Within a few years vaccination became widespread.

Despite massive vaccination programs, in 1967 smallpox was still endemic in 33 countries, and there were 10 million to 15 million cases worldwide. Three facts led the World Health Organization to attempt total eradication of the disease: (1) There are no animal carriers. (2) There is no human chronic carrier state. (3) There exists a safe, effective vaccine. In October 1977, what is hoped to be the last naturally occurring case of smallpox in the world was found in Somalia. No cases have been reported since then.

pacity to introduce such life-saving public health measures. Americans are fortunate that sanitary and nutritional measures have largely eliminated these kinds of infectious diseases in this country. However, it is essential that U.S. citizens take precautions when traveling to other areas of the world, where they can be exposed to unfamiliar infectious organisms.

Fighting Infectious Diseases

Although the great French scientist Louis Pasteur established the germ theory of disease in the late nineteenth century, the medical profession was slow to accept his novel idea that "germs" (microorganisms) were the cause of diseases. Pasteur aroused the anger of many doctors when, in 1874, he advocated sterile surgical techniques:

If I had the honor of being a surgeon, I would never introduce into the human body an instrument without having passed it through boiling water or, better still, through a flame and rapidly cooled right before the operation. (Quoted in Bender, 1966)

The use of antiseptic (sterile) techniques to reduce infections in hospitals was slow to be adopted even though Joseph Lister successfully applied Pasteur's ideas in his hospital ward as early as 1865. Until that time, a broken arm or leg often meant death as a consequence of the infection that usually followed. It wasn't until the late nineteenth and early twentieth centuries, when the ideas of Pasteur and Lister were manifested in large-scale sanitation and public health programs, that the incidence of infectious diseases such as tuberculosis, bubonic plague, cholera, and diphtheria declined dramatically.

In the late 1940's another highly effective method for dealing with infectious diseases was discovered in the form of the antibiotic penicillin, produced by certain species of the mold *Penicillium*. Nowadays, hundreds of different antibiotics are available to combat infections from all kinds of microorganisms—with the general exception of viruses. Antibiotics interfere with functions in living cells. Those used medically are chosen for selective interference, that is, for their ability to kill infectious organisms while doing little or no harm to the patient. Because viruses are not cells, they are not directly affected by antibiotics. However, antibiotics are often prescribed to control a bacterial infection that might follow a viral infection. For example, lung cells frequently are so weakened after a bout with flu that potentially fatal bacterial pneumonia may develop. The administration of an antibiotic to prevent growth of the pneumonia bacterium is often appropriate.

Here are the essential points about infectious diseases:

1. All infections require the presence of a pathogenic organism (virus, bacterium, or parasite), but development of disease and its symptoms depends greatly on one's mental, emotional, immunological, and nutritional state.
2. A healthy environment, adequate nourishment, personal cleanliness, and appropriate immunizations can prevent most infections.
3. Antibiotics are justifiably called "miracle drugs" and are often appropriate treatment for serious infections.
4. The healing process usually can be helped by a "get-well" attitude and positive mental images of health and healing.

LIFESTYLE DISEASES

The majority of diseases that afflict Americans today, such as diabetes, most arthritis, cardiovascular diseases, allergies, ulcers, colitis, and even cancer, have no single principal environmental or genetic cause and are increasingly regarded as *diseases of lifestyle*. This means that factors in our daily lives contribute to the development and progression of the disease. These factors include stress, poor nutrition, weakened immunological defenses, destructive habits such as smoking cigarettes or drinking alcohol, being overweight, and probably many more. Medical science is increasingly aware of the multifactorial nature of many diseases. As Thomas (1978) puts it:

The new theory is that most of today's human illnesses, the infectious aside, are multifactorial in nature, caused by two great arrays of causative mechanisms: the influence of things in the environment; and one's personal lifestyle. For medicine to become effective in dealing with such diseases, it has become common belief that the environment will have to be changed, and personal ways of living will also have to be transformed, and radically.

Most diseases can be regarded as the failure of an organism to adapt to its natural, cultural, and social environment. Furthermore, most lifestyle diseases cannot be cured; at most the doctor and medicines can relieve suffering and alleviate symptoms. Weiner (1978) points out some of the factors of living that increase a person's risk for developing a variety of diseases:

The stress of being an air-traffic controller is associated with an increased incidence of elevated blood pressure, peptic duodenal ulcer, and sometimes, diabetes mellitus. Bereavement that is not coped with and produces the "giving-up, given-up" complex has been estimated to precede different diseases. Bereavement plays an important role in many, if not all, patients with "psychosomatic" diseases. Real or threatened loss has often been cited as a factor contributing to the initiation of other diseases as well: cancer, tuberculosis, diabetes mellitus, lymphomas and leukemias, juvenile diabetes mellitus, and heart failure. Depressive moods, the attitude of giving up, and the loss of all hope also adversely affect the outcome of surgical operations.

THE BODY'S DEFENSES

Most people feel well most of the time. This is because the body contains a remarkable array of defense mechanisms that help keep noxious substances and disease-causing organisms out of the body and help eliminate any diseased cells and infectious organisms found in the body.

Your body provides habitat for a variety of viruses, bacteria, and other pathogens. These microorganisms are always present, yet they rarely make you sick or cause disease. Every day you ingest harmful organisms and toxic substances in the food you eat, the air you breathe, and the water you drink. Yet your body rarely falls prey to these harmful substances. If you become sick, it is probably because you had excessive or prolonged exposure to a harmful substance or because you have become more susceptible to it.

Most of the responses of the body's defense systems, as well as the detoxification of chemicals in the liver and the repair of damage to cells and tissues, are physiological processes regulated automatically by the body itself. These defense mechanisms can be hampered by poor nutrition, stressful environment, emotional upset, and negative attitude. Understanding how the body's defense mechanisms protect you from disease will also help you understand how physical and mental well-being and harmonious interactions with the environment can keep the body's defenses functioning optimally.

The First Line of Defense: Keeping Harmful Substances Out

The best way to prevent disease caused by foreign substances, whether pathogens or poisons, is to exclude them from the body. The skin keeps out most microorganisms and harmful substances (Figure 22.6). In addition, the mildly acid surface of the skin provides a poor habitat for most harmful bacteria, while allowing certain beneficial bacteria to colonize the skin.

The *mucous membranes* provide another vital barrier to disease-causing substances. Our eyes, nose, throat, and breathing passages are protected by membranes that continuously produce secretions that flush away harmful particles. These membranes also secrete enzymes that degrade foreign substances. The mouth, gastrointestinal tract (digestive system), and excretory organs are similarly encased and protected by membranes that guard the body's internal cells and organs.

Tears keep the surface of the eyeball moist and wash foreign particles out of the eye. Earwax protects the delicate hearing apparatus. The mucous coating of the respiratory tract is sticky and provides a trap for irritating particles and organisms; microscopic hairlike fibers called *cilia* keep the mucus of the respiratory tract moving out of the bronchial tubes so that eventually you are able to cough or spit out the irritating substances. Sneezing and blowing the nose eliminate irritating particles that are inhaled.

Enzymes and substances in the blood form a clot that rapidly seals any break in the skin and

FIGURE 22.6

The skin provides the first line of defense in protecting the body from harmful substances. It is a complex organ consisting of several layers of specialized organelles.

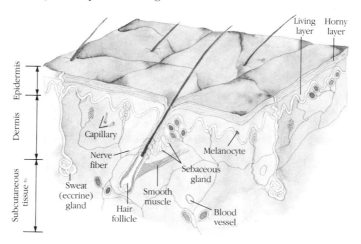

prevents entry of harmful substances and organisms. Still other enzymes and special cells in the blood attack and kill other microorganisms that enter the body through the wound before it is sealed.

If a toxic chemical or pathogen should enter the bloodstream or gastrointestinal tract, other defenses are called into action. In the stomach, strong acid secretions and special enzymes help destroy pathogens. For toxic chemicals, the body has a vast array of enzymes, especially those synthesized in the liver, that *biotransform,* or detoxify, most harmful chemicals. One form of detoxification carried out by liver enzymes is the biotransformation of alcohol, a highly toxic substance that if allowed to accumulate in the body may cause serious disease and even death. Enzymes convert alcohol into carbon dioxide and water. The unpleasant symptoms of alcohol intoxication are felt when the body's enzymes cannot biotransform ingested alcohol fast enough.

Internal Defenses

White Blood Cells and Macrophages

If microorganisms or foreign particles find their way into the blood or accumulate in body tissue, they soon encounter *leukocytes,* or *white blood cells.* Leukocytes engage in *phagocytosis* (eating of cells), in which foreign organisms and particles are engulfed and destroyed. Only about one blood cell in 700 is a leukocyte, but their number can increase dramatically in times of acute infection. That is why the blood is tested for an elevated white blood cell count when an infection is suspected; increased production of white blood cells by the bone marrow is the body's response to the infectious organisms proliferating in the body.

Other specialized phagocytic cells, *macrophages,* are associated with specific organs and tissues and are vital to the body's defense mechanisms. Leukocytes and macrophages have a relatively brief life span, usually a few weeks or months, after which they themselves are destroyed and replaced by new leukocytes and macrophages. Your health depends on the continuous monitoring and removal of foreign material and cellular debris from all regions of the body by phagocytic cells.

The ways in which the body regulates the production of essential white blood cells are not well understood. Occasionally, production of white blood cells goes out of control, and too many white blood cells crowd out other blood substances. The result is *leukemia,* a form of cancer. Leukemia can be either acute or chronic. The acute form is characterized by rapid cell proliferation. Chronic leukemia, the more easily manageable form of the disease, generally cycles through periods of normal and abnormal production of white blood cells. The disease is said to be *in remission* when the white cell level is normal.

Remember, you may be able to influence the course of infectious diseases, and possibly even of cancer, by stimulating or retarding the production of white blood cells. Even though the physiological mechanisms by which the mind affects the production of white blood cells are not yet understood, a person can help healing by using relaxation and visualization techniques to influence the body's physiology and cellular defenses. How the mind affects the immune system is discussed later in this chapter.

Inflammation

One of the body's internal defenses is *inflammation,* a reaction of tissue to injury or the invasion of microorganisms. Inflammation consists of a complex series of events in a wounded or diseased area (Figure 22.7). The damaged cells usually release histamine and related substances that dilate local blood vessels. This often causes swelling and pain. White blood cells are attracted to the wound or diseased region in large numbers to clean away the tissue debris and any foreign matter that has entered the body. A mixture of white blood cells and debris from damaged cells makes up pus, which sometimes accumulates in wounds and infected areas. The existence of pus tells you that your body's defenses are working and that healing is taking place.

FIGURE 22.7

Penetration of the skin by any unsterile sharp object often produces inflammation, the normal response of the body to injury or infection.

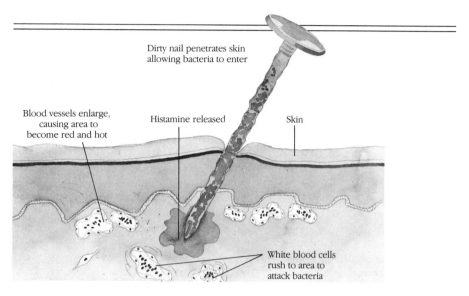

Dirty nail penetrates skin
allowing bacteria to enter

Blood vessels enlarge,
causing area to
become red and hot

Histamine released

Skin

White blood cells
rush to area to
attack bacteria

Interferon

Humans and animals have a special internal defense mechanism that protects them from virus infections. Viruses are particles of genetic material (RNA or DNA) encapsulated in a protein shell. They can only grow and reproduce in cells they infect. Infection of even one cell in the body by a single virus can result in the rapid production of hundreds or thousands of identical new viruses by that cell. The new viruses, released from that cell, attack other cells. That is why viral infections spread so quickly through the body and why viral diseases can make you extremely sick in a short time. To combat virus infections, some of the body's cells, especially the white blood cells called *lymphocytes* because they are found in the lymphatic system, produce *interferon*, which interferes with a virus's growth and its ability to infect cells.

Each animal makes its own special kinds of interferon, which can vary from one tissue to another. Nobody knows exactly how interferon inhibits viruses, but it is clear that viruses do not multiply in cells containing interferon. Even more intriguing is that once interferon production in a cell has been stimulated by viral infection, that cell and others in its neighborhood become resistant to many other kinds of viruses.

Although the use of pure interferon to treat certain viral diseases was predicted soon after its discovery in 1957, until recently it was difficult to obtain enough to conduct clinical studies of its efficacy. Now, however, genetically engineered organisms produce large amounts of interferon, and soon more information about its potential usefulness in treating virus diseases such as herpes infections (cold sores) and the common cold will be at hand. There is also some hope that interferon will treat certain kinds of cancer.

The Final Defense: Immune Responses

When foreign substances such as bacteria, viruses, pollen, cells and molecules from other organisms, and many industrial chemicals enter the body, a complex series of reactions called

ACNE

Acne—pimples, whiteheads, blackheads, or "zits"—on the face and occasionally on the shoulders, chest, and back—afflicts millions of people. Acne is so common among adolescents that many consider it normal for that stage of life. Few of those afflicted with acne agree, however; they spend millions of dollars on acne medications each year.

Acne comes from the blocking of oil-producing glands (sebaceous glands) in the skin. Normally these tiny glands produce an oily substance, sebum, which drains onto the skin through a pore. For reasons that are not understood, sometimes a pore becomes plugged by dead cells, bacteria, and sebum, preventing sebum from getting out. When this material builds up within the gland, along with skin pigment particles (causing the blackhead) and white blood cells, a pus-filled pimple forms.

No one knows what causes the plugging of sebaceous glands in acne. Acne is not caused by overconsumption of chocolate, cola drinks, or greasy foods. Neither is it a bacterial infection of the skin, though it may worsen because of the degradative action of certain bacteria on sebum. Some acne may result from physically covering the pores of sebaceous glands. Athletes and hikers can develop acne in skin areas pressed by their gear. Wearing a hat can lead to acne on the forehead. Even resting your hands on your face while studying can sometimes produce a localized bout of acne. Virtually all cosmetics, especially the pancake type, are likely to worsen acne.

Acne can be affected by hormones. Sebum production increases in response to the sex hormone testosterone. In some women, pregnancy or birth control pills makes acne worse, whereas in others pregnancy or oral contraceptives may clear up acne. Some women have minor flare-ups of acne near the beginning of menstruation.

Because the cause of acne is unknown, there is no known single way to clear it up; neither is there a simple preventive measure. Most dermatologists recommend a combination of cleanliness and certain types of medications to control acne. They especially suggest proper washing that removes surface oils and dirt but that does not irritate the skin. Medicines containing benzoyl peroxide are often useful. Antibiotics, especially tetracycline, may not be the best course of treatment except in severe cases. Disfiguring acne can be treated with a new drug, 13-cis-retinoic acid (trade name: Acutane). Although this drug is very effective, it produces a number of side effects including elevated cholesterol in the blood. This drug should only be used under close medical supervision.

For many, acne is worst in times of emotional turmoil. Some experts in psychosomatic medicine suggest that acne is a response to the anger engendered by the belief that one's sense of independence or individuality is being threatened. More than one person has had acne clear up as soon as he or she moved away from home to go to college. As with many other conditions, the role of the mind in prevention and treatment of acne cannot be ignored.

---

immune responses take place. The outcome is the production of protein molecules, called *antibodies*, and certain kinds of blood cells, called lymphocytes, that attach to the foreign substances and begin to eliminate them from the body. Antibodies and lymphocytes inactivate the foreign material until it can be digested and removed by phagocytic cells in the blood. Any substance that stimulates immune responses is called an *antigen* (*anti*body *gen*erator).

The immune responses provide the body's last defense against disease and are responsible for the immunity that may follow an infection. The other defenses we have mentioned can be regarded as outer defenses that the body uses until the immune system can produce sufficient antibodies to neutralize invading organisms or harmful substances. Typically it takes the body a week or more to develop an immune response to a substance. This is why other, faster-acting defense mechanisms are also needed. For healing to be complete, the body's immune system must respond to infecting organisms and destroy them all.

The Lymphatic System

The cells responsible for the recognition of antigens and the production of antibodies originate mainly in bone marrow and are transported to all parts of the body through the *lymphatic system* (Figure 22.8). The lymphatic vessels contain a circulating fluid called *lymph*. At intervals along the lymphatic vessels are masses of specialized tissue called *lymph nodes,* which filter out bacteria and other foreign particles from the lymph. They also manufacture antibody-producing cells (lymphocytes). "Swollen glands" are enlarged lymph nodes engaged in the removal of the invading organisms from the body.

The tonsils, adenoids, spleen, and thymus are members of the immune system. They carry out several functions in maintaining an effective immune response as well as produce lympho-

cytes. Until recently it was a frequent practice to remove tonsils (tonsillectomy) or adenoids (adenoidectomy) if they became inflamed on the theory that if those organs were removed, they could not become inflamed. Today, however, the importance of these tissues to the defenses of the body is widely recognized, and most health care practitioners agree that no child or adult should have either of these operations performed unless there is compelling medical reason to do so.

The lymphatic cells are called *B lymphocytes* and *T lymphocytes*. B lymphocytes produce specific antibodies (the protein molecules that attach to particular antigens), whereas T lymphocytes attack any foreign substances at once (Figure 22.9).

It is thought that the T lymphocytes play a crucial role in the detection of cancer cells and other abnormal cells. Most scientists believe we produce cancer cells throughout our lives but that their number is small, and when they do arise, the cancer cells are destroyed by vigilant T lymphocytes. If this hypothesis is correct, then lifelong health is highly dependent on the activeness of the immune responses.

FIGURE 22.8

The body's lymphatic system. The principal lymph nodes and other organs of the immune system are shown. The lymphatic system performs many functions in protecting the body from disease.

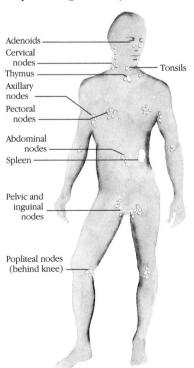

Adenoids
Cervical nodes
Thymus
Axillary nodes
Pectoral nodes
Abdominal nodes
Spleen
Pelvic and inguinal nodes
Popliteal nodes (behind knee)
Tonsils

Recognition of "Self"

So far we have described the ability of the immune system to recognize and destroy virtually any substance or organism that is foreign to the body. What prevents the immune system from turning on your own tissues and cells? By mechanisms yet to be discovered, the immune system is able to distinguish between "self" and all other substances, which are "not self." It is thought that during embryonic development, as tissues are being formed, the antibody-producing cells directed against the body's normal cellular components are destroyed or inactivated, although scientists do not yet know how.

During fetal development, before the child's own immunological system is functional, he or she receives antibodies from the mother's blood. In this way the newborn infant is protected from infections and foreign substances for several months after birth. Antibodies are also passed to the child in the mother's milk, which is one reason that breast-feeding is so beneficial. Eventu-

FIGURE 22.9

The synthesis of all immune system cells begins in bone marrow. Precursor cells are processed in various parts of the body and acquire their specialized functions. Mature T lymphocytes attack and destroy invading microorganisms directly. Mature B lymphocytes manufacture antibody proteins (immunoglobulins) that bind to antigens and inactivate foreign organisms and toxins.

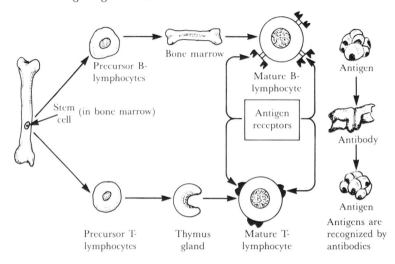

ally the child's own immune system becomes capable of producing antibodies.

One of the principal causes of diseases in infants and young children is malnutrition or starvation, either of which interferes with the immune system. This explains why malnutrition increases the chances of infectious diseases as well as their severity. Poor nutrition and pathogenic organisms are both responsible for disease and childhood mortality in much of the world's undernourished populations (Rosenberg, 1976).

Autoimmune Diseases

The immune system must function with precision to distinguish "self" from "nonself." Any mistake that resulted in antibodies attacking the body's own cells could result in serious disease or death. Such *autoimmune diseases* do exist. Some genetic disorders, fortunately quite rare, may result in loss of immune responsiveness or in a breakdown in the mechanisms responsible for "self" recognition. Other autoimmune disorders may or may not have a genetic basis but still cause serious diseases and even death.

Lupus erythematosus is an autoimmune disorder that mainly affects women 18 to 35. In this disease, for reasons still unknown, autoantibodies are synthesized and directed against the person's own DNA and cell nuclei. Many organs of the body may be affected, and the symptoms—rashes, pain, and anemia—usually flare up and fade away throughout life.

Another serious disease partly caused by an autoimmune response—one that affects millions of people—is *rheumatoid arthritis*. In this disease autoantibodies are directed primarily against the body's joints, producing inflammation, pain, and suffering. There is also evidence that in some people the symptoms of arthritis can be arrested or reversed by nutritional changes or by changes in mental state. However, no single nutritional or mental change—or medical treatment—has been scientifically demonstrated to lead to a cure or to permanent remission of this disease.

An autoimmune disease that affects the central nervous system is *multiple sclerosis*, or MS. Recent research suggests that MS may be initiated by a viral infection that triggers the immune system to produce antibodies directed against myelin, which sheaths and insulates nerve fibers in the brain and spinal cord. Interferon is one of the drugs being tested in patients with MS to see whether it will reduce or eliminate attacks and symptoms.

Some rare genetic immune deficiency disorders such as *agammaglobulinemia* result in inability to produce antibodies. When the mother's antibodies begin to disappear from the newborn's blood, it suffers from recurrent infections. The child's survival depends on antibiotic therapy, injections of antibodies, and, for a few such children, living in an isolated germ-free environment. The most famous case of agammaglobulinemia is David, the "bubble boy," who was delivered under sterile conditions and kept in a germ-free environment for 12 years in a Texas hospital. David was born without a thymus gland, lymph nodes, or tonsils, and he lacked the ability to make any antibodies. Shortly before his twelfth birthday, David's physicians along with David and his family decided to attempt a bone-marrow transplant from his sister in order to provide him with cells capable of producing antibodies. The transplanted tissue was rejected, and David died in 1984.

Blood Transfusions and Rh Factors

Today people are concerned about blood transfusions because of possible contamination with AIDS. In the early part of this century a blood transfusion often led to death because the patient's immune system recognized the donor blood as "foreign" and attacked with phagocytic cells and antibodies. The antibodies cause clumps of blood cells to form in the veins and arteries, impeding the flow of blood, oxygen, and waste products. If oxygen and nutrients are prevented from reaching essential tissues such as the heart or brain, death may occur.

Red blood cells have many potential antigens on their cell surfaces, each of which can evoke an antibody response. However, you do not make antibodies against your own antigens. The two most important groups of human red blood cell antigens are the ABO and Rh-positive/Rh-negative groups. There are many other groups of antigens on red blood cells, but these are by far the most important ones in terms of immune responses that can endanger health. Table 22.3 shows the pattern of donor-recipient ABO blood types that must be matched for a successful transfusion.

People with type O blood have neither A nor B antigens on their red blood cells. Their immune system makes A and B antibodies early in life because these antigens are prevalent in bacteria and food plants. People with type O blood are *universal donors;* their blood cells will not stimulate an antibody response in the recipient, no matter what his or her blood type. People with type AB blood have both antigens present on their red blood cells and do not synthesize A or B antibodies because these antigens are recognized as "self" and those antibody-producing cells are destroyed in the embryo. People with type AB blood are *universal recipients;* they can accept blood from any of the four groups.

The Rh-positive antigen and the antibody that reacts against it cause problems primarily in pregnancy. A woman is termed Rh-negative if her red blood cells do not contain any of this antigen. If the red blood cells of a developing fetus have the Rh-positive antigen (inherited

TABLE 22.3

How Blood Transfusions Are Determined According to ABO Blood Groups

Blood group	Genotype	Antigens on red blood cells	Transfusions cannot be accepted from	Transfusions are accepted from
O (universal donor)	OO	none	A, B, AB	O
A	AA, AO	A	B, AB	A, O
B	BB, BO	B	A, AB	B, O
AB (universal recipient)	AB	A, B	none	A, B, AB, O

from the father), and if any of the fetus's red blood cells enter the mother's blood supply, production of anti-Rh antibodies can result. This usually does not cause any difficulty during the first pregnancy and might even go unnoticed until the woman became pregnant again.

If the second fetus is also Rh-positive, the Rh-positive antibodies synthesized in the mother's blood during the first pregnancy will attack the developing infant's red blood cells, resulting in anemia, brain damage, or even death. Fortunately, doctors can manage this problem. Right after the first child is delivered, the mother is given an injection of anti-Rh antibodies that destroy any fetal blood cells in her blood. Her immune system is prevented from responding to the fetal antigen and producing Rh-positive antibodies that might endanger the fetus during a subsequent pregnancy.

Vaccination: Priming the Immune System

One of the great achievements of modern medical science is the development of vaccinations against serious bacterial and viral diseases, including smallpox, whooping cough, poliomyelitis, measles, diphtheria, and tetanus. Vaccination is the administration of substances called vaccines, usually by injection, that stimulate the immune response to specific infecting organisms if subsequently encountered.

When a person is vaccinated, specific antigens—from inactivated viruses, bacteria, or toxins—are injected into the body. The immune system responds with lymphocytes and antibodies directed against those antigens. If the body later encounters the natural disease-causing agents, it already has immunity and is protected. For example, the polio vaccine developed by Jonas Salk employed a chemically inactivated virus. The polio vaccine currently in use in this country, developed by Albert Sabin, uses genetically inactivated strains of polio virus that cannot cause the disease but can stimulate long-lasting immunity. Genetic inactivation produces a strain of virus that is incapable of causing disease but that has antigens similar to those of the original virus. The antibody made in response is effective against the naturally occurring virus.

In general, vaccination is safe and effective for disease prevention and has resulted in vastly improved human health. The reason that a single—or at most several—inoculation produces long-term immunity is that the immune system, once stimulated by a particular antigen, maintains special white blood cells that "remember" that particular antigen. If the body is again challenged by that antigen, even after many years, those "memory cells" proliferate rapidly and produce sufficient antibodies to combat the disease.

Serious diseases for which vaccines are available are listed in Table 22.4. Vaccination for milder diseases such as influenza is controversial, since it is not clear that the benefits outweigh the risks for all people. Some people may respond adversely to any vaccination because of emotional anxiety or allergic reactions, or may contract the disease because of some unforeseen complication with their own biochemical processes. Most healthy people recover quickly from a bout of flu and probably don't need flu shots. Smallpox immunizations are no longer necessary or recommended; the risks of an adverse reaction from the shot far outweigh the risk of contracting smallpox, since no cases have been reported for a number of years.

The most recent addition to the list of immunizations is *hepatitis B* vaccine. About 200,000 cases of hepatitis B, a serious viral liver disease, are diagnosed in the U.S. each year. Hepatitis B vaccination is recommended for particular groups at high risk—health care workers who are exposed to the disease, heroin addicts, male homosexuals, and sexually promiscuous persons. The original vaccine was made from the blood of human carriers of the virus, but an equally effective vaccine produced by genetic engineering should be available within a few years.

Allergies

Allergies are responses of the immune system to foreign substances called *allergens*. Pollens, grasses, grains, molds, dust, animal hair, foods, and drugs contain allergy-causing antigens. Almost anything containing a foreign substance can be an allergen. The allergic response

TABLE 22.4
Immunizations Available in the United States

Type of immunization	Effectiveness of immunization and frequency of booster doses	Type of immunization	Effectiveness of immunization and frequency of booster doses
Cholera	Only partial immunity; recommended renewal every 6 months for duration of exposure	German measles	Highly effective; need for boosters not established
Diphtheria	Highly effective; recommended renewal every 10 years	Measles	Highly effective; usually produces lifelong immunity
Influenza	Renew every year (because viral strains change easily)	Smallpox	Immunization no longer required
Mumps	Believed to confer lifetime immunity	Spotted fever	Effectiveness not established
Bubonic plague	Incomplete protection; boosters necessary every 3 to 6 months	Tetanus	Very effective; renew every 10 years or when treated for a contaminated wound if more than 5 years have elapsed since last booster
Polio	Long-lasting immunity; no booster necessary unless exposure anticipated	Tuberculosis	Highly effective
		Typhoid fever	About 80 percent effective
Rabies	A vaccination each day for 14 to 21 days beginning soon after the bite (before symptoms appear)	Typhus	Renew every year (if exposed)
		Whooping cough	Highly effective
		Yellow fever	Highly effective; provides long-lasting immunity
		Hepatitis B	Effective; only for individuals at risk

is synthesis of a class of antibodies that are different from the ones that recognize and inactivate bacteria, viruses, and cells. No one is sure what benefit accrues from allergy-related antibodies, called immunoglobulin E, but millions of people can attest to the misery and discomfort caused by this immune response (Figure 22.10).

The allergic reaction is usually accompanied by inflammation, mucus secretion, and the release of histamine, a chemical that is stored in cells that are abundant in the skin, respiratory passages, and digestive tract. It is no coincidence that many allergic reactions are associated with skin (eczema, hives, poison ivy), the respiratory tract (hay fever, asthma), and the digestive tract (vomiting, diarrhea).

Though allergies involve physiological and immunological responses in the body, they are also strongly tied to a person's emotional and psychic state. Asthmatic children are often much improved when separated from their parents. Sometimes skin eruptions are a sign of itching to get away from something or someone. Sneezes may be seasonal or interpersonal.

Allergies are blamed on many substances, yet allergens are but one component of the complex immunological response. Moorefield (1971) has successfully treated asthmatic patients using hypnosis and behavior therapy. It is his view that:

In asthma a conditioned bronchial spasm is the common pathway for a complexity of physical, allergic, and emotional mechanisms. Most studies have shown that even in the presence of allergic conditions, some emotional overlay usually triggers the attack of asthma. It is known that emotional influences are activated through the autonomic nervous system. It is quite likely that emotions acting via the autonomic nervous system produce local conditions in the mucosa of the bronchial tubes, which would make the respiratory system sensitive both to infections and allergens.

FIGURE 22.10
Between a third and half of all Americans suffer from some form of allergy.

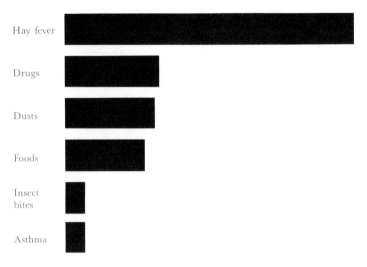

Hay fever

Drugs

Dusts

Foods

Insect bites

Asthma

Millions of allergic people receive inoculations that are supposed to desensitize them to the irritating substances. Some people do get better with desensitizing shots, yet there is scant evidence to substantiate the idea that allergy shots are beneficial. In fact, several studies have shown that placebos can be just as effective as allergens. Fontana (1966) concluded:

A five-year study has been done on children sensitive to ragweed in which a comparison was made between specific hyposensitization injections and placebo injections. Even though the allergen injections may have had some beneficial effect on some children, the amount of benefit was indistinguishable from differences likely to occur in pure randomization experiments. No justification was found for promising any greater benefit to children treated with allergens than they would obtain from placebo injections.

Allergies of all kinds can be caused and cured by a person's beliefs and by suggestion. The human skin is particularly vulnerable to disturbed emotional and mental states. Millions of people suffer from rashes, eczema, acne, and other skin disorders. Bobroff (1962) sums up his unconventional medical view of eczema in strong language:

I now regard every new case of eczema as immediately curable with absolute certainty, provided the patient (or the parent if the patient is a child) is of average intelligence and willing to make a reasonable effort. For I now know that any eczema—regardless of extent, severity, or duration—can, without the slightest doubt, be made to disappear within two weeks by easily mastered procedures which the patient can be taught to perform for himself. At the same time the patient can be trained in the simple preventive measures that will thereafter preclude any recurrence of eczema.

Bobroff argues that the successful treatment of eczema requires (1) elimination of itching and (2) elimination of inflammation. For many patients he recommends applying cold damp compresses for about 20 minutes several times each day. Following this regimen the skin usually clears up within a week or two.

Other patients were cured simply by wrapping the affected area for two weeks to prevent scratching and irritation. Bobroff also dealt with his patients' emotional and personal problems. Their skin eruptions were invariably associated with unresolved personal problems or relationships. Bobroff practiced holistic medicine long before the concept became widely accepted.

Allergies are real. People do not imagine that they are unable to breathe or that their skin itches. But the causes are complex and lie as much within us as in what we are exposed to in the environment. A holistic approach to coping with an allergic problem would begin by determining what has upset a person's mental and emotional tranquility. When harmony is disturbed, the immune responses are affected, and one of the undesirable responses can be allergic reactions.

The Role of Nutrition

Finally, the effect of nutrition on the immune system should be emphasized. It has been known for a long time that nutritional deficiency and susceptibility to disease are closely intertwined. Lack of essential nutrients impairs the body's ability to defend itself against infectious organisms.

Although few people actually starve in the United States, many people are not well nourished. Both undernourished and overnourished people may suffer impairment of their defense mechanisms, especially the ability of the immune system to protect them from infectious organisms and cancer cells. We cannot emphasize often enough that the body needs all of the essential nutrients in order to synthesize the cells and substances that keep a person healthy.

All this means that the more positive your mental attitudes and emotional states, the less you are stressed by your environment; the better your nutrition, the more responsive and functional your immune system will be. A healthy immune response means fewer infections. Allergies may decrease or disappear. You may be less likely to fall victim to any of the autoimmune diseases, and you will probably be less susceptible to cancer.

SUMMARY

Well-being and disease cannot be defined or distinguished in terms of anatomical, physiological, or mental attributes. Their real measure is in the ability of the individual to function acceptably. The criteria for functioning vary with age, conditions of living, and cultural value system. How a young child perceives illness or disease may be very different from how an adolescent or teacher perceives it. Perhaps teachers should perceive illnesses and diseases as at the opposite end of the wellness spectrum. Illnesses and diseases may be a consequence of irresponsible behavior and poor ways of coping with life. Optimal well-being may be interpreted as a consequence of responsible behavior and good ways of coping with problems. Teachers should impress this consequence concept on children, for it ties in harmoniously with ecological and risk-taking behavior themes.

Finally, as our technological lifestyle changes, we can expect to form new habits deleterious to our well-being. Although such habits are initiated early in life, their consequences may remain latent until middle age, when the symptoms become acute and the person becomes prematurely disabled. Heart disease is a good example of this process. A child's overeating; not exercising regularly; academic, social, and emotional stresses; and cigarette smoking form a syndrome predisposing him or her to heart disease later. Many other diseases have similar latent and chronic overtones. Children need to be made aware that new health problems arise from technological progress and social change. They need to be made aware that such problems may start as acute disrupting illnesses and emerge into chronic disabling diseases for which there are as yet no cures. Chronic diseases should be anticipated during the formative years. Prevention against social and chronic diseases of progress must begin with elementary school children, even though chronic diseases are a health problem of later life.

EXEMPLARY LESSON PLANS

In light of our preceding discussion in this chapter, peruse the following lesson plan examples, keeping in mind that they are indicative of the type of lesson plans that you will likely be expected to implement in your classroom. Remember that they are only exemplary in nature and by no means encompass a complete unit of instruction. They are simply offered as a guide or basis for the formation of a comprehensive unit dealing with the topic in question.

TOPIC: HOW TO AVOID CATCHING A COLD

Grade Level: Primary

Concept: Good health habits help prevent colds.

Expected Pupil Outcome: The student will be able to state ways to avoid catching a cold.

Content: Good health habits that help us avoid catching a cold are:

1. Using paper tissue when coughing or sneezing
2. Eating balanced diet regularly
3. Getting proper amount of sleep
4. Drinking plenty of fluids
5. Wearing warm clothes
6. Washing hands before eating
7. Keeping feet dry
8. Getting regular exercise
9. Getting plenty of rest
10. Being cheerful
11. Not playing with someone who has a cold
12. Not using same drinking glass
13. Disposing of paper tissue properly

Learning Experiences

1. *Flannel board—Snoopy Fights a Cold:* Snoopy and various pictorial situations depicting good and bad health habits. Children place Snoopy in situations preventing cold. Let class react to pupil choices
2. *Alternative suggestions:*
   a) *Picture Quiz* on how to avoid a cold (see below).
   b) *Demonstration:* How cold is spread. Place some flour in the palm of a hand and cough. Observe flour dispersing. Flour conceptualized to germs.

Evaluation Procedures With either the flannel board or picture quiz learning experiences the teacher will subjectively evaluate the student responses. If the answers are generally correct the objective will be considered attained.

Picture Quiz

Which picture in each pair shows how to prevent colds? Which picture is incorrect (has something wrong with it)? Circle the correct face.

TOPIC: HOW DISEASES ARE SPREAD

Grade Level: Primary, Intermediate

Concept: Diseases are easily spread.

Expected Pupil Outcome: The student will be able to identify the ways by which disease is spread.

Content: Diseases are spread in following ways:
1. *Through the air:* by coughing and sneezing.
2. *Personal contact:* directly by touching another person or indirectly by touching objects (glass, towel, washcloth, etc.) handled by another.
3. *By insects:* flies, mosquitoes, ticks, etc.

FIGURE 22.11
Determination of sensitivity of bacteria to different antibiotics (single-paper disk-diffusion method). A Petri dish of agar was heavily inoculated with the test organisms. Disks of filter paper impregnated with different antibiotics were dropped on the freshly inoculated surface. Note the white bacterial growth with a zone of no growth around two of the disks. There is no inhibition of growth around the third. A zone of inhibition indicates that the growth of the organism would probably be limited in a patient receiving an antibiotic.

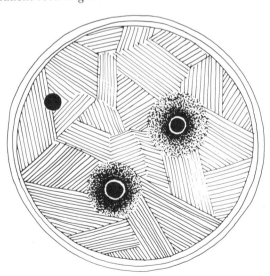

Learning Experiences
1. *Simulate ways* microbes are spread:
   a) *Demonstration:* Place cocoa or flour in palm of hand and cough. Action of flour can be compared to that of microbes.
   b) *Demonstration:* Place red lipstick on palm of hand of student or clean glass. Have another student touch palm or infected glass. Observe for tracings of lipstick on hand of second student.
   c) *Demonstration:* Attach transparent sticky tape to feet of a large model fly. Have fly land on flour, and dust, then on some flat white paper. Observe color tape tracings on white paper.
   d) *Demonstration:* Cultivate culture plates of several foods and observe for bacteria growth.
   e) *Demonstration:* Cultivate culture plates of different samples of water (pond, river, tap) and observe for bacterial growth and contamination.
   f) Refer to demonstration of drinking glass and lipstick.
2. *Alternative learning experience*
   a) *Demonstration:* Plant antibiotic paper disks on jar media inoculated with infectious bacteria. Incubate for 36-48 hours. Observe. (See Figure 22.11.)
   b) *Simulate* bacterial growth needs with several plants. All living things need oxygen, water, food, and warmth.
   c) *Demonstration:* After conceptualizing, by use of flour or lipstick, how germs are spread, have infected student wash hands with soap and water. Do same with use of paper tissue and coughing. Likewise wash dirty glass with soap and water.

4. *In food:* touched by insects and humans.
5. *In water:* drinking infected water.
6. *By animals and pets:* cats, dogs, and birds; ringworm, ticks, fleas.

d) *Pictures simulating* ways of spreading diseases. Add to this a pupil matching bee technique.
e) *Demonstration:* With oral disclosing pill. Red coloring of teeth and gums identifies bacterial plaques.

Evaluation Procedures   Teacher develops a matching bee to be used a day or so following instruction. If the students can successfully complete the matching bee with very few or no mistakes the objective will be attained.

REFERENCES AND BIBLIOGRAPHY

Bender, G. A. "Great Moments in Medicine," Detroit: Northwood Institute Press/Parke Davis Co., 1966.

Bobroff, A. *Eczema: Its Nature, Cure and Prevention* (Springfield, Ill.: Charles C Thomas, 1962).

Dubos, R. *Man, Medicine, and Environment* (New York: Praeger, 1968).

Edlin, G., and E. Golanty. *Health and Wellness: A Holistic Approach,* Third Edition (Boston, Mass.: Jones and Bartlett, 1988).

Fontana, V. J., L. E. Holt, Jr., and D. Mainland. "Effectiveness of Hyposensitization Therapy in Ragweed Hayfever in Children," *Journal of the American Medical Association,* 195 (1966), 109.

Hadler, N. M. "Regional Back Pain," *New England Journal of Medicine,* 315 (1986), 1090-1092.

Hecht, F., B. K. Hecht, and H. A. Bixenman. "Caution About Chorionic Villi Sampling in the First Trimester," *New England Journal of Medicine,* 310 (1984), 1388-1395.

Holmgren, J. "Actions of Cholera Toxin and the Prevention and Treatment of Cholera," *Nature,* 292 (1981), 413-418.

Moorefield, C. W. "The Use of Hypnosis and Behavior Therapy in Asthma," *American Journal of Clinical Hypnosis,* 13 (1971), 162.

Reading, A. "Illness and Disease," *Medical Clinics of North America,* 61 (1977), 703.

Rosenberg, I. H., N. W. Solomons, and D. M. Levin. "Interaction of Infection and Nutrition: Some Practical Concerns," *Ecology of Food and Nutrition,* 4 (1976), 203.

Thomas, L. "On Magic in Medicine," *New England Journal of Medicine,* August 1978.

Thomas, L. *The Medusa and the Snail* (New York: Viking-Penguin, 1979).

Weiner, H. "The Illusion of Simplicity: The Medical Model Revisited," *American Journal of Psychiatry,* 135 (July 1978), supp.

Williams, M. E., and N. M. Hadler, "The Illness as the Focus of Geriatric Medicine," *New England Journal of Medicine,* 308 (1983), 1357-1359.

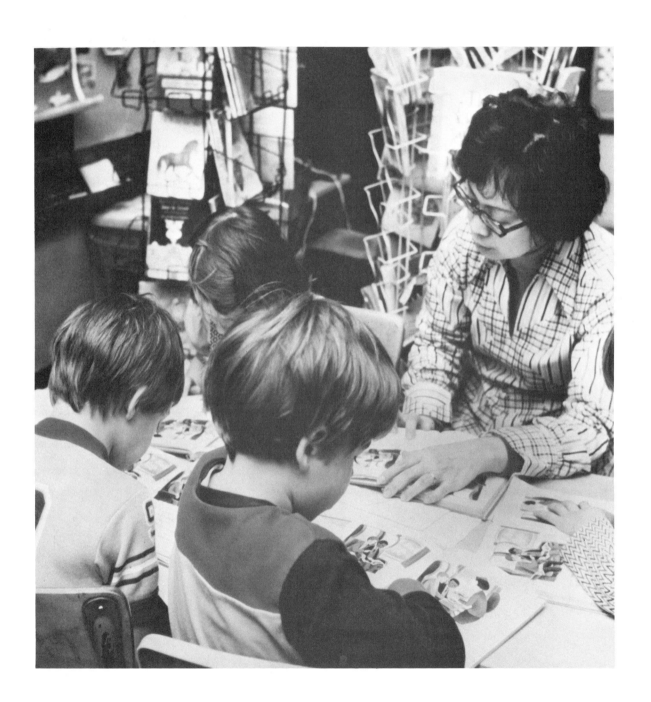

Chapter 23

Teaching About Family Living and Sexuality

INTRODUCTION

Family life is perhaps the most controversial content area of elementary health education. The mere mention of sex education is bound to create conflict in most communities. This is indeed unfortunate.

All of us are potentially capable of mating and reproduction. Closely related to those basic functions are keen passions, satisfaction, and devotion. These feelings range from the primarily physical to the essentially psychic. Psychophysical sexual development is complicated, demanding, and important. It involves emotions, societal influences, parental guidance, information, and experience. Ideally, the end product is a fully functioning person who has a sensible, humane, and healthy attitude toward sex, marriage, and life.

Sex and reproduction are natural and fundamental. However, the range of behavior within this spectrum is most diverse. Sexual behavior can be approached for immediate, selfish, and totally physical gratification or be a harmonious blending of physical and pyschological forces. In the long run, the latter approach will contribute the most to positive and healthy sexual adjustment.

It is unfortunate that society does little to support the premise above. Our culture continues to operate under a double standard of sexual freedom for men and chastity for women.

Our culture continues to encourage the young man to exploit his female counterpart, and yet sexual encounters based solely on physical attraction lack the tenderness and satisfaction of a meaningful relationship. When sex is approached from the purely physical standpoint, it is only a matter of time before the participants lose their ability to give of themselves and find true happiness and peace of mind with their partners. Attitudes toward sex are extremely important; consider the vast number of people who are afflicted with sex-related emotional problems.

Information and the impulses connected with sexual behavior are far too complex and important to personality development to be ignored or left to instinct. As with all other matters, the parents have the prime responsibility for sex education. However, most children receive very little, if any, sexual education at home. Therefore, the school should assist in the development of the child's sexual knowledge. Other agencies, such as the church, can contribute to family living education.

Sexual education should begin at the elementary level because it is the only one that everyone attends and because the subject is far less likely to encounter conflict at the elementary level than at other levels. The elementary school child accepts sexual education readily and naturally. Thus it does not represent the emotional hurdle at the early elementary level that occurs during puberty. More important, most elementary school children are likely to become the victims of inaccurate street information and unwholesome attitudes. Children want answers about reproduction, birth, sex, and family living. They need straightforward, honest information at appropriate times during their lives. The teacher should satisfy the child's immediate curiosity and leave the door open for the child to come back for more information when he or she needs it.

The emphasis at the elementary level should help children to evolve healthy attitudes toward family living. Such attitudes have been referred to as healthy sexuality and are reflected in the degree to which one feels comfortable with (and toward): sexual roles (father, mother, sister, brother); relationships with the same and with the opposite sex; and fulfilling personal, family, and social responsibilities (as a worker, student, family member, housewife). Healthy sexuality is compatible with a healthy attitude toward life. Children need to structure their identity with sexual roles early. They need to appreciate the role of the body in reproduction and to understand the part that emotions play in sexual behavior. They need to learn how to relate to others in positive ways. And they need to learn to assume responsibilities in general. All this is interrelated with emotional and social well-being.

A number of important factors influence the sexual development of children. The following discussion centers on many of the most influential ones.

THE FAMILY*

The family is at various times held sacred and considered a scourge. For many people it is regarded more often as one than the other. It is difficult to cast the contemporary North American family into one mold; although the functions that families perform may be similar, their social and emotional climates can be vastly dissimilar.

A primary function of families is physical care of children. Children require years of feeding, clothing, sheltering, and protecting before they can take care of themselves. A second very important function of families is socialization. Social values and appropriate social behavior must be taught. The family more than any other institution has the responsibility for instilling religious and moral training and for providing discipline. A third important function of families is to provide a sense of belonging. A family connotes ancestors, traditions, intimacy, family rituals, private passwords or jokes. The tie to one's family is enduring, even if family members feud or change frequently or if the home is conflict-ridden and crisis-prone. A fourth function of families is the provision of affection. Parents should be a source of love to each other, to their offspring, and to all those who reside in the household. Provision of a loving, supportive feeling is one of the most important ways in which a family can affect its members.

SIGNIFICANCE OF THE FAMILY IN SOCIAL DEVELOPMENT

The American family has changed profoundly in the last 50 years, from a predominantly rural life to a suburban and urban one. Many people have divorced themselves from the extended family and learned to value the privacy and self-sufficiency of the nuclear unit (father, mother, children) or to rely on themselves alone. With

this emphasis on self-sufficiency has come a hesitancy to ask too much of relatives, friends, or neighbors. Today many American families do not know or care to know the names of the families living next door to them. This tendency is partially due to the high mobility rate of Americans, who are apt to move away and be replaced by strangers rather frequently.

Twenty-five years ago most mothers stayed home to raise their children. Now approximately 60 percent of the mothers in the United States work outside the home. Child-rearing is shared by baby-sitters, by day care centers, by family day care homes, and increasingly by fathers who arrange flexible work schedules to allow them to stay home part time with their children. The family's social network, the school, and the children's peer group join the parents as major socialization influences. How potent the school and the peer group are depends in part on how strict or relaxed the family members are in shaping behavior and on the stoutness of the family's affectionate bond. Children from 6 to 12 identify with and model their behavior after the people they perceive as most nurturant and powerful. Strong family ties relegate peers and school to lesser importance, whereas weak family ties escalate the influence of significant others in the community.

Single Parenting

About half of American children will spend a portion of their childhood in a single-parent family for reasons of divorce, desertion, death, unwed mothering, or single parent adoption. About 40 percent of marriages end in divorce. In about 90 percent of divorces involving children, the mother becomes the custodial parent. Children without fathers generally do less well in school and have poorer impulse control, less ego strength, and lower levels of moral development.

One frequently hears, "kids are resilient" or "children bounce back quickly" to assuage fears about the effects of separation and divorce on them. Are they true? Generalizations are of questionable validity, but researchers are finding that children suffer a great deal of anguish because

---

*From Karen L. Freiberg, *Human Development: A Life-Span Approach,* Third Edition. (Boston: Jones & Bartlett Publishers, 1987).

of the breaking up of the two-parent family, the primary foundation of security. The aftermath is long-lived. In fact, children usually do better during the crisis and have their worst problems with guilt, anger, fear, and depression later. The "bouncing back" seldom occurs until at least a year after the divorce.

When a mother loses her husband, she experiences shock, fears and anxieties, anger, bitterness, and resentment, especially if the husband now enjoys his freedom and/or a new sex partner, and loss of self-esteem. Less than one-third of departing fathers make significant monetary contributions to support their families, so most single-parent mothers must work. Most lose out economically. Many must move to more modest housing and give up luxuries such as a car. The physical and emotional stresses of working, balancing a budget, running the house, functioning as both father and mother, and being solely in charge can exhaust even the best organized and most emotionally stable women. Weinraub (1983) found that many of them work long hours and become socially isolated. They also become more authoritarian and erratic in the ways they discipline their children (Hetherington, 1979).

Single parenting usually becomes easier with time. Mothers learn how to cope by experience and by talking to other single parents in organizations such as Parents Without Partners. Counseling by mental health professionals is also desirable. Single parenting is made easier by sufficient money; help from the ex-husband, parents, neighbors, relatives, or friends; and people with whom to discuss physical, social, and emotional concerns.

When children lose a parent, they commonly experience anger, fears, insecurity, guilt, and depression (Hetherington, 1979). They worry about whether their needs will be met, about the absent parent, and about whether they are still loved. Kalter (1984) found that about one third of children believe their behavior caused the divorce. Most fantasize about, or actively try to negotiate, a reunion. If they must move away from old friends, neighbors, and classmates, or if they see less of their mother as she takes on extra work, they often feel extreme loneliness

and depression. Depression in children often takes the form of school setbacks, uncontrolled temper, destructive acts, and antisocial behavior. Boys seem to have many more problems adjusting to loss of a father than do girls (Hetherington, 1979). They refuse to comply with many of their mother's requests, adding to her stress. In turn, mothers often view their sons in a more negative light than their daughters. There are several things the parents can do to help tensions subside and bring children back to a sense of well being:

- Assure each child that the break-up was not his or her fault.
- Assure each child that he or she is still loved.
- Talk with each child about anger, fear, guilt, and depression.
- Be honest about your own feelings.
- Be honest about the financial situation.
- Don't tear down the reputation of the absent parent.
- Hide any quarrels with the absent parent.
- Encourage frequent contact with the absent parent (if he or she is emotionally well adjusted).
- Discourage fantasies and hopes for reconciliation (unless feasible).
- Discuss and reach agreement with the absent parent on rules of child-rearing and discipline and keep them consistently.
- Keep consistent schedules for meals, school, bedtime, and the like.
- Look to others (parents, siblings, friends, competent housekeeper) for support when stressed.
- Seek professional counseling or therapy for self or children if stressed.

Many mothers are concerned about how their sons will achieve a stable masculine self-concept without a live-in male role model. They should encourage their ex-husband or a trusted uncle, grandfather, brother, neighbor, or other man to interact with the boy(s). They should encourage independence and mastery of tasks, praise the boys' strengths and capabilities, and present maleness in a positive light.

Some mothers overprotect their sons and reward dependence. This may arise from the mothers' own needs for love and attention. Such mothers may encourage physical contact, discourage any signs of aggression, and interfere with the boys' attempts at mastery of tasks. Such boys may become timid and retiring, be underachievers, and have a low sense of worth in terms of their maleness. Some overprotective mothers also add negative comments about men to their tactics. The mother's comments about the inadequacy, incompetence, or worthlessness of men further decreases the son's sense of masculine worth.

Sometimes when the father is absent, the mother withdraws from or neglects her children. This may be especially true of sons, who she expects can take care of themselves and maybe even her. Boys so treated may dramatize their masculinity, toughness, and independence yet have an underlying low sense of worth as males.

Stepparenting

Within five years, most children whose parents break up have to learn to adjust to a stepparent. Approximately one out of eight children in the United States today has a stepparent (Einstein, 1979). It is hard to make generalizations about how children react to a new adult in the home since each situation is different. However, some jealousy and resentment are common. Blending new families is easier if the stepparent does not try to replace the biological parent but rather becomes a third (or fourth) parent. Relationships develop slowly and should not be rushed. The stepparent and biological parent should agree on child-rearing and discipline and be consistent, supporting each other when necessary. Although it is normal for one child to warm up to the stepparent before others, showing favoritism should be studiously avoided. Boys often accept a stepfather sooner than girls (Santrock, 1982). Daughters tend to be angry with their mothers for remarrying and anxious about the new interactions required.

Stepfathers are usually more acceptable to children than are stepmothers, and younger children accept stepparents more easily than do older children (Stapleton, 1981). Initially children may have more behavioral problems in the reconstituted family than in the single-parent family (Nunn, 1983), but over an extended period remarriage can mitigate the negative effects of the divorce and single-parent experience if the new partner is supportive, caring, and willing to work at becoming a parent (Rutter, 1979). Designing workable relationships between children and stepparents can seem overwhelmingly difficult at times. Many families cannot meet the challenge. Over 40 percent of newly blended families end in divorce within five years (Einstein, 1979).

THE SCHOOL'S ROLE IN SOCIALIZATION

A well-liked teacher, especially one who resembles a child in some way (sex, race, religion, ethnicity) may be taken on as a role model by a child. Sometimes a teacher will be aware of the child's modeling; often he or she will not. Consider these examples of teachers' impacts. Conant (1970), who helped develop the atom bomb, attributed his early interest in chemistry to a teacher. In his autobiography he wrote, "I doubt if any schoolteacher has ever had a greater influence on the intellectual development of a youth than Newton Henry Black had on mine." Helen Keller (1954) paid an even greater tribute to her teacher. She wrote, "All the best of me belongs to her—there is not a talent, or an aspiration or a joy in me that has not been awakened by her loving touch."

Lewin (1939) helped make educators aware of the ways a teacher can influence the social behavior of a group. They compared autocratic (dictatorial), democratic, and laissez-faire (let people make or do what they choose) teaching styles. They discovered that although the autocratic teachers ostensibly had good classes, the democratic teachers actually had the better ones. When the autocratic teachers left their groups, fighting broke out immediately. The laissez-faire teachers had fighting in their presence. In the democratic atmosphere policies were established by the group, and the children felt some responsibility for the rules they helped make. They showed little aggression in the teacher's presence or absence. They also liked the democratic leaders and worked harder for them.

The findings of this classic study are not unlike recent research pointing to both greater effectiveness and popularity of authoritative (democratic) parenting styles. More recently, Deci (1981) showed that autonomy-oriented (democratic) teachers contributed to their pupils' desires to learn and to their self-esteem much more than did control-oriented (autocratic) teachers. Autocratic teachers are more apt to engage in stereotypic labeling, which can have the Rosenthal effect, eliciting expected classroom performance. Tom (1984) found that authoritarian (autocratic) teachers have higher grade expectations for girls than for boys, for Asians than for whites, and for middle-class than for lower-class students. Ball (1984) also found that teachers lower their performance expectations for children from divorced single-parent families, especially boys.

While many persons believe that schools do not make a difference, research suggests differently. In an extensive review of the effect of school on the progress of pupils, Rutter (1983) concluded that effective schooling needs to be measured not only by scholastic attainment but also by attitudes toward learning, classroom behavior, social functioning, absenteeism, continuation in education, and ultimate employment. School features that may contribute to beneficial effects include resources, size of class, composition of student body, degree of academic emphasis, classroom management, pupil participation, discipline, and staff. One good teacher, especially in the first grade, can have remarkably persistent positive effects on students (Pedersen, 1978).

The effect of a teacher on in-classroom social behavior is better known than the carryover effect of socialization from class to home life. Much carryover modeling depends on the child's perception of the importance of the teacher's nurturance and power. Much also depends on how well caregivers understand, agree with, and are willing to adopt school socialization practices in their homes. A parent's negative attitude toward a school may contribute to a child's school phobia (box).

Carryover of socialization practices from school to home has been demonstrated more clearly in the Soviet Union than here (Bronfenbrenner, 1970). Character education is considered one of the most important functions of Soviet schools. Parents and community members are duty-bound to uphold the socialization begun in the schools. Children are taught to help each other and work together for the good of the class, the school, and ultimately the community and their country. They learn to praise and criticize their own and others' strengths and shortcomings rather than hide them. The group decides on rewards or punishments for behavior. Selfishness is one of the most serious offenses. A. S. Makarenko is the Soviet equivalent to America's Dr. Spock. Whereas Spock deals predominantly with physical health, Makarenko deals with character education and informs parents how to raise socially upright citizens.

PEER INTERACTIONS

Just as a schoolteacher may affect social development, so too can friends. Peers' influence on a child's behavior can be weak or strong, depending on several factors:

- Age
- Sex
- Self-esteem
- Intelligence
- The amount of time spent with peers
- The stoutness of the affectionate bond between parents and child
- The amount of constructive time spent with the family
- The family's acceptance of peer group members
- The values and activities of the peer group
- The child's position in the peer group

Children use their friends as sounding boards and testing grounds for the values and attitudes

SCHOOL PHOBIA

A fairly prevalent (and disabling) childhood phobia is *school phobia*. It is a condition whose victim develops symptoms of illness when left at school (headache, vomiting, cramps, diarrhea, hysteria, crying). It is most common when a child starts school but may also occur after a trauma, such as the loss of a parent by death or divorce. School-phobic children are typically more dependent, immature, and anxious than nonphobic children (Trueman, 1984). The root of the child's anxiety is not usually the school or the teacher but fear of being separated from the parent(s). However, over time the child may also become fearful of teasing or rejection or of being called on to recite. Symptoms decrease if a parent stays in the classroom. However, this is not a good solution. The immediate goal is to get the child to remain in school without the parent.

To help children overcome school phobia, parents need to be made aware of the ways in which they consciously or unconsciously convey the impression to their child that all will not be well during the separation. School-phobic children may sense that the parent will be lonely without them or that the parent does not believe the school is as safe, healthful, and loving as the home. Parents differ in their readiness to accept their own roles in their child's problem. Many need help in adjusting to their child's being in school all day. In some cases, the mother's taking a job will allow her to untie the apron strings and more willingly send her child to school. In some cases one or both parents need psychotherapy to work out their underlying conflicts about allowing their child autonomy, and about the safety of the school. This can help to prevent recurrences of the phobia.

When a school-phobic child does have physical symptoms in school, he or she should be sent to the nurse's office, not home. As soon as possible, the child should be gently but firmly returned to the classroom. Home teaching should not be prescribed. It creates more psychological invalidism and encourages continuation of the conscious or unconscious domination by the parent.

they have learned at home. In many cases the peer group (groups of persons of equal rank or status) is more democratic than the home. Instead of rules being laid down by authority figures, they are debated, with some or all of the group having a say in what they should be. Home values and attitudes may be upgraded or watered down, depending on the participants in the group.

Children increasingly turn to their peers for assistance. Nelson-LeGall (1984) asked children whom they would seek help from in academic and social contexts and found that their preferences for parental help decrease with age. Peer academic tutoring or collaboration brings with it unique motivational and cognitive benefits for the participating children (Damon, 1984).

During late childhood friendships become more stable. Friends are usually of the same sex and often of the same race, religion, culture, or socioeconomic standing. Organized activities such as scouting, sports, and religious group projects tend to strengthen friendships and add a cohesive element to a group. Little League has been shown to enhance the self-esteem of players (Hawkins, 1982). When children work together, they learn new respect for each other. Occasionally after a group failure or defeat, members will turn against each other, but in general teamwork strengthens friendships.

Children in groups often do things they would never do on their own. This can take the form of increased altruism (for example, visiting nursing homes) or increased delinquency (such as destroying property). Many a quiet, well-behaved child has joined a fight or used vulgar language along with a supporting peer group. Peers can influence each other for good or for bad. Some children are more powerful in influencing others, and some children are more influenced by powerful peers.

Being a member of a minority within a larger community frequently presents special problems for school-age children. If the minority group is large enough so a child can find a cohesive group of same-sex friends, the going is easier. Without other members as friends, it is often difficult for a child to feel worthwhile or acceptable to the mainstream peer groups. By the elementary school years children have learned many prejudices of their parents. Prejudice is an insidious thing. Even members of minority groups may adopt the mainstream culture's prejudice against themselves. Fu (1982) found that both black and white children from the South had a bias in favor of whites and against blacks.

Prejudice can be leveled at religious, language, cultural, and economic groups as well as racial groups. Obese children, chronically ill children, even homely children may find themselves the objects of peer ridicule. Communities and neighborhoods differ in what they find acceptable. Children may be ostracized if they come to school in old fashioned, small, or ragged clothes or without spending money for candy or other things purchased by the majority of the school children.

Children who lack proficiency in English or who speak with an accent are especially vulnerable to rejection by their classmates. The melting pot is not appreciated by many children during late childhood. Unless a child can master English quickly, he or she usually cannot participate fully in the social activities of the English-speaking core group. Unless steps are taken to teach English before other academic subjects are introduced, children fall farther and farther behind and may be classified as retarded in spite of very adequate intelligence. A proposed Bilingual Education Act, to fund school projects to teach English to children before attempting to teach them other academic subjects, was withdrawn by the Reagan administration in 1981. Schools themselves must now set up programs and find teachers to conduct English-language classes in the children's native languages, or else the teaching of English must be done at home or in the community before the child can learn in school.

NEIGHBORHOOD INTERACTIONS

Increasingly, child developmentalists are looking beyond the family, the school, and the peer group for other social influences on growing children. Neighbors are emerging as important sources of support in late childhood. As more mothers work outside the home, more at-home neighbors watch the children after school. Research on latchkey children, who are home alone after school, has suggested that while they tend to be more independent, they may also suffer more fears, loneliness, boredom, and depression (Long, 1983).

Because of increased fears of child abduction and child molestation, many parents make a conscious effort to introduce their children to several trusted neighbors to whom they may run if a stranger or older child bothers them. Many nonworking parents also want their children to know about safe houses, where trusted neighbors will be home, along the route to and from school. If children walk through business areas, parents may also want their children to know about stores, libraries, and the like where the child will be recognized, sheltered, and perhaps allowed to use the telephone. Bryant (1985) found that children who had more identifiable sources of support in their neighborhoods scored higher on several measures of social and emotional functioning. Helping school-age children develop a social network in their neighborhoods has many beneficial effects for safety, socialization, and mental health.

THE EFFECT OF TECHNOLOGY

The influences of parents, schools, peers, and neighbors are modified somewhat by machines of technology available to children. In addition to television, children now increasingly have videocassette recorders (VCRs). These enable them to tape television programs for late replay or to play movies, games, or music videos on their television sets. Children also have easy access to video games in arcades and other public places. Many of them are exposed to computers in school, and many have personal computers at home. The effects of television on children are better known than the effects of computers.

The average North American child is a heavy consumer of television, watching two to four hours a day on school days and more on weekends and school vacations. By completion of high school most children have spent about twice as much time watching television as in classrooms. Researchers have focused more on the negative concepts they acquire (aggression, junk food preferences, and sex role stereotypes) than on positive behavior (obedience to rules, empathy, altruism) they might learn.

Much aggression is shown on television. Networks have kept prime-time evening programs less violent until after 9 P.M. However, many children are allowed to stay up to watch the more violent programs. Pearl (1984) reported that over the past 10 years there has been more violence on children's weekend programs than on prime-time television.

In the past some social scientists believed that watching televised violence would have a cathartic effect and displace or dissipate a child's need to be aggressive. Instead, it has been found that the more violent programming children watch, the more aggressive they become in all aspects of life: conflicts with parents, fighting, and delinquent behavior. They also view the world with more suspicion and distrust and perceive violence as an effective solution to conflict (Pearl, 1984). Cordes (1985) reported that the more children watch TV, the likelier they are to believe it is real. This is true not only for violence but also for the behavior of men and women.

Children also believe in the enormous presence, in all homes except their own, of certain toys and foods. Commercial time on TV is higher than most people imagine, about 22 percent of the broadcast day. Commercials rarely last longer than 60 seconds, but they are skillfully designed to stay on their viewers' minds for much longer. Many commercials hire celebrities to endorse foods or toys for children. Ross (1984) found that 8- to 14-year-olds prefer products promoted by celebrities and fail to see that the ads are staged, especially when the commercial includes live action. Ads for highly sugared or salted foods with low nutritional value are flashed at children frequently, as often as eight times per hour on Saturday mornings. Children beg to be allowed to eat such foods and consider their parents particularly cruel if they deny them the "pleasures" the ad kids have consuming these foods.

Feldstein (1982) analyzed televised toy commercials and found that they not only have more males than females per commercial but also are more likely to put females in passive roles. Prime-time adult-oriented commercials do the same (Mackey, 1982).

Wright (1983) and Greenfield (1984) made it clear that television has a rich, although as yet largely untapped, potential for enhancing the cognitive and psychosocial development of children. Information-processing skills and retention of information can be increased and improved by television. Children can also acquire many positive concepts such as moral and prosocial behavior. It is unfortunate that so few programs have been developed to exploit these possibilities.

Parents can enhance the television viewing time of their children by watching with them, asking questions, explaining concepts, and discussing outcomes and alternatives to outcomes. When used wisely and sparingly, television can be an interactive, educational, and constructive family activity. Heavy viewing is potentially harmful, especially with the paucity of age-specific educational programming for children and the abundance of aggressive, violent, sex-stereotyped programs.

Greenfield (1984) described computer technology as another potentially great tool for enhancing children's cognitive and psychosocial development. While children watching television are passive, children playing video games are active. They must plan moves ahead and develop their fine motor skills to play competently. However, the natures of the video games children play have an effect on their behaviors, just as TV programming does. Some video games are terrifyingly violent, with ultimate goals of destruction and annihilation. Ascione (1985) reported that children who play violent video games are less likely to help other children.

Some people fear that computer games are addictive—that children who play a great deal may feel a compulsive need to continue playing. There is little evidence to support this. Most video games encourage interactions among competitive players. Rather than creating obsessive-compulsive socially isolated children, they often stimulate social involvement. Playing may improve the social acceptance and self-esteem of children who are competent at video games even though they are not good athletes or good scholars. Levin (1985) wrote that mastering a new computer game has much in common with solving a math problem. It absorbs the child's whole attention. The child must modify, augment, delete, or transform behavior in order to succeed.

Many children have computers in their homes. They use them not only to play games but also to create new games or other programs. Many adults who have tried to learn one or more computer languages are amazed at how quickly children learn these languages relative to their own slow progress. Programming requires that the user provide the machine with a carefully thought through series of instructions. This requires patience and willingness to correct one's mistakes. The computer provides precise feedback of what it has been told to do. It cannot be intimidated into doing something else. The user must take full responsibility for any bugs in the program and find out what he or she has done wrong. Levin (1985) writes that this process teaches children humility and personal responsibility. They cannot place the blame for mistakes on others. Many schools have incorporated computer programming courses into their curriculum. It will be years before we have a clear idea of the effects of computers on education and on intellectual, social, and emotional development. However, there is an optimistic sense that this technology can be beneficial. It will not be a substitute for parents and teachers, but used wisely, it can enhance the work of adults who rear children.

GENDER IDENTITY AND SEX ROLE*

Although anatomy and physiology provide the biological bases of human sexuality, most people's sexual experiences also involve beliefs,

thoughts, feelings, and social behavior. Even a person who knows little about reproductive biology is aware of the socially approved behavior for males and females. The awareness of being male or female is called *gender identity,* and gender-specific behavior is referred to as the *sex role.*

How individuals think and behave sexually is almost entirely a product of what they learn as children about gender and the kinds of behavior expected of members of the sexes. Studies of psychosexual development indicate that the development of gender identity and the subsequent expression of sex-specific behavior begins with the sex typing of newborn infants (Hampson, 1961; Money, 1972). When a child is born, almost the first thing noticed is its sex. "It's a boy" or "it's a girl" follows the observation.

Having been sex typed at birth, the infant is thereafter treated by adults as they think appropriate for that gender, and eventually the infant incorporates into its self-image the awareness of being male or female. By about 2, a child's gender identity is fixed for life (Hampson, 1961). How the child acts on the knowledge depends on a variety of factors. Children learn attitudes and behavior by modeling after parents, teachers, celebrities, and fictional characters, and they are also trained by reward and punishment. Whatever the sources of information and influence, children learn early in life which attitudes and behavior are appropriate for boys and which are appropriate for girls. By the age of 3, children are capable of citing a long list of items of behavior that are characteristic of one gender or the other.

Exactly which attitudes and behavior are deemed appropriate for both sexes depends on the culture. In some societies, sex roles are strictly defined, and little deviance from the stereotype is allowed. Our culture possesses a set of stereotypes that includes economic role, dominance or submissiveness in social relationships, responsibilities for home and child care, mode of dress, personal appearance, and the mode of expression of emotions. There is little evidence that our culture's stereotype was ever the predominant behavioral pattern, expect perhaps on television shows and in romantic fiction. Today the American sex role stereotype is a myth: Ap-

---

*From Gordon Edlin and Eric Golanty, *Health & Wellness, A Holistic Approach,* Third Edition. (Boston: Jones & Bartlett Publishers, 1988).

proximately 50 percent of the labor force consists of women; couples in increasing numbers are sharing the responsibilities of family care; women are becoming more assertive about their needs and wants; and men are becoming freer to express their feelings.

Another aspect of our cultural sex role stereotype is that people should be sexual only with members of the opposite sex, and that same-sex (homosexual) relationships are wrong, illegal, immoral, or indicative of psychological illness, although in some cultures homosexuality in some degree is condoned (Ford, 1951).

In spite of this bias, many people have had at least one sexual experience with someone of the same sex (Kinsey, 1948, 1953). Only about a third of the population is thought never to have had a same-sex experience. About 5 percent of the population is exclusively homosexual. The rest have had at least one same-sex experience, probably in childhood, when sexual experimentation is common. As adults, many of these people now define themselves as exclusively heterosexual.

The fact that many people have had some homosexual experience and that many admit to being erotically aroused by individuals of the same sex, even if they do not act on their feelings by having sex with them, supports the idea that homosexuality is not an illness. Moreover, attempts to find some genetic, hormonal, or metabolic explanation of homosexual inclinations have had no success. Psychological explanations proposing some form of psychopathology are also not accepted. The lack of evidence to support the contention that homosexuality is an illness is summed up by the official position of the American Psychiatric Association: "Homosexuality by itself does not necessarily constitute a psychiatric disorder. Homosexuality *per se* is one form of sexual behavior and, like other forms of sexual behavior which are not themselves psychiatric disorders, it is not listed (as one of the) mental disorders."

There is such a strong bias that heterosexuality is natural and homosexuality unnatural that people often wonder why some people are homosexual at all. In light of the lack of evidence that homosexuality is a psychological disorder and because there apparently is no biological explanation for homosexuality, the question is not what makes someone homosexual but rather what factors determine sexual orientation, whether heterosexual, homosexual, or bisexual (preference for members of either sex). Some people believe that humans are, in fact, inherently bisexual and that any preference for sexual partners of one sex or the other is determined by early experiences, as are most other forms of sexual behavior.

The Changes of Puberty*

After a child is born, its reproductive cells secrete low levels of hormones until some unknown factor triggers the final development of the reproductive system. This process—known as *puberty*—usually begins between 8 and 13 in girls and 9 and 14 in boys (Ganong, 1981) and may take several years.

The unknown factor seems to send chemical messages to the *hypothalamus,* a part of the brain that is important to sex hormone regulation. The hypothalamus then apparently sends a chemical-releasing factor to the *pituitary gland,* which lies just below the brain. The pituitary in turn secretes two *gonadotropins* (gonad-stimulating substances)—FSH (follicle-stimulating hormone) and LH (luteinizing hormone)—that stimulate the development of sex hormones in ovaries and testicles. These sex hormones prepare the body for reproduction by creating numerous physical changes (Figure 23.1).

In women the ovaries secrete *estrogens,* hormones that are feminizing in their effects, and *progesterone,* a hormone that prepares the uterus for pregnancy. Women produce small amounts of androgens in their ovaries and adrenal cortex, but it is the estrogens that cause most of the *secondary sex characteristics* that develop at puberty. These include enlargement of the breasts, uterus, and vagina; broadening of the hips; development of fat deposits on the breasts and buttocks; an increase in vaginal secretions; and the onset of menstruation *(menarche)* at a mean age

---

*This material is from Gilbert Nass and Mary Fisher, *Sexuality Today.* (Boston: Jones & Bartlett Publishers, 1988).

FIGURE 23.1
Male and female changes of puberty.

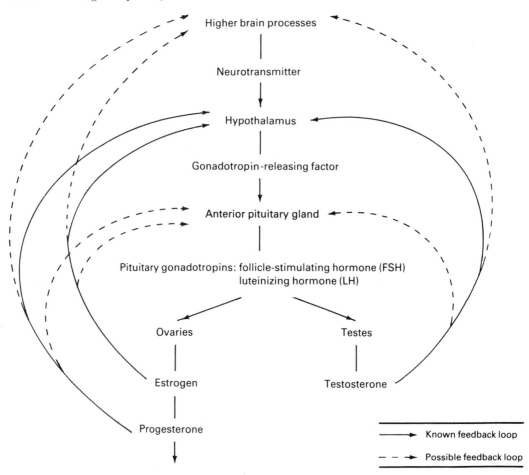

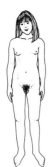
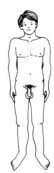

Female

Growth of breasts
Development of fat deposits
Enlargement and preparation of
  uterus for pregnancy
Growth of hair on armpits
  and pubis
Enlargement of vagina, labia,
  and clitoris
Onset of menstruation
Beginning of secretion of
  vaginal fluids

Male

Recession of scalp hair, growth
  of facial hair
Growth of larynx and vocal cords
  (voice pitch deepens)
Development of muscles and bones
Growth of hair on chest, abdomen,
  armpits, and pubis
Enlargement of penis, testes,
  and scrotum
Development of ducts and glands
  that transport and nurture sperm
Beginning of ejaculation

PRECOCIOUS PUBERTY

Although girls often want their first period to come and boys want their growth spurt to begin so they can be like their friends and feel grown-up, puberty occasionally comes so soon to children that it creates terrible problems for them. In 1 out of every 5,000 to 10,000 children (particularly girls), puberty occurs before the age of 8 or 9 in girls and 10 in boys and is therefore classified precocious. Sometimes the changes of puberty occur as early as infancy.

One girl had developed breasts, a slender waist, and mature legs by the time she started menstruating at age three, and she was several inches taller than other children her age. Her mother had to make all her clothes and protect her from public ogling by measures such as not taking her to the beach. With the stares of strangers, the turbulent mood swings of hormonal change, and "teenage" acne, her childhood was hardly a normal one. As Ora Hirsch Pescovitz, a specialist in precocious puberty, put it, "You can imagine what you'd be dealing with if you take a child going through the terrible twos and add the hormones a thirteen-year-old has" (Lehman, 1986a, 47). These children also feel conspicuously different and isolated from their peers, who often tease them or avoid them.

Fortunately, advances in hormonal treatment offer hope of delaying the changes of puberty until the usual age. For some, daily injections of LHRHa, a synthetic version of the chemical message sent from the hypothalamus gland to the pituitary gland, prevent the natural LHRH (or gonadotropin-releasing factor) from reaching the pituitary. These shots stop pubertal growth of breasts and testicles, rapid bone growth, and menstrual periods, all of which seem to recur normally when the shots are stopped. The therapy is too new, though, to know whether it will affect reproductive potential in adulthood.

---

of 12.6 in the United States (Udry, 1986). Girls also begin to grow hair in their pubic area and armpits, a change triggered chiefly by androgens.

In boys large amounts of androgens, principally testosterone, and a small amount of estrogens are secreted by the testes; more androgens and perhaps estrogens are secreted by the adrenal cortex. The androgens create the male secondary sex characteristics. These include growth of muscles and pubic and underarm hair, the beginning of a beard, enlargement of the penis and scrotum, deepening of the voice, maturation of internal sexual organs, and thickening of skin gland secretions that may lead to acne. Ejaculation is now possible and may happen spontaneously as wet dreams (nocturnal emissions). Ejaculations during sleep may be associated with erotic dreams or simply may occur as a release of sexual tensions built up during the day. Girls may experience orgasm during sleep, and both sexes may experience emotional turbulence as their hormonal patterns shift and become temporarily imbalanced. Girls often find themselves crying "for no reason at all," and boys may have explosive sensations of crazy energy. One otherwise gentle 15-year-old skipped classes when he couldn't stand the feeling, explaining, "I was feeling so violent and crazy that I was afraid I'd hurt somebody."

The changes of puberty may be a source of embarrassment or fear to those who don't know that the new things their bodies are doing have a natural, expected biological base. In the past girls who were not taught about menstruation feared that they were bleeding to death. Because they had learned to regard their genital area as taboo, they were afraid to tell anybody and instead secretly suffered, worried, and tried to hide the blood. Today, girls still find the onset of menstruation a significant milestone in their lives, for various reasons: being like (or different from) their friends, seeing menstruation as a badge of maturity or womanhood, being bothered by the inconvenience and messiness of menstrual flow, or feeling new physical discomfort, emotional changes, or restrictions on their activities. The potential for becoming pregnant, as ovulation begins on an erratic basis during the first year of menstruation, is not usually regarded as significant (Ruble, 1982).

Although many girls are now educated to anticipate the beginning of menstrual bleeding, they may be unaware that puberty also means that they will secrete vaginal fluids when they are sexually excited. Young women who do not know that it is natural for lubricating fluids to appear in their vaginal area when they are sexually aroused may think they are wetting their pants, something they were trained from infancy to avoid. It is possible that in trying to inhibit this natural flow of fluids, some may develop holding-in (or tensing) patterns that later interfere with free enjoyment of sex.

For boys, too, absence of talk within the family about sex may lead to embarrassing attempts to conceal the evidence of wet dreams. The spontaneity of erections, which begin to happen at socially awkward times, may also lead to embarrassment. Nevertheless, early pubertal development enhances boys' self-esteem. By contrast, girls who experience the physical changes of puberty early and have begun "dating" are typically, but perhaps temporarily, lower in self-esteem than sixth- and seventh-grade girls who have not (Simmons, 1979). Girls whose breasts swell early may try to hide them because they are disturbed by attention from others who perceive them, on the basis of their changed physical appearance, as being mature and sexually interested.

Female Sexual Anatomy*

A woman's internal sexual organs consist of two *ovaries*, which lie on either side of the abdominal cavity, the *fallopian tubes*, the *uterus*, and the *vagina*; together these structures make up a specialized tube that goes from each ovary to the outside of the body (Figure 23.2). The ovaries produce fertilizable ova and sex hormones, which control the development of the female body type, maintain normal sexual physiology, and help maintain the course of a normal pregnancy. The fallopian tubes gather and transport ova that are released from the ovaries (about one each month). The two fallopian tubes connect to the uterus, an organ about the size of a woman's fist, situated just behind the pelvic bone and the bladder (Figure 23.3). The uterus is part of the

---

*The following material is from Gordon Edlin and Eric Golanty, *Health & Wellness, A Holistic Approach*, Third Edition. (Boston: Jones & Bartlett Publishers, 1988).

FIGURE 23.2
The female sexual and reproductive system.

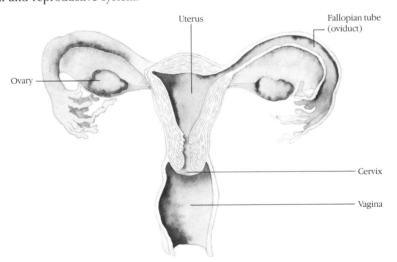

FIGURE 23.3
A side view of the female reproductive and sexual organs.

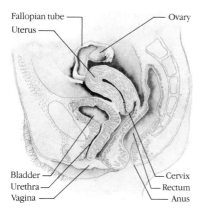

passageway for sperm that move from the vagina to the fallopian tubes; after fertilization, it provides the environment in which the fetus grows. It is the inner lining of the uterus that is shed each month in menstruation.

The lower part of the uterus is the *cervix,* which means "neck." The cavity of the uterus is connected to the vagina by means of a small opening called the cervical os. The cervix secretes mucus, which changes in consistency during the menstrual cycle. Some women learn to estimate the time of *ovulation* (ovum release) by examining their cervical mucus, providing a method of contraception that does not involve pills or mechanical devices.

The vagina is a tube that leads from the cervix to the outside of the body. Normally, the vagina is narrow, but it can readily widen to accommodate the penis during intercourse, a tampon during menstruation, the passage of a baby during childbirth, or a pelvic examination. The vagina possesses a unique physiology that is maintained by the secretions of the vaginal walls. These secretions help control the growth of microorganisms that normally inhabit the vagina and help to cleanse the vagina. Because the vagina is self-cleansing, it is usually unnecessary to employ any extraordinary cleansing measures, such as douching. Very often douching merely upsets the natural chemical balance of the vagina

and increases the risk of vaginal infections, called *vaginitis.*

A woman's external genitals (Figure 23.4) consist of two pairs of fleshy folds that surround the opening of the vagina, and the *clitoris*. The smaller, inner pair of folds are called the *labia minora,* and the larger, outer pair are called the *labia majora.* The clitoris, a highly sensitive sexual organ, is situated above the vaginal opening.

The opening of the *urethra,* the exit tube for urine, is located at the vaginal region just below the clitoris. The fact that the urethra is only about ½ inch long and so close to the vagina makes it susceptible to irritation and infection, called *urethritis,* which is characterized by a burning sensation during urination and usually by a frequent urge to urinate. Occasionally, bacteria introduced into the urethra migrate to the bladder and produce an infection called *cystitis.* The symptoms of cystitis are similar to those of urethritis.

If a woman develops a mild case of urethritis or cystitis, she can often eliminate the irritating

FIGURE 23.4
External female genitals.

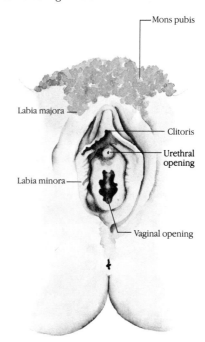

bacteria by drinking a lot of fluids to wash the bacteria from the urinary tract and by making the urine more acidic, either by taking high doses of vitamin C or by drinking acidic fruit juices. It is also advisable not to drink alcohol or ingest caffeine or spices, for these substances may irritate an already inflamed urinary tract. If pain is severe or if there is blood in the urine, a physician should be consulted.

A woman's secondary sex characteristics include the breasts, a network of milk glands and milk ducts embedded in fatty tissue. Breast size among women varies with the amount of fatty tissue in the breasts. There is little variation among women in the amount of milk-producing tissue; thus, a woman's ability to breast-feed is unrelated to the size of her breasts.

The breasts are supplied with nerve endings that are important in the delivery of milk to a nursing baby. These nerves also make the breast highly sensitive to touch, and many women find certain forms of tactile stimulation to be sexually pleasurable. Sexual arousal, tactile stimulation, and cold temperatures can cause small muscles in the nipples to contract, resulting in erection of the nipples.

Male Sexual Anatomy

The principal role of male sexual organs is to make viable sperm cells and to deliver them into the female reproductive tract during sexual intercourse. The male reproductive system consists of two *testes* (singular: testis), the sites of sperm and sex hormone production; a series of sperm ducts that originate at the testes, course through the pelvis, and terminate at the urethra of the penis; glands that produce seminal fluid; and the *penis,* the organ of copulation (Figure 23.5).

The testes are in a flesh-covered sac, the *scrotum,* that hangs outside the man's body. In the embryo, the testes develop inside the body, but just before birth they descend into the scrotum. Inside the scrotum the testes are kept a few degrees cooler than the internal body temperature, a condition that is apparently necessary for the production of fertile sperm. One testis is usually a little higher than the other.

Sperm are deposited in the female reproductive system during sexual intercourse (copulation). At that time, the male and female reproductive tracts form an uninterrupted passageway from the testes to the fallopian tubes,

FIGURE 23.5
The male sexual and reproductive system.

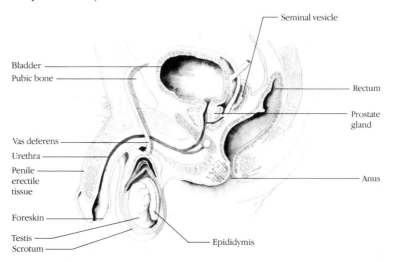

where fertilization of the ovum takes place. When a man ejaculates, sperm are propelled through the sperm ducts and out of the penis by contractions of the smooth muscles that line the ducts and the muscles of the pelvis. As they make their way out of the male body, the sperm mix with fluid from the seminal vesicles, prostate gland, and Cowper's glands to form semen. The semen, the gelatinous milky fluid that is emitted at ejaculation, contains about 300 million sperm cells and about 3 ml to 6 ml of seminal fluid. Seminal fluid contributes 95 percent or more of the volume of semen.

Normally the penis is soft, but when a man becomes sexually aroused, it fills with blood, enlarges, and becomes erect. All men are born with a fold of skin, the *foreskin*, that covers the end of the penis. For centuries Jewish and Muslim families have surgically removed the foreskin from male children for religious reasons. Nowadays, *circumcision*, as this procedure is called, is often carried out routinely on newborn boys regardless of religion. Although there is no clear medical indication that circumcision is beneficial, removal of the foreskin does eliminate the buildup of *smegma*, a white, cheesy substance that can accumulate under the foreskin. Although some scientists have suggested that smegma may contribute to penile and cervical cancer in a few individuals, Wallerstein (1980) points out that the evidence does not support this. The belief that circumcision leads to an increase in sexual arousal because it exposes the glans, and the related belief that circumcision produces inability to delay ejaculation have been shown to be incorrect (Masters and Johnson, 1966). For most men, circumcision has no effect on sexual arousal or sexual activity.

THE DECISION TO BECOME A PARENT

From childhood, almost everyone, particularly women, is instilled with the expectation that to have a child is the purpose of life. Many people never question this. They simply assume that they will have children just as their parents did. It is common for people to believe that having children is a special and rewarding part of life and that it would be a mistake not to do it. Some may see having a child as a way to leave a legacy of themselves to the world—a kind of immortality.

Not everyone is suited for parenthood, however. In spite of our society's values, many people decide that having a child is not best for them or for an overpopulated world. They may see parenthood as an infringement on their career goals or as an unnecessary or unwanted addition to their intimate partnership. Perhaps they have doubts about their psychological or economic abilities to nurture and support a child. Some people refrain from parenthood because they have or may carry a genetic disease.

Rearing a child is an enormous responsibility for both father and mother, and it often requires major adjustments in their personal lives. It certainly requires a change in the way family resources—time, energy, physical space, and money—are distributed. It may involve a change in the career plans of one or both of the parents. Uses of leisure time often change. Travel becomes more difficult. Ditzion (1978) of the Boston Women's Health Book Collective points out:

The decision to parent cannot be taken lightly. As soon as we've decided to become parents through pregnancy, adoption, or step-parenting, we find ourselves confronted with new emotional decisions. We want to develop a strong bond with our child and at the same time maintain our partnership, our adult friendships, as well as our involvements with the outside world. What we discover even before we have a baby is that our lives are thrown off balance once we become parents and we need time to establish a new equilibrium.

The period of parenting is an intense one. Never again will we know such responsibility, such productive and hard work, such potential for isolation in the caretaking role, and such intimacy and close involvement in the growth and development of another human being.

Our children do not ask to be born. We make that decision for them. We must be as certain as we can that our decisions to have children are appropriate for our life goals and that we have the means for caring for our children.

BECOMING PREGNANT

For most people, becoming a parent involves pregnancy—a 40-week period during which a fetus grow inside the mother's uterus and the mother's body undergoes considerable change to nurture the child developing within her. Every pregnancy begins with *fertilization,* the fusion of a father's sperm cell with a mother's ovum to form the first cell of their child, called the *zygote.* When a man ejaculates during sexual intercourse, millions of sperm cells swim with their long tails through the uterus and into the fallopian tubes, the usual site of fertilization (Figure 23.6). Only one of the many sperm cells actually fertilizes the egg. After fertilization, the zygote moves to the uterus, where it implants in the lining and proceeds to develop.

FIGURE 23.6
The joining of sperm and egg in fertilization. After fertilization, the zygote travels down the fallopian tube to the uterus. Implantation of the multicelled organism begins approximately six days after fertilization.

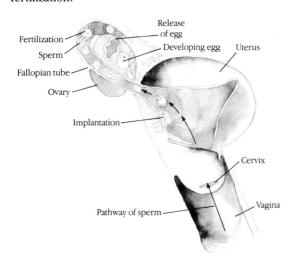

Soon after the zygote implants in the uterus, the mother begins to secrete a unique hormone called *human chorionic gonadotropin,* or HCG. This changes the production of estrogen and progesterone in the mother's ovaries (Figure 23.7). Under the influence of HCG, the ovaries release increasing amounts of these two hormones, which in turn bring about the first noticeable signs and symptoms of pregnancy, the most common of which are absence of menstruation; occasional nausea and vomiting, or morning sickness; enlarged and tender breasts; increased frequency of urination; and enlargement of the uterus. Often these signs and symptoms convince a couple that the woman is pregnant, but proof of pregnancy depends on confirmation of the presence of a fetus in the uterus. This information is most often obtained by analyzing the mother's urine for HCG. Women can now test themselves with home pregnancy kits. After the fetus has grown, it is possible to feel it moving around, to hear its heartbeat, and to see it with ultrasound. X-rays should be avoided except in

FIGURE 23.7
The pattern of human chorionic gonadotropin (HCG) secretion during pregnancy.

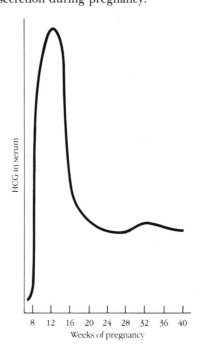

highly unusual cases, as the x-rays can cause birth defects.

FERTILITY AND THE MENSTRUAL CYCLE

Human beings are fertile after puberty, which almost always occurs during adolescence. From the time of sexual maturity men are capable of producing a continuous supply of sperm cells—about 150 million a day—for many years.

Women are neither fertile on a daily basis nor capable of producing ova as late in life as men are capable of producing sperm. From the time of sexual maturity, women usually produce only one fertile ovum each month, and ovum production usually stops altogether between 40 and 55.

The fact that fertile ova are produced about monthly is the basis of a woman's *menstrual cycle.* During each ovulation a woman's body undergoes several hormone changes that prepare her body for pregnancy. One of these changes is the thickening of the lining of the uterus, called the *endometrium,* so as to nurture a zygote during the first stages of pregnancy. Also, certain blood vessels in the uterus increase in size. Their role is to bring maternal nutrients to the fetus via the placenta.

If the ovum is not fertilized, the enlarged endometrium and the blood vessels within it are shed. This produces a loss of about two or three tablespoons of blood and tissue debris, which leaves the body through the vagina over the course of 3 to 6 days during *menstruation.*

The length and regularity of the menstrual cycle vary from woman to woman. Most women's cycle is approximately 28 days, with 24 to 35 days most common. Shorter and longer cycles are possible, and so are cycles that occur nearly monthly but that vary by a few days from cycle to cycle. Irregular cycles are typical at puberty and just before *menopause,* when a woman's menstrual cycle ceases.

The menstrual cycle is controlled by a number of hormones (Figure 23.8). The hypothalamus secretes hormones called *releasing factors,* which influence the release of other hormones, called gonadotropins, from the pituitary gland. Their function is to stimulate the production of a mature ovum, estrogen, and progesterone. These ovarian hormones induce changes necessary to support pregnancy. The preparation of the endometrium for pregnancy is but one function of estrogen and progesterone (Table 23.1). If fertilization does not occur, the hormonal support of tissue growth in the uterus stops and the endometrium is lost in menstruation.

For some women, menstruation is accompanied by unpleasant symptoms. It is estimated that 50 percent of women have abdominal pain, called cramps or *dysmenorrhea,* usually during the first day or so of menstrual flow. Although psychological, anatomical, and hormonal factors can contribute to menstrual cramps, in most cases the likely cause is strong, frequent uterine contractions by *prostaglandins.* Prostaglandins, formed at menstruation, seem to produce uterine contractions so that the menstruate will be completely removed from the uterus. Women who suffer from menstrual cramps tend to produce high levels of prostaglandins during menstruation. In many instances, cramps are reduced or eliminated if no ovum is released during a cycle. This is why many women have no cramps when they take birth control pills. The severity of cramps is sometimes lessened if a woman's body is flexible. Physical exercises can increase flexibility, and relaxation through meditation, autogenic training, image visualization, or any of the several relaxation techniques discussed in previous chapters of this book may also relieve menstrual discomfort. Medications that reduce the effects of prostaglandins can also help relieve cramps.

Another frequent problem is changes in feelings and disposition as menstruation approaches and during the first day or two of flow. Although reliable statistics are unavailable, it is possible that near menstruation approximately half of women undergo distressing physical, psychological, and behavioral changes, collectively known as *premenstrual syndrome* (PMS). These changes may include headache, backache, fatigue, feeling bloated, breast tenderness, depression, irritability, unusually aggressive feelings, and social

FIGURE 23.8

(Below) Hormonal control of the menstrual cycle. Hormones from the hypothalamus control the release of hormones from the pituitary gland, which regulates the production of the ovum and sex hormones from the ovaries. Note how the rise and fall of the hormones is related to the building up and sloughing off of the uterine lining.

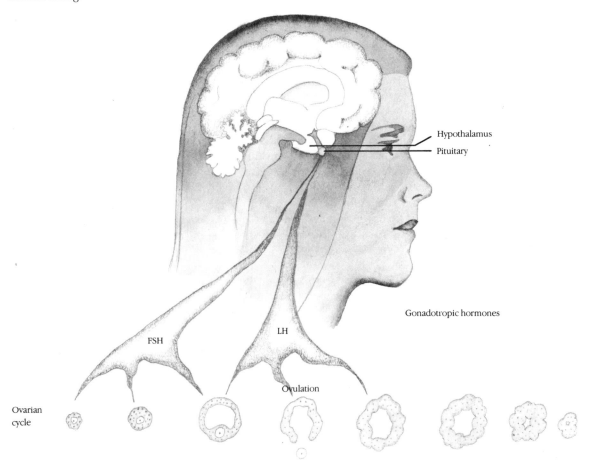

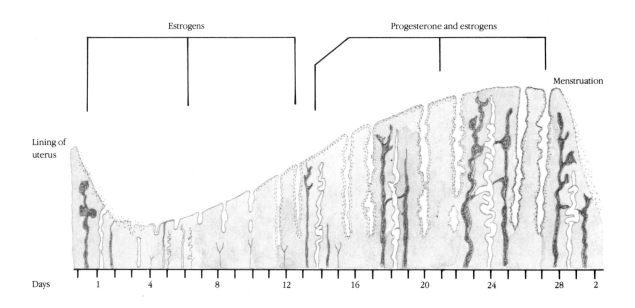

TABLE 23.1
Functions of Estrogen and Progesterone

Organ	Estrogen	Progesterone
Ovary	Increases sensitivity to gonadotropins	
	Stimulates growth in ovarian cells	
Fallopian tubes	Increases motility and secretion	Decreases motility
Uterus	Stimulates proliferation of blood vessels	Increases secretory activity of endo-metrium
	Increases size of muscle cells	Decreases contractions in uterine muscle
	Stimulates production of cervical mucus	Causes changes in viscosity of cervical mucus
Vagina	Stimulates growth and changes in vaginal cells	Causes changes in cells of vagina
	Maintains vaginal secretions	
Breasts	Stimulates growth and development of nipple and milk ducts	
Secondary sex characteris-tics	Stimulates feminine pattern of hair growth	
	Stimulates feminine pattern of fat distribution	

withdrawal. With the onset of menstruation, most sufferers of PMS report prompt relief from the symptoms, although many also get cramps.

Whether PMS is the result of changes in hormone levels or is the manifestation of negative attitudes and experiences with menstruation is uncertain (Parlee, 1982). A number of hypotheses have been proposed, including deficiencies in progesterone or vitamin B_6 (pyridoxine), fluid retention, hypoglycemia, and abnormal changes in endogenous opiate peptides (endorphins) in the late phases of the menstrual cycle (Reid, 1983). So far none of these hypotheses has been proven. However, a number of private clinics treat PMS, often with high doses of progesterone or vitamins. The efficacy of these treatments is uncertain; the greatest benefit may be going to clinics that charge high fees for administering to women with PMS (Eagan, 1983; Heneson, 1984). Many physicians treat PMS with diuretics, tranquilizers, antidepressants, and other drugs, which often only make the symptoms worse (Reid, 1983).

Still another common menstrual difficulty is the unexpected interruption or cessation of menstrual periods, called *amenorrhea*. The most

frequent reason is pregnancy, but the list of factors that can interfere with menstruation is quite long. It includes any kind of psychological stress, such as grief, depression, trauma, marital or sexual problems; excess fatigue; and even the fear of pregnancy. Other reasons menstrual periods stop are nutritional abnormalities (including crash diets), obesity, ingestion of drugs such as chlorpromazine or heroin, and taking the Pill.

Although there may be a physiological basis for some menstrual disorders and discomforts, often the problems have a psychological origin. Impressionable young girls are "forewarned" by friends or relatives; they may be told that the menstrual discharge is unclean, or that they will feel uncomfortable and irritable.

The hormones and reproductive system are particularly sensitive to a woman's mental state and beliefs about menstruation. Often a reexamination of any negative programming stemming from childhood or adolescence can release some fear and tension that may be associated with menstruation. Positive, comfortable suggestions given to oneself during relaxation exercises and mentally visualizing the menstrual cycle as a natural, biologically normal process can sometimes reduce and perhaps even eliminate cramps and other menstrual problems.

A woman can also try to ameliorate menstrual distress by attending to her diet and exercise patterns near the time of menstruation. To help reduce fluid retention, she can limit salt intake. To help maintain emotional stability, she can cut down on or eliminate the use of caffeine and sugar, especially in large doses. Vigorous exercise can promote endorphin release, which may modulate any tendency toward mood swings and possibly relieve physical discomforts.

INFERTILITY

Ten percent to 15 percent of couples who want to have children have difficulty doing so. These couples may be *infertile,* particularly if they have not been able to achieve a pregnancy after a year without using a contraceptive. In about half of infertile couples the reason for infertility is discovered and there is some way to overcome the problem. Occasionally, couples are infertile simply because they are not having intercourse at ovulation. The rhythm method of contraception (calendar rhythm, recording of the basal body temperature, or observation of cervical mucus) can also be used to determine the time of ovulation to help the woman get pregnant. Infertility may also result from ill health. Diabetes, hepatitis, chronic alcoholism, malnutrition, anxiety, stress, and fatigue can lessen fertility. Medical management of a problem or a change in lifestyle can often restore fertility.

In about 40 percent of infertile couples, the problem stems from low numbers of living sperm. From puberty, when a man becomes sexually and reproductively capable, he can produce about 150 million sperm cells daily—unless there is some problem. Injury, disease, drug and alcohol abuse, stress, and genetic or developmental problems can reduce the sperm count below the level necessary for fertility. It is thought that conception is highly improbable unless about 20 million healthy sperm are present. Difficulty in getting and maintaining an erection or ejaculating in the vagina can also inhibit fertility.

Infertility stems from the female partner about as often as from the male one. The most frequent factor in feminine infertility is preventing sperm from meeting the ovum. In some instances a benign growth in the uterus or cervix blocks the fallopian tubes. Sometimes cervical mucus is too thick or voluminous to allow sperm entry into the uterus. Infections of the female reproductive tract, especially untreated gonorrhea and chlamydia, can cause permanent scarring that blocks the tubes. A variety of hormonal imbalances can upset the growth, development, and release of fertile ova. In some cases, surgery to remove physical blocks or hormone therapy can overcome the problem, and the couple will be able to conceive.

CHILDBIRTH

Few human events are as dramatic as childbirth. We can only surmise what a new baby feels during the hours-long journey from the uterus to the outside world (Figure 23.9). Whether painful, frightening, or exhilarating, it must be intense. For parents, childbirth brings exaltation and relief that the pregnancy and waiting are over. For onlookers and family members, childbirth elicits wonder, sometimes reverence, and concern for the condition of the mother and baby. Childbirth, with its nakedness, blood, mess, effort, sweat, and tears of pain and joy, exposes our primal humanness like nothing else.

The release of intense emotions in childbirth is heightened by the inherent risk of danger to mother and baby. In a small percentage of births, certain life-threatening complications do arise. The mother can bleed extensively, infection may occur, or the baby's oxygen supply can be cut off as it makes the transition from the amniotic fluid to air. If the air supply is cut off too long, brain damage and even death can result. The goal of childbirth is to make the experience as rewarding as possible and to make the event safe.

Not many years ago, many expectant mothers and their families feared childbirth. They knew it was painful, that the baby could be stillborn, that the mother could die (see Figure 23-10). The high risks led to the development of a

NEW WAYS TO OVERCOME INFERTILITY

At the moment of her birth in the summer of 1978, Louise Brown became a celebrity, not because her parents were famous but because Louise was the first "test tube baby"—the first child to be conceived outside the mother's body. Like millions of other couples, Louise's parents are infertile. The revolutionary medical procedure that helped bring Louise into the world, *in vitro* fertilization, is only one of several new methods infertile couples are using, or soon will use, to have children.

In vitro fertilization is used when a woman's fallopian tubes are obstructed. The woman can produce eggs, but the blocked tubes prevent the meeting of egg and sperm. To overcome this problem, a doctor removes eggs from the woman's ovaries and places them in a laboratory dish (the "test tube"), where they are bathed with sperm donated by the husband. Fertilization takes place in the dish. Then the fertilized egg is inserted into the mother's uterus, where it develops into a baby in the normal way.

Hundreds of children so conceived have been born, and many more are likely to be born as more medical specialists learn the procedure. The few specialists who have been successful with it are deluged with pleas for help from infertile couples.

Whereas *in vitro* fertilization raises some ethical questions for a few, most people seem to be enthralled rather than worried. Acceptance of new medical technologies for overcoming infertility may open the door for more unusual methods of treatment.

For example, if a woman cannot have a normal pregnancy, she and her husband can hire a surrogate mother to have the child for them. A woman is chosen from a group of consenting candidates to be artificially inseminated by the husband's sperm. The surrogate receives a fee for carrying and giving birth to the couple's child.

Another possible way for surrogates to be used is to combine *in vitro* fertilization with surrogate motherhood. That is, the infertile couple donates egg and sperm, which are brought together in the laboratory to form a fertilized egg. But instead of putting the embryo back into the donor's uterus, it is implanted in the surrogate's uterus, where it develops into a child.

Yet another possibility is prenatal adoption. An egg donated by a surrogate is fertilized *in vitro* with the husband's sperm. The resulting embryo is then placed inside the wife's uterus.

Couples who overcome their infertility problem, whatever the procedure, are grateful that they can have children. Those who donate eggs and sperm to others, or who serve as surrogate mothers, usually feel special because they are helping to give life and are helping others to fulfill important life goals. As for the children brought into the world with these unusual techniques, most experts believe that a child's well-being is determined not by where conception takes place, or by who carries the baby to term, but by the quality of the love and care they receive after birth.

---

specialized type of medical practice—obstetrics—dedicated to controlling the complications of pregnancy and childbirth. With the advent of anesthesia, antibiotic therapy, identification of high-risk mothers, fetal monitoring, and trained birth attendants, the degree of maternal and infant mortality and the incidence of maternal and infant illness are quite low. Serious complications arise in about 5 percent of unaided pregnancies and childbirths. With obstetric help, however, the complication rate is 1 or 2 in 10,000.

Until the recent past, nearly all births were managed the same way: Mother begins rhythmic uterine contractions and tells her husband it's

time to go to the hospital. He rushes her to the hospital, where she is taken to a room and put to bed to deliver. The husband goes to a waiting room to pace nervously. The baby is born and put in a small crib in a nursery filled with other newborns. Father looks at the babies from behind a glass partition, trying to determine which is his.

Less familiar procedures are prepping the mother with an enema and giving a tranquilizer or anesthetic. When the baby is about to emerge, the mother is transferred to a delivery room, where her doctor and the nursing attendants assist with the remainder of the birth. It is likely

FIGURE 23.9
Childbirth.

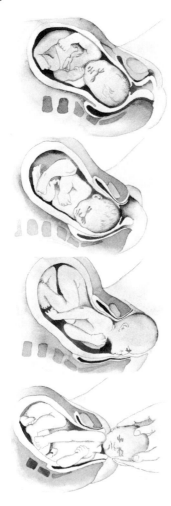

that the doctor will perform an *episiotomy*, a surgical incision between the vagina and the anus that helps prevent tears to the vagina and the perineum by enlarging the vaginal exit. The mother may hold the baby immediately after it is born. The baby is then taken to a nursery and mother to a recovery room.

One of the characteristics of the traditional hospital birth is that the families have little control over the procedure. Once the obstetrician is selected, virtually all decisions about how the birth is carried out are left to the doctor and the obstetrical assistants in the hospital. Many families prefer this, for they trust the doctor and hospital staff to make decisions that they feel

unqualified to make. Other families want to participate in the birthing. They might find a traditional hospital setting too cold for what they feel is a joyous, warm occasion, and consequently may want to have their baby in an alternative birth center or at home. Because unforeseen medical emergencies can occur during childbirth, the birthing room—a hospital-based delivery room with a homelike atmosphere where the husband or entire family can participate in the birth—is preferable to birthing at home, where no medical help is on hand.

Couples may want to make other decisions about the birth. The mother may want to be awake and in full control of her body, which means that she receives no anesthesia or only minor pain relief. The mother may not want to have an episiotomy unless the birth is difficult. The couple may want low lighting and perhaps music to make the mother more comfortable, and to make the birth less traumatic for the baby (Leboyer, 1975).

Several programs and organizations teach families how to prepare for childbirth. These "natural childbirth," classes include the Lamaze course, named after a French doctor who developed a popular program. Almost all childbirth preparation courses teach the biology of pregnancy and childbirth as well as breathing and relaxation exercises to help the delivery proceed smoothly. While attending the six- to eight-week courses, parents-to-be meet other expectant couples with whom they can share anxieties and experiences. In the class couples learn of the many choices they have about childbirth and how to find the setting and professional help they prefer.

Stages of Labor and Delivery*

Women typically begin labor with uterine contractions that are fifteen to twenty minutes apart and that gradually increase in strength and frequency. During this *first stage* of labor, the length-

---

*The following material is from Gilbert Nass and Mary Fisher, *Sexuality Today* (Boston: Jones & Bartlett Publishers, 1988).

FIGURE 23.10

a, Incidence of maternal mortality in the United States, 1940 to 1980. b, Incidence of infant mortality in the United States, 1930 to 1980. (Data from National Center for Health Statistics.)

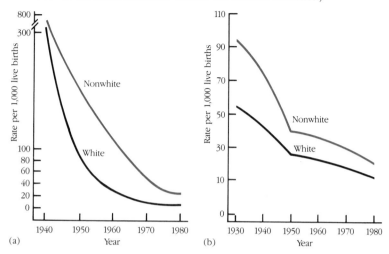

wise muscles of the cervix are working to enlarge *(dilate)* and thin *(efface)* the opening of the cervix (Figure 23.11).

During this stage, which may last from two hours to a day or more, the health care practitioner monitors the baby's life signs. When the baby's head begins to move through the dilated cervix into the birth canal, most women feel a tremendous urge to push, or bear down, with all their strength. This period is the *second stage* of labor. It is usually much shorter than the first stage, and most women become more actively involved during this phase of the birth. Because they grimace with the strain of each push, onlookers often assume that they are in pain, when in fact such expressions may be as much the result of extreme physical and emotional concentration as much as from pain. Muscular, breathing, and relaxation exercises or medication can help women cope with the intensity of second stage labor.

As the woman begins to bear down, if she is in a hospital, she is typically brought to a delivery room, where she is placed on a table flat on her back with her feet held apart in stirrups. This traditional procedure is a necessity when the mother is medicated, but many hospitals have modified the procedure, for in a flat position gravity works against outward passage of the

baby. If the woman is allowed to sit with her legs spread, she can push more easily. If she squats, she can help the baby pass through by altering the position of her pelvic bones.

Accordingly, many birth settings accommodate the individual needs of the laboring woman. Depending on the progress of labor and comfort of the woman, various positions may be used throughout labor and delivery. The woman may spend the early part of the second stage in a semiupright position and then, as the bearing down becomes more intense, be more comfortable lying on her side for delivery so that the baby exerts less pressure on her spine.

The second stage of labor ends when the baby is delivered and the umbilical cord is severed. During the *third stage* of labor, the placenta separates from the uterine wall. Uterine contractions continue until the placenta is expelled through the vagina, thus ending labor.

Intervention Techniques

During the second stage of labor, the doctor may perform an episiotomy—to allow the baby to pass through without tearing the perineum. This procedure is sometimes necessary even though the incision that results may cause discomfort

FIGURE 23.11

The three stages of labor. The baby is slowly pushed toward and through the birth canal by intermittent contractions of the muscular uterus. *First stage* contractions thin and stretch the cervix by pulling it open and pushing the baby (encased in the amniotic membrane, which eventually ruptures) against it. The *second stage* of labor begins when the cervix is fully dilated to 10 centimeters, large enough to allow the baby's head to pass through. At this point the mother feels the urge to push with her abdominal muscles with each contraction. This action soon results in birth of the baby if it is in the normal position, shown here. Other presentations, such as *breech* (buttocks-first) or *posterior* (head facing up rather than down), usually take longer and may require active assistance from birth attendants.

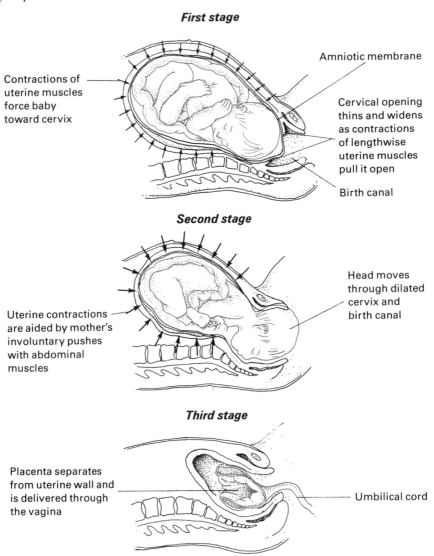

First stage

Amniotic membrane

Contractions of uterine muscles force baby toward cervix

Cervical opening thins and widens as contractions of lengthwise uterine muscles pull it open

Birth canal

Second stage

Head moves through dilated cervix and birth canal

Uterine contractions are aided by mother's involuntary pushes with abdominal muscles

Third stage

Placenta separates from uterine wall and is delivered through the vagina

Umbilical cord

after delivery and in rare cases even long-lasting numbness. If the doctor sews the incision too tightly—a procedure called "husband's knot" because it increases the vaginal grip on the penis—the tightness may make intercourse painful for the woman for some time. Many care providers are now avoiding episiotomies by providing gentle massaging and stretching of the perineal area as the baby's head emerges.

If the baby has difficulty coming out, the doctor may decide to use *forceps*, a metal tonglike device used to pull the baby from the birth canal. This procedure is becoming less common, as it may cause discomfort and damage both the mother's tissues and the baby's head. In recent years some doctors have switched to a suction-cup device—a *vacuum extractor*—applied to the baby's head.

If neither of these methods is judged adequate for a vaginal delivery and if monitoring devices indicate that the baby's life signs are slowing, the doctor may elect to deliver the baby by *caesarean section*—that is, an incision in the mother's abdomen. The procedure is expensive major surgery, and the mother's recovery is much slower than in vaginal births. Nevertheless, 20 percent of all births were caesarean deliveries in 1983.

Doctors elect caesarean section for four major reasons. One is that the labor is not progressing or the birth canal is too small. A second is breech presentation, in which the fetus has its feet instead of its head nearest the cervical canal. A third is fetal distress as determined by electronic monitoring or stethoscopes. Finally, if a woman has previously had a caesarean section birth some doctors prefer to repeat so that the "weakened" uterus will not rupture during labor. This fourth reason is being reexamined.

Breast-feeding or Bottle-feeding

Another choice is whether to breast-feed or bottle-feed. Although an estimated 95 percent of women are physically capable of breast-feeding, many choose not to. In the late 1920s about 80 percent of first-time mothers nursed their babies, but a change favoring bottle-feeding occurred in the following decades. By 1962 only 11 percent of mothers nursed their babies (Weiss 1986).

The radical decline in breast-feeding is thought to have several causes. One is vigorous promotion of prepared milk formulas and supplemental foods by commercial interests. Another is lack of support for breast-feeding from medical personnel.

A third reason centers on a social taboo. Despite its biological function—milk production—the breast is defined as a potent sex symbol; aversion to its open use for nursing infants is often linked to general sexual embarrassment and dislike of nudity. Even today 27 percent of Americans think that a mother should not nurse in public (Weiss 1986).

Fourth, the decline in breast-feeding is linked to the increased number of mothers who return to work after the baby is born. Many companies find it inconvenient to provide on-site day care so that nursing mothers can breast-feed their babies every few hours. Nevertheless, by 1984, 60 percent of American mothers were breast-feeding (Weiss 1986).

Mother's milk is more economical and more convenient than prepared formulas. It is highly nutritious and safe from spoilage. Advocates of breast milk further point out that it contains antibodies to protect the baby from disease and that it has a distinct advantage if the baby shows allergic tendencies.

Breast-feeding also helps the uterus return to its former shape and delays the return of menstruation, augmenting but not providing reliable conception control. Another benefit is the emotional and sensual satisfaction it may give both mother and baby. Ideally nursing provides a time for caressing and enjoying each other, not merely an easy way of transferring milk to the baby.

Organizations such as La Leche League, a breast-feeding support group, have provided immeasurable help to new mothers who breast-feed their babies. In 1978 the American Academy of Pediatrics recommended breast-feeding—an indication of a more positive attitude on the part of the medical community. In addition many hospitals now encourage breast-feeding by informing prospective parents of its benefits at childbirth classes and by offering a number of other supportive options.

For example, some hospitals now encourage a new mother to breast-feed immediately after birth. Such early nursing helps stimulate production of prolactin, a hormone required for milk release. Many hospitals offer a rooming-in plan whereby a newborn spends its hospital stay (or selected parts) in its mother's room rather than in the nursery so that the mother may breast-feed on demand or whenever she and her baby find appropriate.

To counteract the persistent taboo on sensual touching between parents and children, a number of observers are now insisting that cuddly contact is essential to the formation of warm family bonds and the emotional and physical health of the infant. Bottle-feeding can satisfy these needs, but only if the baby is lovingly held and cuddled instead of being left alone in a crib with a propped-up bottle. Fathers may be as responsive to infants as mothers are (Chodorow 1978); bottle-feeding may give them a special time for being close to their babies and for sharing the baby with the mother. Whether parents choose breast-feeding or bottle-feeding, they have the opportunity to mold in the child from birth the idea of loving as central to living.

LESSON PLANS

In light of this discussion, peruse the following lesson plans, keeping in mind that they are the type you will likely be expected to implement in your classroom. Remember that they by no means encompass a complete unit of instruction. They are basis for the formation of a comprehensive unit.

TOPIC: THE BIRTH PROCESS

Grade level: Primary

Concept: Birth is a natural process.

**Expected Pupil
Outcome:** The student will be able to describe where babies come from.

Content: All mothers have babies (for example):
1. Baby chick comes from egg of the hen.
2. Baby kitten comes from mother cat.
3. Baby fish come from mother fish
4. Human babies come from mother.

Learning Experiences
1. *Demonstration:* Pupils and teacher raise guppies in a fish bowl.
   Alternative learning experiences
   a) *Demonstration:* Incubate some chicken eggs. If electricity is available in your classroom, a simple incubator can be made at a very low cost. Obtain two cardboard boxes, one large and one small. (Figure 23.12). Cut one end from the small box and cut a six-inch-square window in a side of the large box. Next, cut a slit in the top of the smaller box and suspend an electric lamp in it. There should be a long cord attached to the lamp.

   Place the small box inside the large box and pack crumpled newspaper between the boxes on all side. Be sure the open end of the small box fits against the side of the large box in which the window was cut. Place a thermometer in the box so that you can read it through the window. A glass plate is fitted over the window.

   Now you are ready to begin the experiment. It is necessary to have a constant temperature of 103°F (40°C) night and day for 21 days. By using different bulbs and by changing the amount of newspaper you will be able after a few days to regulate your incubator to this temperature. A small dish of water should be placed in the incubator.

   Now obtain a dozen fertile eggs. Place the eggs in the incubator and leave them. At the end of three days, remove one of the eggs and carefully crack it into a shallow saucer. A three-day embryo will usually show the heart already beating. It may continue to beat for half an hour. Remove

FIGURE 23.12

Plans for a classroom egg incubator.

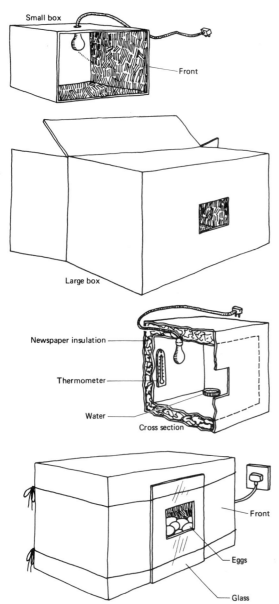

an egg every three days and observe the development of the embryo. Some of the eggs can be left for the full 21 days to see if any of them will hatch.

b) *Demonstration:* Raise gerbils

Purpose: To explain reproduction in mammals and to make children aware of the animal family unit.

Procedure: Purchase a pair of gerbils 9 to 12 weeks prior to begining of unit. Sexual maturity occurs between 11 and 12 weeks. This gives the gerbils time to get used to each other. Gerbils will mate by 14 weeks. The gestation period is 24 to 30 days. Since the pregnant gerbil gains very little weight, it is often difficult to tell whether a gerbil is pregnant.

Both mother and father are affectionate toward the babies, and there is no reason to separate the parents. A hamster cage may be used. Use hamster litter or cedar shavings as a floor cover for the cage. Gerbils are very clean, hence odorless. The cage needs to be cleaned about every two weeks. They nibble on sunflower seeds and corn. Carrots, celery, and lettuce may also be included in the diet. Keep the diet high in protein and low in fat. Add a little evaporated milk to the diet during pregnancy and nursing. Gerbils drink very little water, but water should be provided in a trough so that they can drink standing upright.

Do not handle gerbils after a litter is born or attempt to clean the cage, as they are very sensitive at this time.

For more insight on raising gerbils in the classroom, refer to: D. G. Robinson, *How to Raise and Train Gerbils*, T.F.H. Publications Inc., New Jersey City, 1967.

Evaluation Procedures   The teacher will subjectively evaluate the students' understanding of the birth process via a series of key questions:

Key Questions   These are broken down into three sequences so that they can be used to guide pupil observation and help children to discover for themselves:

1st day (two weeks before birth):

1. Which is the mother guppy?
2. What part of her body is the largest?
3. Is the mother guppy the same color as the father guppy?
4. Can you see through the mother's stomach?

2nd day (day or two just before birth):

1. Is the mother's body bigger now than before?
2. Can you still see through the mother's body?
3. What can you see?
4. Can you see any dark spots?
5. Where are these black spots?

3rd day (baby guppies are born):

1. Is the mother's body as big as it was several days ago?
2. What color is the mother's stomach?
3. Where did the dark spots in the mother's stomach go?
4. How many baby guppies are there?
5. Where do babies come from?

   If the students display a clear understanding of the birth process based upon their answers to the key questions, the objective will be considered accomplished. Similar key questions should be developed for the chicken egg and gerbil alternative learning experiences.

TOPIC: MENSTRUATION

Grade level: Intermediate

Concept: Menstruation is a normal body function.

Expected Pupil Outcome: The student will be able to outline the process of menstruation.

Content

1. The menstruation process:
   a. Thick inner lining does not receive a fertilized egg.
   b. Thick lining is made up of endometrial cells and rich supply of blood vessels.
   c. Cells and blood vessels discarded as flow.
   d. Menstrual flow occurs for several days, hence menstrual period.

Learning Experiences

1. *Film: The Story of Menstruation,* by Walt Disney. Order from Association Films (10 min, color).
   Teacher should first introduce film by suggesting what pupils should look for the in the film. This may be done by listing key words on the blackboard:
   pituitary gland
   ovaries
   fallopian tubes
   uterus
   ovulation
   menstruation
2. *Worksheet:* To accompany film showing. Worksheet may be used by pupils during the film or as a quiz or review after the film.

Menstruation Worksheet/Quiz

Directions: Select the best answer.

1. The pituitary gland
   a) sends out growth hormones
   b) is located in the upper arm
   c) affects the ovaries
   *d) a and c
2. Ovulation
   a) occurs every other week
   b) is when the uterus lining is discarded
   *c) is the process in which a ripe egg leaves the ovary
   d) involves the liver and the small intestine
3. Menstruation occurs
   a) every 14 days
   b) every other week
   *c) about every 28 days
   d) every three months
4. What is the correct sequence of passage for the egg?
   a) ovary, uterus, fallopian tubes, vagina
   *b) ovary, fallopian tubes, uterus, vagina
   c) uterus, ovary, vagina, fallopian tubes

---

*Correct answer is marked with the asterisk.

5. A special lining of blood and tissue builds up in the
   *a) uterus
   b) ovaries
   c) fallopian tubes
6. The menstrual period usually lasts
   a) 3 to 10 days
   *b) 4 to 5 days
   c) 10 to 15 days
   d) 28 days

The four seasons compared to menstruation

Seasons	Tree (one-year cycle)	Menstruation in young girl (28-day cycle)
Winter	During the winter the tree is dormant, but while it is dormant it prepares for spring internally.	During this time of the month the ovaries receive a hormone that triggers the production and maturation of an egg.
Spring	During the spring the tree begins to grow, and new leaves appear.	At this stage the egg is beginning to mature. Nature prepares the uterus for it with a lining called the endometrium.
Summer	In the summer the tree continues to grow, and to prepare for fall and the onset of winter.	The egg matures and is released from the ovaries into the fallopian tubes. If the egg is not fertilized, it disintegrates.
Fall	During the fall the tree begins to shed its leaves and prepare for winter.	After the egg disintegrates, the endometrium is shed and passes through the vagina. The cycle is ended and the body begins it again.

7. Menstruation is
   a) a basic part of growing up for a girl
   b) one long, natural, continuous cycle of life
   c) should be regular within each girl
   *d) all of above
8. Suggest five ways a woman can take care of herself during the menstrual days.

Suggestion: teacher may stop the film to emphasize or clarify a point or to direct student's attention to an answer on the worksheet.

3. *Alternative suggestion:* Should film not be available, menstruation should be explained by the Story of the Four Seasons (compare the process of menstruation to nature's cycle of the seasons).

Evaluation Procedures   If the class average on the menstruation worksheet quiz is 80% or better, the objective will be considered accomplished.

REFERENCES AND BIBLIOGRAPHY

Ascione, F. R., and Chambers, J.H. Videogames and pro-social behavior: The effects of prosocial and aggressive video games on children's donating and helping. Paper presented at the meeting of the Society for Research in Child Development, Toronto, April 1985.

"Avoiding Unnecessary Repeat Cesarean Deliveries May Help Stem Overall Rise in C-Section Rates." 1985. *Family Planning Perspectives* 17, no. 3:125-127.

Ball, D. W., Newman, J.M., and Scheuren, W.J. Teachers' generalized expectations of children of divorce. *Psychological Reports*, 1984, *54*, 347-353.

Boston Women's Health Book Collective. *Ourselves and Our Children.* New York: Random House, 1978.

Bronfenbrenner, U. *The Worlds of Childhood: US-USSR* (New York: Russell Sage Foundation, 1970).

Bryant, B. K. The neighborhood walk: Sources of support in middle childhood. *Monographs of the Society for Research in Child Development*, 1985, *50*(3, Serial No. 210).

Conant, J. *My Several Lives* (New York: Harper & Row, 1970): 160.

Cordes, C. Kids who watch more found more likely to believe TV. *APA Monitor*, 1985, *16*(11), 35.

Damon, W. Peer education: The untapped potential. *Journal of Applied Developmental Psychology*, 1984, *5*, 331-343.

Deci, E. L., Schwaratz, A.J., Sheinman, L., and Ryan, R.M. An instrument to assess adults' orientations toward control versus autonomy with children: Reflections on intrinsic motivation and perceived competence. *Journal of Educational Psychology*, 1981, *73*, 642-650.

Eagan, A. "The Selling of Premenstrual Syndrome," *Ms* 11 (1983): 24-31.

Einstein, E. "Stepfamily Lives," *Human Behavior* (April 1979): 63-68.

Edlin, G., and Golanty, E. *Health and Wellness*, 3rd. ed. (Boston, MA: Jones and Bartlett, 1988).

Feldstein, J. H., and Feldstein, S. Sex differences on televised toy comercials. *Sex Roles*, 1982, *8*, 581-587.

Freiberg, K. L. *Human Development: A Life-Span Approach*, 3rd ed. (Boston, MA: Jones and Bartlett. 1987).

Ford, C. S., and Beach, A. *Patterns of Sexual Behavior* (New York: Harper & Row, 1951).

Fu, V. R., and Fogel, S. W. Prowhite/antiblack bias among southern preschool children. *Psychological Reports*. 1982, *51*, 1003-1006.

Ganong, W. F. *Review of Medical Physiology* (Los Altos, CA: Large Medical Publications, 1981).

Greenfield, P. M. *Mind and media: The effects of television, video games, and computers.* Cambridge, Mass.: Harvard University Press, 1984.

Hampson, J. L., and Hampson, I. G. "The Ontogenesis of Sexual Behavior in Men." In W. C. Young (ed.): *Sex and Internal Secretions*, 3rd ed. (Baltimore: Williams & Wilkins, 1961).

Hawkins, D. B., and Gruber, J. J. Little League baseball and players' self-esteem. *Perceptual and Motor Skills*, 1982, *55*, 1335-1340.

Heneson, N. "The Selling of P.M.S.," *Science 84* (May 1984): 67-71.

Hetherington, E. M. "Divorce: A Child's Perspective," *American Psychologist*, 34:10 (1979): 851-858.

Hetherington, E. M., Cox, M., and Cox, R. "The Aftermath of Divorce." In J. Stevens and M. Mathews (eds.): *Mother/child, Father/child Relationships* (Washington, D.C.: National Association for the Education of Young Children, 1978).

Kalter, N., and Plunkett, J. W. Children's perceptions of the causes and consequences of divorce. *Journal of the American Academy of Child Psychiatry*, 1984, *23*, 326-334.

Keller, H. *The Story of My Life* (New York: Doubleday, 1954): 46.

Kinsey, A. C., W. Pomeroy, and C. Martin. *Sexual Behavior in the Human Male* (Philadelphia: Saunders, 1948).

Kinsey, A. C., et al. *Sexual Behavior in the Human Female* (Philadelphia: Saunders, 1953).

Leboyer, F. *Birth Without Violence* (New York: Alfred A. Knopf, 1975).

Lehman, B. A. Early puberty curbed by shots of new hormone. *Boston Globe*, 1986 (March 17, pg. 47).

Levin, G. Computers and kids: The good news. *Psychology Today*, 1985, *19*(8), 50-51.

Lewin, K., R. Lippitt, and White, R. "Patterns of Aggression in Experimentally Created Social Climates," *Journal of Social Psychology*, 10 (1939): 271-299.

Long, T., and Long, L. *The handbook for latchkey children and their parents.* New York: Arbor House, 1983.

Mackey, W. D., and Hess, D. J. Attention structure and stereotype of gender on television: An empirical analysis. *Genetic Psychology Monographs*, 1982, *106*, 199-215.

Masters, W. H., and Johnson, V. E. *Human Sexual Response.* Boston: Little, Brown, 1966.

Money, J., and Ehrhardt, A. *Man and Woman: Boy and Girl* (Baltimore: Johns Hopkins University Press, 1972).

Nelson-LeGall, S. A., and Gumerman, R. A. Children's perceptions of helpers and helper motivation, *Journal of Applied Developmental Psychology*, 1984, *5*, 1–12.

Nunn, G. D., Parish, T. S., and Worthing, R. J. Perceptions of personal and familial adjustment by children from intact, single-parent, and reconstituted families. *Psychology in the Schools*, 1983, *20*, 166-174.

Parlee, M. B. "New Findings: Menstrual Cycles and Behavior," *Ms*, 10 (1982): 126-127.

Pearl, D. Violence and aggression. *Society*, 1984, *21*(6), 17-22.

Pedersen, E., Faucher, T. A., and Eaton, W. W. A new perspective on the effects of first grade teachers on children's subsequent adult status. *Harvard Educational Review*, 1978, *48*, 1-1.3.

Reid, R. L., and Yen, S. S. C. "The Premenstrual Syndrome," *Clinical Obstetrics and Gynecology*, 26 (1983): 710-717.

Ruble, Diane N., and Jeanne Brooks-Gunn. 1982. "The Experience of Menarche." *Child Development* 53:1557-1566.

Rutter, M. Protective factors in children's response to stress and disadvantage. In M.W. Kent and J.E. Rolf (Eds.) *Primary prevention of psychopathology, vol. 3: Social competence in children.* Hanover, N.H.: University Press of New England, 1979.

Rutter, M. School effects on pupil progress: Research findings and policy implications. *Child Development*, 1983, *54*, 1-29.

Santrock, J. W., Warshak, R. A., Lindbergh, C., and Meadows, L. Children's and parents' observed social behavior in stepfather families. *Child Development*, 1982, *53*, 472-480.

Stapleton, C., and MacCormack, N. When parents divorce, DHHS Publication No. (ADM) 81-1120. Washington, D.C.: U.S. Government Printing Office, 1981.

Tom, D. Y. H., Cooper, H., and McGraw, M. Influences of student background and teacher authoritarianism on teacher expectations. *Journal of Educational Psychology*, 1984, *76*, 259-265.

Trueman, D. What are the characteristics of school phobic children? *Psychological Reports*, 1984, *54*, 191-202.

Udry, J. Richard, Luther M. Talbert, and Naomi M. Morris. 1986. "Biosocial Foundations for Adolescent Female Sexuality." *Demography* 23, no. 2:217-227.

Wallerstein, E. *Circumcision: An American Health Fallacy.* New York: Springer, 1980.

Weinraub, M., and Wolf, B. M. Effects of stress and social supports on mother-child interactions in single- and two-parent families. *Child Development*, 1983, *54*, 1297-1311.

Wright, J. C., and Huston, A. C. A matter of form: Potentials of television for young viewers. *American Psychologist*, 1983, *38*, 835-843.

Appendix A

U.S. Recommended Daily Allowances of Nutrients

TABLE A.1
U.S. Recommended Daily Allowance (U.S. RDA)*

Nutrient	Adults and children 4 years or older	Infants birth to 1 year	Children under 4 years	Pregnant or lactating women
Protein (g)	45 or 65	18 or 25	20 or 28	45 or 65
Vitamin A (IU)	5,000	1,500	2,500	8,000
Vitamin C (mg)	60	35	40	60
Thiamin (mg)	1.5	0.5	0.7	1.7
Riboflavin (mg)	1.7	0.6	0.8	2.0
Niacin (mg)	20	8	9	20
Calcium (mg)	1,000	600	800	1,300
Iron (mg)	18	15	10	18
Vitamin D (IU)	400	400	400	400
Vitamin E (IU)	30	5	10	30
Vitamin B_6 (mg)	2.0	0.4	0.7	2.5
Folic acid (mg)	0.4	0.1	0.2	0.8
Vitamin B_{12} (µg)	6	2	3	8
Phosphorus (mg)	1,000	500	800	1,300
Iodine (µg)	150	45	70	150
Magnesium (mg)	400	70	200	450
Zinc (mg)	15	5	8	15
Copper (mg)	2	0.6	1	2
Biotin (mg)	0.3	0.05	0.15	0.3
Pantothenic acid (mg)	10	3	5	10

*Source: *Recommended Dietary Allowances,* 9th edition (Washington, DC: National Academy of Sciences, 1980).

Note: Recommendations of the 1985 Food and Nutrition Board were rejected by the National Academy of Sciences. Thus, the 1980 RDAs remain in effect.

TABLE A.2
Estimated Safe and Adequate Daily Dietary Intakes of Additional Selected Vitamins and Minerals

	Age (years)	Vitamins			Trace elements[b]						Electrolytes		
		Vitamin K (μg)	Biotin (μg)	Pantothenic acid (mg)	Copper (mg)	Manganese (mg)	Fluoride (mg)	Chromium (mg)	Selenium (mg)	Molybdenum (mg)	Sodium (mg)	Potassium (mg)	Chloride (mg)
Infants	0-0.5	12	35	2	0.5-0.7	0.5-0.7	0.1-0.5	0.01-0.04	0.01-0.04	0.03-0.06	115-350	350-925	275-700
	0.5-1	10-20	50	3	0.7-1.0	0.7-1.0	0.2-1.0	0.02-0.06	0.02-0.06	0.04-0.08	250-750	425-1275	400-1200
Children	1-3	15-30	65	3	1.0-1.5	1.0-1.5	0.5-1.5	0.02-0.08	0.02-0.08	0.05-0.1	325-975	550-1650	500-1500
and	4-6	20-40	85	3-4	1.5-2.0	1.5-2.0	1.0-2.5	0.03-0.12	0.03-0.12	0.06-0.15	450-1350	775-2325	700-2100
Adolescents	7-10	30-60	120	4-5	2.0-2.5	2.0-3.0	1.5-2.5	0.05-0.2	0.05-0.2	0.1 -0.3	600-1800	1000-3000	925-2775
	11 +	50-100	100-200	4-7	2.0-3.0	2.5-5.0	1.5-2.5	0.05-0.2	0.05-0.2	0.15-0.5	900-2700	1525-4575	1400-4200
Adults		70-140	100-200	4-7	2.0-3.0	2.5-5.0	1.5-4.0	0.05-0.2	0.05-0.2	0.15-0.5	1100-3300	1875-5625	1700-5100

Source: Recommended Dietary Allowances, 9th edition. (Washington, DC: National Academy of Sciences).

Because there is less information on which to base allowances, these figures are not given in the main table of the RDA and are provided here in the form of ranges of recommended intakes.

Since the toxic levels for many trace elements may be only several times usual intakes, the upper levels for the trace elements given in this table should not be habitually exceeded.

Appendix B

Mean Heights and Weights and Recommended Energy Intakes

TABLE B.1
Mean Heights and Weights and Recommended Energy Intakes for the United States

Category	Age (years)	Weight (kg)	Weight (lb)	Height (cm)	Height (in.)	Energy needs (with range) (kcal)	Energy needs (with range) (MJ)
Infants	0.0- 0.5	6	13	60	24	kg × 115 (95-145)	kg × .48
	0.5- 1.0	9	20	71	28	kg × 105 (80-135)	kg × .44
Children	1- 3	13	29	90	35	1,300 (900-1,800)	5.5
	4- 6	20	44	112	44	1,700 (1,300-2,300)	7.1
	7-10	28	62	132	52	2,400 (1,650-3,300)	10.1
Males	11-14	45	99	157	62	2,700 (2,000-3,700)	11.3
	15-18	66	145	176	69	2,800 (2,100-3,900)	11.8
	19-22	70	154	177	70	2,900 (2,500-3,300)	12.2
	23-50	70	154	178	70	2,700 (2,300-3,100)	11.3
	51-75	70	154	178	70	2,400 (2,000-2,800)	10.1
	>76	70	154	178	70	2,050 (1,650-2,450)	8.6
Females	11-14	46	101	157	62	2,200 (1,500-3,000)	9.2
	15-18	55	120	163	64	2,100 (1,200-3,000)	8.8
	19-22	55	120	163	64	2,100 (1,700-2,500)	8.8
	23-50	55	120	163	64	2,000 (1,600-2,400)	8.4
	51-75	55	120	163	64	1,800 (1,400-2,200)	7.6
	>76	55	120	163	64	1,600 (1,200-2,000)	6.7
Pregnancy						+300	
Lactation						+500	

Source: Recommended Dietary Allowances, 9th ed. (Washington, D.C.: National Academy of Sciences, 1980).

Notes: The data in this table have been assembled from the observed median heights and weights of children together with desirable weights for adults for the mean heights of men (70 in.) and women (64 in.) between the ages of 18 and 34 years as surveyed in the U.S. population (Health, Education and Welfare/National Center for Health Statistics data).

The energy allowances for the young adults are for men and women doing light work. The allowances for the two older age groups represent mean energy needs over these age spans, allowing for a 2% decrease in basal (resting) metabolic rate per decade and a reduction in activity of 200 kcal d for men and women between 51 and 75 years, 500 kcal for men over 75 years, and 400 kcal for women over 75. The customary range of daily energy output is shown for adults in parentheses, and is based on a variation in energy needs of ±400 kcal at any one age emphasizing the wide range of energy intakes appropriate for any group of people.

Energy allowances for children through age 18 are based on median energy intakes of children these ages followed in longitudinal growth studies. The values in parentheses are 10th and 90th percentiles of energy intake, to indicate the range of energy consumption among children of these ages.

Appendix C

Acquired Immune Deficiency Syndrome (AIDS)*

AIDS
AIDS Caused by Virus

The letters A-I-D-S stand for Acquired Immune Deficiency Syndrome. When a person is infected with AIDS, he or she is in the final stages of a series of problems caused by a virus (germ) that can be passed from one person to another chiefly during sexual contact and through the sharing of intravenous drug needles used for "shooting" drugs. Scientists have named this virus "HIV or HTLV-III or LAV."[1] These abbreviations stand for information denoting a virus that attacks cells (T-Lymphocytes) in the human blood. Throughout this publication, we will call the virus the "AIDS virus." Aids virus attacks a person's immune system and damages his/her ability to fight other disease. Without a functioning immune system to ward off other germs, he/she now becomes vulnerable to becoming infected by bac-

teria, protozoa, fungi, and other viruses and malignancies, which may cause life-threatening illness, such as pneumonia, meningitis, and cancer.

No Known Cure

There is presently no cure for AIDS. There is presently no vaccine to prevent AIDS.

Virus Invades Blood Stream

When the AIDS virus enters the blood stream, it begins to attack certain white blood cells (T-Lymphocytes). Substances called antibodies are produced by the body. These antibodies can be detected in the blood by a simple test, usually two weeks to three months after infection. Even before the antibody test is positive, the victim

---

[1]These are different names given to AIDS virus by the scientific community: HIV, Human Immunodeficiency Virus; HTLV-III, Human T-Lymphotropic Virus Type III; LAV, Lymphadenopathy Associated Virus.

*This material is from the Surgeon General's Report on Acquired Immune Deficiency Syndrome.

can pass the virus to others by methods that will be explained.

Once an individual is infected, there are several possibilities. Some people may remain well but even so they are able to infect others. Others may develop a disease that is less serious than AIDS referred to as AIDS Related Complex (ARC). In some people the immune system may be destroyed by the virus and then other germs (bacteria, protozoa, fungi and other viruses) and cancers that ordinarily would never get a foothold cause "opportunistic diseases"—using the *opportunity* of lowered resistance to infect and destroy. Some of the most common are *Pneumocystis carinii* pneumonia and tuberculosis. Individuals infected with the AIDS virus may also develop certain types of cancers such as Kaposi's sarcoma. These infected people have classic AIDS. Evidence shows that the AIDS virus may also attack the nervous system, causing damage to the brain.

SIGNS AND SYMPTOMS
No Signs

Some people remain apparently well after infection with the AIDS virus. They may have no symptoms of illness. However, if proper precautions are not used with sexual contacts and/or intravenous drug use, these infected individuals can spread the virus to others. Anyone who thinks he or she is infected or involved in high risk behaviors should not donate his/her blood, organs, tissues, or sperm because they may now contain the AIDS virus.

ARC

AIDS-Related Complex (ARC) is a condition caused by the AIDS virus in which the patient tests positive for AIDS infection and has a specific set of clinical symptoms. However, ARC patients' symptoms are often less severe than those with the disease we call classic AIDS. Signs and symptoms of ARC may include loss of appetite, weight loss, fever, night sweats, skin rashes, diarrhea, tiredness, lack of resistance to infection, or swollen lymph nodes. These are also signs and symptoms of many other diseases and a physician should be consulted.

AIDS

Only a qualified health professional can diagnose AIDS, which is the result of a natural progress of infection by the AIDS virus. AIDS destroys the body's immune (defense) system and allows otherwise controllable infections to invade the body and cause additional diseases. These opportunistic diseases would not otherwise gain a foothold in the body. These opportunistic diseases may eventually cause death.

Some symptoms and signs of AIDS and the "opportunistic infections" may include a persistent cough and fever associated with shortness of breath or difficult breathing and may be the symptoms of *Pneumocystis carinii* pneumonia. Multiple purplish blotches and bumps on the skin may be a sign of Kaposi's sarcoma. The AIDS virus in all infected people is essentially the same; the reactions of individuals may differ.

Long Term

The AIDS virus may also attack the nervous system and cause delayed damage to the brain. This damage may take years to develop and the symptoms may show up as memory loss, indifference, loss of coordination, partial paralysis, or mental disorder. These symptoms may occur alone or with other symptoms mentioned earlier.

AIDS: THE PRESENT SITUATION

The number of people estimated to be infected with the AIDS virus in the United States is about 1.5 million. All of these individuals are assumed to be capable of spreading the virus sexually (heterosexually or homosexually) or by sharing needles and syringes or other implements for intravenous drug use. Of these, an estimated 100,000 to 200,000 will come down with AIDS Related Complex (ARC). It is difficult to predict the number who will develop ARC or AIDS because symptoms sometimes take as long as nine years to show up. With our present knowledge, scientists predict that 20 to 30 percent of those infected with the AIDS virus will develop an illness that fits an accepted definition of AIDS within five years. The number of persons known to have AIDS in the United States to date is over 25,000; of these, about half have died of the disease. Since there is no cure, the others are expected to also eventually die from their disease.

The majority of antibody-positive individuals who carry the AIDS virus show no symptoms and may not come down with the disease for many years, if ever.

No Risk from Casual Contact

There is no known risk of non-sexual infection in most of the situations we encounter in our daily lives. We know that family members living with individuals who have the AIDS virus do not become infected except through sexual contact. There is no evidence of transmission (spread) of AIDS virus by everyday contact even though these family members shared food, towels, cups, razors, even toothbrushes, and kissed each other.

Health Workers

We know even more about health care workers exposed to AIDS patients. About 2,500 health workers who were caring for AIDS patients when they were sickest have been carefully studied and tested for infection with the AIDS virus. These doctors, nurses and other health care givers have been exposed to the AIDS patients' blood, stool and other body fluids. Approximately 750 of these health workers reported possible additional exposure by direct contact with a patient's body fluid through spills or being accidentally stuck with a needle. Upon testing these 750, only 3 who had accidentally stuck themselves with a needle had a positive antibody test for exposure to the AIDS virus. Because health workers had

much more contact with patients and their body fluids than would be expected from common everyday contact, it is clear that the AIDS virus is not transmitted by casual contact.

Control of Certain Behaviors Can Stop Further Spread of AIDS

Knowing the facts about AIDS can prevent the spread of the disease. Education of those who risk infecting themselves or infecting other people is the only way we can stop the spread of AIDS. People must be responsible about their sexual behavior and must avoid the use of illicit intravenous drugs and needle sharing. We will describe the types of behavior that lead to infection by the AIDS virus and the personal measures that must be taken for effective protection. If we are to stop the AIDS epidemic, we all must understand the disease—its cause, its nature, and its prevention. *Precautions must be taken.* The AIDS virus infects persons who expose themselves to known risk behavior, such as certain types of homosexual and heterosexual activities or sharing intravenous drug equipment.

Risks

Although the initial discovery was in the homosexual community, AIDS is not a disease only of homosexuals. AIDS is found in heterosexual people as well. AIDS is not a black or white disease. AIDS is not just a male disease. AIDS is found in women; it is found in children. In the future AIDS will probably increase and spread among people who are not homosexual or intravenous drug abusers in the same manner as other sexually transmitted diseases like syphilis and gonorrhea.

Sex Between Men

Men who have sexual relations with other men are especially at risk. About 70 percent of AIDS victims throughout the country are male homosexuals and bisexuals. This percentage probably will decline as heterosexual transmission increases. *Infection results from a sexual relationship with an infected person.*

Multiple Partners

The risk of infection increases according to the number of sexual partners one has, *male or female*. The more partners you have, the greater the risk of becoming infected with the AIDS virus.

How Exposed

Although the AIDS virus is found in several body fluids, a person acquires the virus during sexual contact with an infected person's blood or semen and possibly vaginal secretions. The virus then enters a person's blood stream through their rectum, vagina or penis.

Small (unseen by the naked eye) tears in the surface lining of the vagina or rectum may occur during insertion of the penis, fingers, or other objects, thus opening an avenue for entrance of the virus directly into the blood stream; therefore, the AIDS virus can be passed from penis to rectum and vagina and vice versa without a visible tear in the tissue or the presence of blood.

Prevention of Sexual Transmission—Know Your Partner

Couples who maintain mutually faithful monogamous relationships (only one continuing sexual partner) are protected from AIDS through sexual transmission. If you have been faithful for at least five years and your partner has been faithful too, neither of you is at risk. If you have not been faithful, then you and your partner are at risk. If your partner has not been faithful, then your partner is at risk which also puts you at risk. This is true for both heterosexual and homosexual couples. Unless it is possible to know with *absolute certainty* that neither you nor your sexual partner is carrying the virus of AIDS, you must use protective behavior. *Absolute certainty* means not only that you and your partner have maintained a mutually faithful monogamous sexual relationship, but it means that neither you nor your partner has used illegal intravenous drugs.

AIDS: YOU CAN PROTECT YOURSELF FROM INFECTION

Some personal measures are adequate to safely protect yourself and others from infection by the AIDS virus and its complications. Among these are:

- If you have been involved in any of the high risk sexual activities described above or have injected illicit intravenous drugs into your body, you should have a blood test to see if you have been infected with the AIDS virus.
- If your test is positive or if you engage in high risk activities and choose not to have a test, you should tell your sexual partner. If you jointly decide to have sex, you must protect your partner by always using a rubber (condom) during (start to finish) sexual intercourse (vagina or rectum).
- If your partner has a positive blood test showing that he/she has been infected with the AIDS virus or you suspect that he/she has been exposed by previous heterosexual or homosexual behavior or use of intravenous drugs with shared needles and syringes, a rubber (condom) should always be used during (start to finish) sexual intercourse (vagina or rectum).
- If you or your partner is at high risk, avoid mouth contact with the penis, vagina, or rectum.
- Avoid all sexual activities which could cause cuts or tears in the linings of the rectum, vagina, or penis.
- Single teenage girls have been warned that pregnancy and contracting sexually transmitted diseases can be the result of only one act of sexual intercourse. They have been taught to say *NO* to sex! They have been taught to say *NO* to drugs! By saying *NO* to sex and drugs, they can avoid AIDS which can *kill* them! The same is true for teenage boys who should also

not have rectal intercourse with other males. It may result in AIDS.

- Do not have sex with prostitutes. Infected male and female prostitutes are frequently also intravenous drug abusers; therefore, they may infect clients by sexual intercourse and other intravenous drug abusers by sharing their intravenous drug equipment. Female prostitutes also can infect their unborn babies.

Intravenous Drug Users

Drug abusers who inject drugs into their veins are another population group at high risk and with high rates of infection by the AIDS virus. Users of intravenous drugs make up 25 percent of the cases of AIDS throughout the country. The AIDS virus is carried in contaminated blood left in the needle, syringe, or other drug related implements and the virus is injected into the new victim by reusing dirty syringes and needles. Even the smallest amount of infected blood left in a used needle or syringe can contain live AIDS virus to be passed on to the next user of those dirty implements.

No one should shoot up drugs because addiction, poor health, family disruption, emotional disturbances and death could follow. However, many drug users are addicted to drugs and for one reason or another have not changed their behavior. For these people, the only way not to get AIDS is *to use a clean, previously unused* needle, syringe or any other implement necessary for the injection of the drug solution.

Hemophilia

Some persons with hemophilia (a blood clotting disorder that makes them subject to bleeding) have been infected with the AIDS virus either through blood transfusion or the use of blood products that help their blood clot. Now that we know how to prepare safe blood products to aid clotting, this is unlikely to happen. This group represents a very small percentage of the cases of AIDS throughout the country.

Blood Transfusion

Currently all blood donors are screened and blood is *not* accepted from high-risk individuals. Blood that has been collected for use is tested for the presence of antibody to the AIDS virus. However, some people may have had a blood transfusion prior to March 1985, before we knew how to screen blood for safe transfusion and may have become infected with the AIDS virus. Fortunately, there are not now a large number of these cases. With routine testing of blood products, the blood supply for transfusion is safer than it has ever been with regard to AIDS.

Persons who have engaged in homosexual activities or have shot street drugs within the last 10 years should *never* donate blood.

Mother Can Infect the Newborn Child

If a woman is infected with the AIDS virus and becomes pregnant, she is more likely to develop ARC or classic AIDS, and she can pass the AIDS virus to her unborn child. Approximately one third of the babies born to AIDS-infected mothers will also be infected with the AIDS virus. Most of the infected babies will eventually develop the disease and die. Several of these babies have been born to wives of hemophiliac men infected with the AIDS virus by way of contaminated blood products. Some babies have also been born to women who became infected with the AIDS virus by bisexual partners who had the virus. Almost all babies with AIDS have been born to women who were intravenous drug users or the sexual partners of intravenous drug users who were infected with the AIDS virus. More such babies can be expected.

Think carefully if you plan on becoming pregnant. If there is any chance that you may be in any high-risk group or that you have had sex with someone in a high-risk group, such as homosexual and bisexual males, drug abusers and their sexual partners, see your doctor.

Summary

AIDS affects certain groups of the population. Homosexual and bisexual males who have had sexual contact with other homosexual or bisexual males as well as those who "shoot" street drugs are at greatest risk of exposure, infection and eventual death. Sexual partners of high-risk individuals are at risk, as well as any children born to women who carry the virus. Heterosexual persons are increasingly at risk.

AIDS: WHAT IS SAFE?
Most Behavior Is Safe

Everyday living does not present any risk of infection. You *cannot* get AIDS from casual social contact. Casual social contact should not be confused with casual *sexual* contact, which is a major cause of the spread of the AIDS virus. Casual *social* contact such as shaking hands, hugging, social kissing, crying, coughing or sneezing, will not transmit the AIDS virus. Nor has AIDS been contracted from swimming in pools or bathing in hot tubs or from eating in restaurants (even if a restaurant worker has AIDS or carries the AIDS virus). AIDS is not contracted from sharing bed linens, towels, cups, straws, dishes, or any other eating utensils. You cannot get AIDS from toilets, doorknobs, telephones, office machinery, or household furniture. You cannot get AIDS from body massages, masturbation or any non-sexual contact.

Donating Blood

Donating blood is *not* risky at all. *You cannot get AIDS by donating blood.*

Receiving Blood

In the U.S. every blood donor is screened to exclude high-risk persons and every blood donation is now tested for the presence of antibodies to the AIDS virus. Blood that shows exposure to the AIDS virus by the presence of antibodies is not used either for transfusion or for the manufacture of blood products. Blood banks are as safe as current technology can make them. Because antibodies do not form immediately after exposure to the virus, a newly infected person may unknowingly donate blood after becoming infected but before his/her antibody test becomes positive. It is estimated that this might occur less than once in 100,000 donations.

There is no danger of AIDS virus infection from visiting a doctor, dentist, hospital, hairdresser or beautician. AIDS cannot be transmitted nonsexually from an infected person through a health or service provider to another person. Ordinary methods of disinfection for urine, stool and vomitus used for non-infected people are adequate for people who have AIDS or are carrying the AIDS virus. You may have wondered why your dentist wears gloves and perhaps a mask when treating you. This does not mean that he has AIDS or that he thinks you do. He is protecting you and himself from hepatitis, common colds or flu.

There is no danger in visiting a patient with AIDS or caring for him or her. Normal hygienic practices, like wiping of body fluid spills with a solution of water and household bleach (1 part household bleach to 10 parts water), will provide full protection.

Children in School

None of the identified cases of AIDS in the United States are known or are suspected to have been transmitted from one child to another in school, day care, or foster care. Transmission would necessitate exposure of open cuts to the blood or other body fluids of the infected child, a highly unlikely occurrence. Even then routine safety procedures for handling blood or other body fluids (which should be standard for all children in school or day care setting) would be effective in preventing transmission from children with AIDS to other children in school.

Children with AIDS are highly susceptible to infections, such as chicken pox, from other children. Each child with AIDS should be examined by a doctor before attending school or before returning to school, day care or foster care settings after an illness. No blanket rules can be made for all school boards to cover all possible cases of children with AIDS and each case should be considered separately and individualized to the child and the setting, as would be done with any child with a special problem, such as cerebral palsy or asthma. A good team to make such decisions with the school board would be the child's parents, physician and a public health official.

Casual social contact between children and persons infected with the AIDS virus is not dangerous.

Insects

There are no known cases of AIDS transmission by insects, such as mosquitoes.

Pets

Dogs, cats and domestic animals are not a source of infection from AIDS virus.

Tears and Saliva

Although the AIDS virus has been found in tears and saliva, no instance of transmission from these body fluids has been reported.

AIDS comes from sexual contacts with infected persons and from the sharing of syringes and needles. There is no danger of infection with AIDS virus by casual social contact.

Testing of Military Personnel

You may wonder why the Department of Defense is currently testing its uniformed services personnel for presence of the AIDS virus antibody. The military feel this procedure is necessary because the uniformed services act as their own blood bank in a time of national emergency. They also need to protect new recruits (who unknowingly may be AIDS virus carriers) from receiving live virus vaccines. These vaccines could activate disease and be potentially life-threatening to the recruits.

AIDS: WHAT IS UNDERSTOOD

Although AIDS is still a mysterious disease in many ways, our scientists have learned a great deal about it. In five years we know more about AIDS than many diseases that we have studied for even longer periods. While there is no vaccine or cure, the results from the health and behavioral research community can only add to our knowledge and increase our understanding of the disease and ways to prevent and treat it.

In spite of all that is known about transmission of the AIDS virus, scientists will learn more. One possibility is the potential discovery of factors that may better explain the mechanism of AIDS infection.

Why are the antibodies produced by the body to fight the AIDS virus not able to destroy that virus? The antibodies detected in the blood of carriers of the AIDS virus are ineffective, at least when classic AIDS is actually triggered. They cannot check the damage caused by the virus, which is by then present in large numbers in the body. Researchers cannot explain this important observation. We still do not know why the AIDS virus is not destroyed by the immune system.

Summary

AIDS no longer is the concern of any one segment of society; it is the concern of us all. No American's life is in danger if he/she or their sexual partners do not engage in high-risk sexual behavior or use shared needles or syringes to inject illicit drugs into the body.

People who engage in high-risk sexual behavior or who shoot drugs are risking infection with the AIDS virus and are risking their lives and the lives of others, including their unborn children.

We cannot yet know the full impact of AIDS on our society. From a clinical point of view, there may be new manifestations of AIDS—for example, mental disturbances due to the infection of the brain by the AIDS virus in carriers of the virus. From a social point of view, it may bring to an end the free-wheeling sexual lifestyle which has been called the sexual revolution. Economically, the care of AIDS patients will put a tremendous strain on our already overburdened and costly health care delivery system.

The most certain way to avoid getting the AIDS virus and to control the AIDS epidemic in the United States is for individuals to avoid promiscuous sexual practices, to maintain mutually faithful monogamous sexual relationships and to avoid injecting illicit drugs.

LOOK TO THE FUTURE
The Challenge of the Future

An enormous challenge to public health lies ahead of us, and we would do well to take a look at the future. We must be prepared to manage those things we can predict as well as those we cannot.

At the present time there is no vaccine to prevent AIDS. There is no cure. AIDS, which can be transmitted sexually and by sharing needles and syringes among illicit intravenous drug users, is bound to produce profound changes in our society, changes that will affect us all.

Information and Education Only Weapons Against AIDS

It is estimated that in 1991 54,000 people will die from AIDS. At this moment, many of them are not infected with the AIDS virus. With proper information and education, as many as 12,000 to 14,000 people could be saved in 1991 from death by AIDS.

AIDS Will Impact All

The changes in our society will be economic and political and will affect our social institutions, our educational practices, and our health care. Al-

though AIDS may never touch you personally, the societal impact certainly will.

Be Educated—Be Prepared

Be prepared. Learn as much about AIDS as you can. Learn to separate scientific information from rumor and myth. The Public Health Service, your local public health officials and your family physician will be able to help you.

Concern About Spread of AIDS

While the concentration of AIDS cases is in the larger urban areas today, it has been found in every state. With the mobility of our society, it is likely that cases of AIDS will appear far and wide.

Special Educational Concerns

There are a number of people, primarily adolescents, that do not yet know they will be homosexual or become drug abusers and will not heed this message; there are others who are illiterate and cannot heed this message. They must be reached and taught the risk behaviors that expose them to infection with the AIDS virus.

High Risk Get Blood Test

The greatest public health problem lies in the large number of individuals with a history of high-risk behavior who have been infected with and may be spreading the AIDS virus. Those with high-risk behavior must be encouraged to protect others by adopting safe sexual practices and by the use of clean equipment for intravenous drug use. If a blood test for antibodies to the AIDS virus is necessary to get these individuals to use safe sexual practices, they should get a blood test. Call your local health department for information on where to get the test.

Anger and Guilt

Some people afflicted with AIDS will feel a sense of anger and others a sense of guilt. In spite of these understandable reactions, everyone must join the effort to control the epidemic, to provide for the care of those with AIDS, and to do all we can to inform and educate others about AIDS and how to prevent it.

Confidentiality

Because of the stigma that has been associated with AIDS, many afflicted with the disease or the AIDS virus are reluctant to be identified with AIDS. Because there is no vaccine to prevent AIDS and no cure, many feel there is nothing to be gained by revealing sexual contacts that might also be infected with the AIDS virus. When a community or a state requires reporting of those infected with the AIDS virus to public health authorities in order to trace sexual and intravenous drug contacts—as is the practice with other sexually transmitted diseases—those infected with the AIDS virus go underground out of the mainstream of health care and education. For this reason current public health practice is to protect the privacy of the individual infected with the AIDS virus and to maintain the strictest confidentiality concerning his/her health records.

State and Local AIDS Task Forces

Many state and local jurisdictions where AIDS has been seen in the greatest numbers have AIDS task forces with heavy representation from the field of public health joined by others who can speak broadly to issues of access to care, provision of care and the availability of community and psychiatric support services. Such a task force is needed in every community with the power to develop plans and policies, to speak, and to act for the good of the public health at every level.

State and local task forces should plan ahead and work with other jurisdictions to reduce transmission of AIDS by far-reaching informational and educational programs. As AIDS impacts more strongly on society, they should be charged with making recommendations to provide for the needs of those afflicted with AIDS. They also will be in the best position to answer the concerns and direct the activities of those who are not infected with the AIDS virus.

The responsibility of state and local task forces should be far-reaching and might include the following areas:

- Insure enforcement of public health regulation of such practices as ear piercing and tattooing to prevent transmission of the AIDS virus.
- Conduct AIDS education programs for police, firemen, correctional institution workers and emergency medical personnel for dealing with AIDS victims and the public.
- Insure that institutions catering to children or adults who soil themselves or their surroundings with urine, stool, and vomitus have adequate equipment for cleanup and disposal and have policies to insure the practice of good hygiene.

School

Schools will have special problems in the future. In addition to the guidelines already mentioned in this pamphlet, there are other things that should be considered such as sex education and education of the handicapped.

Sex Education

Education concerning AIDS must start at the lowest grade possible as part of any health and hygiene program. The appearance of AIDS could bring together diverse groups of parents and educators with opposing views on inclusion of sex education in the curricula. There is now no doubt that we need sex education in schools and that it must include information on heterosexual and homosexual relationships. The threat of AIDS should be sufficient to permit a sex education curriculum with a heavy emphasis on prevention of AIDS and other sexually transmitted diseases.

Handicapped and Special Education

Children with AIDS or ARC will be attending school along with others who carry the AIDS virus. Some children will develop brain disease which will produce changes in mental behavior. Because of the right to special education of the handicapped and the mentally retarded, school boards and higher authorities will have to provide guidelines for the management of such children on a case-by-case basis.

Labor and Management

Labor and management can do much to prepare for AIDS so that misinformation is kept to a minimum. Unions should issue preventive health messages because many employees will listen more carefully to a union message than they will to one from public health authorities.

AIDS Education at the Work Site

Offices, factories, and other work sites should have a plan in operation for education of the work force and accommodation of AIDS or ARC patients *before* the first such case appears at the work site. Employees with AIDS or ARC should be dealt with as are any workers with a chronic illness. In-house video programs provide an excellent source of education and can be individualized to the needs of a specific work group.

Strain on the Health Care Delivery System

The health care system in many places will be overburdened, as it is now in urban areas, with large numbers of AIDS patients. It is predicted that during 1991 there will be 145,000 patients requiring hospitalization at least once and 54,000 patients who will die of AIDS. Mental disease (dementia) will occur in some patients who have the AIDS virus before they have any other manifestation such as ARC or classic AIDS.

State and local task forces will have to plan for these patients by utilizing conventional and time-honored systems but will also have to investigate alternate methods of treatment and alternate sites for care, including home care.

The strain on the health system can be lessened by family, social, and psychological support mechanisms in the community. Programs are needed to train clergy, social workers, and volunteers to deal with AIDS. Such support is particularly critical to the minority communities.

Mental Health

Our society will also face an additional burden as we better understand the mental health implications of infection by the AIDS virus. Upon being informed of infection with the AIDS virus, a young, active, vigorous person faces anxiety and depression brought on by fears associated with social isolation, illness, and dying. Dealing with these individual and family concerns will require the best efforts of mental health professionals.

Issues

A number of controversial AIDS issues have arisen and will continue to be debated largely because of lack of knowledge about AIDS, how it is spread, and how it can be prevented. Among these are the issues of compulsory blood testing, quarantine, and identification of AIDS carriers by some visible sign.

Compulsory Blood Testing

Compulsory blood testing of individuals is not necessary. The procedure could be unmanageable and cost-prohibitive. It can be expected that many who *test* negatively might actually be positive due to *recent* exposure to the AIDS virus and give a false sense of security to the individual and his/her sexual partners concerning necessary protective behavior. The prevention behavior described in this report, if adopted, will protect the American public and contain the AIDS epidemic. Voluntary testing will be available to those who have been involved in high-risk behavior.

Quarantine

Quarantine has no role in the management of AIDS because AIDS is not spread by casual contact. The only time that some form of quarantine might be indicated is in a situation where an individual carrying the AIDS virus knowingly and willingly continues to expose others through sexual contact or sharing drug equipment. Such circumstances should be managed on a case-by-case basis by local authorities.

Identification of AIDS Carriers by Some Visible Sign

Those who suggest the marking of carriers of the AIDS virus by some visible sign have not thought the matter through thoroughly. It would require testing of the entire population, which is unnecessary, unmanageable and costly. It would miss recently infected individuals, who would test negative but be infected. The entire procedure would give a false sense of security. AIDS must and will be treated as a disease that can infect anyone. AIDS should not be used as an excuse to discriminate against any group or individual.

Updating Information

As the Surgeon General, I will continually monitor the most current and accurate health, medical, and scientific information and make it available to you, the American people. Armed with this information you can join in the discussion

and resolution of AIDS-related issues that are critical to your health, your children's health, and the health of the nation.

ADDITIONAL INFORMATION
Telephone Hotlines (Toll Free)

PHS AIDS Hotline
800-342-AIDS
800-342-2437

National Sexually Transmitted Diseases Hotline/
American Social Health Association
800-227-8922

National Gay Task Force
AIDS Information Hotline
800-221-7044
(212) 807-6016 (NY State)

Information Sources

U.S. Public Health Service
Public Affairs Office
Hubert H. Humphrey Building, Room 725-H
200 Independence Avenue, S.W.
Washington, D.C. 20201
Phone: (202) 245-6867

Local Red Cross or American Red Cross
AIDS Education Office
1730 D Street, N.W.
Washington, D.C. 20006
Phone: (202) 737-8300

American Association of Physicians for Human Rights
P.O. Box 14366
San Francisco, CA 94114
Phone: (415) 558-9353

AIDS Action Council
729 Eighth Street, S.E., Suite 200
Washington, D.C. 20003
Phone: (202) 547-3101

Gay Men's Health Crisis
P.O. Box 274
132 West 24th Street
New York, NY 10011
Phone: (212) 807-6655

Hispanic AIDS Forum
  c/o APRED
  853 Broadway, Suite 2007
  New York, NY 10003
  Phone: (212) 870-1902 or 870-1864

Los Angeles AIDS Project
  1362 Santa Monica Boulevard
  Los Angeles, CA 90046
  (213) 871-AIDS

Minority Task Force on AIDS
  c/o New York City Council of Churches
  475 Riverside Drive, Room 456
  New York, NY 10115
  Phone: (212) 749-1214

Mothers of AIDS Patients (MAP)
  c/o Barbara Peabody
  3403 E Street
  San Diego, CA 92102
  (619) 234-3432

National AIDS Network
  729 Eighth Street, S.E., Suite 300
  Washington, D.C. 20003
  (202) 546-2424

National Association of People with AIDS
  P.O. Box 65472
  Washington, D.C. 20035
  (202) 483-7979

National Coalition of Gay Sexually Transmitted Disease Services
  c/o Mark Behar
  P.O. Box 239
  Milwaukee, WI 53201
  Phone: (414) 277-7671

National Council of Churches/AIDS Task Force
  475 Riverside Drive, Room 572
  New York, NY 10115
  Phone: (212) 870-2421

San Francisco AIDS Foundation
  333 Valencia Street, 4th Floor
  San Francisco, CA 94103
  Phone: (415) 863-2437

Appendix D

Elementary Health Education Computer Software

RESOURCE LIST OF AVAILABLE HEALTH EDUCATION SOFTWARE (GRADES 3-8)

The following programs are available for specific computer models and specific computer operating systems (DOS versions). The authors do not make any claim for the programs nor their teaching effectiveness. It is up to the instructor to validate the claims of the software program.

Before purchasing software, you should do the following:

1. View the program if possible. Ask the dealer to demonstrate the program. See it run.
2. Match the software with the make of computer you have. The program must be compatible with your hardware.
3. Match the software operating system with that of your personal computer.
4. Match relevancy of software to your needs.
5. Ask about Lab-pack deal for classroom multiset use.
6. Review manual or documentation.

Program	Description	Level Approp.	Memory Needed	Computer Model	Cost	Manufacturer
BODY TRANSPAR-ENT	Several games about anatomy & body parts, bones/organs functions, diseases	Grade 4+	48K 64K 64K 64K	Apple Comm64 IBM-XT IBM-AT	$ 44.95 44.95 44.95 44.95	DesignWare 185 Berry St San Francisco, Ca. 94107 Tel: 415-546-1866
DENTAL HEALTH	Dental hygiene inventory Asks questions about 10 major risks, analyzes & gives recommendations to lower high risks (printout) For teachers, dentists	Grade 3+	64K 128K	Kaypro IBM-XT	$150.00 $150.00	Alpha Health P.O. Box 21153 El Cajon, Ca. 92021 Tel: 619-447-6925
DIET ANALYSIS	Health promotion software Database 840 foods, fats, CHO, proteins, sugar, chol, fiber, caffeine, alcohol, cal balan, 10 vits, 10 min, identifies high risk foods, recommends best food sources, body wt	Grade 5+	64K 128K	Kaypro IBM-XT	$250.00 $250.00	Alpha Health P.O. Box 21153 El Cajon, Ca. 92021 Tel: 619-447-6925
DIET PARTNER	Series of M-Basic programs that may need modification: food & activity calculator; predict ideal wt, menus	Grade 4+	64K	Apple IBM-XT IBM-AT	$ 10.00 10.00 10.00	Elliam Associates (Public Domain Software) 24000 Bessemer St. Woodland Hills, Ca. 91367 Tel: 818-348-4278
FEELING BETTER	Information about feelings	Grade 3+	16K	Apple	$ 37.00	CTRL Health Software 18653 Ventura Blvd. #348 Tarzana, Ca. 91356 Tel: 818-788-0888
FIVE SENSES & YOU	Factual	Grade 3+	64K	Apple Comm64 Texas	$ 59.90 $ 49.90 $ 59.90	Eyegate Media P.O. Box 303 Jamaica, NY 11435 Tel: 212-291-9100
FOOD FOR THOUGHT	Game: learn nutrients of various foods;	Grade 5+	64K	Apple	$ 59.00	Sunburst Rm #GM20 39 Washington Av. Pleasantville, NY 10570

Program	Description	Level Approp.	Memory Needed	Computer Model	Cost	Manufacturer
	Database: 300 foods & 11 nutrients					Tel: 800-431-1934
EPIDEMIC	Simulation game: You try to deal with heart epidemic	Grade 6+		Apple IBM-PC	$ 31.00 $ 31.00	CTRL Health Software
HEALTHAIDE	Nutritional analysis Database: 800 foods, 33 nutrients, amino acids Energy exp for 150 activities	Grade 6+	48K 128K	Apple IBM-PC	$ 74.00 $ 74.00	CTRL Health Software
HOME SAFETY	Fire, electrical & poison hazards, falls	Grade 2+		Apple	$165.00	MCE 157 S. Kalamazoo Mall Kalamazoo, Mi. 49007 Tel: 616-345-8681
HUMAN PUMP	Anatomy, function, risk factors & simulation	Grade 4+	48K	Apple	$ 59.00	Sunburst
GOOD HEALTH HABITS	Factual: uses humor to teach about habits	Grade 3+	64K	Apple Comm64	$ 18.00	Right on programs P.O. Box 977 Huntington, NY 11743
LEARNING TO COPE WITH PRESSURE	Use of biofeedback to teach stress reduction/relaxation Galvanic skin resistance monitor supplied	Grade 3+	48K	Apple	$ 99.00	Sunburst
MAKE IT CLICK	Facts, decisions, re use of seatbelts	Grade 5+	48K	Apple	$ 59.00	Sunburst
REPRODUCTION	Human reproductive process	Grade 4+		Apple	$ 44.50	Eyegate Media
RISKO-HEART HEALTH	Risk questions analyzed	Grade 5+		IBM-PC	$140.00	CTRL Health Software
STANDING ROOM ONLY	Study population dynamics	Grade 8+	128K	IBM-AT	$ 59.00	Sunburst
STRESS MANAGEMENT	Measures stress in life, graphs it, suggests coping	Grade 5+		Apple	$ 29.00	CTRL Health Software
THE PUPPET	Narrative puppet show about assuming responsibility	Grade 1+	48K	Apple	$ 19.00	CTRL Health Software

Program	Description	Level Approp.	Memory Needed	Computer Model	Cost	Manufacturer
THE SMOK-ING DECI-SION	Facts given to rein-force students not to smoke	Grade 5+	48K	Apple	$ 59.00	Sunburst
TRAINS	Simulation game about managing business and working with people (success)	Grade 5+	64K	Apple Comm64 IBM-PC	$ 29.95 $ 26.95 $ 29.95	L.F. Garlinghouse Co. 34 Industrial Parl Place P.O. Box 1717 Middletown, Ct. 06457

Appendix E

Eating Disorders

ANOREXIA AND BULIMIA

What Is Anorexia Nervosa?

It is a life-threatening disorder of deliberate self-starvation with wide-ranging physical and psychiatric factors. Anorexia nervosa is a misnomer, as it means lack of appetite due to nerves. The reverse is true. The person is obsessed with the idea of eating, but because of emotional problems, she denies her hunger and does not eat, or binges, then vomits or takes laxatives.

What Are the Symptoms?

1. 20% to 25% body weight loss
2. Lack of menstrual periods
3. Hyperactivity
4. Distorted body image
5. Food binges followed by fasting, vomiting, or using laxatives
6. Excessive constipation
7. Depression
8. Loss of hair (head)
9. Growth of fine body hair
10. Intolerance to cold
11. Low pulse rate

What Is Bulimia?

Recurrent episodes of binge eating, followed by self-induced vomiting or purge by laxatives and diuretics.

What Are the Symptoms?

1. Inconspicuous binge eating
2. Menstrual irregularities
3. Swollen glands
4. Frequent significant weight fluctuations due to alternating binges and fasts
5. Fear of inability to stop eating voluntarily

Who Is Susceptible?

The illness usually occurs during adolescence and young adulthood and is the aftermath of a diet. It mainly affects white females from middle and upper class families. The parents are usually conscientious, educated, well-meaning people who are high achievers themselves. In many cases, one of the parents is overconcerned about eating patterns and is likely to be a perfectionist.

What Are the Consequences?

Some recover completely, some lead a borderline existence, and some die.

What Is the Treatment?

The best approach is the combination of medical treatment and psychotherapy for the patient as well as counseling for parents, spouses, and siblings. Participation in a self-help group is an adjunct to medical and psychiatric care.

OVERWEIGHT AND OBESITY

What Is the Difference Between Overweight and Obesity?

Technically speaking, when you weigh more than your ideal, you are overweight. The excess weight can be in the form of fat, cell solids, or muscle mass.

One is obese when the excess weight is clearly fat as opposed to water, muscle, or bone and the ideal body weight is exceeded by 15 percent to 25 percent. The term grossly obese is used when ideal body is exceeded by 25 percent or more.

Obesity results from a long period of overeating. To prevent obesity, calories consumed must equal energy expended. Studies indicate that approximately one fourth of Americans over 30 are 10 percent to 25 percent above their ideal body weight.

What Are the Consequences of Obesity?

Potential medical complications of obesity:

1. Shorter lifespan
2. Frequent sickness
3. Respiratory difficulties
4. Increased incidence of hypertension, heart attack, and stroke
5. Diabetes
6. Gallbladder problems
7. Hernia
8. Arthritis
9. Complicated pregnancy
10. Chronic illness

In addition to medical complications, psychological problems can occur. Obese children are often the target of ridicule, which can generate significant unhappiness. Social rejection can lead the obese individual to eat more for the sense of comfort food provides.

What Makes a Person Fat?

There probably is no single satisfactory answer beyond the rare clinical disorder. Some of the theories of obesity:

Some Proposed Causes of Obesity

Factor	Analysis
Genetics	
Body build by birth	All types: round, plump, thin, fragile, heavily muscular. For example, a person born thin, fragile, and linear may grow up to be a small person and underweight.
Familial traits	If parents are obese, their children have a higher chance of being obese.
Defective hunger and satiety center	Hypothalamus does not respond normally. Usually, it responds to hunger and informs the person to stop eating when full. Its failure to do so results in obesity.
Defective body metabolism	Defects in an obese person: inability to release energy efficiently (from ATP, for example), reduced lipase (enzyme) activity to mobilize fat, and overactive fat storage enzyme system.

Some Proposed Causes of Obesity—Cont'd

Factor	*Analysis*
Body fat cell type	An obese person may be born with a large number of fat cells or a special type of fat cell that can hypertrophy easily.
Anthropological factors	
Cultural acceptance	Obesity is considered good fortune or a beautiful attribute in many countries.
Food and hospitality	The expression of hospitality through food and drink makes food more available. In an affluent society like the United States, this increases food consumption.
Eating habits	
Overeating	Obese people like to eat. They eat more calories than they expend.
Meal pattern	Eating three meals a day may predispose some individuals to deposit more fat. Nibbling the same quantity of food throughout the day may enable the body enzyme system to use the calories more efficiently, and less fat is deposited.
Childhood conditioning	
Infancy eating maladjustment	Solid foods given too early, excess high caloric-density milk, and excess food consumption all may result in large weight gain. A big baby (from too much fat) is not necessarily a healthy baby.
Overeating	A fat child can grow into an obese adult.
Psychological factors	
Eating as an emotional outlet	If the person wants to stay away from food, he or she must be persuaded to use another means of emotional support.
Eating to allay anxiety, tension, frustration, and insecurity	The greater the anxiety, tension, frustration, or insecurity, the more food a person eats and the more likely he or she is to gain weight.
Eating as a substitute or demonstration of love and affection	The relationship between family members is expressed with food. To show love and affection, one person serves more food to another. Or to replace loss of love and affection, a person eats more or is served more food.
Eating as a substitute for whatever is missing (e.g., no job)	In this context, food is similar to excess alcohol drinking and heavy smoking.
Physiological factors	
Hormones	Hypothyroidism or decreased metabolism may result in weight gain and therefore obesity.
Basal metabolic rate	BMR decreases with age, while the caloric consumption is undiminished and there is a decrease (or no increase) in daily activity.
No exercise or activity	Eating a lot of foods without a good exercise program results in obesity.
Environmental factors	
Trauma and emotion	Certain individuals are susceptible to traumatic and emotional experiences and will eat more.
Family eating habits	One develops an overeating habit if parents and other members in the family eat too much.
Sedentary job	A job requires constant sitting, with minimal movement.
Abundance of foods	Obesity is more common in affluent societies.
Advertisements	A person is conditioned to the type of foods advertised on television and in magazines, most of which are high in calories.
Living comfort	Comfortable ambient temperature, light clothing, minimal shivering, and lack of heavy work all contribute to reduced expenditure of calories.
Convenience of food preparation	Minimal preparation time and labor. Less activity, more food consumed.
Smoking or alcohol	When a person tries to stop smoking or drinking, he or she may eat more and gain weight.

Appendix F

Emergency Care*

---

*The material on choking and CPR is provided courtesy of Fitnus® for Life. The flowcharts on first aid procedures are from Alton L. Thygerson, *First Aid and Emergency Care Workbook* (Boston: Jones and Bartlett, 1987).

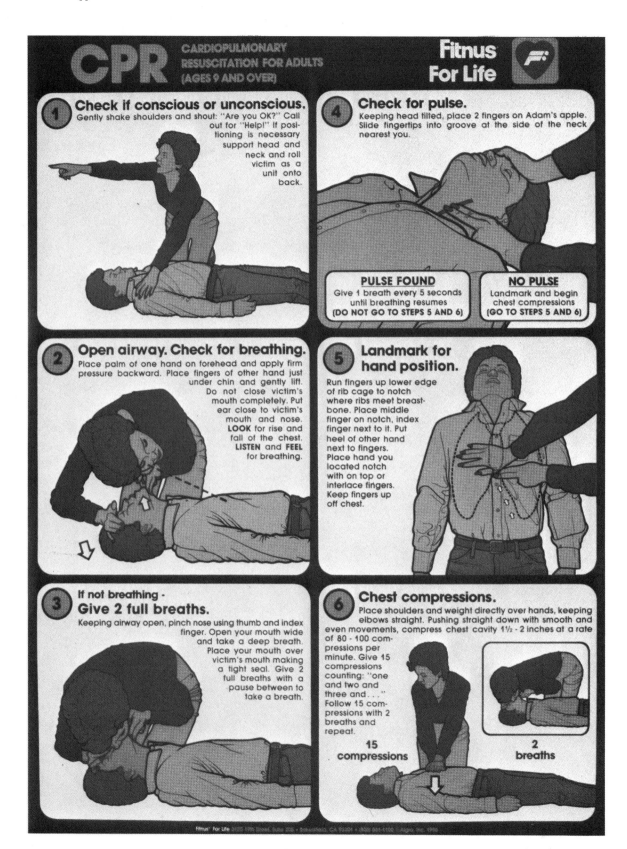

FIRST-AID FOR CHOKING
OBSTRUCTED AIRWAY TECHNIQUES FOR ADULTS (AGES 9 AND OVER)

Fitnus For Life

Conscious Victim Standing

1 Recognize choking signs.

Choking victim will have severe difficulty speaking, breathing, coughing and may be clutching throat between thumb and fingers (Universal Distress Signal). Ask if he or she is choking. If able to speak or cough effectively, do not interfere.

2 If choking—Give 6-10 abdominal thrusts.

Stand behind victim and wrap arms around his or her waist. Make a fist with one hand. Place thumb side of fist into abdomen above navel and below rib cage. Grasp fist with other hand and press inward and upward with 6-10 quick thrusts.

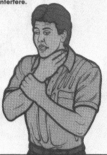

3 If pregnant or obese—Give 6-10 chest thrusts.

Stand behind victim, placing your arms under victims armpits, and encircle chests. Place thumb side of fist on the middle of the breastbone. Grasp fist with other hand and press backward with 6-10 quick thrusts.

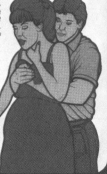

Victim Lying Conscious or Unconscious

1 Check if conscious or unconscious.

Gently tap and shake shoulders to determine if victim is ok. If unresponsive call out for "Help!"

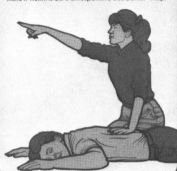

2 Position victim carefully on back.

If lying face down, roll victim flat onto back. Supporting head, neck, and torso carefully turn victim as a unit without twisting.

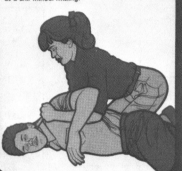

3 Open airway. Check for breathing.

Apply downward pressure with hand on forehead and gently lift with other hand just under chin. Place ear close to victim's mouth and nose. **LOOK** for rise and fall of chest. **LISTEN** and **FEEL** for breathing.

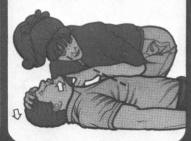

4 Attempt to ventilate.

Keeping head tilted and airway open, pinch victim's nose with thumb and index finger. Cover victim's mouth and attempt to get air into the lungs.

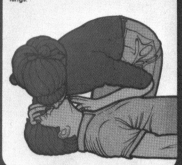

5 If unsuccessful—Give 6-10 abdominal thrusts.

Kneeling close to victim's hips, place heel of hand on victim's abdomen above navel and below rib cage. Put other hand on top of first, and press into abdomen with 6-10 quick inward and upward thrusts.

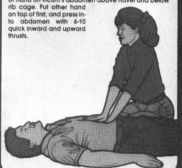

6 Finger sweep for foreign object.

Open victim's mouth by grasping tongue and lower jaw, and lift. Insert index finger of other hand deep into mouth along the cheek. Using hooked finger try to dislodge object.

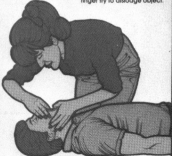

▪ If unsuccessful reattempt to ventilate ▪

Fitnus' For Life 3135 19th Street, Suite 305 • Bakersfield, CA 93301 • (805) 861-1100 Algra, Inc. 1986

Fainting

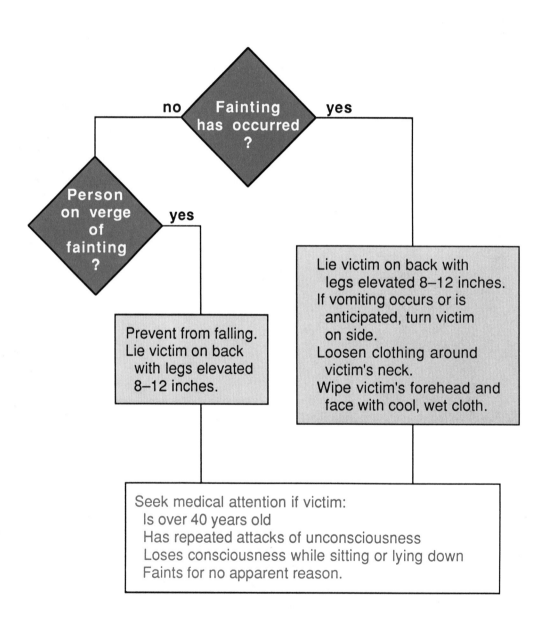

Fainting has occurred ? no / yes

Person on verge of fainting ? yes

Prevent from falling.
Lie victim on back
with legs elevated
8–12 inches.

Lie victim on back with
legs elevated 8–12 inches.
If vomiting occurs or is
anticipated, turn victim
on side.
Loosen clothing around
victim's neck.
Wipe victim's forehead and
face with cool, wet cloth.

Seek medical attention if victim:
Is over 40 years old
Has repeated attacks of unconsciousness
Loses consciousness while sitting or lying down
Faints for no apparent reason.

Nosebleeds

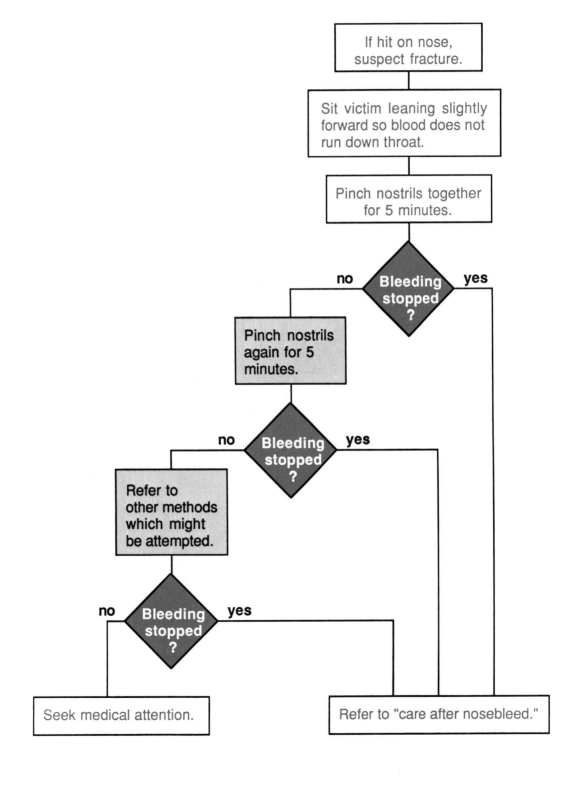

Insect Stings (Flying Insects)

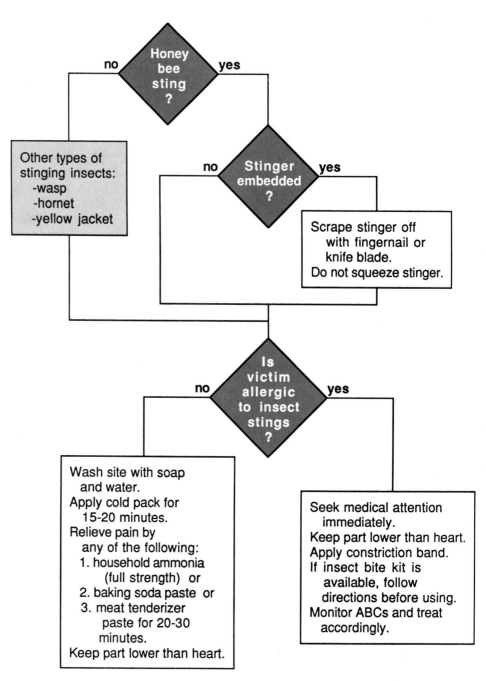

Poison Ivy, Poison Oak, and Poison Sumac

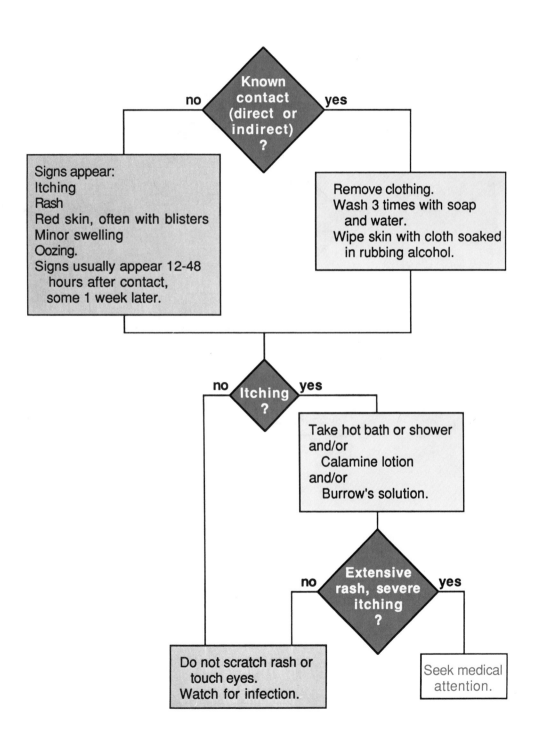

Sprains, Strains, Contusions, Dislocations

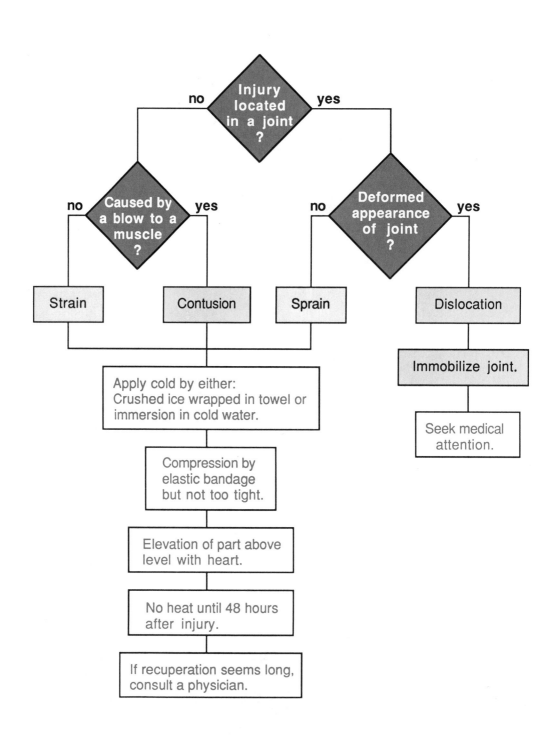

Diabetic Emergencies

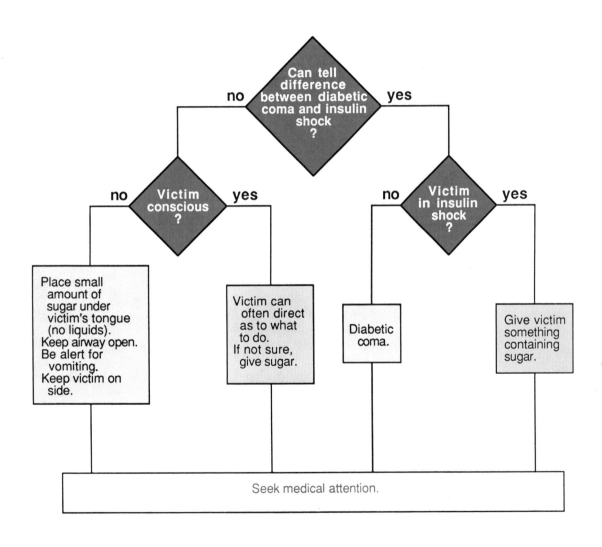

Seizures

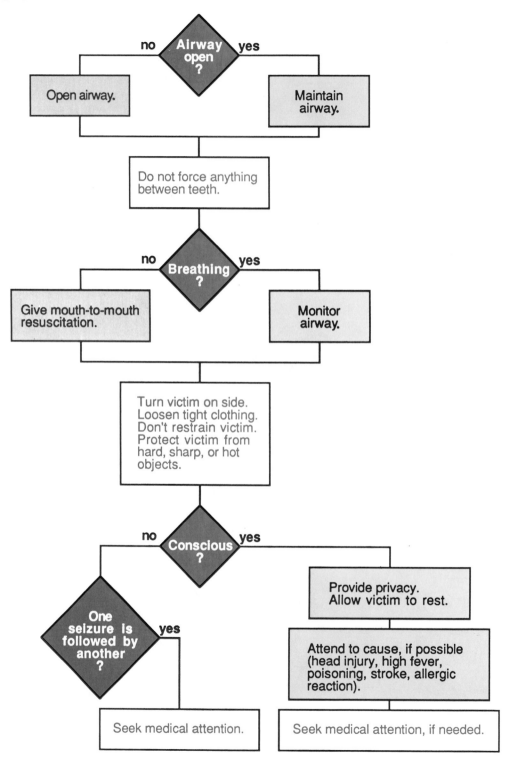

Earache

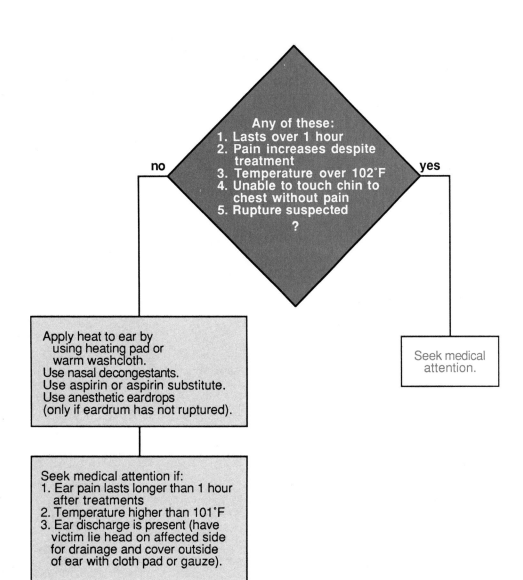

Any of these:
1. Lasts over 1 hour
2. Pain increases despite treatment
3. Temperature over 102°F
4. Unable to touch chin to chest without pain
5. Rupture suspected
?

no

yes

Apply heat to ear by
  using heating pad or
  warm washcloth.
Use nasal decongestants.
Use aspirin or aspirin substitute.
Use anesthetic eardrops
(only if eardrum has not ruptured).

Seek medical attention if:
1. Ear pain lasts longer than 1 hour after treatments
2. Temperature higher than 101°F
3. Ear discharge is present (have victim lie head on affected side for drainage and cover outside of ear with cloth pad or gauze).

Seek medical attention.

Index